Prosthodontic Treatment for Edentulous Patients

Complete Dentures and Implant-Supported Prostheses

Prosthodontic Treatment for Edentulous Patients

Complete Dentures and Implant-Supported Prostheses

Twelfth Edition

SENIOR EDITORS

George A. Zarb, BChD (Malta), DDS, MSc (Michigan), MSc (Ohio State), FRCD (C)
Professor, and Head of Prosthodontics
Department of Clinical Sciences
Faculty of Dentistry
University of Toronto
Toronto, Ontario, Canada

Charles L. Bolender, DDS, MS
Professor Emeritus and Former Chairman
Department of Prosthodontics
School of Dentistry
University of Washington
Seattle, Washington

ASSOCIATE EDITORS

Steven E. Eckert, DDS, MS
Associate Professor
Department of Dental Specialties
Mayo Graduate School of Medicine
Consultant in Prosthodontics
Division of Prosthodontics
Mayo Clinic
Rochester, Minnesota

Rhonda F. Jacob, DDS, MS
Professor of Dental Oncology and Maxillofacial
   Prosthodontics
Department of Head and Neck Surgery
M.D. Anderson Cancer Center
University of Texas
Houston, Texas

Aaron H. Fenton, DDS, MS, FRCD (C)
Associate Professor
Department of Graduate Prosthodontics and
   Qualifying Program Director
Faculty of Dentistry
University of Toronto
Toronto, Ontario, Canada

Regina Mericske-Stern, DrMedDent
Head, Department of Prosthodontics
School of Dental Medicine
University of Bern
Bern, Switzerland

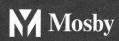

Mosby
An Affiliate of Elsevier

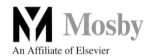
An Affiliate of Elsevier

11830 Westline Industrial Drive
St. Louis, MO 63146

Previous editions copyrighted 1940, 1947, 1953, 1959, 1964, 1970, 1975, 1980, 1985, 1990, 1997

International Standard Book Number 0-323-02296-0

Publishing Director: Linda Duncan
Executive Editor: Penny Rudolph
Developmental Editor: Courtney Sprehe
Publishing Services Manager: Melissa Lastarria
Project Manager: Joy Moore
Design Manager: Bill Drone

Printed in the United States of America

Last digit is the print number: 9   8   7   6   5   4   3   2   1

This text is dedicated to the memory of Carl O. Boucher and to Judson Hickey. It is also dedicated to Gunnar E. Carlsson, who continues to be our discipline's best global ambassador. We remain grateful to these extraordinary friends for their legacy of clinical scholarship in all its aspects—education, research, and service.

George A. Zarb
Charles L. Bolender
Steven E. Eckert
Rhonda F. Jacob
Aaron H. Fenton
Regina Mericske-Stern

Contributors

Tomas Albrektsson, MD, PhD
Professor and Head
Department of Biomaterials/Handicap Research
Institute of Surgical Sciences
Göteborg University
Göteborg, Sweden

James D. Anderson, BSc, DDS, MScD
Professor of Prosthodontics
Department of Clinical Sciences
Faculty of Dentistry
University of Toronto
Toronto, Ontario, Canada
Director, Craniofacial Prosthetic Unit
Toronto Sunnybrook Regional Cancer Centre
Toronto, Ontario, Canada

Nancy S. Arbree, DDS, MS
Associate Dean of Academic Affairs and Professor
Department of Administration
Department of Restorative Dentistry
Tufts University School of Dental Medicine
Boston, Massachusetts

Nikolai Attard, BChD, MSc
Research Associate in Prosthodontics
Faculty of Dentistry
University of Toronto
Toronto, Ontario, Canada

S. Ross Bryant, BSc, DDS, MSc, PhD, FRCD(C)
Assistant Professor
Department of Oral Health Sciences
Faculty of Dentistry
University of British Columbia
Vancouver, British Columbia, Canada

Ejvind Budtz-Jørgensen, DDS, DrOdont
Professor
Department of Gerodontology and Removable
    Prosthodontics
Section of Dental Medicine
University of Geneva
Geneva, Switzerland

Alan B. Carr, DMD, MS
Professor of Dentistry
Department of Dental Specialties
Mayo Clinic
Rochester, Minnesota

Douglas V. Chaytor, DDS, MS, MEd
Professor of Prosthodontics and Director of
    Implant Dentistry
Department of Dental Clinical Sciences
Faculty of Dentistry
Dalhousie University
Halifax, Nova Scotia, Canada

Thuan Dao, DMD, MSc, Dip Prostho, PhD
Associate Professor of Prosthodontics
Department of Clinical Sciences
Faculty of Dentistry
University of Toronto
Toronto, Ontario, Canada

David M. Davis, PhD, FDSRCS (Eng), BDS
Senior Lecturer and Honorary Consultant
Department of Prosthetic Dentistry
Guy's, Kings, St. Thomas' Dental Institute
London, England

Randa R. Diwan, BDS, PhD
Assistant Professor of Prosthodontics
Department of Clinical Sciences
Faculty of Dentistry
University of Toronto
Toronto, Ontario, Canada

Emad S. Elsubeihi, BDS, MSc, Dip Prosth, PhD

Assistant Professor of Prosthodontics
Department of Clinical Sciences
Faculty of Dentistry
University of Toronto
Toronto, Ontario, Canada

Mary P. Faine, MS, RD

Associate Professor Emeritus
Department of Prosthodontics
School of Dentistry
University of Washington
Seattle, Washington

Yoav Finer, BSc, MSc, DMD, PhD

Research Associate in Prosthodontics
Faculty of Dentistry
University of Toronto
Toronto, Ontario, Canada

Stig L. Karlsson, DDS, Odont Dr

Professor and Head
Department of Prosthetic Dentistry and Dental
    Materials Science
Faculty of Odontology
Göteborg University
Göteborg, Sweden

Howard M. Landesman, DDS, MEd

Dean and Professor
Department of Restorative Dentistry
School of Dentistry
University of Colorado Health Sciences Center
Denver, Colorado

Michael I. MacEntee, LDS(I), Dip Prosth, FRCD(C)

Professor
Department of Oral Health Sciences
University of British Columbia
Vancouver, British Columbia, Canada

Kenneth Shay, DDS, MS

Adjunct Associate Professor
Department of Periodontics,
    Prevention, and Geriatric Dentistry
School of Dentistry
University of Michigan
Ann Arbor, Michigan
Director of Geriatrics and Extended Care Service
    Line
Veterans Integrated Service Network #11
U.S. Department of Veterans Affairs
Ann Arbor, Michigan
Chief of the Section of Dental Geriatrics and
    Affiliated Investigator of the Geriatrics
    Research, Education, and Clinical Center
Ann Arbor VA Healthcare System
Ann Arbor, Michigan

Ann Wennerberg, LDS, PhD

Professor
Department of Biomaterials/Handicap Research
Institute of Surgical Sciences
Göteborg University
Göteborg, Sweden

John P. Zarb, DDS, MSc

Clinical Assistant Professor
Department of Restorative Dentistry
School of Dentistry
University of Illinois at Chicago
Chicago, Illinois

Preface

This twelfth edition of *Prosthodontic Treatment for Edentulous Patients: Complete Dentures and Implant-Supported Prostheses* seeks to assist dental students, dentists, and prosthodontists to make informed clinical decisions on the optimal management of edentulous patients. In correlating basic and behavioral sciences with technical skills, ours is an effort to balance the art of patient treatment with the physical and biological sciences involved in prostheses fabrication. As active academic clinicians, we continue to seek educational formats that reconcile clinical research development with a provocative pedagogic approach, one which never loses sight of those who should benefit most from our service—our patients or clients. Each patient/client in today's practice is increasingly aware of his or her right to efficacious and effective dental therapy—hence this text, which provides a basis for a participatory partnership between patient and dentist.

Impact of Clinical Research on Text's Content and Organization

The prosthodontic educational and research focus has evolved dramatically in recent years. This progress resulted from three major initiatives. First, materials research has simplified impression-making protocols and denture relining techniques. Second, understanding of the role and particularly the limitations of mechanical analogues for the masticatory system (i.e., articulators) has improved. Both of these lateral shifts in traditional prosthodontic thinking have reduced the self-imposed technique burden that characterized denture fabrication in so many teaching institutions. The third initiative, arguably the most compelling advance in the management of edentulism, is implant prosthodontics. Osseointegration has had a profound impact on research and education in virtually all of our clinical endeavors. As a result, the consequences of an aging edentulous environment or a terminal dentition have been more successfully addressed than ever before and many clinicians even began to forecast the demise of the complete denture technique.

Optimal management of the edentulous predicament in virtually all its forms is now seen in a broader and more rational context, and there is clearly still a major ongoing role for complete denture therapy. In fact, the cost effectiveness, simplicity, efficacy, and effectiveness of this treatment technique is virtually universal. However, long-term adverse sequelae of denture wearing or behavioral problems associated with the experience no longer militate against our traditional efforts to cope with chronic and unsolvable clinical problems. Implant support, be it of the fixed or over-denture variety, has enlarged and enriched the therapeutic scope of a previously limited prosthodontic paradigm. Furthermore, the conviction has reemerged that basic principles of managing edentulism with complete denture fabrication are more necessary than ever, since implant-supported treatment remains an outgrowth of traditional prosthodontic protocols.

We have chosen an eclectic approach to the topic and invited leading international educators to join us in articulating a strong case for understanding the edentulous predicament and its management. Our contributors remain committed to optimal patient therapy but never lose sight of the total picture of the biological underpinnings of the edentulous milieu. This is where the twelfth edition's thrust and novelty lies—an enriched and integrated interpretation of what it means to be edentulous plus ways and means of addressing its consequences.

Acknowledgments

We readily acknowledge our indebtedness to the many teachers and colleagues whose influence over the years enabled us to both enjoy and grow in our discipline. They, together with our secretaries, dental technicians, assistants, and photography personnel, are the ones who really made this text possible. While they are too numerous to mention, they continue to occupy a very special place in our hearts.

We are also grateful to past contibutors of this text—notably, Gunnar Carlsson, Warner Kalk, Brien Lang, and Adrianne Schmitt.

Janet deWinter's indispensable organizational role throughout the preparation of this text demands a very special mention. Her diligence, tenacity, and, above all, her sense of humor continue to be appreciated.

Contents

Prosthodontic Treatment for Edentulous Patients

Complete Dentures and Implant-Supported Prostheses

part **1** one

ON BEING EDENTULOUS

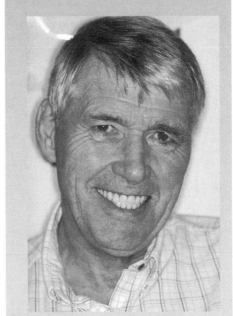

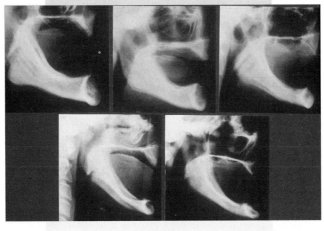

CHAPTER 1

The Edentulous Predicament

George A. Zarb

Loss of teeth causes adverse esthetic and biomechanical sequelae, a predicament that is worse when the patient is completely edentulous and the entire periodontal ligament is lost. This leads to drastic changes in the potential support for any planned prosthesis because the residual ridges are a poor substitute for the missing periodontal ligament support. Until recently, prosthodontic therapy focused mainly on the technical skills and clinical judgment expertise required to fabricate complete dentures. Such knowledge helped nurture the development of new materials and knowledge about the relationships among esthetics, occlusion, and patients' expectations. This, in turn, led to strong convictions about the inherent merits of complete denture treatment as dentists all over the world presumed that their prosthodontic endeavors could meet the gold standard of healthy intact dentitions. Most denture-wearing patients appear to have benefited from this professional attitude, and compromised oral health and esthetic appearance were treated with extractions and complete denture replacements. Regrettably, partial and entire dentitions were sometimes needlessly sacrificed because the complete denture prescription often was regarded as an alternative to, or a solution for, expensive periodontal and restorative therapy or an unesthetic dentition.

History supports the conviction that the skills and ingenuity of complete denture fabrication have contributed to a better quality of life for edentulous patients. The passage of time allowed dentists to refine requisite technical skills and to develop scientifically based rationales for their use. As a result, the complete denture treatment method became, and indeed remains, an integral and important part of dental education and practice. As a clinical teaching and professional activity, it demands knowledge of applied basic sciences, biomaterials, occlusion, and esthetics. In fact, the basis for most of the esthetic clues or decisions currently used to improve the appearance of the natural smile is an extension of complete denture esthetic principles described in Part 3 of this text. It provides, above all else, the challenge and satisfaction of managing patients' behavioral and age-related concerns and infirmities. In a public-health context, complete denture prosthodontics remains a relatively simple and inexpensive treatment method, one that offers scope for virtual universal application. Nevertheless, it is not a panacea for the edentulous predicament (Plate 1-1).

Many health care professionals may forget that although much research and attention have been devoted to various forms of organ loss, such as mastectomies and hysterectomies, the edentulous state has received relatively little psychological attention. Only a few authors have acknowledged the fact that it is a serious emotional life issue, albeit not a life-threatening one. Furthermore, outcome measures of health care treatment are only partially defined by technical excellence and are not exclusively dentist determined. Patient perceptions and responses to health care measures are now regarded as an integral part of the clinical decision-making paradigm. It is therefore not surprising to note that many edentulous patients may be described as unable to adapt to complete dentures and are described as prosthetically "maladaptive." The term is used in this very specific context

3

in this text. We recognize the fact that such patients perceive their denture-wearing experience as one they cannot adapt to and that this can occur despite the dentist's skills and humanitarian concerns. Most dentists have been inclined to regard maladaptive denture wearing as a result of anatomical or physiological causes. They have treated such patients with technique (and hopefully improved) modifications and with occasional surgical attempts to enlarge the denture-bearing areas, even if the latter measures proved to be palliative at best. These patients have also received a diagnosis and been dismissed as long-term complainers, and even regarded as needing psychiatric help to cope with their maladaptation. Regrettably, the poignant consequences of such patients' edentulous predicament were overlooked.

Clinical experience also has demonstrated that patients who are initially adaptive may indeed become maladaptive in the end. The reason is that regressive, or degenerative, changes in the supporting tissues and neuromuscular control militate against a continuum of an adaptive functional and esthetic experience. In fact, it must be admitted that the field of complete denture prosthodontic research has been characterized by a lack of methodological rigor in developing treatment outcome measures. As a result, practical, useful results from studies involving presumed determinants of prosthetic success underscore the unpredictability of the complete denture service. Furthermore, quantifiable measurements of patients' quality of life after undergoing prosthodontic treatment are still evolving.

IMPLANT PROSTHODONTICS

The objective of stabilizing replacement or prosthetic dentitions with endosseous anchorage went through numerous pioneering efforts. However, predictable time-dependent and morbidity-free documented outcomes proved to be elusive until the publication of Per Ingvar Brannemark's seminal research on the technique of osseointegration. In 1982 the Toronto Conference on Tissue Integrated Prostheses introduced the concept of inducing a controlled interfacial osteogenesis between dental implant and host bone to the dental academic community. The ability to safely locate alloplastic tooth

roots in the jawbones had finally become a reality. This was soon followed by an international research endorsement of the merits of the technique for maladaptive edentulous patients who could be treated with both implant-retained fixed or removable overdenture prostheses.

In subsequent publications implant prosthodontics was demonstrated as a valid treatment option for any adaptive denture-wearing patient as well. The proviso would, of course, be that the patient should be willing to undergo the required preprosthetic surgical procedures and incur the necessary additional expenses (Plate 1-2).

In preparing the twelfth edition of this text, we continue a half-century-old tradition of describing the objectives and methods of making complete dentures. We also have acknowledged the impact of implant-supported prostheses on clinical decision making for managing the edentulous patient. Since 1985 we have recognized the merits of an applied scientific concept that can place the required number of implants in all edentulous jaws to "cure" the edentulous predicament. Nevertheless, we assert that this approach is clearly neither realistic nor desirable for all patients because traditional complete denture therapy has compellingly already proven its merits. We also remain convinced that the clinical skills and judgment required to make complete dentures are essential to the osseointegration technique. They are the two sides of the same coin—the treatment currency that ensures optimal prosthodontics therapy for edentulous patients.

Because of these requirements, there is a need for this text and its increasingly dual purpose. Today's dentist can offer all edentulous patients two treatment options: complete dentures or implant-retained or implant-supported prostheses (Table 1-1). Choosing the best form of therapy is not always a clear-cut selection. The clinical decision should ideally reflect the dentist's knowledge of the selected treatment efficacy and effectiveness, as well as a patient's understanding of treatment risks and cost-effectiveness. Biological, functional, personality, and fiscal considerations may preclude one option or the other. Admittedly, the complete denture option lends itself to more frequent application than a fixed implant-supported prosthetic one, with costs being a major determinant of patient choice. On the other hand, an implant-supported

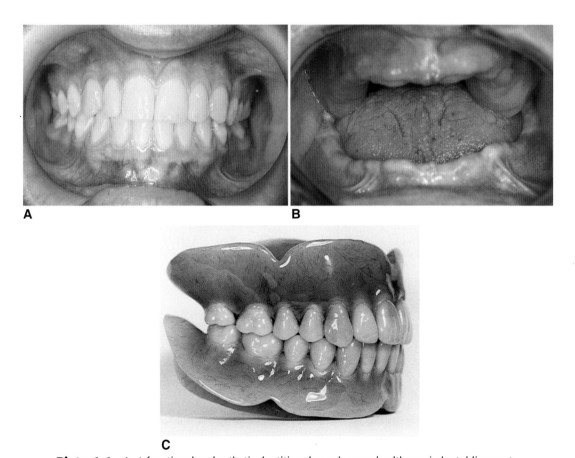

Plate 1-1   **A,** A functional and esthetic dentition depends upon healthy periodontal ligament support. **B,** The edentulous state reflects a serious deficit in the qualitative and quantitative roles of the residual tissue's mechanism of support for complete dentures (**C**), which are a compromised substitute for the natural dentition.

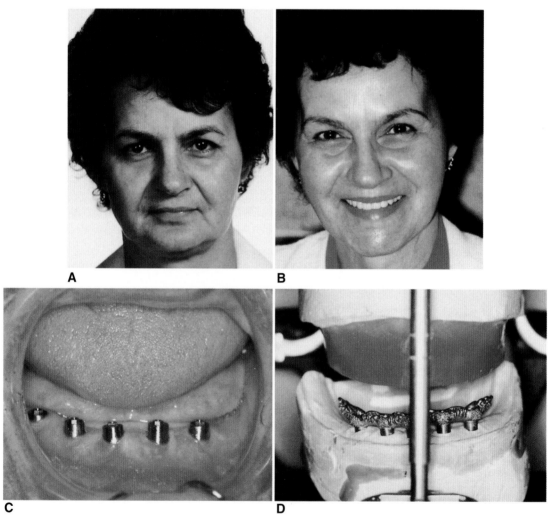

A **B**

C **D**

Plate 1-2 Pre- and postprosthodontic photographs, **A** and **B,** of a woman who exhibited chronic maladaptive complete denture behavior. Although this gratifying esthetic result might have been readily achieved with conventional complete dentures, in the present case, a more stable support mechanism was required for the mandibular prosthesis, which was attained by the use of five osseointegrated implants, whose transepithelial abutment components are shown in **C.** The articulated working cast (**D**) incorporated implant abutment analogues to support a custom-designed, rigid, silver-palladium framework.

Continued

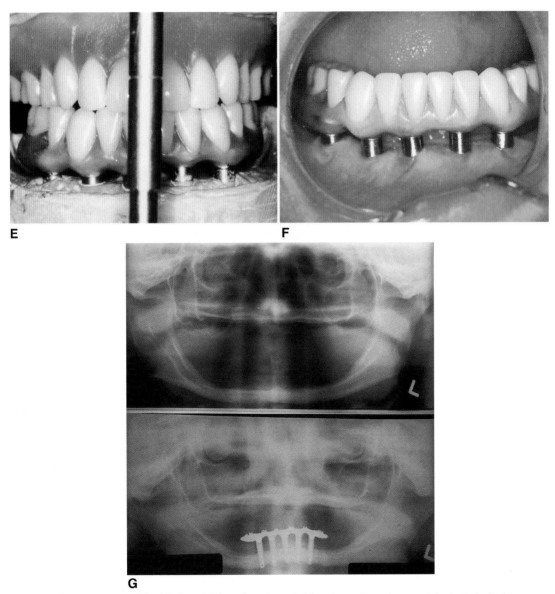

E

F

G

Plate 1-2 *cont'd* With the addition of stock teeth (**E**) and a resin replacement for lost gingival tissues (**F**) a design was created that both facilitated home care procedures and enhanced the cosmetic effect. **G,** Pre- and post-implant placement radiographs. It should be noted that a porcelain baked to metal framework is an alternative to this laboratory protocol.

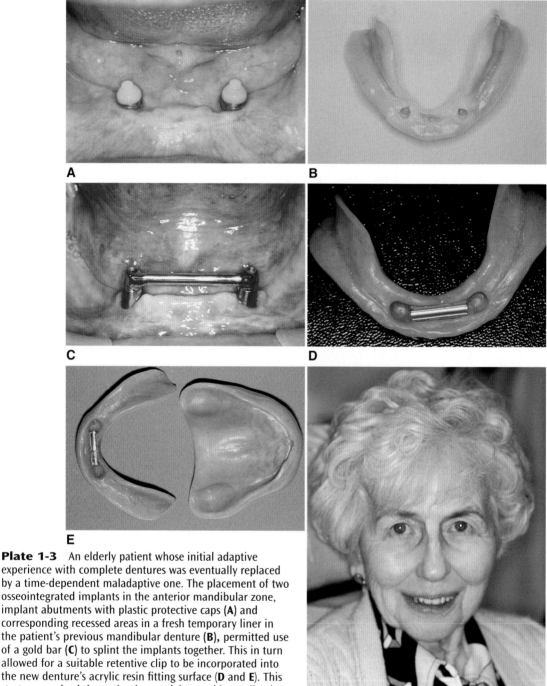

Plate 1-3 An elderly patient whose initial adaptive experience with complete dentures was eventually replaced by a time-dependent maladaptive one. The placement of two osseointegrated implants in the anterior mandibular zone, implant abutments with plastic protective caps (**A**) and corresponding recessed areas in a fresh temporary liner in the patient's previous mandibular denture (**B**), permitted use of a gold bar (**C**) to splint the implants together. This in turn allowed for a suitable retentive clip to be incorporated into the new denture's acrylic resin fitting surface (**D** and **E**). This strategy resolved the patient's complaints and immediately restored her adaptive prosthetic experience (**F**). Note that numerous variations on the retentive method employed are available for the dentist to choose from.

Table 1-1 Treatment Options for Edentulous Patients		
Diagnosis	**Evidence-Based Treatment Choices**	**Burden of Illness**
Edentulous in one or both arches	A. Complete dentures or B. Implant-supported overdentures or C. Implant-supported fixed prosthesis	Functional esthetic and perceptual consequences that are encountered on a time-dependent and escalating basis
I. Without prior denture experience	A, B, or C	
II. With an adaptive complete denture experience	A, B, or C	
III. With a current history of maladaptive denture-wearing experience	B or C	

Treatment choice is influenced by both patient and dentist-mediated concerns. However, the impact of time-dependent regressive changes in the prosthodontic adaptive experience can be significantly reduced through an implant-supported/retained prosthesis.

overdenture appears to combine the best of both options without either method's restrictions. Functional and esthetic requirements are better achieved and maintained, with the risk of time-dependent supporting tissue morbidity compellingly reduced. We therefore endorse the emerging clinical educational conviction that the current standard of complete denture service for prosthodontically maladaptive patients should be an implant-supported overdenture, particularly in the mandible (Plate 1-3).

Osseointegration has ushered in a new scientific era for the management of edentulous patients. Reconciliation of the technique's potential with the proven merits and ingenuity of complete denture fabrication can only improve dentists' ability to resolve the edentulous predicament.

CHAPTER 2

Biomechanics of the Edentulous State

George A. Zarb

It would be inaccurate to state that disease factors such as caries or periodontal disease are the sole causes of patients' edentulism. Some authors actually argue that tooth loss does not bear even a close relationship to the prevalence of dental disease. Although the latter viewpoint is probably equally inaccurate, research has demonstrated that several nondisease factors such as attitude, behavior, dental attendance, and characteristics of the health care system play an important role in the decision to become edentulous. In addition, a significant relationship exists between the edentulous state and fiscal concerns usually associated with low occupational levels. It is therefore reasonable to conclude that edentulism is due to various combinations of cultural, financial, and dental disease attitudinal determinants, as well as to treatment received in the past.

The heterogeneous etiology of edentulism has been tackled on several worldwide fronts by the dental profession, resulting in a reported decrease in the numbers of edentulous persons. More recent reviews of tooth loss and edentulism in various parts of North American and European countries predict that treatment of patients with complete dentures will continue to decline in the future while the needs for partial tooth replacement will likely increase in the short term (see Chapter 3). Although these observations may suggest the need for a reduced dental educational commitment to treatment of edentulous patients, some very compelling points must be underscored:

1. Documented evidence reveals that despite projections of declining edentulism, the unmet need for complete denture treatment will remain high.
2. Predictions from several surveys regarding a healthy elderly population indicate that a high percentage of older people will be edentulous. Therefore the effective demand for prosthetic care for this population is likely to increase.
3. The impact of longevity on edentulism has not been fully ascertained. Clinical experience suggests that the cumulative consequences of biological and chronological aging will likely confront dentists with a significant increase in the number of difficult edentulous mouths that require treatment.

Irrespective of precise future population needs, the psychological and biomechanical consequences of tooth loss must never be overlooked. Most patients regard tooth loss as mutilation and as a strong incentive to seek dental care for the preservation of a healthy dentition and socially acceptable appearance. Dentists, on the other hand, also regard tooth loss as posing the additional hazard of an even greater mutilation: the destruction of part of the facial skeleton with the accompanying distortion of soft tissue shape, together with varying degrees of functional discomfort (Figure 2-1).

The edentulous state represents a compromise in the integrity of the masticatory system. It is frequently accompanied by adverse functional and esthetic sequelae, which are varyingly perceived by the affected patient. Perceptions of the edentulous state may range from feelings of inconvenience to feelings of severe handicap

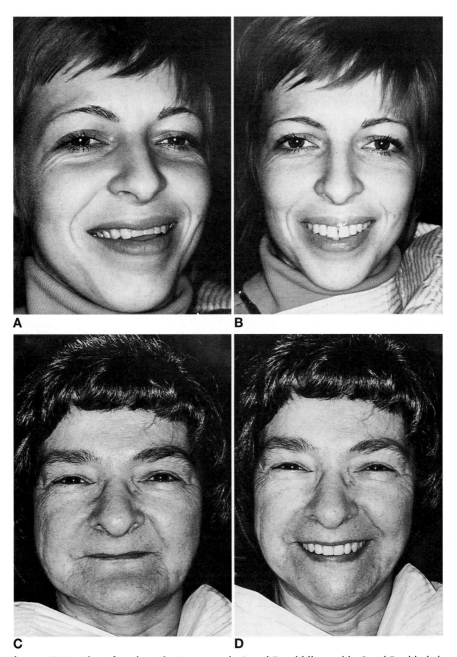

Figure 2-1   Three female patients—young in **A** and **B**, middle-aged in **C** and **D**, elderly in **E** and **F**—whose edentulous state is reflected in a range of circumoral changes that are more overt as a result of both chronological and biological aging determinants. Note the effect of well-designed dentures on varying degrees of recovery of soft tissue support with pleasing esthetic treatment outcomes.

Continued

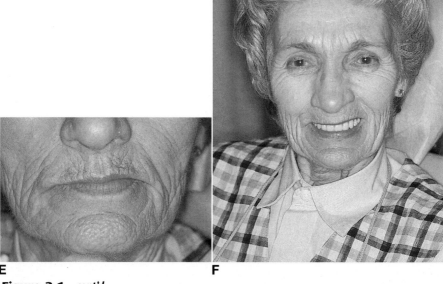

Figure 2-1   *cont'd*

because many regard total loss of teeth as equivalent to the loss of a body part. Consequently, the required treatment addresses a range of biomechanical problems that involve a wide range of individual tolerances and perceptions.

This text seeks to provide an understanding of the effects of the edentulous condition and to describe its clinical management.

SUPPORT MECHANISM FOR THE NATURAL DENTITION

The natural or prosthetic dentition and its supporting mechanism are the most visible and frequently managed parts of the masticatory system. The masticatory system is made up of closely related morphological, functional, and behavioral components. Their interactions are affected by changes in the mechanism of support for a dentition when natural teeth are replaced by artificial or prosthetic ones. An understanding of the many subtleties associated with the transition from a dentulous to an edentulous state demands a comparison of the mechanisms of both natural teeth and complete denture support (Figure 2-2).

The masticatory apparatus is involved in the trituration of food. Direct responsibility for this task falls on the teeth and their supporting tissues. The attachment of teeth in sockets is but one of many important modifications that took place during the period when the earliest mammals were evolving from their reptilian predecessors. The success of this modification is indicated by the fact that it appears to have been rapidly adopted throughout the many different groups of emerging Mammalia. Teeth function properly only if adequately supported, and this support is provided by the periodontium, an organ composed of soft and hard connective tissues.

The periodontium attaches the teeth to the bone of the jaws, providing a resilient suspensory apparatus resistant to functional forces. It allows

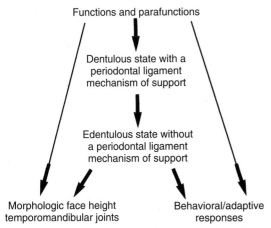

Figure 2-2   Possible interactions among the various components of the masticatory system in the context of a change in the mechanism of occlusal support.

the teeth to adjust their position when under stress. The periodontium comprises hard connective tissues (cementum and bone) and soft connective tissues (the periodontal ligament and the lamina propria of the gingiva), which are covered by epithelium. The periodontium is regarded as a functional unit and is attached to the dentin by cementum and to the jawbone by the alveolar process. The periodontal ligament and the lamina propria maintain continuity between these two hard tissue components.

The periodontal ligament provides the means by which force exerted on the tooth is transmitted to the bone that supports it. The two principal functions of the periodontium are support and positional adjustment of the tooth, together with the secondary and dependent function of sensory perception. The patient who needs complete denture therapy is deprived of periodontal support, and the entire mechanism of functional load transmission to the supporting tissues is altered.

The occlusal forces exerted on the teeth are controlled by the neuromuscular mechanisms of the masticatory system. Reflex mechanisms with receptors in the muscles, tendons, joints, and periodontal structures regulate mandibular movements. Through normal function, the periodontal structures in a healthy dentition undergo characteristic mechanical stress. The most prominent feature of

physiological occlusal forces is their intermittent, rhythmic, and dynamic nature.

The greatest forces acting on the teeth are normally produced during mastication and deglutition, and they are essentially vertical in direction. Each thrust is of short duration, and for most people, chewing is restricted to short periods during the day. Deglutition, on the other hand, occurs about 500 times a day, and tooth contacts during swallowing are usually of longer duration than those occurring during chewing. Loads of a lower order but longer duration are produced throughout the day by the tongue and circumoral musculature. These forces are predominantly in the horizontal direction. Estimates of peak forces from the tongue, cheeks, and lips have been made, and lingual force appears to exceed buccolabial force during activity. During rest or inactive periods, the total forces may be of similar magnitude.

During mastication, biting forces are transmitted through the bolus to the opposing teeth whether or not the teeth make contact. These forces increase steadily (depending on the nature of the food fragment), reach a peak, and abruptly return to zero. The magnitude, rise time, and interval between thrusts differ among persons and depend on the consistency of the food, the point in the chewing sequence, and the dental status. The direction of the forces is principally perpendicular to the occlusal plane in normal function, but the forward angulation of most natural teeth leads to the introduction of a horizontal component that tends to tilt the teeth medially as well as buccally or lingually. Upper incisors may be displaced labially with each biting thrust, and these tooth movements probably cause proximal wear facets to develop.

In healthy dentitions, teeth are in occlusion only during the functional movements of chewing and deglutition and during the movements associated with parafunction (i.e., clenching and grinding). It has been calculated that the total time during which the teeth are subjected to functional forces of mastication and deglutition during an entire day amounts to approximately 17.5 minutes (Box 2-1). More than half of this time is attributable to jaw-closing forces applied during deglutition. Therefore the total time and the range of forces seem to be well within the tolerance level of healthy periodontal tissues. It must be emphasized

Box 2-1

Calculation of Total Time during 24 Hours When Direct Functional Occlusal Force Is Applied to the Periodontal Tissues

Chewing

Actual chewing time per meal	450 sec
Four meals per day	1800 sec
One chewing stroke per sec	1800 strokes
Duration of each stroke	0.3 sec
Total chewing forces per day	540 sec (9 min)

Swallowing

Meals

Duration of one deglutition	1 sec
During chewing, three deglutitions per min, one third with occlusal force	30 sec (0.5 min)

Between meals

Daytime: 25/hr (16 hr)	400 sec (6.6 min)
Nighttime: 10/hr (8 hr)	80 sec (1.3 min)
Total	1050 sec = 17.5 min

From Graf H: *Dent Clin North Am* 13:659-665, 1969.

that the collective forces acting on a prosthetic occlusion are not likely to be controlled or attenuated as effectively as they appear to be by the natural dentition. Consequently, the time-dependent response of complete denture tissue support will manifest itself differently from those changes observed in the natural dentition.

SUPPORT MECHANISM FOR COMPLETE DENTURES

The basic challenge in the treatment of edentulous patients lies in the nature of the difference between the ways natural teeth and their artificial replacements are supported. The previous section empha-

sized the superbly evolved quantitative and qualitative aspects of periodontal ligament support for a functioning dentition. The approximate area of 45 cm^2 in each arch combines with viscoelasticity, sophisticated sensory mechanisms, and osteogenesis regulation potential to cope with the diverse directions, magnitudes, and frequencies of different forms of occlusal loading. On the other hand, the unsuitability of the tissues supporting complete dentures for load-bearing function must be immediately recognized because the mucous membrane is forced to serve an identical purpose as the periodontal ligaments.

Mucosal Support and Masticatory Loads

The area of mucosa available to receive the load from complete dentures is limited when compared with the corresponding areas of support available for natural dentitions. Researchers have computed the mean denture-bearing area to be 22.96 cm^2 in the edentulous maxillae and approximately 12.25 cm^2 in an edentulous mandible. These figures, particularly the mandibular ones, are in dramatic contrast with the 45-cm^2 area of periodontal ligament available in each dental arch (Figure 2-3). It also must be remembered that the denture-bearing area (basal seat) becomes progressively smaller as residual ridges resorb. Furthermore, the mucosa demonstrates little tolerance or adaptability to denture wearing. This minimal tolerance can be reduced still further by the presence of systemic diseases such as anemia, hypertension, or diabetes, as well as nutritional deficiencies. In fact, any disturbance of the normal metabolic processes may lower the upper limit of mucosal tolerance and initiate inflammation.

Masticatory loads are much smaller than those that can be produced by conscious effort and are in the region of 44 lb (20 kg) for the natural teeth. Maximum forces of 13 to 16 lb (6 to 8 kg) during chewing have been recorded with complete dentures, but the average loads are probably much less than these. In fact, maximal bite forces appear to be five to six times less for complete denture wearers than for persons with natural teeth. Moreover, the forces required for chewing vary with the type of food being chewed. Patients with prostheses frequently limit the loading of

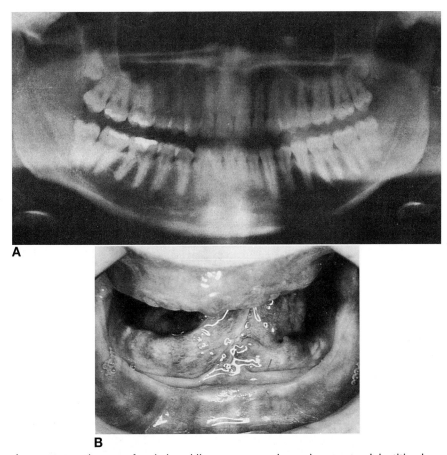

Figure 2-3 The area of periodontal ligament supporting an intact natural dentition has been computed to be approximately 45 cm² in each arch **(A)**. When teeth are lost, and a patient becomes edentulous **(B)**, aspects of support for an occlusion are severely compromised both qualitatively and quantitatively.

supporting tissues by selecting food that does not require masticatory effort exceeding their tissue tolerance.

Residual Ridge

The residual ridge consists of denture-bearing mucosa, the submucosa and periosteum, and the underlying residual alveolar bone. Residual bone is that bone of the alveolar process that remains after teeth are lost. When the alveolar process is made edentulous by loss of teeth, the alveoli that contained the roots of the teeth fill in with new bone.

This alveolar process becomes the residual ridge, which is the foundation for dentures. A variety of changes occur in the residual bone after tooth extraction and use of complete dentures. Alveolar bone supporting natural teeth receives tensile loads through a large area of periodontal ligament, whereas the edentulous residual ridge receives vertical, diagonal, and horizontal loads applied by a denture with a surface area much smaller than the total area of the periodontal ligaments of all the natural teeth that had been present. Clinical experience underscores the frequently remarkable adaptive range of the masticatory system. On the other hand, edentulous patients demonstrate very little adaptation of the supporting tissues to functional requirement.

One of the few firm facts relating to edentulous patients is that wearing dentures is almost invariably accompanied by an undesirable and irreversible bone loss. The magnitude of this loss is extremely variable, and little is known about which factors are most important for the observed variations (Figure 2-4). Two concepts have been advanced concerning the inevitable loss of residual bone: One contends that as a direct consequence of loss of the periodontal structures, variable progressive bone reduction occurs. The other maintains that residual bone loss is not a necessary consequence of tooth removal but depends on a series of poorly understood factors.

Clinical experience strongly suggests a definite relationship between healthy periodontal ligaments and maintained integrity of alveolar bone, thus the dentist's commitment to the preservation and protection of any remaining teeth to minimize or avoid advanced residual ridge reduction. The tissue support for complete dentures is conspicuously limited in both its adaptive ability and inherent capability of

simulating the role of the periodontium. This compromised support is further complicated because complete dentures move in relation to the underlying bone during function. This movement is related to the resiliency of the supporting mucosa and the inherent instability of the dentures during functional and parafunctional movements. Almost all "principles" of complete denture construction have been formulated to minimize the forces transmitted to the supporting structures or to decrease the movement of the prostheses in relation to them. Because movement of denture bases on their basal seats can cause tissue damage, it is tempting to conclude that the particularly recurrent movements of removable prostheses during parafunctional movements may be a major factor contributing to residual ridge reduction.

There are two physical factors involved in denture retention that are under the control of the dentist and are technique driven. One is the maximal extension of the denture base; the other is the maximal intimate contact of the denture base and its basal seat.

Muscular factors can be used to increase retention (and stability) of dentures. In fact, the buccina-

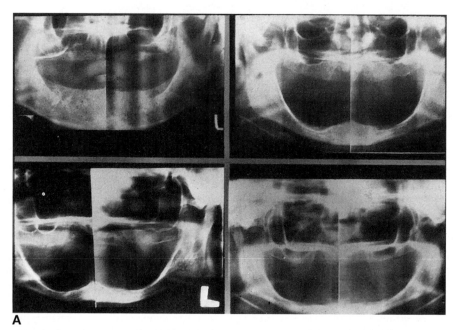

A

Figure 2-4   **A,** Panoramic radiographs showing the jaws of four edentulous patients. Residual ridge reduction has occurred to variable extents.

Continued

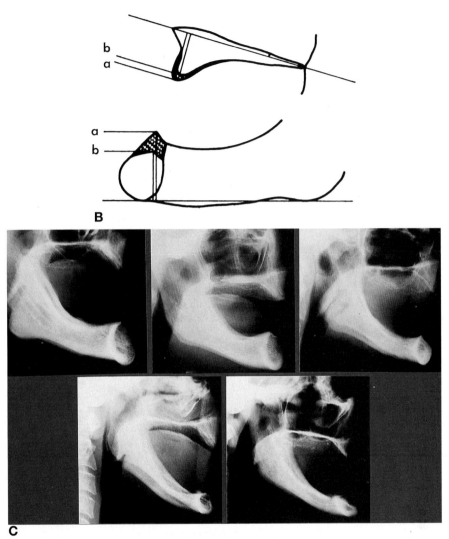

Figure 2-4 *cont'd* **B,** The rate of ridge reduction is quantified between two stages of observation (*a* and *b*). The difference between *a* and *b* represents the reduction in height of the alveolar ridges between stages of observation. The shaded area denotes resorption. **C** is a reproduction of progressive residual ridge reduction as reflected in a composite of five different lateral cephalograms. (**B,** Modified from Tallgren A: *J Prosthet Dent* 27:120-132, 1972.)

tor, the orbicularis oris, and the intrinsic and extrinsic muscles of the tongue are key muscles that the dentist harnesses to achieve this objective by means of impression techniques. Furthermore, the design of the labial, buccal, and lingual polished surfaces of the denture and the form of the dental arch are considered in balancing the forces generated by the tongue and perioral musculature.

As the form and size of the denture-supporting tissues (the basal seat) change, harnessing muscular forces in complete denture design becomes particularly important for denture retention.

Psychological Effect on Retention

The dentures may have an adverse psychological effect on some patients, and the nervous influences that result may affect salivary secretions that affect retention. Eventually, most patients seem to acquire an ability to retain their dentures by means of their oral muscle control. This muscular stabilization of dentures is probably also accompanied by a reduction in the actual physical forces used in retaining their dentures. Clearly, the physical forces of retention can be improved and reestablished, up to a point, by careful and frequent attention to the denture status. Periodic inspection, including relining procedures, will help prolong the usefulness of the prosthesis.

OCCLUSION: FUNCTIONAL AND PARAFUNCTIONAL CONSIDERATIONS

The masticatory system appears to operate best in an environment of continuing functional equilib-rium. This equilibrium depends on the interactions of the many components represented in Figure 2-2. The substitution of a complete denture for the teeth/periodontium mechanism alters this equilib-rium. An analysis of this alteration is the basis for understanding the significance of the edentulous state.

The primary components of human dental occlusion are (1) the dentition, (2) the neuromus-cular system, and (3) the craniofacial structures. The development and maturation of these compo-nents are interrelated so that growth, adaptation, and change actively participate in the develop-ment of an adult occlusion. Dentition develop-ment is characterized by a period of dental alveolar and craniofacial adaptability (Figure 2-5), which is also a time when motor skills and neuro-muscular learning are developing. Clinical treat-ment at this time may take advantage of such responsive adaptive mechanisms; for example, teeth can be guided into their correct alignment by orthodontic treatment.

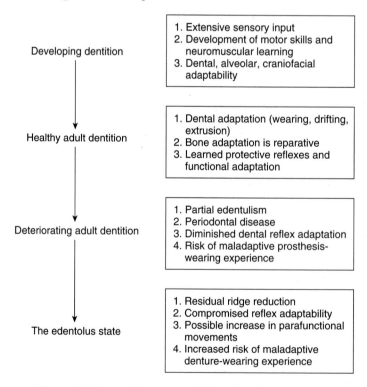

Figure 2-5 Development and adaptation of the occlusion.

In a healthy adult dentition, dental adaptive mechanisms are restricted to wear, extrusion, and drifting of teeth. Bony adaptations are essentially of a reparative nature and are slow in their operation. Protective reflexes are learned so one can avoid pain and inefficiency of the masticatory system. If and when an adult dentition begins to deteriorate, the dentist resorts to fixed or removable prosthodontic therapy in attempts to maintain a functional occlusal equilibrium. This period is characterized by greatly diminished dental and reflex adaptation and by bone resorption. Obviously, the presence of tooth loss and disease and the depletion of reparative processes pose a major prosthodontic problem. Finally, in the edentulous state, there are few natural adaptive mechanisms left. The prosthesis rests on tissues that will change progressively and irreversibly, and the artificial occlusion serves in an environment characterized by constant change that is mainly regressive.

Design and fabrication of prosthetic occlusions have led to fascinating controversies. Dental occlusion was studied first in the field of complete dentures and then in other disciplines. Early workers encountered enormous mechanical difficulties in constructing reasonably well-fitting dentures that would be both durable and esthetic. Inevitably, these dentists had to be mechanically minded. Because anatomy was the first of the biological basic sciences to be related to prosthodontic services, its application dominated prosthodontic protocol. Later, histology, physiology, and bioengineering were recognized as having essential roles in the treatment of edentulous patients. The emphasis on and application of these basic sciences lifted prosthodontics from the early mechanical art to the applied clinical science it is today.

The modern complete denture service is characterized by an integration of biological information with instrumentation materials and clinical techniques. Complete dentures are designed so that their occlusal surfaces permit multidirectional contact movements of the mandible. Orofacial and tongue muscles play an important role in retaining and stabilizing complete dentures. This is accomplished by arrangement of the artificial teeth to occupy a "neutral zone" in the edentulous mouth so the teeth will occupy a space determined by the functional balance of the orofacial and tongue musculature.

Function: Mastication and Other Mandibular Movements

Mastication consists of a rhythmic separation and apposition of the jaws and involves biophysical and biochemical processes, including the use of the lips, teeth, cheeks, tongue, palate, and all the oral structures to prepare food for swallowing. During masticatory movements, the tongue and cheek muscles play an essential role in keeping the food bolus between the occlusal surfaces of the teeth. The control of mastication within the narrow limits of tolerance of the mouth requires considerable sensory information because deviations from the normal path of mandibular movement can injure the tongue, buccal mucosa, and even the teeth and their supporting tissues. Here again, the reader's attention must be drawn to the importance of the placement of the arch of artificial teeth in the making of complete dentures. The teeth must be placed within the confines of a functional balance of the musculature involved in controlling the food bolus between the occlusal surfaces of the teeth.

The comminution of much twentieth-century food does not demand a vigorous masticatory performance. Mastication has other functions, however. It is necessary for a full appreciation of the flavor of foods and is therefore indirectly involved in the excitation of salivary and gastric secretions. Because mastication results in the mixing of food with saliva, it facilitates not only the swallowing but the digestion of carbohydrates by amylase as well. Amylase activity, of minor importance while food is in the mouth, is responsible for the continuation of carbohydrate digestion in the stomach, and this phase can account for as much as 60% of the total carbohydrate digestion. Although no reports of quantitative tests on the importance of chewing on the various stages of digestion have appeared, it has been concluded that masticatory efficiency as low as 25% is adequate for complete digestion of foods. Other investigators have noted that loss of teeth can lead to a diminished masticatory efficiency. Patients do not compensate for the smaller number of teeth by more prolonged or a larger number of chewing strokes—they merely swallow larger food particles. Although it appears that the importance of a good dentition or denture in promoting digestion and use of food has not been adequately demonstrated, clinical experience suggests that the quality of the prosthetic service may have a direct bearing on the denture wearer's masticatory performance.

As mentioned previously, the maximal bite force in denture wearers is five to six times less than in edentulous subjects. Edentulous patients are clearly handicapped in masticatory function, and even clinically satisfactory complete dentures are a poor substitute for natural teeth.

The results of studies of mandibular movement patterns of complete denture patients indicate that these movements are similar in denture-wearing patients and persons with natural teeth. Therefore treatment of partially edentulous and edentulous patients might improve their chewing efficiency and masticatory muscle activity, which would be accompanied by a decreased duration of the occlusion phase and contribute to a lessening of elevator muscle activity.

Chewing occurs chiefly in the premolar and molar regions, and both right and left sides are used to about the same extent. The position of the food bolus during mastication is dependent on the consistency of the food, and the tougher the consistency the greater is the person's preference for using the premolar region. The latter observation is apparent even in patients who have worn bilateral, soft-tissue–supported, mandibular partial dentures opposing complete upper dentures. There is an obvious advantage that the patient accrues with the replacement of missing premolar and molar segments, and these patients do not chew predominantly in the segments where natural teeth are present.

The pronounced differences between persons with natural teeth and patients with complete dentures are conspicuous in this functional context: (1) the mucosal mechanism of support as opposed to support by the periodontium; (2) the movements of the dentures during mastication; (3) the progressive changes in maxillomandibular relations and the eventual migration of dentures; and (4) the different physical stimuli to the sensor motor systems.

The denture-bearing tissues are constantly exposed to the frictional contact of the overlying denture bases. Dentures move during mastication because of the dislodging forces of the surrounding musculature. These movements manifest themselves as displacing, lifting, sliding, tilting, or rotating of the dentures. Furthermore, opposing tooth contacts occur with both natural and artificial teeth during function and parafunction when the patient is both awake and asleep.

Apparently, tissue displacement beneath the denture base results in tilting of the dentures and tooth contacts on the nonchewing side. In addition, occlusal pressure on the dentures displaces soft tissues of the basal seat and allows the dentures to move closer to the supporting bone. This change of position under pressure induces a change in the relationship of the teeth to each other.

Parafunctional Considerations

Nonfunctional or parafunctional habits involving repeated or sustained occlusion of the teeth can be harmful to the teeth or other components of the masticatory system. There are no compelling epidemiological studies about the incidence of parafunctional occlusal stress in populations with natural dentition or with dentures. Nevertheless, clinical experience indicates that teeth clenching is common and is a frequent cause of the complaint of soreness of the denture-bearing mucosa. In the denture wearer, parafunctional habits can cause additional loading on the denture-bearing tissues (Table 2-1). The unsuitability of the mechanism of denture support has already been recognized and described.

The neurophysiological basis underlying bruxism has been studied experimentally both in animals and in human beings, and part of its mechanism can be explained by an increase in the tonic activity in the jaw muscles. It is a very complex area of research and has been shown to result from psychosocial factors (such as stress or anxiety) or to be a reaction to strong emotions (e.g., anger, frustration). It may be associated with specific medical conditions (oral tardive dyskinesia, Parkinson's disease) or with sleep parasomnia (e.g., bruxism [tooth grinding], rapid eye movement [REM] behavior disorders, oromandibular myoclonus) or sleep disorders (apnea). It may also be found concomitantly with certain intraoral conditions such as pain, oral lesions, xerostomia, and discomfort with prostheses or occlusion.

The initial discomfort associated with wearing new dentures is known to evoke unusual patterns of

Table 2-1		
Direction, Duration, and Magnitude of the Forces Generated during Function and Parafunction		

	Force Generated	
	Direction	**Duration and Magnitude**
Mastication	Mainly vertical	Intermittent and light
		Diurnal only
Parafunction	Frequently horizontal as well as vertical	Prolonged, possibly excessive
		Both diurnal and nocturnal

behavior in the surrounding musculature. Frequently, the complaint of a sore tongue is related to a habit of thrusting the tongue against the denture. The patient usually is unaware of the causal relationship between the painful tongue and its contact with the teeth. Similarly, patients tend to occlude the teeth of new dentures frequently at first—perhaps to strengthen confidence in retention until the surrounding muscles become accustomed or to provide some accommodation in the chewing pattern—and experimental closure of the teeth is part of the process of adaptation. A strong response of the lower lip and mentalis muscle has been observed electromyographically in long-term complete denture wearers with impaired retention and stability of the lower denture. It is feasible and probable that the tentative occlusal contacts resulting may trigger the development of habitual nonfunctional occlusion.

The mechanism whereby pressure causes soreness of the mucous membrane is probably related to an interruption or a diminution of the blood flow in the small blood vessels in the tissues. These vascular changes could very well upset the metabolism of the involved tissues. The relationship between parafunction and residual ridge reduction has not been investigated. Nevertheless, it is tempting to include parafunction as a possible significant prosthetic variable that contributes to the magnitude of ridge reduction.

CHANGES IN MORPHOLOGICAL FACE HEIGHT AND THE TEMPOROMANDIBULAR JOINTS

The terminal stage of skeletal growth is usually accepted as being at 20 to 25 years of age. It is also recognized that growth and remodeling of the bony skeleton continue well into adult life and that such growth accounts for dimensional changes in the adult facial skeleton. It has been reported that morphological face height increases with age in persons possessing an intact or relatively intact dentition. Nevertheless, a premature reduction in morphological face height occurs with attrition or abrasion of teeth. This reduction is even more conspicuous in edentulous and complete denture-wearing patients. Figure 2-5 presents a flow chart of the presumed range of changes that take place during the development and adaptation of the occlusion. It also serves to underscore the resiliency of the masticatory system as it adapts to changes associated with disease and attendant teeth loss.

Maxillomandibular morphological changes take place slowly over a period of years and depend on the balance of osteoblastic and osteoclastic activity. The articular surfaces of the temporomandibular joints (TMJs) are also involved, and at these sites, growth and remodeling are mediated through the proliferative activity of the articular cartilages. In the facial skeleton, any dimensional changes in morphological face height or the jawbones because of the loss of teeth are inevitably transmitted to the TMJs. It is not surprising, then, that these articular surfaces undergo a slow but continuous remodeling throughout life. Such remodeling is probably the means whereby the congruity of the opposing articular surfaces is maintained, even in the presence of dimensional or functional changes in other parts of the facial skeleton.

The reduction of the residual ridges under complete dentures and the accompanying reduction in vertical dimension of occlusion tend to cause reduction in total face height and a resultant mandibular prognathism. In fact, in complete denture wearers, the mean reduction in height of the mandibular process measured in the anterior region may be approximately four times greater than the mean reduction occurring in the maxillary process (Figure 2-6). Furthermore, longitudinal studies support the hypothesis that the vertical dimension of rest position of the jaws (which is allegedly not teeth related) does not remain stable and can change over time. This clinical fact contradicts the previously popular and convenient concept of a stable vertical dimension of rest position throughout the patient's lifetime.

Obviously, complete dentures constructed to conform to clinical decisions regarding jaw-relation records are placed in an environment that retains considerable potential for change. Therefore concepts of reproducible and relatively unchangeable mandibular border movements may not apply as closely to edentulous patients as they do to persons with a healthy dentition. Practical methods that recognize these facts are described in subsequent chapters. Nevertheless, it must be reemphasized that the recognition that jaw relations are not immutable does not invalidate the clinical requirement of using a centric relation record as a starting point for developing a prosthetic occlusion.

Centric Relation

Concepts of centric relation of the upper and lower jaws have been a dominant factor in prosthodontic thinking on occlusion. *Centric relation* is defined as the most posterior position of the mandible relative to the maxillae at the established vertical dimension. Centric relation coincides with a repro-

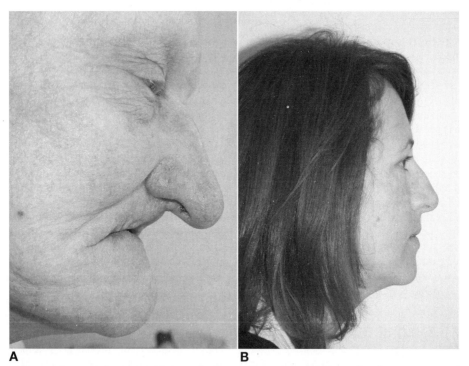

Figure 2-6   **A,** A 67-year-old man who has worn unserviced dentures for almost 20 years. Notice the reduction in total face height and the increased mandibular prognathism. **B,** Contrast his appearance with that of a 24-year-old woman who recently acquired complete dentures but posed for this picture with her dentures out of her mouth.

ducible posterior hinge position of the mandible, and it may be recorded with a high degree of accuracy. It is regarded as a very useful reference or starting point for establishing jaw relationships in any prosthodontics treatment, particularly in complete denture fabrication.

The use of centric relation has its physiological justification as well. In the vast majority of patients, unconscious swallowing is carried out with the mandible at or near the centric relation position. The unconscious or reflex swallow is important in the developing dentition. The act and frequency of swallowing are important influences in the movement of teeth within the muscle matrix, and this movement determines the tooth position and occlusal relations. The erupting teeth are guided into occlusion by the surrounding musculature (the muscle matrix), whereas the position of the mandible is determined by its location in space during the act of unconscious swallowing. The contacts of inclined planes of the teeth aid in the alignment of the erupting dentition. During this developmental period most of the mandibular activities have not yet been learned, at least not in their adult form.

The occlusion of complete dentures is designed to harmonize with the primitive and unconditioned reflex of the patient's unconscious swallow. Tooth contacts and mandibular bracing against the maxillae occur during swallowing by complete denture patients. This suggests that complete denture occlusions must be compatible with the forces developed during deglutition to prevent disharmonious occlusal contacts that could cause trauma to the basal seat of dentures. During swallowing, the mandible is close to, in centric relation, or the position of maximum mandibular retrusion relative to the maxillae at the established vertical dimension of occlusion. It is conceded, nevertheless, that most functional natural tooth contacts occur in a mandibular position anterior to centric relation, a position referred to as *centric occlusion*.

However, in complete denture prosthodontics, the position of planned maximum intercuspation of teeth is established to coincide with the patient's centric relation. The coincidence of centric relation and centric occlusion is consequently referred to as centric relation occlusion (CRO).

The centric occlusion position occupied by the mandible in the dentate patient cannot be registered with sufficient accuracy when the patient becomes edentulous. Consequently, clinical experience suggests that the recording of centric relation is the starting point in the design of an artificial occlusion.

Nevertheless, one must realize that an integral part of the definition of centric relation—at the established vertical dimension—has potential for change. This change is brought about by alterations in denture-supporting tissues and facial height, as well as by morphological changes in the TMJs. An appreciation for the dynamic nature of centric relation in denture-wearing patients, particularly in an aging context, recognizes the changing functional requirements of the masticatory system. It also accounts for different concepts and techniques of design of occlusions.

Temporomandibular Joint Changes

Numerous descriptions of TMJ function have evolved because of several research methods. The basic physiological relationship among the condyles, the disks, and their glenoid fossae appears to be maintained during maximal occlusal contacts and during all movements guided by occlusal elements. It seems logical that in the treatment with complete dentures, the dentist should seek to maintain or restore this basic physiological relation. The border movements of the mandible are reproducible, and all other movements take place within the confines of the classic "envelopes of motion." Researchers have concluded that the passive hinge movement tends to have a constant and definite rotational and reproducible character. The reproducibility of the posterior border path is of tremendous practical significance in the treatment of patients undergoing prosthodontics, but this reproducibility has been established in healthy young persons only. It must be recalled that most edentulous patients have experienced a spectrum of variations on the theme of a mutilated dentition. In the course of such periods, pathological or adaptive structural alterations or changes of the TMJs may have occurred. These investigations are mainly based on autopsy studies; thus the results are only speculative.

It has also been reported that impaired dental efficiency resulting from partial tooth loss and absence of or incorrect prosthodontic treatment can influence the outcome of temporomandibular disorders (TMDs). This is thought to be particularly the case when arthritic or degenerative changes have occurred. The hypothesis has been advanced that degenerative joint disease is a process rather than a disease entity. The process involves joint changes that cause an imbalance in adaptation and a degeneration that results from alterations in functional demands on or the functional capacity of the joints. However, because the onset of degenerative conditions is frequently encountered in the adult years, and because the greater number of denture wearers are older patients who are edentulous, the treatment of such conditions is very much the concern of the dentist. Clinical experience and long-term studies indicate that a combination of adjunctive prosthodontic protocols, and appropriate pharmacological and supportive therapy, are usually adequate to provide these patients with comfort.

One of the difficulties in managing degenerative joint involvement is achieving joint rest. Because of the necessity for mastication and for the avoidance of parafunctional habits, voluntary or even enforced rest may be difficult to achieve.

ESTHETIC, BEHAVIORAL, AND ADAPTIVE RESPONSES

Esthetic Changes

There is little doubt that tooth loss can adversely affect a person's appearance. Patients seek dental treatment for both functional and esthetic or cosmetic reasons, and dentists have been successful in restoring or improving many a patient's appearance.

Box 2-2 lists some of the conspicuous and clinically challenging features that frequently accompany the edentulous state. It must be emphasized that one or more of these items are also frequently encountered in persons with intact dentitions because the compromised facial support of the edentulous state is not the exclusive cause of the morphological changes. In clinical practice, we frequently encounter situations in which factors such as a patient's weight loss, age, and heavy tooth

---

Box 2-2

Morphological Changes Associated with the Edentulous State

1. Deepening of nasolabial groove
2. Loss of labiodental angle
3. Decrease in horizontal labial angle
4. Narrowing of lips
5. Increase in columella-philtral angle
6. Prognathic appearance

---

attrition manifest orofacial changes suggestive of compromised, or absent, dental support for the overlying tissues. Some patients fail to appreciate the fact that aspects of their facial appearance for which they are seeking a solution are merely magnified perceptions or are unrelated to their edentulous predicament. In recent years, numerous plastic surgical interventions, which address facial cosmetic issues, have been popularized. One or more of the available techniques may provide the sort of solution desired by the patient, and which is not the dentist's remit. In such a context, the dentist must be prepared to guide the patient with a referral to an experienced specialist in the field of cosmetic surgery.

These patients can cause the dentist considerable frustration. Experience suggests that early communication about a patient's cosmetic expectations should be established to avoid later misunderstanding. Patients should be asked to provide photographs of their preedentulous appearance, and relevant details from these photographs should be carefully analyzed and discussed with the patient. If this is not possible, photographs of siblings or of children who resemble the patient may be helpful.

Careful explanation of prosthodontic objectives and methods is the basis for good communication with all patients. This is the case when the patient's cosmetic desires exceed morphological or functional realities.

Behavioral and Adaptive Responses

The process whereby an edentulous patient can accept and use complete dentures is complex. It requires adaptation of learning, muscular skill, and motivation and is related to the patient's expectations. The patient's ability and willingness to accept and learn to use the dentures ultimately determine the degree of success of clinical treatment. Helping a patient adapt to complete dentures can be one of the most difficult but also one of the most rewarding aspects of clinical dentistry. The presence of inanimate foreign objects (dentures) in an edentulous mouth is bound to elicit different stimuli to the sensorimotor system, which in turn influences the cyclic masticatory stroke pattern. Both exteroceptors and proprioceptors are probably affected by the size, shape, position, pressure from, and mobility of the prostheses. The exact role and relative importance of mucosal stimuli in the control of jaw movements need clarification, but it has been clearly demonstrated that control of dentures by muscle activity is reduced if surface anesthetic is applied to the oral mucous membrane. Although it is tempting to assume that there is a correlation between oral stereognosis and purposeful oral motor activity, the results of most investigations up to now indicate that successful denture wearing possibly involves factors other than oral perception and oral performance. It therefore remains very difficult to apply learning theory concepts to the presumed process, which a patient undergoes while learning to wear complete dentures.

Learning means the acquisition of a new activity or change of an existing one. *Muscular skill* refers to the capacity to coordinate muscular activity to execute movement. The acceptance of complete dentures is accompanied by a process of habituation, which is defined as a "gradual diminution of responses to continued or repeated stimuli." The tactile stimuli that arise from the contact of the prosthesis with the richly innervated oral cavity are probably ignored after a short time. Because each stage of the decrease in response is related to the memory trace of the previous application of the stimulus, storage of information from the immediate past is an integral part of habituation. Difficulty in the storage of information of this type accompanies older age, and this is the reason why older patients have difficulties becoming comfortable with dentures. Furthermore, stimuli must be specific and identical to achieve habituation. This is what probably prevents the transfer of habituation

evoked by an old familiar denture to a new denture, which inevitably gives rise to a new range of stimuli, and several clinical applications of adaptation problems may be encountered. The patient who has worn a complete upper denture opposing a few natural anterior mandibular teeth usually will find a complete lower denture difficult to adapt to. Such a patient has to contend with altered size and orientation of the tongue. The tongue frequently responds to the loss of posterior teeth and alveolar bone by changing size to bring its lateral borders into contact with the buccal mucosa. The insertion of a new denture introduces a new environment for the tongue, and the intrinsic tongue musculature reorganizes the shape of the tongue to conform to the altered space available. A degree of retraining tongue activity also takes place. Furthermore, the posterior residual ridges are exposed to new sensations from the overlying prosthesis. Pressures transferred through the denture base replace tactile stimuli from the tongue and frictional contact with food. In addition, control of the upper denture frequently must be unlearned because the posterior part of the tongue is no longer required to counter the dislodging effect on the denture produced by the remaining mandibular dentition.

Edentulous patients expect, and are expected, to adapt to the dentures more or less instantaneously. That adaptation must take place in the context of the patient's oral, systemic, emotional, and psychological states.

The facility for learning and coordination appears to diminish with age. Advancing age tends to be accompanied by progressive atrophy of elements in the cerebral cortex, and a consequent loss in the facility of coordination occurs. Certainly, patient motivation dictates the speed with which adaptation to dentures takes place. It is imperative that the dentist determine the patient's motivation in seeking treatment, cultivate this motivation, and seek to foster it if it is lacking or absent.

A distinct need exists for dentists to be able to understand a patient's motivation in seeking prosthodontic care and to identify problems before starting treatment. Emotional factors are known to play a significant role in the etiology of dental problems. The interview and clinical examination are obvious ways to observe the patient and form the best treatment relationship. Successful management begins with identification of anticipated difficulties before treatment starts and with careful planning to meet specific needs and problems. Dentists must train themselves to reassure the patient, to perceive the patient's wishes, and to know how and when to limit the patient's expectations. An essential accompaniment of a denture design that is physically compatible with the oral complex is a good interpersonal relationship between dentist and patient. It is up to the dentist to explore the patient's symptoms and tensions. The way the patient handles other illnesses and dental situations will aid in the prediction of future problems. It has been observed that the secure patient will adjust readily, cope with discomfort, and be cooperative.

It has also has been reported that when a complete denture population was examined for depression most of the depressive symptoms were found to coincide with age groups that included the greatest proportion of denture wearers. Awareness by the dentist of high-risk groups for depression within the patient pool may help explain difficulties in achieving patient satisfaction with dentures, facilitate recognition of a problem, and make possible appropriate referral for diagnosis and treatment of the patient's depression.

The whole area of prosthodontist/patient interpersonal relationships has not been adequately studied or emphasized by the dental profession. Recently, educational programs to modify the often-unrealistic expectations of patients who wear dentures have shown favorable results. Similarly, programs to modify the knowledge, skills, and habits of patients who wear dentures may assist them to adapt more successfully to denture wearing. Although the taking of a health history can be effective, a great deal of experience and training are necessary to conduct a patient interview effectively and profitably. Unfortunately, the rigors of dental practice prevent most dentists from taking the time to carry out a thorough patient interview. Because a connection between emotional problems and denture problems may exist, a health questionnaire should be used as a guide for a structured personal interview with the patient. It is a useful adjunct to establishing a prognosis for the proposed treatment.

Finally, the absence of a yardstick to gauge a patient's adaptive potential to wearing a prosthesis is one of the most challenging facets of treating edentulism. The success of prosthetic treatment is predicated not only on the dentist's manual dexterity but also on the ability to relate to patients and to understand their needs. The importance of empathy and correct clinical judgment on the part of the dentist can hardly be overemphasized. The dentist's ability to understand and recognize the problems of edentulous patients, to select the proper course of required treatment, and to reassure them has proven to be of greatest clinical value.

Bibliography

Arendorf TM, Walker DM: Denture stomatitis; a review, *J Oral Rehabil* 14:217-227, 1987.

Atwood DA: A cephalometric study of the clinical rest position. II. The variability in the rate of bone loss following the removal of occlusal contacts, *J Prosthet Dent* 7:544-552, 1957.

Atwood DA: The future of prosthodontics, *J Prosthet Dent* 51:262-267, 1984.

Berry DC, Mahood M: Oral stereognosis and oral ability in relation to prosthetic treatment, *Br Dent J* 120:179-185, 1966.

Blomberg S, Lindquist L: Psychological reactions to edentulousness and treatment with jawbone anchored bridges, *Acta Psychiatr Scand* 68:252-256, 1983.

Bolender CL, Swoope CC, Smith DE: The Cornell Medical Index as a prognostic aid for complete denture patients, *J Prosthet Dent* 22:20-29, 1969.

Bouma J: *On becoming edentulous: an investigation into the dental and behavioral reasons for full mouth extractions,* thesis, Groningen, 1987, University of Groningen.

Brill N: Factors in the mechanism of full denture retention, *Dent Pract* 18:9-19, 1967.

Brisman AS: Esthetics: a comparison of dentists' and patients' concepts, *J Am Dent Assoc* 100:345, 1980.

Carr L, Wolfaardt JF, Haitas GP: Speech defects in prosthetic dentistry. (ii) Speech defects associated with removable prosthodontics, *J Dent Assoc S Afr* 40:387-390, 1985.

Chamberlain BB, Chamberlain KR: Depression: a psychological consideration in complete denture prosthodontics, *J Prosthet Dent* 53:673-675, 1985.

Cohen LK: Dental care delivery in seven nations: the International Collaborative Study of Dental Manpower Systems in relation to oral health status. In Ingle JI, Blair P, editors: *International dental care delivery systems: issues in dental health policies*, Cambridge, Mass, 1978, Ballinger Publishing.

Douglass CW, Gammon MD, Atwood DA: Need and effective demand for prosthodontic treatment, *J Prosthet Dent* 59: 94-99, 1988.

Eichner FKW: Recent knowledge gained from long-term observations in the field of prosthodontics, *Int Dent J* 34:35-40, 1984.

Ettinger RL, Beck JD, Jakobsen J: Removable prosthodontic treatment needs a survey, *J Prosthet Dent* 51:419-427, 1984.

Glaser EM: *The physiological basis of habituation*, New York, 1966, Oxford University Press.

Graf H: Bruxism, *Dent Clin North Am* 13:659-665, 1969.

Hammond J, Thomson JC: Diagnosis of complete denture difficulties, *Dent Update* 9:35-40, 1982.

Hannam AG, De Cou RE, Scott TD, Wood WW: The relationship between dental occlusion, muscle activity and associated jaw movements in man, *Arch Oral Biol* 22:25-32, 1977.

Haraldsson T, Karlsson U, Carlsson GE: Bite force and oral function in complete denture wearers, *J Oral Rehabil* 6:41-48, 1979.

Jacobson TE, Krol AJ: A contemporary review of the factors involved in complete denture retention, stability and support, *J Prosthet Dent* 49:5-15, 165-172, 306-313, 1983.

Jooste CH, Thomas CJ: Complete mandibular denture stability when posterior teeth are placed over a basal tissue incline, *J Oral Rehabil* 19:441-448, 1992.

Kuebker WA: Denture problems: causes, diagnostic procedures, and clinical treatment. (I) Retention problems, *Quintessence Int* 10:1031-1044, 1984; (II) Patient discomfort problems, *Quintessence Int* 11:1131-1141, 1984; (III/IV) Gagging problems and speech problems, *Quintessence Int* 12:1231-1238, 1984.

Kydd WL, Daly CH, Wheeler JB: The thickness measurement of masticatory mucosa in vivo, *Int Dent J* 21:430-441, 1971.

McCord JF, Grant AA, Quayle AA: Treatment options for the edentulous mandible, *Euro J Prosthodontic Restor Dent* 1:19-23, 1992.

Redford M, Drury TF, Kingman A, Brown LJ: Denture use and the technical quality of dental prostheses among persons 18-74 years of age: United States, 1988-1991, *J Dent Res* 75:714-725, 1996.

Sandström B, Lindquist LW: The effect of different prosthetic restorations on the dietary selection in edentulous patients: a longitudinal study of patients initially treated with optimal complete dentures and finally with tissue-integrated prostheses, *Acta Odontol Scand* 45(6):423-428, 1987.

Speirs RL: The sense of taste, *Dent Update* 15:82-87, 1988.

Tallgren A: The continuing reduction of the residual alveolar ridges in complete denture wearers: a mixed-longitudinal study covering 25 years, *J Prosthet Dent* 27:120-132, 1972.

Tourne LP, Luc PM, Fricton JR: Burning mouth syndrome, *Oral Surg Oral Med Oral Pathol* 74:158-167, 1992.

Weintraub J, Burt B: Oral health status in the United States: tooth loss and edentulism, *J Dent Educ* 49:368-376, 1985.

Yemm R: Stress-induced muscle activity: a possible etiologic factor in denture soreness, *J Prosthet Dent* 28:133-140, 1972.

Zarb GA: Oral motor patterns and their relation to oral prostheses, *J Prosthet Dent* 47:472, 1982.

CHAPTER 3

The Effects of Aging on the Edentulous State

Michael I. MacEntee

THE AGING POPULATION

The global population is aging at an unprecedented rate (Table 3-1). This change is noticeable, particularly in Japan and in some European countries where almost 2 in 10 residents are older than 65 years of age (Anderson & Hussey, 2000). The demographic scenario is similar in most industrialized countries, and is remarkable particularly among the "middle-old" (age 75 to 84) and "old-old" (age 85+) populations. In Canada, for example, about half (45.2%) of the elderly population is older than 75 years of age (Statistics Canada, 2001), and in Japan the number of persons older than 80 years will more than double (from 3.7% to 7.5%) between 2000 and 2020 (Anderson & Hussey, 2000). The expansion of the geriatric population has been growing rapidly over the last quarter of a century and will increase further probably by at least one third within the next 20 years or so. The result has already produced a major shift in health care away from the cure of acute diseases and disorders to the management of chronic illness (Bury, 2001). The impact of this demographic change causes great concern generally because of the potential increase in health care costs, although the correlation currently between health care spending and an aging population is weak (Anderson & Hussey, 2000).

Cardiovascular disease, cancer, and cirrhosis of the liver were particularly hazardous to men during the early part of the twentieth century, in large part because of industrial pollutants, smoking, and alcohol abuse. Women seem to have benefited more from improved health care, especially in obstetrics.

Consequently, there are nearly twice as many older women than older men simply because women live longer, with an average life expectancy of 80 years versus 73 years for men. The reason for the prolonged life expectancy of women is not fully understood, and it is not at all certain that women will continue to outlive men in the future.

A small but internationally consistent proportion (~6%) of persons 65 years of age and older live in long-term care facilities, but of course the proportion of older persons who are institutionalized increases dramatically with advancing age. By age 75 nearly everyone is burdened by at least one chronic disorder that limits access to dental care and influences dental treatment. Furthermore, most older persons believe that they have very little flexibility with their income, and a large proportion of them, in North America at least, receive an income that is below the poverty line. In 1995 nearly one fifth (17%) of the total Canadian population and more than one third (36%) of unattached Canadian residents were attempting to live on incomes below the poverty line (National Council of Welfare, 1999). Another perspective on poverty defines it as a lack of resources "for achieving self-respect, taking part in the life of the community, (and) appearing in public without shame," all influenced directly by oral health and a comfortable dentition (Sen, 1999). Consequently, there are many older people who are likely to be very concerned by unexpected dental costs, unless the need for treatment is explicit and reasonable to them.

Table 3-1
Current (2002) and Expected (2020) Distribution of the Population 65 Years of Age and Older in Eight Countries (2000)

	Percentage					
	Age 65 + yr			**Age 80 + yr**		
Country	**2000**	**2020**	**Increase**	**2000**	**2020**	**Increase**
Australia	12.1	16.8	39	2.8	3.7	30
Canada	12.8	18.2	43	3.1	4.4	42
France	15.9	20.1	26	3.8	5.5	45
Germany	16.4	21.6	32	3.6	6.3	76
Japan	17.1	26.2	54	3.7	7.5	107
New Zealand	11.6	15.6	34	2.8	3.5	24
United Kingdom	16.0	19.8	24	4.2	5.1	22
United States	12.5	16.6	33	3.3	3.7	14

From Anderson GF, Hussey PS: Population aging: a comparison among industrialized countries, *Health Affairs* 19:191-203, 2000.

DISTRIBUTION AND IMPACT OF EDENTULISM IN OLD AGE

Distribution

The prevalence of edentulism is declining. Today, about one third to one half of the population 65 years of age and older in most industrialized countries are edentate, but there are large regional and age-related variations (Table 3-2). More older men than women are likely to have teeth, probably because many women have had unsightly teeth removed earlier in life. The loss of natural teeth is also associated with less affluent people. For example, in the United States within the last two decades about half (51%) of the less educated population were edentate, compared with about one quarter (29%) of the more highly educated population (Burt, 1992), which most likely reflects the scope of health services accessible to individuals. Quite simply, those who have less education and less money are less exposed to preventive dental information and are unable to afford restorative treatment when needed (Dharamsi & MacEntee, 2002).

Despite the benefits of water fluoridation and dentistry, about three of four older persons within the last decade were using complete dentures in at least one jaw (Mojon and MacEntee 1992; MacEntee, Stolar, and Glick, 1993), but even this is substantially lower than the prevalence of complete edentulism reported only a few decades ago from many countries (MacEntee, 1985). The decrease in total tooth loss in the United States, for example, has dropped by about 10% each decade for the last 30 years, although there will be a net increase in the number of edentulous people for the foreseeable future with the growing numbers of older people overall (Douglass, Shih, and Ostry, 2002).

Impact

Residual alveolar ridges continue to resorb for several decades after extraction of teeth, yet older persons rarely seek treatment for problems with dentures, possibly because many of them have been dissatisfied with previous treatment (MacEntee et al., 1991). Moreover, older people usually adapt poorly to new dentures, which probably explains why they seldom return to have old but familiar dentures replaced. When they do complain, it is usually about the pain of chewing hard foods with uncomfortably loose dentures on flat residual ridges.

THE IMPACT OF AGE ON THE EDENTULOUS MOUTH

Mucosa

Stomatitis and other mild inflammations are the mucosal lesions encountered most frequently in older edentulous mouths, especially of older men

Table 3-2
The Distribution of Edentulism in Old Age

Country	Year	Reference	Age Group (yr)	Percent Edentate
Australia	1987/1988	DHHLGCS (1993)	>65	50
			>75	62
	1999	DSRU (2001)	>65	33
United Kingdom	1988	Todd & Lader (1991)	>65	69
	1998	Walls & Steele (2001)	65-74	39
			75+	60
Canada	1990	Charette (1993)	>65	50
	1992	Hawkins, Main and Locker (1998)	85+	66
Denmark	1982	Ainamo & Österberg (1992)	65-81	60
Finland	1990	Ainamo & Österberg (1992)	>65	46
Germany	1997	Nitschke (2001)	65-74	25
Ireland	1990	O'Mullane and Whelton (1990)	>65	48
Japan	1993	Ministry Hlth and Welfare (1993)	>65	30
Norway	1989	Ainamo & Österberg (1992)	>65	29
Spain	1989	Bourgeois, Nihtila, and Mersel (1998)	65-74	40
	1999	The Spanish Geriatric Oral Health Research Group (2001)	>65	31
Sweden	1988/1989	Ainamo & Österberg (1992)	65-74	29
			75-84	50
United States	1985	Miller et al. (1987)	>65	41
	1988-91	Marcus et al. (1996)	65-74	29
			75+	43
	1990	Douglass et al. (1993)	>70	38
	1999	MMWR (1999)	>65	29

who wear dentures, smoke tobacco, and drink alcohol excessively (MacEntee, Glick, and Stolar, 1998). Oral cancer or precancerous lesions are unusual in Western countries, although they are the most common forms of cancer on the Indian subcontinent and in other parts of Asia. It is reasonably clear that the incidence of oral cancer is higher among African Americans than among the rest of the U.S. and Canadian populations of other races and that the prognosis is also poorer among African Americans, which probably reflects the influence of low socioeconomic status more than genes or culture (Arbes et al., 1999; Skarsgard et al., 2000). External carcinogens, such as nicotine and alcohol, should be more damaging to the oral mucosa in old age because of atrophy, increased mitosis with slow turnover of cells, and increased number of elastic fibers. Therefore it is likely that the risk of oral cancer is increased among edentulous denture wearers, especially among those who drink alcohol to excess and smoke tobacco, simply because many of them are poor and they make little use of screening services for early detection.

Bone

Bone mass is at its maximum in midlife, with substantially more in men than in women, and in some racial groups more than others. However, even within individuals, the quality of bone in all parts of the skeleton, including the jaws, varies greatly and decreases with age (Esteves, 1994). The decrease occurs because osteoblasts are less efficient, estrogen production declines, and there is an overall reduction of calcium absorption from the intestine in old age.

The turnover and metabolism of bone are influenced by many factors, including exercise, genes, hormones and nutrition, but usually resorption surpasses formation somewhere around midlife in both men and women. The jaws of both sexes also become more porous with time probably because of metabolic rather than functional changes in the bone.

Osteoporosis is a disorder caused by an accelerated loss of trabecular bone. It happens usually, but not exclusively, in women after menopause, and is discovered frequently when an older person breaks a vertebra, hip, or forearm. It has primary and secondary forms that are difficult to diagnose. The more prevalent Type I (postmenopausal) form affects women for a decade or so after menopause, whereas the Type II (senile or idiopathic) form can attack men and women alike at any age for no obvious reason. Actually, the Type II form can develop as a consequence of any disease, such as hyperparathyroidism, and induce bone loss. Residual ridge resorption may be a manifestation of primary Type I osteoporosis, but there is very little evidence to show that the two conditions are associated (Esteves, 1994). Estrogen replacement therapy, bisphosphonates, or other systemic treatments for osteoporosis do affect the density and content of jawbones as in other skeletal bone, but the extent of the effect varies considerably at different sites, and the preventive attributes of the treatments are unknown (von Wowern, 2001).

Saliva

The role of saliva as a lubricant and as a chemical buffer is central to the comfort and function of the mouth. The electrolytes, glycoproteins, and enzymes of mucous saliva lubricate, cleanse, and protect the mucosa, and they ease the passage of food around the mouth while contributing to the sense of taste. Inadequate quality or quantity of saliva is particularly difficult for complete denture wearers because mucous saliva produced by the minor glands of the palatal helps to retain and lubricate the dentures. We do not know whether the quantity or quality of saliva in healthy individuals is disturbed by age, but we do know that older persons take a vast array of potentially xerostomic medications for depression, sleeping disorders,

hypertension, allergies, heart problems and many other geriatric problems. Indeed, stress, depression, tobacco use, and abuse of alcohol alone can disturb salivary flow, whereas hyposalivation of the minor salivary glands of the palate, which disturbs denture retention, is a common side effect of digitalis preparations, tranquillizers, and polycyclic antidepressants (Niedermeier et al., 2000). Pharmacological side effects, especially on submandibular glands, are complicated further by the biochemical interactions of multiple medications (Wu et al., 1993). Sjögren's syndrome and radiation treatment also cause dry mouth. Food may have a metallic or salty taste, and an unpleasant sensitivity to bitter and sour foods increases when salivary flow is poor, whereas reduced sensitivity to sweet tastes can generate an unhealthy craving for sugar. A change in the quality of saliva might not be obvious clinically, but it should be suspected as a cause of denture intolerance when a patient is taking multiple medications. Management of hyposalivation is difficult, but recent evidence indicates that secretion of mucous saliva from the palate improves measurably after drinking 2 L of water, when chewing or exercising vigorously, or when taking estrogen or pilocarpine (Niedermeier et al., 2000).

JAW MOVEMENTS IN OLD AGE

People chew more slowly as they get older. Although the duration of the total chewing cycle does not appear to change, it does seem that the vertical displacement of the mandible is shortened (Karlsson and Carlsson, 1990). Movements of the mandible are governed by a generator in the brain stem influenced by proprioceptors in muscles, joints, and mucosa. Advancing age may delay the central processing of nerve impulses, impede the activity of striated muscle fibers, and inhibit decisions. It can also reduce the number of functional motor units and fast muscle fibers, and decrease the cross-sectional area of the masseter and medial pterygoid muscles (Newton et al., 1987). Consequently, older people tend to have poor motor coordination and weak muscles. Muscle tone can decrease by as much as 20% to 25% in old age, which probably explains the shorter chewing strokes and prolonged chewing time (Sonies,

1992). Older persons also have a less coordinated chewing stroke close to maximum intercuspation, probably because of a general deficit in the central nervous system, and some individuals who assume the characteristic stoop of old age experience pain on swallowing because of osteophytes and spurs growing on the upper spine adjacent to the pharynx. A noticeable change in swallowing strongly suggests that there might be an underlying pathosis, such as Parkinson's disease or palsy that is not a part of normal aging (Sonies, 1992).

TASTE AND SMELL

Taste and smell are frequently confused because the sensory mechanisms are closely related and dependent. The sensation of "tasting" rarely occurs in isolation, but results from the interaction of proprioception, taste, and smell. Texture is felt, chemical constituents stimulate taste, and aromatic gases smell. Bitter, sweet, sour, and salty tastes stimulate receptors independently, so one may be damaged without disturbing the others. Olfactory cells send projections directly to the brain so they can be traumatized anywhere along the way.

Sensitivity to taste declines with age, and especially in older persons with Alzheimer's disease (Murphy, 1993). Also, the preference for specific flavors changes over time to favor higher concentrations of sugar and salt. Complaints of an impairment affecting the sense of taste at any age should be investigated thoroughly because they forebode an upper respiratory infection or a serious neurological disorder. The three cranial nerves (VI, IX, and X) carrying sensations of taste can be disturbed and damaged by tumors, viruses (e.g., Bell's palsy and herpes zoster), and trauma (e.g., head injury and ear washing), but, fortunately, damage in one part of the system can be compensated readily by increased sensitivity elsewhere.

NUTRITION

There is some evidence, largely from animal studies, that diet influences longevity and aging, with the weight of evidence favoring restrictions on fat and protein. The relationship between diet and prolonged life in human beings is complex and, as yet, inadequately explained. Currently, the recom-

mended daily allowances for the various vitamins, minerals, fats, carbohydrates, and proteins are probably inaccurate because most of the data on intake of specific nutrients have been estimated for young adults. Nevertheless, the elderly population is at particular risk for malnutrition because of a variety of factors that range from socioeconomic stress to an overconsumption of drugs, and including, to some extent, the state of the dentition. A national survey in the United States around 1970 (Rhodus and Brown, 1990) revealed that older people frequently had inadequate calories or calcium in their diet and that many of them absorbed vitamins (notably A, B, and C) and minerals poorly (Figure 3-1).

The role of the dentition in mastication and food selection is complex. Some edentulous persons with faulty dentures restrict themselves to a soft diet high in fermentable carbohydrates, whereas others, even with uncomfortable and well-worn dentures, can eat nearly all of the food available to them (Millwood and Heath, 2000). A recent population-based study in the United Kingdom found that edentulous older persons, compared with older persons with natural teeth, had significantly lower levels of plasma ascorbate and plasma retinol, which could disturb their skin and eyesight (Sheiham and Steele, 2001).

AGING SKIN AND TEETH

Skin

The scars of a lifetime are revealed dramatically on the skin as wrinkles, puffiness, and pigmentations, but the changes are not all manifestations of degeneration. For example, fewer Langerhans' cells in older skin can prevent undesirable immunological responses, whereas mottling of the skin protects against the sun. The leathery look characteristic of the older sun worshipper is caused by epidermal growths with large melanocytes—*solar lentigines*—that thicken in the epidermis. Gradually the dermis thins, enzymes dissolve collagen and elastin, and wrinkles appear when layers of fat are lost.

Age reduces the concavity and "pout" of the upper lip, and it flattens the philtrum. The nasolabial grooves deepen, which produces a sagging look to the middle third of the face, whereas

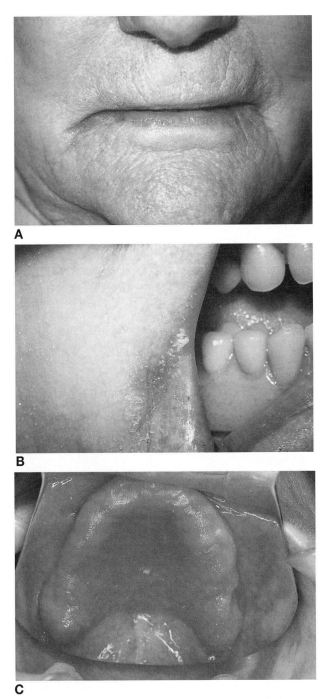

Figure 3-1 Angular cheilitis (**A** and **B**) and stomatitis (**C**) in an elderly man caused by malnutrition and/or liver dysfunction (white blood cell count, 3.19; hemoglobin, 12.4; hematocrit, 36.3; vitamin B_{12}, 203).

atrophy of the subcutaneous and buccal pads of fat hallows the cheeks. Subsequently, as the loss of fat continues, support for the presymphyseal pad of fat disappears, and the upper lip droops (cheiloptosis) over the maxillary teeth (Figure 3-2). Of course, these changes are accentuated even more dramatically when teeth are missing or when there is a loss of occlusal vertical dimension (Figure 3-3).

Teeth

The color of healthy, natural teeth ranges in hue from yellow to orange, with large variation in chroma and value (MacEntee and Lakowski, 1981). The chroma, and occasionally the hue, will change as the enamel is abraded, exposing the underlying dentine to extrinsic stains. The chroma may also deepen by a systemic distribution of various medications, particularly those containing heavy metals. Ultimately, natural teeth take on the jagged brownish appearance of an aging dentition when the incisal edges break and the exposed dentine gathers extrinsic stains. It is not always easy to reproduce this rugged appearance in artificial teeth. In fact, some patients in conflict with the esthetic sense of their dentist prefer to have complete dentures with teeth that are smaller, straighter, and whiter than natural teeth.

CONCERNS FOR PERSONAL APPEARANCE IN OLD AGE

Older persons worry about their self-image as much, if not more, than at any other stage of life. They may be ambivalent about growing old, but typically they attempt to strike a psychosocial balance between the good and the bad effects. Unfortunately, the respect afforded occasionally to older people can be diminished by feelings of social rejection and physical collapse compounded by the stigma of inadequate dentures (Goffman, 1963).

The profits of the cosmetic industry, including plastic surgery and esthetic dentistry, and the popularity of the keep-fit industry, attest to a widespread concern that wrinkles, shifting body fat, and other "disfigurements" may inhibit or damage personal relationships. Concealment of age has become a preoccupation of the Western world, a fixation that seems to disturb women more directly than men. The aging woman is considered unattractive and judged, even by other women, more harshly than the aging man, whereas women in general seem less repelled by the graying or "mature look" of the older man.

Society frowns on anyone, young or old, (but especially on elderly men) who use cosmetics or

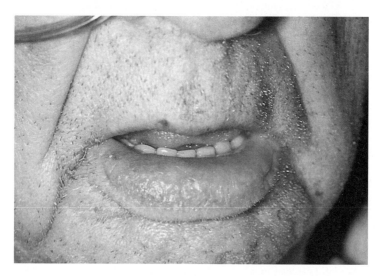

Figure 3-2   Appearance of the lower two thirds of an elderly person's face demonstrating the typical droop of the upper lip that accentuates the mandibular incisors.

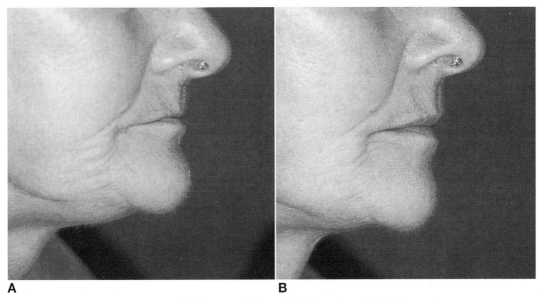

A   B

Figure 3-3   **A** and **B,** The influence of the vertical dimension of occlusion on the "youthful" appearance of the face.

other concealments of age. Apparently, we admire those who do not have to cover up their defects. Consequently, men are more furtive than women about seeking improvements to their appearance. Furthermore, age concealment is acceptable for oneself but not for others, a clear indication that there are double standards operating on the public image.

An attractive appearance is considered important to self-satisfaction. Healthy older persons frequently admit that they try hard to feel and look young. A healthy person will accept the natural consequences of aging without undue disturbance, although psychosocial pressures can cause an unhealthy obsession with appearance, even to the point of anorexia surfacing for the first time in old age (Nicholson and Ballance, 1998). Unusual requests for alterations to appearance should be managed with caution and related directly to the psychosocial status of the patient. Indeed, expectations that seem to be in any way unrealistic, particularly if the patient is depressed or deluded, should be offered a very guarded prognosis. Actually, a marked discrepancy between the assessment of the clinician and the patient offers a valuable diagnostic clue to a problem, assuming of course that the

clinician has a rational rather than a distorted view of aging.

SUMMARY

The need for complete dentures in the Western world will increase over the next quarter of a century despite the current successes of preventive dentistry and the apparent affluence of contemporary society. Management of edentulous elderly patients involves a constant sensitivity to the potential impact of a multitude of medical disorders. There are few disorders that are exclusive to older individuals; nevertheless, the mouth is a fine sensor of systemic stability, and occasionally it offers the first physical manifestation of a disease. For example, the edentulous mouth can suffer from a very painful attack of shingles involving sensory nerves of the face, neck, and trunk, or display angular cheilitis with a denture-induced stomatitis usually without symptoms. Wounds heal more slowly and possibly less effectively in old age because of decreased turnover of cells or poor blood circulation. Consequently, the mucosa and underlying bone supporting complete dentures heal more slowly from the trauma of ill-fitting dentures.

Prosthodontic treatment for older people requires accurate diagnoses of systemic and local problems before attending to the design of dentures. Systemic problems, including psychological distress and physiological disturbances, are frequently complicated by inappropriate use of prescribed medications. Local inflammation of the alveolar mucosa is caused usually by unhygienic and structurally defective dentures and can be corrected relatively easily by relining and repairing the dentures. Subsequently, mucosal inflammation should resolve after improved hygiene.

New dentures are not accepted easily by older patients, so, whenever possible, modify dentures that are familiar to the patient rather than make new dentures. However, if the denture must be replaced, it is preferable when possible to duplicate the general shape and tooth arrangement of the old denture. Lastly, every denture should have the patient's identity embedded visibly but inconspicuously in the acrylic resin.

Overall, the management of problems encountered in an aging population can seem like a series of objectionable compromises, but adaptation is the hallmark of successful aging, and coping with difficulties is an acceptable part of everyday life. Life at any age does have pleasant surprises and rewards.

References

Ainamo A, Österberg T: Changing demographic and oral disease patterns and treatment needs in the Scandinavian populations of old people, *Int Dent J* 42:311-322, 1992.

Anderson GF, Hussey PS: Population aging: a comparison among industrialized countries, *Health Affairs* 19:191-203, 2000.

Arbes SJ Jr, Olshan AF, Caplan DJ, Schoenbach VJ, Slade GD, Symons MJ: Factors contributing to the poorer survival of black Americans diagnosed with oral cancer (United States), *Cancer Causes & Control* 10:513-523, 1999.

Bourgeois D, Nihtila A, Mersel A: Prevalence of caries and edentulousness among 65-74-year-olds in Europe, *Bull World Health Org* 76:413-417, 1998.

Burt BA: Epidemiology of dental diseases in the elderly, *Clinics in Geriatric Med* 8:447-459, 1992.

Bury M.: Illness narratives: fact or fiction? *Sociol Health Illn* 25:263-285, 2001.

Charette A: Dental health. In Stephens T, Graham DF editors: *Canada's Health Promotion Survey 1990: technical report*. Health and Welfare Canada. Ottawa: Minister of Supply and Services Canada. Chap. 15: 210-218, 1993.

Dharamsi S, MacEntee MI: Dentistry and distributive justice, *Soc Sci Med* 55(4):55: 323-329, 2002.

DHHLGCS: *National Oral Health Survey Australia 1987-88*. Department of Health, Housing, Local Government and Community Services. Canberra: Australian Government Publishing Service, 1993.

Douglass CW, Jette AM, Fox CH, Tennstedt SL, Joshi A, Feldman HA, McGuire SM, McKinlay JB: Oral health status of the elderly in New England, *Journals of Gerontol* 48:M39-46, 1993.

Douglass CW, Shih A, Ostry L: Will there be a need for complete dentures in the United States in 2020, *J Prosthet Dent* 87:5-8, 2002.

DSRU: Australian Institute of Health & Welfare Dental Statistics and Research Unit. Oral health and access to dental care—1994-96 and 1999. Research Report AIHW [Den 73], March: 1-6, 2001.

Esteves APZ: The relationship between systemic metabolism and the structure and deposition of human jaw bone, a thesis submitted in partial fulfillment of the requirements for the degree of M.Sc., Vancouver, 1994, The University of British Columbia.

Goffman E: *Stigma: notes on the management of spoiled identity*, Englewood Cliffs, NJ, 1963, Prentice Hall.

Hawkins RJ, Main PA, Locker D: Oral health status and treatment needs of Canadian adults aged 85 years and over, *Spec Care Dent* 18:164-169, 1998.

Karlsson S, Carlsson GE: Characteristics of mandibular masticatory movement in young and elderly dentate subjects, *J Dent Res* 69:473-476, 1990.

MacEntee MI: The prevalence of edentulism and diseases related to dentures: a literature review, *J Oral Rehabil* 12:195-207, 1985.

MacEntee MI, Glick N, Stolar E: Age, gender, dentures and oral mucosal disorders, *Oral Dis* 4:32-36, 1998.

MacEntee MI, Hill PM, Wong G, Mojon P, Berkowitz J, Glick N: Predicting concerns for oral health among institutionalized elders, *J Public Health Dent* 51:82-91, 1991.

MacEntee MI, Lakowski R: An instrumental colour analysis of vital and extracted human teeth, *J Oral Rehabil* 8:203-208, 1981.

MacEntee MI, Stolar E, Glick N: The influence of age on the oral health of an independent elderly population, *Community Dent Oral Epidemiol* 21:234-239, 1993.

Marcus SE, Drury TF, Brown LJ, Zion GR: Tooth retention and tooth loss in the permanent dentition of adults: United States, 1988-91, *J Dent Res* 75:684-695, 1996.

Miller AJ, Brunelle JA, Carlos JP, Brown LJ, Löe H: Oral health of United States adults: national findings. US Dept. of Health and Human Services, National Institute of Health (USA), Bethesda, 1987.

Millwood J, Heath MR: Food choice by older people: the use of semi-structured interviews with open and closed questions, *Gerodontol* 17:25-32, 2000.

Ministry of Health and Welfare: Report on the survey of dental disease. Tokyo: Health Policy Bureau, Ministry of Health and Welfare, 1993.

Mojon P, MacEntee MI: Discrepancy between need for prosthodontic treatment and complaints in an elderly edentulous population, *Community Dent Oral Epidemiol* 20:48-52, 1992.

Murphy C: Nutrition and chemosensory perception in the elderly, *Critical Reviews in Food Sci & Nutr* 33:3-15, 1993.

National Council of Welfare: Poverty in Canada. In Curtis J, Grabb E, Guppy N, editors. *Social inequality in Canada: patterns, problems, policies*, ed 3, Scarborough, Ontario, 1999, Prentice-Hall Canada Inc.

Newton JP, Abel RW, Robertson EM, Yemm R. Changes in human masseter and medial pterygoid muscles with age: a study by computed tomography, *Gerodontics* 3:151-154, 1987.

Nicholson SD, Ballance E: Anorexia nervosa in later life: an overview, *Hospital Med (London)* 59:268-72, 1998.

Niedermeier W, Huber M, Fischer D, Beier K, Muller N, Schuler R, Brinninger A, Fartasch M, Diepgen T, Matthaeus C, Meyer C, Hector MP: Significance of saliva for the denture-wearing population, *Gerodontol* 17:104-118, 2000.

Nitschke I: Geriatric oral health issues in Germany, *Int Dent J* 51:235-246, 2001.

O'Mullane D, Whelton H. *National survey of adults' dental health 1989/'90: preliminary report*, Cork, 1990, University College Cork, Oral Health Services Research Unit.

Rhodus NL, Brown J: The association of xerostomia and inadequate intake in older adults, *J Amer Dietic Assoc* 90: 1688-1692, 1990.

Sen A: *Development as freedom*, Oxford, 1999, Oxford University Press.

Sheiham A, Steele J: Does the condition of the mouth and teeth affect the ability to eat certain foods, nutrient and dietary intake and nutritional status amongst older people? *Public Health Nutrition* 4:797-803, 2001.

Skarsgard DP, Groome PA, Mackillop WJ, Zhou S, Rothwell D, Dixon PF, O'Sullivan B, Hall SF, Holowaty EJ: Cancers of the upper aerodigestive tract in Ontario, Canada, and the United States, *Cancer* 88:1728-1738, 2000.

Sonies BC: Oropharyngeal dysphagia in the elderly, *Clinics Geriatric Med* 8: 569-576, 1992.

Statistics Canada: Canadian Statistics: The People: Population, 2001. http://www.statcan.ca/english/Pgdb/People/popula.htm

The Spanish Geriatric Oral Health Research Group: Oral health issues of Spanish adults aged 65 and over, *Int Dent J* 51:228-234, 2001.

Todd JE, Lader D: *Adult dental health 1988 United Kingdom*, London, 1991, HMSO.

Total tooth loss among persons aged ≥65 years—selected states, 1995-1997, US Dept. of Health & Human Services, *MMWR (1999) Morb Mortal Wkly Rep* 48:206-210, 1999.

von Wowern N: General and oral aspects of osteoporosis: a review, *Clinic Oral Investigat* 5:71-82, 2001.

Walls AWG, Steele JG: Geriatric oral health issues in the United Kingdom, *Int Dent J* 51:183-187, 2001.

Wu AJ, Atkinson JC, Fox PC, Baum BJ, Ship JA: Cross-sectional and longitudinal analyses of stimulated parotid salivary constituents in healthy, different-aged subjects, *Journals of Gerontol* 48: M219-224, 1993.

CHAPTER 4

Sequelae Caused by Wearing Complete Dentures

Ejvind Budtz-Jørgensen

THE DENTURE IN THE ORAL ENVIRONMENT

Placement of a removable prosthesis in the oral cavity produces profound changes of the oral environment that may have an adverse effect on the integrity of the oral tissues (Box 4-1). Mucosal reactions could result from a mechanical irritation by the dentures, an accumulation of microbial plaque on the dentures, or, occasionally, a toxic or allergic reaction to constituents of the denture material. The continuous wearing of dentures may have a negative effect on residual ridge form because of bone resorption. Furthermore, wearing complete dentures that function poorly and that impair masticatory function could be a negative factor with regard to maintenance of adequate muscle function and nutritional status, particularly in older persons.

There are several aspects of the interaction between the prosthesis and the oral environment.

Surface properties of the prosthetic material may affect plaque formation on the prosthesis; however, the original surface chemistry of the prosthetic material is modified by the acquired pellicle and thus is of minor importance for the establishment of plaque (Box 4-2). On the contrary, surface irregularities or microporosities greatly promote plaque accumulation by enhancing the surface area exposed to microbial colonization and by enhancing the attachment of plaque. Furthermore, plaque formation is greatly influenced by environmental conditions such as the design of the prosthesis, health of adjacent mucosa, composition of saliva, salivary secretion rate, oral hygiene, and denture-wearing habits of the patient.

The presence of different types of dental materials in the oral cavity may give rise to electrochemical corrosion, but changes in the oral environment due to bacterial plaque may constitute an important cofactor in this process. Corrosive galvanic currents have been implicated in the burning mouth syndrome (BMS), oral lichen planus, and altered taste perception. Most often it is difficult to establish a definite causal relationship because mechanical irritation or infection may also be involved. For instance, local irritation of the mucosa by the dentures may increase mucosal permeability to allergens or microbial antigens. This makes it difficult to distinguish between a simple irritation and an allergic reaction against the prosthetic material, microbial antigens, or agents absorbed to the prosthesis capable of eliciting an allergic response. The matter is further complicated by the fact that certain microorganisms (e.g., yeasts) are able to use methylmethacrylate as a carbon source, thereby causing a chemical degradation of the denture resin.

In the interface between a prosthesis and the oral mucosa, microbial plaque may have important negative or harmful effects (Figure 4-1). Thus a prosthesis may promote infection of the underlying mucosa, caries, and periodontal disease adjacent to overdenture abutments, periimplant gingivitis, and chemical degradation or corrosion of prosthetic materials.

Box 4-1

Direct Sequelae Caused by Wearing Removable Prostheses: Complete or Partial Dentures

Mucosal reactions
Oral galvanic currents
Altered taste perception
Burning mouth syndrome
Gagging
Residual ridge reduction
Periodontal disease (abutments)
Caries (abutments)

Box 4-2

Interaction of Prosthetic Materials and the Oral Environment

Surface Properties: Plaque Accumulation
Chemical stability
Adhesiveness
Texture
Microporosities
Hardness

Chemical Properties
Corrosion
Toxic reactions
Allergic reactions

Physical Properties
Mechanical irritation
Plaque accumulation

Changes of Environmental Conditions
Plaque microbiology

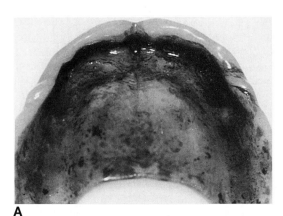

A

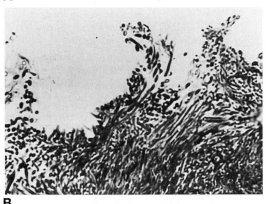

B

Figure 4-1   A, Microbial plaque on the fitting denture surface visualized with the stain erythrosin. **B,** Section of a denture showing microbial deposits penetrating into irregularities of the fitting denture surface.

DIRECT SEQUELAE CAUSED BY WEARING DENTURES

Denture Stomatitis

The pathological reactions of the denture-bearing palatal mucosa appear under several titles and terms such as *denture-induced stomatitis, denture sore mouth, denture stomatitis, inflammatory papillary hyperplasia*, and *chronic atrophic candidosis*. In the following sections, the term *denture stomatitis* will be used with the prefix *Candida*-associated if the yeast *Candida* is involved. In the randomized populations, the prevalence of denture stomatitis is about 50% among complete denture wearers.

Classification   According to Newton's classification, three types of denture stomatitis can be distinguished.

Type I   A localized simple inflammation or pinpoint hyperemia (Figure 4-2).

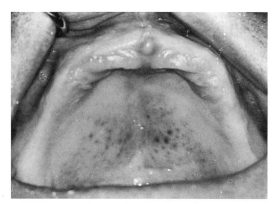

Figure 4-2   Pinpoint hyperemia, a characteristic feature of type I denture stomatitis.

Type II   An erythematous or generalized simple type seen as more diffuse erythema involving a part or the entire denture-covered mucosa (Figure 4-3).

Type III   A granular type (inflammatory papillary hyperplasia) commonly involving the central part of the hard palate and the alveolar ridges. Type III often is seen in association with type I or type II (Figure 4-4).

Strains of the genus *Candida*, in particular *Candida albicans*, may cause denture stomatitis. Still, this condition is not a specific disease entity because other causal factors exist such as bacterial infection, mechanical irritation, or allergy. Type I most often is trauma induced, whereas types II and

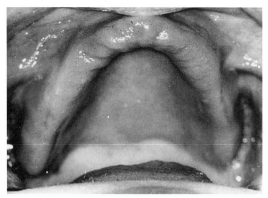

Figure 4-3   Type II denture stomatitis showing erythema of the entire mucosa in contact with the fitting denture surface.

III most often are caused by the presence of microbial plaque accumulation (bacteria or yeasts) on the fitting denture surface and the underlying mucosa. The often relative association of *Candida*-associated denture stomatitis with angular cheilitis or glossitis indicates a spread of the infection from the denture-covered mucosa to the angles of the mouth or the tongue, respectively (Figure 4-5).

Diagnosis   The diagnosis of *Candida*-associated denture stomatitis is confirmed by the finding of mycelia or pseudohyphae in a direct smear or the isolation of *Candida* species in high numbers from the lesions ($\geq$50 colonies) (Figure 4-6). Usually, yeasts are recovered in higher numbers from the fitting surface of the dentures than from corresponding areas of the palatal mucosa. This indicates that *Candida* residing on the fitting surface of the denture is the primary source of the infection.

Etiology and Predisposing Factors   The direct predisposing factor for *Candida*-associated denture stomatitis is the presence of the dentures in the oral cavity (Box 4-3). Thus the infection prevails in patients who are wearing their dentures both day and night; the infection will disappear if the dentures are not worn. It is likely that bacteria, which constitute the major part of the microorganisms of the denture plaque, are also involved in the infection. In addition, trauma could stimulate the turnover of the palatal epithelial cells, thereby reducing the degree of keratinization and the barrier function of the epithelium; thus the penetration of fungal and bacterial antigens can take place more easily.

The colonization of the fitting denture surface by *Candida* species depends on several factors, including adherence of yeast cells, interaction with oral commensal bacteria, redox potential of the site, and surface properties of the acrylic resin. The pathogenicity of denture plaque can be enhanced by factors stimulating yeast propagation, such as poor oral hygiene, high carbohydrate intake, reduced salivary flow, and continuous denture wearing. The more important factors that can modulate the host-parasite relationship and increase the susceptibility to *Candida*-associated denture stomatitis may be aging, malnutrition, immunosuppression, radiation therapy, diabetes mellitus, and possibly treatment with antibacterial antibiotics.

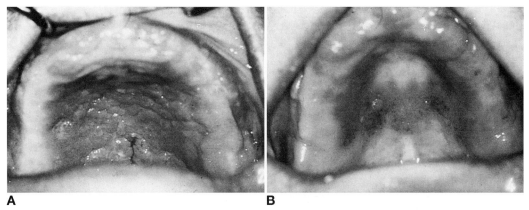

A   B

Figure 4-4 **A,** Type III denture stomatitis, papillary hyperplasia, the nodular type. **B,** Type III denture stomatitis, papillary hyperplasia, the mossy type.

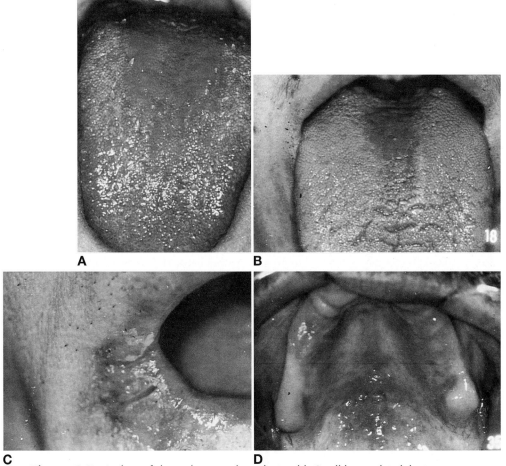

C   D

Figure 4-5 Lesions of the oral mucosa in patients with *Candida*-associated denture stomatitis. **A,** Diffuse atrophic glossitis. **B,** Median rhomboid glossitis. **C,** Angular cheilitis. **D,** Erythema of the soft palate.

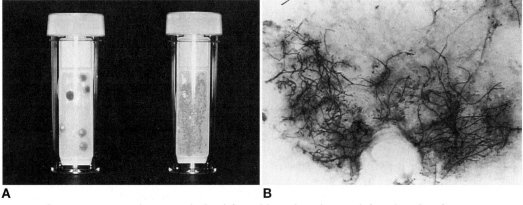

Figure 4-6   A, Culture on Oriculty: *left,* positive culture in a noninfected carrier of *Candida*; *right,* high number of yeast colonies from a patient with denture stomatitis indicates a *Candida* infection. **B,** Smear from the fitting denture surface yielded pseudomycelium.

Evidence supports that unclean dentures and poor hygiene care are major predisposing factors because healing of the lesions is often seen after meticulous oral and denture hygiene is instituted. However, the tissue surface of the dentures usually

---

Box 4-3

Factors Predisposing to *Candida*-Associated Denture Stomatitis

Systemic Factors

Old age
Diabetes mellitus
Nutritional deficiencies (iron, folate, or vitamin B_{12})
Malignancies (acute leukemia, agranulocytosis)
Immune defects
Corticosteroids, immunosuppressive drugs

Local Factors

Dentures (changes in environmental conditions, trauma, denture usage, denture cleanliness)
Xerostomia (Sjögren's syndrome, irradiation, drug therapy)
High-carbohydrate diet
Broad-spectrum antibiotics
Smoking tobacco

---

shows micropits and microporosities that harbor microorganisms that are difficult to remove mechanically or by chemical cleansing. According to several in vitro studies, the microbial contamination of denture acrylic resin occurs very quickly, and yeasts seem to adhere well to denture base materials.

Angular cheilitis is often correlated to the presence of *Candida*-associated stomatitis, and it is thought that the infection may start beneath the maxillary denture and from that area spread to the angles of the mouth (see Figure 4-5). It seems, however, that this infection results from local or systemic predisposing conditions such as overclosure of the jaws, nutritional deficiencies, or iron deficiency anemia. Frequently, a secondary infection caused by *Staphylococcus aureus* could be present. It must be recognized that visible infection by *Candida* species can be an early indicator of immune dysfunction and the discovery of such should prompt a review of the patient's clinical background.

Although denture stomatitis and angular cheilitis usually do not reflect a serious predisposing disease or abnormality, with denture wearing as the direct cause of the lesions, it should be realized that severe infections by *Candida* species may occur in the immunocompromised host (Figure 4-7).

Management and Preventive Measures   Because of the diverse possible origins of denture stomatitis, several treatment procedures could be used, including antifungal therapy, correction of ill-fitting dentures, and efficient plaque control.

The most important therapeutic and preventive measures are the institution of efficient oral and denture hygiene and correction of the denture-wearing habits because the major etiological factor is the presence of the denture. The patient should be instructed to remove the dentures after the meal and scrub them vigorously with soap before reinserting them. The mucosa in contact with the denture should be kept clean and massaged with a soft toothbrush. Patients with recurrent infections should be persuaded not to use their dentures at night but rather leave them exposed to air, which seems to be a safe and efficient means of preventing microbial colonization. The dentures often may cause trauma because they are old and ill fitting or because there are faults in the design. Rough areas on the fitting surface should be smoothed or relined with a soft tissue conditioner. About 1 mm of the internal surface being penetrated by microorganisms should be removed and relined frequently. A new denture should be provided only when the mucosa has healed and the patient is able to achieve good denture hygiene.

There is no substantial evidence that harmless commercial denture cleansers are efficient in preventing colonization of the dentures by microorganisms. Polishing or glazing of the tissue surface of removable dentures should be considered a routine step in prosthodontic treatment to facilitate denture cleansing by brushing.

Antifungal drugs could be used to remove *Candida albicans* residing on oral mucosa and the fitting denture surface, but recurrence of the infection is often observed if the hygiene is not improved. Treatment with antifungal agents should be used mainly in the following patients:

1. In patients after the clinical diagnosis has been confirmed by a mycological examination.
2. In patients with associated burning sensations from the oral mucosa.
3. In patients in whom the infection has spread to other sites of the oral cavity or the pharynx.
4. In patients with an increased risk of systemic mycotic infections due to debilitating diseases, drugs, or radiation therapy.

Local therapy with nystatin, amphotericin B, miconazole, or clotrimazole should be preferred to systemic therapy with ketoconazole or fluconazole because resistance of *Candida* species to the latter drugs occurs regularly. For a reduction in the risk of relapse, the following precautions should be taken:

1. Treatment with antifungals should continue for 4 weeks (Figure 4-8).
2. When lozenges are prescribed, the patient should be instructed to take out the dentures during sucking.
3. The patient should be instructed in meticulous oral and denture hygiene; the patient should be told to wear the dentures as seldom as possible and to keep them dry or in a disinfectant solution of 0.2% to 2.0% chlorhexidine during nights.

Surgical elimination of deep crypt formations in type III denture stomatitis usually is a prerequisite for effective mucosal hygiene. This could preferably be achieved with cryosurgery.

It must be emphasized that the interrelationship between host status and the clinical presentations of oral candidiasis means that the dentist can gain useful insight into the patient's overall health. In addition to suggesting appropriate antifungal treatment, such insights may also help in the early diagnosis and treatment of more serious and underlying disease.

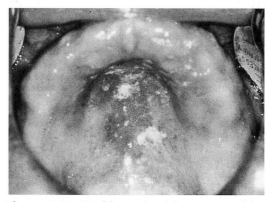

Figure 4-7 *Candida*-associated denture stomatitis in an immunocompromised patient. There is evidence of thrush on the hard palate.

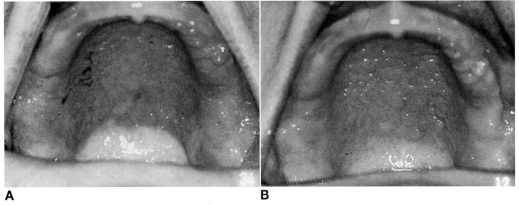

A   **B**

Figure 4-8 **A,** Type III denture stomatitis showing modular hyperplasia with severe inflammation. **B,** After only a 2-week treatment with amphotericin B lozenges, which are usually prescribed for 4 weeks, the erythema has declined, but the hyperplasia has persisted.

Flabby Ridge

Flabby ridge (i.e., mobile or extremely resilient alveolar ridge) is due to replacement of bone by fibrous tissue. It is seen most commonly in the anterior part of the maxilla, particularly when there are remaining anterior teeth in the mandible, and is probably a sequela of excessive load of the residual ridge and unstable occlusal conditions (Figure 4-9). Results of histological and histochemical studies have shown marked fibrosis, inflammation, and resorption of the underlying bone. Flabby ridges provide poor support for the denture, and it could be argued that the tissue should be removed surgically to improve the stability of the denture and to minimize alveolar ridge resorption. However, in a situation with extreme atrophy of the maxillary alveolar ridge, flabby ridges should not be totally removed because the vestibular area would be eliminated. Indeed the resilient ridge may provide some retention for the denture.

Denture Irritation Hyperplasia

A common sequela of wearing ill-fitting dentures is the occurrence of tissue hyperplasia of the mucosa in contact with the denture border (Figure 4-10). The lesions are the result of chronic injury by unstable dentures or by thin, overextended denture flanges. The proliferation of tissue may take place relatively quickly after

placement of new dentures and is normally not associated with marked symptoms. The lesions may be single or quite numerous and are composed of flaps of hyperplastic connective tissue. Inflammation is variable; however, in the bottom of deep fissures, severe inflammation and ulceration may occur.

After replacement or adjustment of the dentures, the inflammation and edema may subside and produce some clinical improvement of the condition. After surgical excision of the tissue and replacement of the denture, the lesions are unlikely to recur.

When pressure ulcerations develop and irritation from microbial products is severe, the patient may experience marked discomfort. If lymphadenopathy is present, the denture irritation hyperplasia may simulate a neoplastic process.

Traumatic Ulcers

Traumatic ulcers or sore spots most commonly develop within 1 to 2 days after placement of new dentures. The ulcers are small and painful lesions, covered by a gray necrotic membrane and surrounded by an inflammatory halo with firm, elevated borders (Figure 4-11). The direct cause is usually overextended denture flanges or unbalanced occlusion. Conditions that suppress resistance of the mucosa to mechanical irritation are predisposing (e.g., diabetes mellitus, nutritional deficiencies, radi-

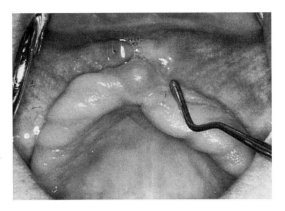

Figure 4-9 Flabby ridge (or hyperplastic replacement) of the anterior part of the maxilla.

ation therapy, or xerostomia). In the systemically noncompromised host, sore spots will heal a few days after correction of the dentures. When no treatment is instituted, the patient will often adapt to the painful situation, which subsequently may develop into a denture irritation hyperplasia.

Oral Cancer in Denture Wearers

An association between oral carcinoma and chronic irritation of the mucosa by the dentures has often been claimed, but no definite proof seems to exist (Figure 4-12). Case reports have detailed the development of oral carcinomas in patients who wear ill-fitting dentures. However, most oral cancers do develop in partially or totally edentulous patients. The reasons appear to include an association with

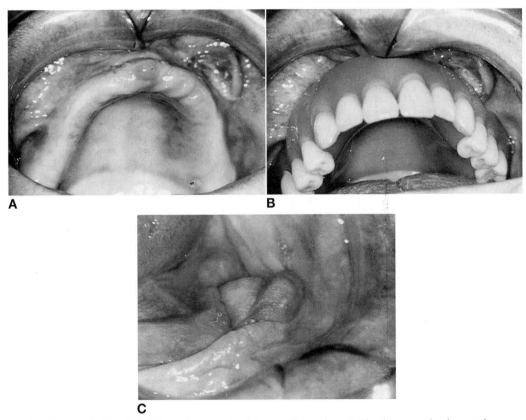

Figure 4-10 **A,** Soft tissue hyperplasia of the maxillary sulcus. **B,** The tissue reaction is caused by chronic irritation by the denture flange. **C,** Fibroma produced by the lingual denture flange.

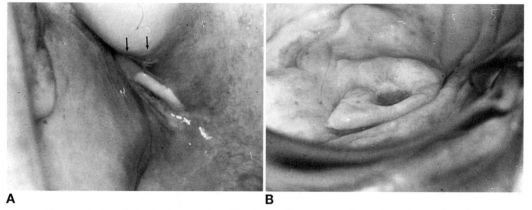

Figure 4-11   **A,** Acute ulcer produced by the maxillary denture in the hamular notch region distal to the tuberosity *(arrows)*. **B,** Chronic ulcer produced by the lingual denture flange.

more heavy alcohol and tobacco use, less education, and lower socioeconomic status, which predispose to oral cancer as well as to poor dental health, including tooth extraction and denture wearing. This underlines the necessity of strict and regular recall visits at 6-month to 1-year intervals for comprehensive oral examinations. The opinion is still valid that if a sore spot does not heal after correction of the denture, malignancy should be suspected. Patients with such cases and clinically aberrant manifestations of denture irritation hyperplasia should be referred immediately to a pathologist. It should be recognized that the prognosis is poor for oral carcinomas, especially for those in the floor of the mouth.

BURNING MOUTH SYNDROME

BMS could be a sequela of denture wearing and is characterized by a burning sensation in one or several oral structures in contact with the dentures. It is relevant to differentiate between burning mouth sensations and BMS. In the former group, the patient's oral mucosae are often inflamed because of mechanical irritation, infection, or an allergic reaction. In patients with BMS, the oral mucosa usually appears clinically healthy. The vast majority of those patients affected by BMS is older than 50 years of age, is female, and wears complete dentures. In the edentulous

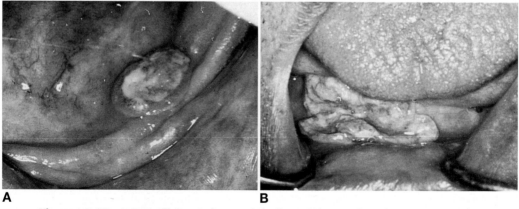

Figure 4-12   **A,** Basocellular carcinoma of the floor of the mouth, early stage. **B,** Carcinoma involving the alveolar ridge and the vestibule.

patient wearing complete dentures, burning sensations from the supporting tissues or the tongue are common complaints, particularly in postmenopausal women. Usually, there are no overt clinical signs, but the symptoms often appear for the first time in association with the placement of new dentures.

Characteristically, the symptoms have a gradual onset, and the pain is often present in the morning and tends to become aggravated during the day. The quality of pain is a burning sensation associated with a feeling of dry mouth and persistent altered taste sensation. Other associated symptoms may include headache, insomnia, decreased libido, irritability, or depression. Aggravating factors include tension, fatigue, and hot or spicy foods, whereas sleeping, eating, and distraction reduce pain intensity.

Etiological Factors

A multitude of causative factors have been described for BMS, which can be classified in three main categories: local, systemic, or psychogenic (Box 4-4).

Local   In denture wearers, a coincidence has been observed between the wearing of faulty dentures and burning symptoms from the underlying mucosa and the tongue. The causative factors could be instability of the dentures, prolonged period of masticatory muscle activity, parafunctional activity of the tongue, and undue friction on the mucosa. Candidal infections or allergic reactions may produce the symptoms related to burning mouth sensations but seldom to BMS.

Systemic   The relatively high prevalence of BMS in menopausal women is difficult to explain because there is no evidence of a direct hormonal effect on the oral mucosa. Thus the oral discomfort is independent of the hormonal level measured, and results of well-controlled clinical trials have shown no clinical effects of systemic or local treatment with estrogen. Vitamin (B_{12}, folic acid) or iron hematological deficiencies are thought to be etiological factors in a varying number of patients with BMS. Furthermore, replacement therapy usually is successful in patients with vitamin deficiency but not

---

Box 4-4

Documented Possible Causes of Burning Mouth Syndrome

Local Factors
Mechanical irritation
Allergy
Infection
Oral habits and parafunctions
Myofascial pain

Systemic Factors
Vitamin deficiency
Iron deficiency anemia
Xerostomia
Menopause
Diabetes
Parkinson's disease
Medication

Psychogenic Factors
Depression
Anxiety
Psychosocial stressors

---

in patients without vitamin deficiency who have BMS. Xerostomic conditions induced by radiation therapy, systemic disease, or drugs are often associated with a burning sensation of the oral tissues, but there is no direct evidence that these conditions are etiologically important for BMS.

Psychogenic   With the use of objective psychometric methods to assess the psychological status of patients with BMS, anxiety and depression were the most frequent diagnoses. Generally, patients with BMS were more concerned with bodily functions and more depressed, emotionally repressed, distrustful, anxious, and socially isolated. It is not quite clear, however, whether these psychopathological factors are causative of the oral complaints or merely the result of chronic pain.

Management   A priori, none of the proposed etiological factors can be ruled out. As a consequence, a systematic approach is necessary to identify the possible causes. In denture wearers in whom no organic basis for the complaints is identified, the approach of the prosthodontist should be very careful. The situation may be further complicated by the fact that the patients often claim that their psychiatric disorders are due to the poor dentures and the inadequate prosthetic treatment they have received. It is important, with appropriate counseling of the patient, to help the patient understand the benign nature of the problem, with subsequent elimination of the fears. The patient's symptoms should always be taken seriously, but any comprehensive prosthetic treatment, including treatment with implant-supported overdentures, should be carried out only as a collaborative effort of psychiatrist and prosthodontist.

Gagging

The gag reflex is a normal, healthy defense mechanism. Its function is to prevent foreign bodies from entering the trachea. Gagging can be triggered by tactile stimulation of the soft palate, the posterior part of the tongue, and the fauces. However, other stimuli such as sight, taste, noise, as well as psychological factors, or a combination of these, may trigger gagging. In sensitive patients, the gag reflex is easily released after placement of new dentures, but it usually disappears in a few days as the patient adapts to the dentures. Persistent complaints of gagging may be due to overextended borders (especially the posterior part of the maxillary denture and the distolingual part of the mandibular denture) or poor retention of the maxillary denture. However, the condition is often due to unstable occlusal conditions or increased vertical dimension of occlusion because the unbalanced or frequent occlusal contacts may prevent adaptation and trigger gagging reflexes. In wearers of old dentures, gagging may be a symptom of diseases or disorders of the gastrointestinal tract, adenoids or catarrh in the upper respiratory passages, alcoholism, or severe smoking.

Residual Ridge Reduction

Longitudinal studies of the form and weight of the edentulous residual ridge in wearers of complete dentures have demonstrated a continuous loss of bone tissue after tooth extraction and placement of complete dentures. The reduction is a sequel of alveolar remodeling due to altered functional stimulus of the bone tissue. It follows a chronic progressive and irreversible course that often results in severe impairment of prosthetic restoration and oral function (Figure 4-13). The process of remodeling is particularly important in areas with thin cortical bone (e.g., the buccal and labial parts of the maxilla and the lingual parts of the mandible). During the first year after tooth extraction, the reduction of the residual ridge height in the midsagittal plane is about 2 to 3 mm for the maxilla and 4 to 5 mm for the mandible. After healing of the residual ridge, the remodeling process will continue but with decreased intensity. In the mandible, the annual rate of reduc-

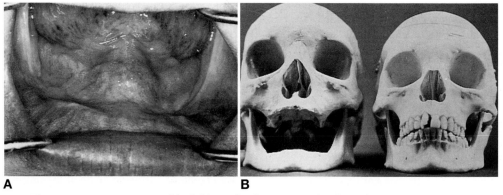

A   **B**

Figure 4-13 **A,** Severe residual ridge reduction—a sequela of wearing complete dentures over several years. **B,** Note the location of the mental foramina near the top of the residual ridge.

tion in height is about 0.1 to 0.2 mm and in general four times less in the edentulous maxilla. However, the intraindividual variations are very important.

The pathogenesis of residual ridge reduction is not well understood (Box 4-5). It is assumed that the degree of residual ridge reduction results from a combination of anatomical, metabolic, and mechanical determinants. For example, severe residual ridge reduction of the mandible has been related to a small gonial angle (i.e., a marked mandibular base bend and a posterior position of the lower incisal edges in relation to the mandibular body). Women are particularly affected by the frequency and extent of residual ridge reduction, and it has been suggested that progressive loss of bone under dentures is a manifestation of osteoporosis. In fact, there is a strong association between the skeletal bone density and bone density of the mandible, and the mandible is also affected by osteoporosis. Recently, it has been shown that low bone mineral content and osteoporotic changes predispose to a more rapid residual ridge reduction, particularly in the maxilla.

The mechanical factors (i.e., masticatory or parafunctional forces) transmitted by the denture or the tongue to the residual ridge are assumed to be important factors in the remodeling process. Thus a correlation exists between the years of denture wearing and the severity of atrophy, and the atrophy also is more important in day-and-night wearers of dentures than in day wearers. Apart from these observations, there is no direct evidence that the design of the dentures or that functional or parafunctional forces are related to the degree of residual ridge reduction.

The consequences of residual ridge reduction are apparent loss of sulcus width and depth, with displacement of the muscle attachment closer to the crest of the residual ridge; loss of the vertical dimension of occlusion, reduction of the lower face height, an anterior rotation of the mandible, and increase in relative prognathia; changes in interalveolar ridge relationship after progression of the residual ridge reduction, which is essentially centripetal in the maxilla and centrifugal in the mandible; and morphological changes of the alveolar bone such as sharp, spiny, uneven residual ridges and location of the mental foramina close to the top of the residual ridge.

A close correlation between a patient's satisfaction with dentures and the anatomical conditions of the residual ridges is not always present. However, in long-term complete denture wearers, the morphological changes and the reduction of the residual ridges present serious problems to the clinician on how to provide adequate support, stability, and retention of new dentures. Traditionally, these problems were approached by prescribing preprosthetic surgical initiatives such as vestibuloplasties with skin or mucosal grafts or, in severe situations, by performing ridge augmentation procedures. These techniques have been virtually eclipsed by the introduction of the osseointegration technique, which is discussed in Part 4.

Overdenture Abutments: Caries and Periodontal Disease

The retention of selected teeth to serve as abutments under complete dentures is an excellent prosthodontic technique (see Chapter 10) (Figure 4-14). In this simple method, a few teeth in a strategically good position are preserved and are treated

---

Box 4-5

Some Proposed Etiological Factors of Reduction of Residual Ridges

Anatomical Factors

More important in the mandible versus the maxilla

Short and square face associated with elevated masticatory forces

Alveoloplasty

Prosthodontic Factors

Intensive denture wearing

Unstable occlusal conditions

Immediate denture treatment

Metabolic and Systemic Factors

Osteoporosis

Calcium and vitamin D supplements for possible bone preservation endodontically before the crown is modified. The exposed root surface and canal are filled with amalgam or a composite restoration. In this way, even periodontally affected teeth can be maintained for several years in a relatively simple way.

Overdenture treatment does not necessarily increase the risk of technical failures such as denture fractures or loss of denture teeth. However, the wearing of overdentures is often associated with a high risk of caries and progression of periodontal disease of the abutment teeth. One of the reasons for this is that the bacterial colonization beneath a close-fitting denture is enhanced, and good plaque control of the fitting denture surface is generally difficult to obtain. One reason is that the species of *Streptococcus* and *Actinomyces* predominating in denture plaque are well known for their major contributions to dental plaque on smooth enamel sur-faces, as well as on root cementum. The inflamma-tory potential of these species is illustrated by the finding that early dentogingival plaque (in which they also predominate) initiates gingivitis after 1 to 3 days of plaque accumulation when oral hygiene is discontinued. This could explain why it is difficult to maintain healthy periodontal conditions adjacent to overdenture abutments. Another outstanding fea-ture of denture plaque flora is its high proportions of lactobacilli and *Streptococcus mutans*, which could explain why caries is difficult to control because caries rates of up to 30% after 1 year have been observed in patients wearing overdentures.

For the success of overdentures to be improved, effective prevention of caries and periodontal dis-eases is necessary. The principal aim of the preven-tive measures should be to control accumulation of plaque on the exposed dentin of the abutment teeth

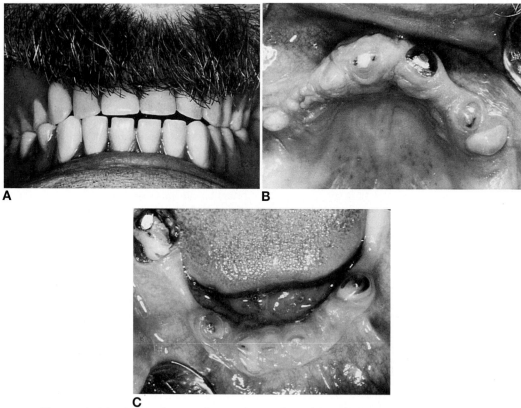

A **B** **C**

Figure 4-14 **A,** Complete overdentures in a patient with multiple aplasia. **B** and **C,** The dentures have been in place for 25 years, and the remaining teeth/roots have prevented residual ridge reduction.

as well as the root surface. The preventive measures include mechanical and chemical plaque control and introduction of adequate denture-wearing habits.

Longitudinal studies indicate that it is generally possible to obtain reasonable oral and denture hygiene in overdenture wearers. However, it is necessary to motivate the patient and to introduce regular follow-up examinations at intervals of 3 to 6 months. Despite these efforts, caries-susceptible patients will have root or dentin caries, and progression of periodontal disease is also likely to take place.

The effect of daily application of gels containing fluoride or fluoride plus chlorhexidine has been assessed in comparative studies. Patients were instructed to put a drop of the gel in the prosthesis at the abutment site and to insert the prosthesis for at least 30 minutes once a day. With the fluoride gel, there was no marked caries reduction when compared with the placebo gel and no effect on periodontal health. On the other hand, use of the fluoride-chlorhexidine gel controlled caries development and maintained healthy periodontal conditions.

The introduction of adequate denture-wearing habits (e.g., to abstain from wearing the denture during the night) is another efficient way to control caries and development of periodontal disease in overdenture wearers. In this way, the microbial plaque is less readily established, and saliva with its buffering capacity, antibacterial systems, and antibodies has free access to the abutments.

Treatment of superficial caries of the overdenture abutments includes application of fluoride-chlorhexidine gel and polishing, and not exclusive placement of fillings, which could result in recurrent caries. The placement of copings that cover the exposed dentin and root surface is indicated only where caries is more deeply penetrating. This is also a way to minimize the risk of new or recurrent caries. Periodontal pockets greater than 4 to 5 mm should be eliminated surgically because they present a high risk of acute periodontal complications.

INDIRECT SEQUELAE

Atrophy of Masticatory Muscles

It is essential that the oral function in complete denture wearers is maintained throughout life. The masticatory function depends on the skeletal muscular force and the facility with which the patient is able to coordinate oral functional movements during mastication. Maximal bite forces tend to decrease in older patients. Furthermore, computed tomography studies of the masseter and the medial pterygoid muscles have demonstrated a greater atrophy in complete-denture wearers, particularly in women. This indicates that reduced bite force and chewing efficiency are sequelae caused by wearing complete dentures, resulting in impaired masticatory function. There is little evidence that the placement of a new denture significantly improves masticatory efficiency. Indeed, elderly denture wearers often find that their chewing ability is insufficient and that they are obliged to eat soft foods.

Diagnosis Direct measurement of the capacity to reduce test food to small particles has verified that chewing efficiency decreases as the number of natural teeth is reduced and is worse for subjects wearing complete dentures. One of the consequences is that wearers of conventional complete dentures need approximately seven times more chewing strokes than subjects with a natural dentition to achieve an equivalent reduction in particle size. As a consequence, complete-denture wearers prefer food that is easy to chew, or they swallow large food particles.

Preventive Measures and Management To some extent, the retention of a small number of teeth used as overdenture abutments seems to play an important role in the maintenance of oral function in elderly denture wearers. Therefore treatment with overdentures has particular relevance in view of the increasing numbers of older people who are retaining a part of their natural dentition later in life.

In the completely edentulous patients, placement of implants is usually followed by an improvement of the masticatory function and an increase of maximal occlusal forces. This improvement may persist in a long-term perspective, and maximal occlusal forces may even increase with the years of denture wearing.

There is no evidence of a similar benefit after a preprosthetic surgical intervention to improve the anatomical conditions for wearing complete dentures.

Nutritional Deficiencies

Epidemiology (see Chapter 6)   Aging is often associated with a significant decrease in energy needs as a consequence of a decline in muscle mass and decreased physical activity. Thus a 30% reduction in energy needs should be and usually is accompanied by a 30% reduction of food intake. However, with the exception of carbohydrates, the requirement for virtually all other nutrients does not decline significantly with age. As a consequence, the dietary intake by elderly individuals frequently reveals evidence of deficiencies, which is clearly related to the dental or prosthetic status. Severe nutritional deficiencies are rare among healthy individuals, even with poor masticatory function. However, in chronically ill or hospitalized patients nutritional deficiencies are frequent. In these patients, factors such as ill-fitting dentures, salivary gland hypofunction, or altered taste perception may have a negative effect on the dietary habits and the nutritional status.

Masticatory Ability and Performance   One of the strong indications for prosthodontic treatment is to improve masticatory function. In this context, the term *masticatory ability* is used for an individual's own assessment of his or her masticatory function, whereas *efficiency* is to be understood as the capacity to reduce food during mastication. As previously mentioned, the wearing of complete dentures greatly compromises both masticatory ability and performance as compared with a situation with natural teeth present. There is no striking evidence that malnutrition could be a direct sequela of wearing dentures. However, edentulous women have a higher intake of fat and a higher consumption of coffee and a lower intake of ascorbic acid compared with dentate subjects within the same age group.

Nutritional Status and Masticatory Function
Four factors are related to dietary selection and the nutritional status of wearers of complete dentures: masticatory function and oral health, general health, socioeconomic status, and dietary habits. In healthy individuals there is no evidence that the nutritional intake is impaired in wearers of complete dentures or that replacement of ill-fitting dentures with well-fitting new dentures will cause

a major improvement of nutrition. In institutionalized patients, some amelioration of the nutritional intake could take place after prosthetic treatment because some patients are likely to start eating hard bread and to choose new food items such as vegetables and fruits.

The principal causes of protein energy malnutrition among elderly denture wearers are associated primarily with poor general health: poor absorption; intestinal, metabolic, and catabolic disturbances; or anorexia. Also, reduced salivary secretion rate during mastication has a negative effect on masticatory ability and efficiency (Box 4-6).

For the improvement and maintenance of the nutritional status it is often necessary to modify dietary habits. This reeducation of elderly denture wearers may be very difficult because their dietary habits are often firmly fixed and because they have a decreased appetite. In addition, poorly adapted dentures prevent patients from achieving improved dietary habits. Mechanical preparation of food before eating will help mastication and reduce its influence on food selection. However, it will not stimulate appetite and increase life quality. The maintenance or reestablishment of oral health and masticatory function remains an integral part of

---

Box 4-6

Associations among Xerostomia, Denture Wearing, Impaired Masticatory Function, and Undernutrition in Frail and Dependent Older Persons

Reduced Stimulated Salivary Flow Rate Associated with:

Complaints of xerostomia
Chewing difficulties
Complaints related to wearing complete dentures
Increased number of chewing cycles before swallowing
Loss of appetite
Reduced serum albumin level
Reduced body mass index
Reduced skinfold thickness

medical health care of the elderly patient who is medically compromised.

CONTROL OF SEQUELAE WITH THE USE OF COMPLETE DENTURES

The essential consequences of wearing complete dentures are reduction of the residual ridges and pathological changes of the oral mucosae. This often results in poor patient comfort, destabilization of the occlusion, insufficient masticatory function, and esthetic problems. Ultimately, the patient may not be able to wear dentures and will receive a diagnosis of prosthetically maladaptive.

For the adverse sequelae of residual ridge resorption to be reduced, the following should be considered:

1. Restoration of the partially edentulous patient with complete dentures should be considered if this is the only alternative as a result of poor periodontal health, unfavorable location of the remaining teeth, and economic limitations. In this situation, every effort should be made to retain some teeth in strategically good positions to serve as overdenture abutments. The maintenance of tooth roots in the mandible is particularly important.
2. The patient with complete dentures should follow a regular control schedule at yearly intervals so that an acceptable fit and stable occlusal condition can be maintained.
3. Edentulous patients should be aware of the benefits of an implant-supported prosthesis (see Part 4). In young patients, the primary advantage would be reduced residual ridge reduction. In elderly patients, the main advantages are improved comfort and maintenance of masticatory function.

The following precautions should be taken to preclude development of soft tissue disease:

1. Patients wearing overdentures supported by natural roots or implants should follow a program of recall and maintenance for continuous monitoring of the denture and the oral tissues. If patient compliance is difficult to obtain, this might indicate that it is necessary to see the patient every 3 to 4 months.
2. The patient should be motivated to practice proper denture-wearing habits such as not wearing dentures during the night.

Finally, it is important to remind and to explain to our patients that treatment with complete dentures is not a "definitive" treatment and that their collaboration is important to prevent the long-term risks associated with the consequences of wearing complete dentures.

Bibliography

Budtz-Jørgensen E: Oral mucosal lesions associated with the wearing of removable dentures, *J Oral Path* 10:65-80, 1981.

Budtz-Jørgensen E: Prognosis of overdenture abutments in the aged: effect of denture wearing habits, *Community Dent Oral Epidemiol* 20:302-306, 1992.

Budtz-Jørgensen E: Prognosis of overdenture abutments in elderly patients with controlled oral hygiene: a 5 year study, *J Oral Rehabil* 22:3-8, 1995.

Budtz-Jørgensen E: Ecology of *Candida*-associated denture stomatitis, *Microb Ecol Health Dis* 12:170-185, 2000.

Budtz-Jørgensen E, Chung JP, Mojon P: Successful aging—the case for prosthetic therapy, *J Publ Health Dent* 60:308-312, 2000.

Canon RD, Holmes AR, Mason AB et al: Oral *Candida*: clearance, colonization or candidiasis? *J Dent Res* 74(5):1152-1161, 1995.

Carlsson GE, Lindquist LW: Ten-year longitudinal study of masticatory function in edentulous patients treated with fixed complete dentures on osseointegrated implants, *Int J Prosthodont* 7:448-453, 1994.

Clifford TJ, Warsi MJ, Burnett SA et al: Burning mouth in Parkinson's Disease sufferers. *Gerodontology* 15:73-78, 1998.

Conny DJ, Tedesco LA: The gagging problem in prosthodontic treatment. Part I: Description and causes, *J Prosthet Dent* 49:601-606, 1983.

Fenlon MR, Sherriff M, Walter JD: Factors associated with the presence of denture related stomatitis in complete denture wearers: a preliminary investigation, *Eur J Prosthodont Rest Dent* 6:145-147, 1998.

Grushka M: Insights into burning mouth syndrome, PhD thesis, Toronto, 1986, University of Toronto.

Guggenheimer J, Hoffman RD: The importance of screening edentulous patients for oral cancer, *J Prosthet Dent* 74:141-143, 1994.

Hillerup S: Preprosthetic surgery in the elderly, *J Prosthet Dent* 72:551-558, 1994.

Jahangiri L, Devlin H, Ting K et al: Current perspectives in residual ridge remodeling and its clinical implications: a review, *J Prosthet Dent* 80:224-237, 1998.

Lombardi T, Budtz-Jørgensen E: Treatment of denture-induced stomatitis: a review, *Eur J Prosthodont* Rest Dent 2:17-22, 1993.

Main DMG, Basker RM: Patients complaining of a burning mouth, *Br Dent J* 154:206-211, 1983.

Mercier P, Vinet A: Factors involved in residual alveolar ridge atrophy of the mandible, *J Can Dent Assn* 5:339-343, 1983.

Mericske-Stern R: Overdentures with roots or implants for elderly patients: a comparison, *J Prosthet Dent* 72:543-550, 1994.

Newton AV: Denture sore mouth, *Br Dent J* 112:357-360, 1962.

Newton JP, Yemm R, Abel RW et al: Changes in human jaw muscles with age and dental state, *Gerodontology* 10:16-22, 1993.

Ortman LF, Hausmann E, Dunford RG: Skeletal osteopenia and residual ridge resorption, *J Prosthet Dent* 61:321-325, 1989.

Reichart PA: Oral mucosal lesions in a representative cross-sectional study of aging Germans, *Community Dent Oral Epidemiol* 28:390-398, 2000.

Tallgren A: The continuing reduction of the residual alveolar ridges in complete denture wearers: a mixed longitudinal study covering 25 years, *J Prosthet Dent* 27:120-132, 1972.

Theilade E, Budtz-Jørgensen E: Predominant cultivable microflora of plaque on removable dentures in patients with denture-induced stomatitis, *Oral Microbiol Immunol* 3:8-13, 1988.

Theilade J, Budtz-Jørgensen E: Electron microscopic study of denture plaque, *J Biol Buccale* 8:287-297, 1980.

Tourne LPM, Fricton JR: Burning mouth syndrome, *Oral Surg* 74:158-167, 1992.

CHAPTER 5

Temporomandibular Disorders in Edentulous Patients

Thuan Dao

Temporomandibular disorders (or TMDs) is a collective term that is used to designate a group of musculoskeletal conditions affecting the temporomandibular area. These include muscular conditions, such as myofascial pain, and disorders affecting the temporomandibular joint complex, such as disc displacement disorders and arthritic diseases. The term *TMDs* was introduced by Dworkin and LeResche (1992) and replaces numerous misleading terms that were previously used.

EPIDEMIOLOGY OF TEMPOROMANDIBULAR DISORDERS IN EDENTULOUS POPULATIONS

The reported prevalence of TMDs in edentulous populations appears to vary considerably, ranging from 0% (Loiselle, 1969) to 94% (Agerberg and Viklund, 1989). The wide discrepancies observed are largely due to differences in the criteria, or the lack of specific criteria, that were used to define TMDs. Although the prevalence of TMDs in the edentulous population still needs to be ascertained, an appraisal of the epidemiological literature on TMDs and related symptoms from different population-based studies reveals consistently that it is primarily a condition of young and middle-age adults (mainly female) and that its prevalence tends to diminish in the older-age group (LeResche, 1997), where partial or complete edentulism prevails (MacEntee, 1985; Warren, Watkins, and Cowen, 2002). These observations suggest that TMDs are encountered in elderly and edentulous subjects, but it is certainly not of the epidemic proportions reported in earlier studies.

ETIOLOGICAL FACTORS

The presumed association between edentulism and TMDs resulted from the traditional mechanistic notions that tooth loss is a predisposing factor to mandibular dysfunction. This association has been further reinforced by reports that the severity of such dysfunction is positively correlated with the loss of occlusal support and the number of remaining teeth or occluding pairs of teeth. It is therefore not surprising to see that the loss of vertical dimension of occlusion has also been assumed to play an important role in the etiology of TMDs in elderly and edentulous patients. However, if tooth loss or edentulism is a direct cause of TMDs, the prevalence of TMDs should be higher in the edentulous population as compared with the dentate one. This is clearly not the case, and in the last decade numerous reports have refuted this assumption (Bibb, Atchison, Pullinger et al., 1995; De Kanter, Truin, Burgersdijk et al., 1993; Gray, McCord, Murtaza et al., 1997). In addition, the lack of correlation between the number of remaining teeth and the prevalence or severity of TMDS has been repeatedly reported (Bibb, Atchison, Pullinger et al., 1995; Tervonen and Knuuttila, 1988).

Although the effect of the dentition and edentulism on changes in the temporomandibular joints (TMJs) has been questioned, an age-related increase in the prevalence of degenerative diseases is a well-known fact, whether in the TMJs per se (Pereira, Lundh, and Westesson, 1994) or in other body joints (Sowers, 2001). Therefore because edentulism is most prevalent among older persons, it is reasonable to assume that the presence of degenerative diseases in the edentulous population is more likely to be associated with age than with edentulism itself.

A few studies have reported a higher prevalence of TMDs in edentulous versus dentate subjects. However, the data either were not substantiated by statistical analysis (Tervonen and Knuuttila, 1988), or group differences failed to reach statistical significance (Harriman, Snowdon, Messer et al., 1990). There are also compelling data that TMD-related signs and symptoms are mild in edentulous subjects (Bergman and Carlsson, 1985; Lundeen, Scruggs, McKinney et al., 1990; Raustia, Peltola, and Salonen, 1997; Wilding and Owen, 1987) and are relatively low in those who do not wear dentures (Wilding and Owen, 1987). A lack of correlation between the severity or presence of TMDs and edentulism-related factors (duration, age, quality and number of complete prostheses, centric occlusion–centric relation coincidence, and denture retention and stability) has also been frequently reported in the literature (Bibb, Atchison, Pullinger et al., 1995; MacEntee, Weiss, Morrison et al., 1987; Raustia, Peltola, and Salonen, 1997). For instance, MacEntee (1987) reported no association between the clinical signs of dysfunction and occlusal instability or denture quality. In their search for etiological factors for TMDs in edentulous denture-wearing patients, Faulkner and Mercado (1990) failed to show significant association between the number of years that patients wore complete dentures, the age of the denture, the centric occlusion–centric relation coincidence, and denture retention and stability. Their result is consistent with the current evidence-based view that questions the role of occlusion in the pathophysiology of TMDs (Greene, 2001).

Mechanistic etiological concepts have now been eclipsed by biological variables, which include cellular, molecular, neurophysiological, neuroendocrinological, immunological, and genetic mechanisms of joint diseases. Chronic orofacial and muscle pains as unique foci for study have emerged from the related clinical and basic science research. The role of neuroendocrine peptides, cytokines, and local cell-derived mediators of pain and inflamma-

tion in arthritic pain and inflammation in the TMJs has received increasing attention (Kopp, 2001). Proposed neural mechanisms for TMD pain now include impairments in central inhibitory mechanisms, disorders in pathways modulated by peripheral baroreceptor afferent input, and alteration in central nervous system processes that regulate the temporal processing of pain (Maixner, Fillingim, Booker et al., 1995). In the case of muscle-related TMDs, sensitization of peripheral tissues, neuroplasticity in pronociceptive and antinociceptive circuits, and behavioral sensitization associated with increased emotionality and with pain-specific neuroendocrine and autonomic responsivity have been also been reviewed (Stohler, 1999). Some newer lines of evidence also suggest that the above pain systems may be modulated by the female hormones. One such example is the interaction between estrogen and neuroactive agents implicated in both peripheral and central pain processing mechanisms (Dao, Knight, and Ton-That, 1998; Dao and LeResche, 2000). Moreover, the use of exogenous hormones (e.g., oral contraceptives and hormone replacement therapies) has also been reported to be associated with increased risks for TMDs, and a dose-response relationship was also evident (LeResche, Saunders, Von Korff et al., 1997). The role of female hormones in the pathophysiology of TMDs is an exciting research area; however, it must be recognized that the etiology of TMD conditions is still unclear.

MANAGEMENT OF TEMPORO-MANDIBULAR DISORDERS IN THE EDENTULOUS PATIENT

The dental approach to TMD treatment in the edentulous patient has traditionally consisted of optimizing the stability, retention, and occlusion of the complete prostheses. This is still a valid approach to the adjunctive management of the TMDs. However, this does not imply a presumed occlusal etiology. Management of TMDs should primarily be directed toward palliation of the condition. The guidelines for management are well summarized in the official Scientific Information Statement published by the American Association of Dental Research (Greene, 2001).

Based on the evidence from clinical trials [of TMDs] . . . it is strongly recommended that, unless there are specific and justifiable indication to the contrary, treatment be based on the use of conservative and reversible therapeutic modalities. While no specific therapies have been proven to be uniformly effective, many conservative modalities have provided at least palliative relief from symptoms without producing harm.

In the absence of true understanding of the condition and until development of specific therapies, correct and prudent conservative symptomatic management of TMDs in denture wearers should be similar to the management strategies prescribed for most TMD patients. This includes patient education and reassurance about the benign nature of the condition, self-care, short-term pharmacotherapy (Dionne, 1997), physical modalities (Feine and Lund, 1997), and cognitive and behavioral intervention (Dworkin, 1997).

REASSURANCE AND SELF-CARE REGIMEN

Although patients should be informed about the limited knowledge of etiological factors, together with reassurance about the relative frequent occurrence of TMDs in the population, the good prognosis of the condition, and the merits of prudent management strategies. In addition, the patient should be instructed to follow a home care program to promote tissue rest and self-healing that includes the following: application of moist heat (10 to 20 minutes, 4 times a day) or cold application (5 minutes each time), soft diet, avoidance of muscle strain (e.g., avoid gum chewing or clenching), and identification and avoidance of events that can trigger pain or discomfort. Encouraging patients to actively participate in the control of their condition should be an integral part of the management strategies because committed patients usually do better than passive recipients of care. This is supported by recent evidence showing that when patients who participated in tailored self-care programs were compared with patients who received the usual TMDs treatment (e.g., physiotherapy,

patient education, medications, oral splints), the former patients showed significantly decreased pain, decreased pain-related activities, a reduced number of painful masticatory muscles, and reduced additional visits for TMDs treatment (Dworkin, Huggins, Wilson et al., 2002).

PHARMACOTHERAPY

Pharmacotherapy may be required when the previous strategies fail to increase the patient's comfort level. For acute pain states, dentists most commonly prescribe medications with analgesic properties, as well as muscle relaxants, nonsteroidal anti-inflammatory drugs (NSAIDs), and the recently introduced selective cyclooxygenase-2 (COX-2) inhibitor. These medications are particularly useful for the treatment of arthritic conditions involving the TMJs. Patients should be followed closely for the titration of the medication, to ensure adequate pain control and minimize unwanted side effects. It is important to note that although the short-term efficacy of these medications is well established, their long-term efficacy is not well documented. For persistent and neuropathic orofacial pain, management with antidepressants and opioids may play an important role. As for other medications that are prescribed on a long-term basis, however, the balance between their therapeutic benefit and toxicity should be carefully weighed, and their administration should be supported and coordinated with the family physician or a pain specialist. The dentist should additionally be aware of the potential interactions of the prescribed medications with other drugs that are used by the patient for comorbid conditions.

PHYSICAL MODALITIES

A wide range of physical modalities can be suggested to patients, including the use of heat and cold therapies, ultrasound, massage, joint mobilization, and passive stretching, and can be administered either by the patient or by a clinician. Although local heat application is widely used for pain relief, its benefit has been questioned because raised temperature increases tissue inflammation. On the other hand, the superiority of cold over heat therapy for reducing inflammation and swelling has been documented (see review by Feine and Lund, 1997). Although the long-term efficacy of physical modalities for musculoskeletal pain conditions has not been established, their safety, low cost, and short-lived benefit in providing pain relief justify their use as palliative measures for TMDs.

BIOBEHAVIORAL MODALITIES

Among the biobehavioral therapies prescribed for chronic pain, the most commonly studied include biofeedback, stress management, relaxation, hypnosis, and education. As proposed by Dworkin, "The label 'biobehavioral' refers to proven, safe methods that emphasize self-management and acquisition of self-control over not only pain symptoms but also their cognitive attributions or meanings and maintaining a productive level of psychosocial function, even if pain is not totally absent" (1997). In addition to modifying maladaptive habits, lifestyle patterns, and behaviors that may contribute to the perception of pain, biobehavioral therapies can also provide patients with coping skills for the control of pain and related disabilities. The efficacy of behavioral therapies in producing long-term relief has been suggested for many persistent pain conditions, and these therapies continue to be part of nearly all chronic pain treatment programs (Dworkin, 1997). However, their long-term efficacy in the management of TMDs has not been established.

SUMMARY

TMDs can affect the edentulous and elderly population, although their prevalence and severity do not exceed those of the dentate subjects in a lower-age range. The shift from a mechanical etiological view to a biological one, including emphasis on the possible etiological role of female hormones, has also resulted in a shift in treatment focus. Although prosthodontic treatment aims at achieving optimal prostheses and improvement of the patient's orofacial comfort and function, the intervention per se is not a specific therapy for TMDs.

References

Agerberg G, Viklund L: Functional disturbances in complete denture patients, *Int J Prosthodont* 2:41-50, 1989.

Bergman B, Carlsson GE: Clinical long-term study of complete denture wearers, *J Prosthet Dent* 53:56-61, 1985.

Bibb CA, Atchison KA, Pullinger AG et al: Jaw function status in an elderly community sample, *Community Dent Oral Epidemiol* 23:303-308, 1995.

Dao TT, Knight K, Ton-That V: Modulation of myofascial pain by the reproductive hormones: a preliminary report, *J Prosthet Den* 79:663-670, 1998.

Dao TT, LeResche L: Gender differences in pain, *J Orofac Pain* 14:169-184; discussion 184-195, 2000.

De Kanter RJ, Truin GJ, Burgersdijk RC et al: Prevalence in the Dutch adult population and a meta-analysis of signs and symptoms of temporomandibular disorder, *J Dent Res* 72:1509-1518, 1993.

Dionne RA: Pharmacologic treatments for temporomandibular disorders, *Oral Surg Oral Med Oral Pathol Oral Radiol Endod* 83:134-142, 1997.

Dworkin SF: Behavioral and educational modalities, *Oral Surg Oral Med Oral Pathol Oral Radiol Endod* 83:128-133, 1997.

Dworkin SF, Huggins KH, Wilson L et al: A randomized clinical trial using research diagnostic criteria for temporomandibular disorders-axis II to target clinic cases for a tailored self-care TMDs treatment program, *J Orofac Pain* 16:48-63, 2002.

Dworkin SF, LeResche L: Research diagnostic criteria for temporomandibular disorders: review, criteria, examinations and specifications, critique, *J Craniomandib Disord Facial Oral Pain* 6:301-355, 1992.

Faulkner KD, Mercado MD: Aetiological factors of craniomandibular disorders in completely edentulous denture-wearing patients, *J Oral Rehabil* 18:243-251, 1990.

Feine JS, Lund JP: An assessment of the efficacy of physical therapy and physical modalities for the control of chronic musculoskeletal pain, *Pain* 71:5-23, 1997.

Gray RJ, McCord JF, Murtaza G et al: The incidence of temporomandibular disorder signs in patients wearing complete dentures compared to patients with a natural dentition, *Eur J Prosthodont Restor Dent* 5:99-103, 1997.

Greene CS: The etiology of temporomandibular disorders: implications for treatment, *J Orofac Pain* 15:93-105; discussion 106-116, 2001.

Harriman LP, Snowdon DA, Messer LB et al: Temporomandibular joint dysfunction and selected health parameters in the elderly, *Oral Surg Oral Med Oral Pathol* 70:406-413, 1990.

Kopp S: Neuroendocrine, immune, and local responses related to temporomandibular disorders, *J Orofac Pain* 15:9-28, 2001.

LeResche L: Epidemiology of temporomandibular disorders: implications for the investigation of etiologic factors, *Crit Rev Oral Biol Med* 8:291-305, 1997.

LeResche L, Saunders K, Von Korff MR et al: Use of exogenous hormones and risk of temporomandibular disorder pain, *Pain* 69:153-160, 1997.

Loiselle RJ: Relation of occlusion to temporomandibular joint dysfunction: the prosthodontic viewpoint, *J Am Dent Assoc* 79:145-146, 1969.

Lundeen TF, Scruggs RR, McKinney MW et al: TMDs symptomology among denture patients, *J Craniomandib Disord* 4:40-46, 1990.

MacEntee MI: The prevalence of edentulism and diseases related to dentures–a literature review, *J Oral Rehabil* 12:195-207, 1985.

MacEntee MI, Weiss R, Morrison BJ et al: Mandibular dysfunction in an institutionalized and predominantly elderly population, *J Oral Rehabil* 14:523-529, 1987.

Maixner W, Fillingim R, Booker D et al: Sensitivity of patients with painful temporomandibular disorders to experimentally evoked pain, *Pain* 63:341-351, 1995.

Pereira FJ Jr, Lundh H, Westesson PL: Morphologic changes in the temporomandibular joint in different age groups: an autopsy investigation, *Oral Surg Oral Med Oral Pathol* 78:279-287, 1994.

Raustia AM, Peltola M, Salonen MA: Influence of complete denture renewal on craniomandibular disorders: a 1-year follow-up study, *J Oral Rehabil* 24:30-36, 1997.

Sowers M: Epidemiology of risk factors for osteoarthritis: systemic factors, *Curr Opin Rheumatol* 13:447-451, 2001.

Stohler CS: Muscle-related temporomandibular disorders, *J Orofac Pain* 13:273-284, 1999.

Tervonen T, Knuuttila M: Prevalence of signs and symptoms of mandibular dysfunction among adults aged 25, 35, 50 and 65 years in Ostrobothnia, Finland, *J Oral Rehabil* 15:455-463, 1988.

Warren JJ, Watkins CA, Cowen HJ et al: Tooth loss in the very old: 13-15-year incidence among elderly Iowans, *Community Dent Oral Epidemiol* 30:29-37, 2002.

Wilding RJ, Owen CP: The prevalence of temporomandibular joint dysfunction in edentulous non-denture wearing individuals, *J Oral Rehabil* 14:175-182, 1987.

CHAPTER 6

Nutrition Care for the Denture-Wearing Patient

Mary P. Faine

Enjoyment of food is regarded as an important determinant of an adult's quality of life. Loose teeth, edentulism, or ill-fitting dentures may preclude eating favorite foods, as well as limit the intake of essential nutrients. Decreased chewing ability, fear of choking while eating, and irritation of the oral mucosa when food particles get under dentures may influence food choices of the denture wearer. Conversely, the nutritional status of a patient with dentures affects the health of the oral tissues and the patient's adaptation to a new prosthesis. In fact, well-designed and constructed dentures or an implant-supported prosthesis may prove to be unsatisfactory for a patient because of poor tolerance by the underlying tissues and bone. Hence, denture failures can be due not only to imperfect design, but also to poorly nourished tissues.

Clinical symptoms of malnutrition are often observed first in the oral cavity. Because of rapid cell turnover (every 3 to 7 days) in the mouth, a regular, balanced intake of essential nutrients is required for the maintenance of the oral epithelium. Inadequate long-term nutrition may result in angular cheilitis, glossitis, and slow tissue healing. The amount of alveolar bone resorption that occurs after tooth extractions may be exacerbated by low calcium and vitamin D intakes.

Nearly half of older individuals have clinically identifiable nutrition problems. Undernutrition increases with advancing age. Persons older than 70 years of age are more likely to have nutritionally poor diets. Dentate status can affect eating ability and thus the diet quality. In elderly persons, oral health problems may contribute to involuntary weight loss and a lower body mass index. Because most edentulous adults are of advanced age, a large number of patients with dentures can be expected to have nutritional deficits. The nutritional status of a denture wearer also is influenced by economic hardship, social isolation, degenerative diseases, medication regimens, and dietary supplementation practices (Figure 6-1). An understanding of the nutritional requirements, symptoms of malnutrition, and environmental factors that influence food choices will assist dental clinicians in identifying denture-wearing patients at risk for malnutrition. Dietary guidance, based on the assessment of the edentulous patient's nutrition history and diet, should be an integral part of comprehensive prosthodontic treatment. Nutrition support will improve the tolerance of the oral mucosa to new dentures and prevent rejection of dentures. Because denture fabrication requires a series of appointments, dietary analysis and counseling can be easily incorporated into an edentulous patient's treatment plan.

THE IMPACT OF DENTAL STATUS ON FOOD INTAKE

The food choices of older adults are closely linked to dental status and masticatory efficiency. Although an intact dentition is not a necessity for maintaining nutritional health, the loss of teeth often leads adults to select diets that are lower in nutrient density. Investigators in the United States and Sweden have reported that adults with compromised

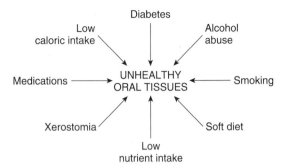

Figure 6-1 Maladaptive denture-wearing signs and symptoms may include unhealthy oral tissues such as cracking at the corners of the lips and persistent soreness of the tongue and oral mucosa. These may be related to a low intake of essential nutrients, reduced nutrient absorption, or altered nutrient metabolism due to medications or alcohol abuse.

dentitions are overrepresented in groups with nutritionally poor diets. Furthermore, denture wearers report that food such as raw carrots, lettuce, corn on the cob, raw apples with peels, steaks, and chops are difficult to chew.

When compared to peers with 25 teeth or more, edentulous male health professionals consumed fewer vegetables, less fiber and carotene, and more cholesterol, saturated fat, and calories. Denture wearers had lower serum β-carotene and ascorbic acid levels than dentate subjects. A large number of denture wearers were among the 691 healthy older persons studied by researchers at the United States Department of Agriculture's (USDA) Human Nutrition Research Center on Aging in Boston. Nutritionally poorer diets were reported by adults who had low educational attainment, who had low family income, or who wore partial or complete dentures. Male denture wearers had poorer nutrient intakes than female denture wearers. Specifically, mean intakes of calories, protein, vitamin A, ascorbic acid, vitamin B_6, and folic acid were lower in male denture wearers than in dentate men. Calcium and protein intakes of female denture wearers were inferior to those of dentate women. In a subset of the USDA subjects, the nutrient intake of those who had one or two complete dentures was about 20% lower than that of dentate subjects.

Age, oral motor function, adequate saliva, and the number of occluding pairs of teeth in the mouth mainly determine an individual's masticatory ability. When compared to those with natural dentition, persons with removable complete dentures had greatly reduced chewing ability. Denture wearers must complete a greater number of chewing strokes to prepare food for swallowing. Even with additional chewing, the average denture does not reduce foods to as small a particle size as does natural dentition. The chewing ability of individuals with a complete denture in only one arch, opposed by a natural dentition, appears to be reduced to nearly the same extent as persons with complete dentures in both arches. In a Veteran's Administration longitudinal study, dentition status and nutrient intakes were significantly related to masticatory function. When new complete dentures replace old ones that had poor retention, patients subjectively reported that masticating performance improved; they chewed better and chewed different foods. However, nutrient intake was not improved. Chewing efficiency is determined by measuring particle size after subjects have chewed a test food as long as necessary to prepare the sample for swallowing.

Texture and hardness, rather than taste and smell, determine acceptability of a food for many patients with dentures. Generally, the intake of hard foods (raw vegetables or fruits, fibrous meats, hard breads, seeds, and nuts) is reduced, whereas the intake of soft foods (ground beef, breads, cereals, pastries, and canned fruits and vegetables) is increased. Whether these changes in food selection negatively affect nutritional status depends on nutrient density of the food substituted, but soft foods are often lower in nutrient density and fiber. For example, replacing steak with ground beef provides similar nutrients, but substituting applesauce for a green salad results in lower nutrient intake.

Replacing a complete denture with osseointegrated implants results in significant improvement in masticatory function. Increased intake of fresh fruits and crisp bread was reported by a small group of Swedish adults who received tissue-integrated prostheses in the lower jaw. Others who previously wore dentures reported that their chewing ability was markedly improved after insertion of a mandibular fixed prosthesis on osseointegrated dental implants. However, improved oral function does not lead to selection of a higher quality diet. Some individuals will eat a more varied diet and increase their intake of fruits and vegetables, but nutrient intake of implant wearers is generally similar to complete denture subjects. To improve diet quality, individual patients undergoing prosthodontics need dietary counseling.

The inability to distinguish the sensory qualities of food reduces a patient's enjoyment of eating and may lead to reduced calorie intake. Because a decrease in taste and smell acuity frequently accompanies aging, it is difficult to separate the effects of aging and denture wearing on sensory acuity. Nearly all denture wearers report a transient decline in taste acuity when dentures are first inserted. This is usually attributed to denture base coverage of the hard palate. However, the ability to taste usually improves as the patient adapts to the dentures. When compared with the sensory perceptions of dentate adults or partial denture wearers, subjective estimates of taste, texture acceptability of test foods, and perceived ease of chewing (by complex denture wearers) were rated the lowest. In blind tests, denture wearers are significantly less able to detect differences in texture and sweetness of certain foods than dentate subjects can.

Dehydration is a major problem for seniors because the ability to sense thirst is reduced in the elderly population. Hypotension, elevated body temperature, and mental confusion may occur when fluid intake is inadequate. The comfort of wearing dentures is dependent on the lubricating ability of saliva in the mouth. If the oral mucosa is dry, chewing is difficult, denture retention is compromised, and mucosal soreness or ulcerations develop. Because salivary flow facilitates mastication, formation of the food bolus, swallowing, and digestion, it is a major contributor to the pleasure of eating.

Xerostomia, more commonly called *dry mouth,* is a clinical manifestation of salivary gland dysfunction. Xerostomia may contribute to geriatric malnutrition. There are several causes of dry mouth: the use of medications, therapeutic radiation to the head and neck, diabetes, depression, alcoholism, pernicious anemia, menopause, vitamin A or vitamin B complex deficiency, HIV infection, and autoimmune diseases such as Sjögren's

syndrome. Aging as the sole cause of decreased salivary flow is unproven. The most common cause of dry mouth is the use of drugs to manage chronic diseases. Xerostomia is a possible side effect associated with more than 400 drugs including antihypertensives, antidepressants, antihistamines, bronchodilators, antiparkinsonians, antispasmodics, anticholinergics, and sedatives. Mouthwashes, alcohol, tobacco, and caffeine may alter salivary flow or cause dryness of the oral mucosa.

Management of xerostomia depends on the cause of the condition. If a drug is suspected to be the cause, consulting with the patient's physician may result in prescription of an alternate drug or modification of the dosage schedule. Saliva substitutes provide temporary relief but have not proven to be acceptable for many patients, and they are expensive. Milk has been proposed as a saliva substitute. Milk not only aids in lubricating the tissues and increasing the pleasure of eating, but also has buffering capacity. This buffering capacity may be an important benefit if overdenture abutment teeth are present. Because dry mouth may result in inadequate nutritional intake, the use of milk not only serves as a saliva substitute but also is an excellent source of nutrients.

Sialogogues (agents that stimulate salivary flow) such as sugar-free gum, lozenges, or sugar-free candies containing citric acid may be recommended. Sorbitol- or xylitol-sweetened products may decrease the risk of candidiasis developing in susceptible adults. Additional recommendations include beverages that may produce more saliva such as water with a slice of lemon, lemonade, or limeade. Carrying a sport bottle when leaving home will allow for frequent sips of water. Sucking Popsicles or ice chips will increase comfort and provide lubrication; sauces, gravies, and dressings will moisten foods and make them easier to swallow. Chewing fibrous foods such as celery or whole grain breads will also increase saliva production. Making a conscious effort to consume at least eight glasses of water, juice, or milk daily is the most important measure to relieve dry mouth.

GASTROINTESTINAL FUNCTIONING

Little research exists on the effect of tooth loss on gastrointestinal function or the likelihood of choking on food. The purpose of mastication is to reduce food particles in size so they can be swallowed and to increase the surface area of food exposed to digestive juices and enzymes. Individuals with poor masticatory ability often swallow large pieces of food. Investigators have proposed that accidental deaths occurring in restaurants have been inaccurately attributed to the "café coronary" when the true cause was choking on food. A review of autopsies performed on adults who died suddenly while eating showed that the ratio of deaths due to food asphyxiation to coronary disease was 55:1. When a denture covers the upper palate, it is difficult to detect the location of a food in the mouth. Adults with such dentures are at a greater risk of having a large piece of food or a bone lodge in the air or food passage.

Inadequate mastication appears to cause gastrointestinal disturbances. For example, the use of laxatives, antacids, antireflux drugs, and antidiuretics was significantly higher in elderly edentulous Canadians with poor masticatory performance. Gastric distress and the use of laxatives in Finnish adults were reportedly reduced when ill-fitting dentures were replaced with well-fitting ones. Although a diet high in fiber helps prevent constipation, edentulous patients may avoid whole-grain breads, fruits with skins, and vegetables.

NUTRITIONAL NEEDS AND STATUS OF OLDER ADULTS

There is a great diversity in the eating habits and food intake of older adults. The nutrient needs of older persons vary depending on health status and level of physical activity. Thus it is difficult to generalize about energy and vitamin and mineral requirements appropriate for all older adults. Depending on body metabolism, an individual may need more, or less of, nutrients proposed in the Dietary Reference Intakes (DRIs), which are quantitative estimates of nutrient intakes for the individual's chronological age.

Energy needs decline with age because of a decrease in basal metabolism and decreased physical activity. With aging, lean body mass is replaced by fat; this leads to a decrease in metabolic rate. The onset of chronic disease usually leads to a decline in physical exercise. Cross-sectional surveys show that the average energy consumption is about 1300 kilocalories (kcal) for 65- to 74-year-old women and 1800 kcal for men of the same ages. This is lower than the caloric recommendation for adults 51 years of age and older (1900 kcal for women and 2300 kcal for men) but may be appropriate if body weight is being maintained. When calorie intake is low, consumption of foods of high nutrient density such as legumes, vegetable soups, meat casseroles, fruit desserts, low-fat dairy foods, and whole-grain breads and cereals is important.

The best means of reducing calorie intake is to replace foods high in fat and sugar with complex carbohydrates, and these should be the mainstay for the elderly person's diet. In contrast to pastries, whole-milk cheeses, luncheon meats, salad dressings, and frozen desserts, the choice of nonfat dairy products, whole-grain breads, cereals, pasta, fruits, vegetables, beans, and legumes will provide important amounts of vitamins, minerals, and fiber. Patients with dentures who prefer soft foods such as doughnuts, pastries, cakes, and cookies, which are high in simple sugars and fat, should be advised of the value of fruits, vegetables, grains, and cereals. An important component of complex carbohydrates is fiber, which promotes normal bowel function, lowers glycemic response, may reduce serum cholesterol, and is thought to prevent diverticular disease.

Fats contribute about 33% of total calories in the diet of the average adult. Because of growing epidemiological evidence of the link between dietary intake of saturated fat, cholesterol, and occurrence of hyperlipidemias, heart disease, certain cancers, and obesity, adults are advised to maintain their dietary fat intake at 20% to 35% of total calories. Because physiological stresses are associated with age-related degenerative diseases, protein needs of older adults are thought to be slightly higher than those of younger persons. It is recommended that 10% to 35% of total calories or 1 g/kg of body weight come from protein. This conclusion is based on studies of serum albumin levels and nitrogen balance studies in older adults. Surveys show that protein intake declines with age; in one national survey one third of seniors did not meet the recommended intake. The protein intake of denture wearers is lower than that of dentate adults but is often adequate. If calorie or protein intake is reduced, protein metabolism is compromised.

Vitamin deficiencies in the elderly population are apt to be subclinical, but any body stress may result in an individual having detectable symptoms. Individuals who have low-calorie intakes, ingest multiple drugs, or have disease states that cause malabsorption are at greatest risk for hypovitaminosis. Free-living older persons often report low dietary intakes of vitamin D, vitamin E, folic acid, calcium, and magnesium. Oral symptoms of malnutrition are usually due to a lack of the vitamin B complex, vitamin C, iron, or protein (Table 6-1). In one study, clinical symptoms of burning mouth syndrome (BMS) were resolved in 24 of 28 patients with proven vitamin deficiency when vitamin B complex supplementation was given. Folic acid plays an important role in cell division and in red blood cell formation; anemia results from an inadequate folate intake. Many drugs and alcohol affect folic acid absorption and metabolism. Individuals with a marginal intake of folic acid who are undergoing long-term drug therapy are at greatest risk of

developing a deficiency of this vitamin. Oranges, cantaloupe, broccoli, spinach, asparagus, and dried beans are good sources of folic acid.

With the measurement of serum metabolites of vitamin B_{12}, a high prevalence of undiagnosed vitamin B_{12} deficiency has been noted among the elderly population. Protein-bound vitamin B_{12} malabsorption leads to a vitamin B_{12} deficiency more often than a low vitamin B_{12} intake or lack of intrinsic factor. A vitamin B_{12} deficiency may lead to problems with dementia in older adults. Vitamin B_{12} is found only in animal products. Synthetic vitamin B_{12} obtained from fortified foods or vitamin supplements is better absorbed than protein-bound vitamin B_{12}.

Because of its role in collagen synthesis, ascorbic acid (vitamin C) is essential for wound healing. There is a wide variation in vitamin C intakes of adults. In one survey, low ascorbic acid intakes associated with low plasma levels were reported in one fourth of older individuals. Heavy smokers, alcohol abusers, or persons with high aspirin intake have a higher daily requirement for ascorbic acid. The denture-wearing patient should be encouraged to consume foods rich in vitamin C daily such as citrus fruits, peppers, melons, kiwifruit, mangos, papaya, and strawberries.

Vitamin E functions as an antioxidant in cell membranes. By acting as a scavenger of free radicals, vitamin E prevents oxidation of unsaturated cell phospholipids. Dietary sources of vitamin E include vegetable oils, nuts, margarines, and mayonnaise.

Magnesium is a component of the body skeleton, is a cofactor for more than 300 enzymes, and plays a role in neuromuscular transmission. The highest amounts of magnesium are found in vegetables and unrefined grains. Milk is a moderately good source.

Alcohol abuse appears to be a serious health problem among some older persons. Although the actual incidence of alcoholism is unknown, estimates of alcohol abuse in independent-living older persons are 1% to 8% of those older than 60 years of age. Alcoholism often is undetected and untreated. The loss of a spouse, loneliness, depression, retirement, loss of status, and reduced income all contribute to excess alcohol intake by older adults. Elderly persons tend to drink a smaller volume of alcohol but drink more frequently. The substitution of

Table 6-1	
Oral Signs of Nutrient Deficiencies	

Nutrient Lacking	Oral Symptom
Protein	Decreased salivary flow
	Enlarged parotid glands
Vitamin B complex,	Lips:
* iron, protein	Cheilosis
	Angular stomatitis
	Angular scars
	Inflammation
	Tongue:
	Edema
	Magenta tongue
	Atrophy of filiform papillae
	Burning sensation
	Soreness
	Pale, bald
Vitamin C	Edematous oral mucosa
	Tender gingiva
	Spontaneous bleeding of gingival
	Hemorrhages in interdental
	papillae

*Vitamin B complex includes thiamin, riboflavin, niacin, pyridoxine, folic acid, and vitamin B_{12}.

alcoholic drinks, which contain no nutrients, for food usually results in multiple nutrient deficits. Deficiencies of thiamine, niacin, pyridoxine, folate (all B-complex vitamins), and ascorbic acid are commonly seen in alcoholics. Osteopenia in males without a history of bone disease may be due to long-term alcohol intake. When efforts to resolve tissue intolerance to a prosthesis are unsuccessful, the misuse of alcohol should be considered.

CALCIUM AND BONE HEALTH

Bone loss is a normal part of aging that affects the maxilla and mandible, as well as the spine and long bones. Skeletal sites where trabecular bone (the alveolar bone, vertebrae, wrist, and neck of the femur) is more prominent than cortical bone are affected first. In a large screening study of healthy U.S. women age 50 or older, 40% had low bone mass. Several factors are thought to contribute to age-related bone loss that leads to osteoporosis: genetic background, hormonal status, bone density at maturity, a disturbance in the bone remodeling process, a low exercise level, and inadequate nutrition. Low calcium intake throughout life is a contributor to osteoporosis. Osteopenia, loss of bone, affects women earlier than men because of loss of estrogen at menopause and a smaller skeleton. In women, bone loss begins during the fourth decade of life or whenever estrogen secretion declines or ceases. In 329 healthy postmenopausal women, a positive linear relationship between the number of teeth and bone mineral density at the spine was reported.

Trabecular bone in the alveolar process is a source of calcium that can be used to meet other tissue needs. It has been proposed that alveolar bone loss may precede loss of mineral from the vertebrae and long bones; thus the dentist may therefore be the first health care provider to detect loss of bone mass. Mandibular bone mass has been positively correlated with total body calcium and the bone mass of the vertebrae and wrist of healthy, dentate postmenopausal and edentulous women with osteoporosis by some investigators, but not all bone researchers concur. In edentulous persons, local factors may have a greater influence on alveolar bone resorption than systemic factors linked to bone loss at other body sites. This area of basic and clinical research is clearly still developing.

Resorption of the alveolar ridge is a widespread problem among denture-wearing patients and results in unstable dentures. Some remodeling of the alveolar processes occurs in response to occlusal forces associated with chewing. With loss of teeth the alveolar bone is no longer needed for tooth support; as a consequence, resorption is accelerated and bone height is diminished. A greater degree of residual ridge resorption is observed in women than in men. Bone loss is accelerated in the first 6 months after tooth extractions, and resorption is much greater in the mandible than in the maxilla. The loss of alveolar bone frequently makes it more difficult to construct a mandibular denture that has good stability and retention.

Dietary calcium intake is critical to maintaining the body skeleton. The most important means of preventing metabolic bone disease is acquiring a dense skeleton by the time bone maturation occurs between 30 and 35 years of age. A woman who has a dense skeleton at 35 years of age will retain proportionately more skeletal mineral content and be less susceptible to fracture after menopause. Calcium intake of postmenopausal women is correlated with mandibular bone mass. Patients with dentures who have excessive ridge resorption report lower calcium intakes. After age 35, about 75% of U.S. women have inadequate calcium intakes. A chronically low calcium intake results in a negative calcium balance. For serum calcium levels to be maintained, calcium will be mobilized from bone, and this leads to demineralization of the skeleton. Although a generous calcium intake by older adults will not result in restoration of bone mass, it will improve calcium balance and slow the rate of bone loss.

In 1997 the National Academy of Sciences recommended that an adequate calcium intake for men and women 19 to 50 years of age is 1000 mg and 1200 mg for adults 51 years of age or older (Table 6-2). This recommendation far exceeds the usual calcium intake of U. S. women and men, 470 and 610 mg/day, respectively. Both aging and menopause lead to reduced calcium absorption and less body adaptation to changes in dietary intake in women. Oxalates found in rhubarb and spinach and phytates found in whole-grain products and legumes may form insoluble complexes with calcium, thereby reducing the amount of calcium absorbed. High intakes of sodium, animal protein, and alcohol increase calcium losses in the urine. A moderate caffeine intake (300 mg or less per day) is recommended to prevent bone loss.

About three fourths of the calcium found in the American diet is obtained from dairy foods. Major sources of calcium are milk, cheese, yogurt, and ice cream. Dairy foods are also a source of protein, riboflavin, vitamin A, and vitamin D. Collard greens, kale, broccoli, oysters, canned salmon, sardines, calcium, fortified fruit juices and cereals, and tofu made with a calcium coagulant are nondairy foods containing substantial amounts of calcium. To receive 1000 to 1200 mg of calcium, adults must drink three or four glasses of low-fat milk per day, eat 5 to 7 oz of hard cheeses, or consume very large quantities of nondairy foods. Lactose-intolerant adults who avoid milk may find yogurt or cheese acceptable. This amount of dairy foods represents a significant number of calories. Women with low calorie intakes should be encouraged to obtain at least half their calcium needs from food sources and the balance from calcium supplements.

Poor vitamin D status is an important public health problem. Adequate intake of vitamin D enhances calcium absorption in the intestine. Low dietary intake, minimal exposure to sunlight, and a lower rate of conversion to the active metabolite in the liver and kidney are responsible for low plasma levels of vitamin D in the elderly population. The primary dietary source of vitamin D is fortified dairy products. To promote bone health, postmenopausal women and andropausal men ages 51 to 70 should strive to obtain 10 µg of vitamin D (400 IU) and increase intake to 15 µg at age 71 (600 IU).

If an individual lacks sun exposure, is lactose intolerant, or dislikes dairy foods, a vitamin D supplement of 10 µg is desirable.

For those women who consume minimal amounts of dairy products, have lactose intolerance, or have allergies to dairy foods, calcium supplementation may be appropriate. Supplements are well tolerated, are inexpensive, and have few side effects. The most common forms of supplements are calcium carbonate, calcium citrate, calcium lactate, calcium gluconate, and calcium diphosphate. Calcium carbonate contains the highest concentration of elemental calcium (40%), but in older women, body absorption of calcium citrate is better. However, less elemental calcium is obtained from each calcium citrate tablet. Calcium supplements that contain vitamin D to enhance absorption of calcium in the gut are useful if vitamin D is not obtained from other sources. A dose of 1000 mg of elemental calcium taken with meals is commonly prescribed. Chemically derived calcium carbonate or calcium citrate is the safest source; bone meal, oyster shell, and dolomite calcium supplements should be avoided because they may be contaminated with heavy metals such as lead or mercury.

Few adverse affects of calcium supplementation have been observed. Some older women have reported nausea, bloating, or constipation. Increasing calcium intake results in higher urinary levels of calcium. A small percent of the population, mainly men, are susceptible to forming kidney stones; however, a high intake of dairy foods does not appear to affect stone formation. A physician should monitor the use of calcium supplements by these persons. The maximum calcium intake that poses no risk of adverse effects is 2.5 g.

VITAMIN AND HERBAL SUPPLEMENTATION

Consuming a variety of foods is considered the best means of obtaining the balance of nutrients required for good health. A varied diet also reduces the risk of chronic disease. The widespread use of vitamin-mineral and herbal supplements among North Americans, especially among elderly persons, is due partly to promotion efforts of the nutrient supplement industry. At least 50% of persons older

Table 6-2
The 1997 Dietary Reference Intake Values for Calcium and Vitamin D*

Age (yr)	Calcium (µg)	Vitamin D (µg)
31-50	1000	5
51-70	1200	10
>70	1200	15

*Adequate intakes.

than 65 years of age report using vitamin-mineral supplements, and one fourth of adults use herbal supplements. Persons who have high incomes and are well educated and those who perceive themselves to be in good health are more likely to use dietary supplements. Many reasons are reported for using nutritional supplements: to increase energy level, to extend life, to prevent the onset of degenerative diseases, to relieve the symptoms of chronic diseases, and to make up deficits caused by unbalanced diets. A large percentage of the supplements ingested are self-prescribed and unrelated to any specific physiological need. In fact, self-medication by individuals may result in toxicity to the tissues or in a delay in seeking diagnosis and treatment for a curable condition. The U.S. Congress has restricted the Food and Drug Administration's role in the regulation of dietary supplements and the claims that can be made on labels.

Vitamin-mineral supplements without energy or fiber and only one third of the essential micronutrients may foster a false sense of security in the patient undergoing prosthodontics. Older adults often select a supplement that does not include nutrients most likely to be missing in their diet. Although the average adult intake of vitamin C seems to be adequate, supplementation with ascorbic acid is common. In contrast, low intakes of calcium, vitamin D, folate, and magnesium are reported among seniors. If clinical signs of malnutrition are detected in the oral tissues of denture-wearing patients, referral to a physician for definitive diagnosis should occur (see Table 6-1).

In 1997, for the first time, the Food and Nutrition Board of the National Academy of Sciences recommended that supplements or fortified foods could help some people meet their nutritional needs. Individuals who are at a greater risk for the development of malnutrition and who may benefit from taking a low-dose vitamin-mineral supplement (≤100% of recommended daily allowances [RDAs] or adequate intakes [AIs]) include those consuming less than 1200 kcal/day or those eating an unbalanced diet that lacks fruits, vegetables, or protein foods, and seniors with low incomes or physical disabilities that hinder mobility may limit access to food. Bioavailability of vitamins and minerals also is affected by preexisting disease, medications, fiber intake, emotional sta-

tus, and environmental stress. Digestion and absorption is negatively affected in older persons taking several over-the-counter or prescription medications. The person ingesting aspirin several times a day may need more iron, vitamin C, and folic acid. Individuals taking corticosteroids and certain diuretics have increased calcium needs. Frequent use of laxatives and antacids results in increased urinary excretion of minerals. For the older person, synthetic vitamin B_{12} and folic acid have higher bioavailability than those vitamins in foods. Supplemental sources of calcium and vitamin D will be needed by many seniors to ensure adequate intake.

For nutrients to be present in the proper ratio to one another, a multivitamin-mineral supplement is preferable to single-nutrient tablets. For patients at risk of nutritional deficits, the American Dietetic Association recommends a multivitamin-mineral supplement that does not exceed the RDAs or AIs. On the basis of nutrient deficiencies reported in denture-wearing patients, it may be reasonable to prescribe a low-dose multivitamin-mineral supplement for certain patients even though clinical signs of a nutrient deficiency are lacking. For patients receiving dentures, a generic one-a-day vitamin tablet that includes vitamin D, folic acid, and vitamin B_{12} may be recommended. If intake of dairy foods cannot be increased to meet daily needs, a calcium supplement is advised; because it is bulky, calcium must be taken in a separate tablet.

The use of megadoses of vitamins or minerals by the elderly persons is a practice of great concern. When a high dose of a vitamin is taken, it no longer functions as a vitamin but becomes a chemical with pharmacological activity. Adverse reactions from megadoses of nutrients are more likely in the older adult because they are metabolized less efficiently and excretion occurs more slowly. High doses of any nutrient are potentially toxic, but because the fat-soluble vitamins A and D are stored in the body, they are considered toxic at lower levels of intake. Megadoses of vitamin D can disturb calcium metabolism, leading to calcification of soft tissues. High doses of dietary retinol (vitamin A) accelerate bone resorption, thereby increasing the risk of hip fracture. The maximum level of nutrient intake (Tolerable Upper Intake Level [UL]) that is unlikely to pose adverse health effects has been determined for some vitamins and minerals. The upper tolerable intake of vitamin D is 50 μg, and the UL for preformed vitamin A is 3000 μg per day.

Although water-soluble vitamins are considered nontoxic, well-documented toxicity syndromes are associated with megadoses of the water-soluble vitamins, niacin, vitamin B_6, and ascorbic acid. Long-term intake of megadoses of vitamin C can induce copper deficiency anemia, cause false-positive readings for glucose in the urine, and increase the risk of urinary stone formation in susceptible individuals. A high niacin intake may result in flushing, headaches, and itching skin. Peripheral neuropathies have resulted from high vitamin B_6 intakes for long periods. Thus the denture-wearing patient should be cautioned against indiscriminate use of megadoses of any nutrient or fiber.

Herbal supplements may have direct effects on the outcome of oral surgery to remove remaining teeth before denture insertion. Herbs are medications that may have adverse pharmacological side effects and should be used with caution. Herbs may increase the risk of bleeding, potentiate the action of anesthetic agents, cause hypotension, or increase the metabolism of drugs being taken concomitantly. Herbal preparations are not standardized; thus the amount of active ingredient may vary among products. Dentists should query patients about their use of herbal supplements and recommend they discontinue the use of herbals before surgery.

DIETARY COUNSELING OF PATIENTS UNDERGOING PROSTHODONTIC TREATMENT

The quality of a denture-wearing patient's diet can be improved with nutrition counseling. One expectation of patients seeking new dentures is that they will be able to eat a greater variety of foods. Such patients often are receptive to suggestions aimed at improving their diet composition. The long-term relationship dentists establish with their patients can create an ideal situation for the identification of older patients at nutritional risk, increasing nutrition awareness, and referral to a physician or dietitian. However, a single structured nutritional

interview is not likely to result in much change in choice of foods.

It often is difficult, based on a visual inspection or an interview, to identify patients in need of nutritional care. Most patients will tell the dentist that they eat a healthy diet. Patients receiving dentures should be carefully screened for nutritional risk factors at the first appointment so that counseling and follow-up can occur during the course of treatment. The dentist and dental hygienist who have backgrounds in basic nutrition can provide nutrition care. In the United States, clinical signs of frank malnutrition are not seen very often. However, certain denture-wearing patients are known to be at greater risk for malnourishment (Box 6-1). Dietary evaluation and counseling should be included in treatment if patients have any of the following physical or social conditions: older than 75 years of age, low income, little social contact, involuntary weight loss, daily use of multiple drugs, or assistance required with daily self-care.

The main objective of diet counseling for patients undergoing prosthodontics care is to correct imbalances in nutrient intake that interfere with body and oral health. The dentist is not expected to diagnose specific nutrient deficiencies, but to determine the general adequacy of the diet. If the patient reports involuntary weight loss or gain greater than 10 lb during the past 6 months, untreated hypertension, a diabetic state, or demonstrated oral tissue changes suggestive of malnutri-

---

Box 6-1

Risk Factors For Malnutrition in Patients with Dentures

Eating less than two meals per day
Difficulty chewing and swallowing
Unplanned weight gain or loss of more than 10 lb in the last 6 months
Undergoing chemotherapy or radiation therapy
Loose denture or sore spots under denture
Oral lesions (glossitis, cheilosis, or burning tongue)
Severely resorbed mandible
Alcohol or drug abuse
Unable to shop for, cook for, or feed oneself

tion, referral to a physician should be made. Patients who express concern about obesity or low body weight or who report poor adherence to a diabetic, reduced sodium, or low cholesterol diet can be referred to a consulting dietitian.

Providing nutrition care for the denture-wearing patient entails the following steps:

- Obtain a nutrition history and an accurate record of food intake over a 3- to 5-day period or complete a food frequency form
- Evaluate the diet; assess nutritional risk
- Teach about the components of a diet that will support the oral mucosa, bone health, and total body health
- Help patient establish goals to improve the diet
- Follow-up to support patient in efforts to change food behaviors

Dietary questions can be incorporated into the medical history form or presented in a separate nutrition questionnaire administered at the first appointment (Figure 6-2). Patients reporting nutritional risk factors are then instructed to prepare a food record. The dental counselor records the past 24-hour food intake on the record. The patient is instructed to record food intake for 2 or more days, which should include a weekend day at home. If a food frequency form is used, the counselor and patient should complete it together. Patients must clearly understand the purpose of diet counseling. Patients' cooperation can be gained by advising them that dietary habits influence how well their oral tissues will adjust to the new denture. The food record is returned by mail or brought to the next appointment.

When the record is received, the actual food intake and quality of a patient's diet is assessed. If a detailed food record is obtained, nutrient analysis can be accomplished on the computer with a dietary analysis software program, or reported foods can be classified into the five basic food groups described in the Food Guide Pyramid. The total reported servings of each food group can be compared with the recommended number of servings in the Food Guide Pyramid (Figure 6-3). The minimum recommendations are three to four servings from the dairy group, two servings each from the meat and fruit groups, three from the vegetable

group, and six from the bread-cereal group. The minimum recommended number of servings of each food group will provide about 1600 kcal. Servings of processed foods high in sodium and fat should be noted. Fish, ground meat, poultry, peanut butter, soups, or casseroles made with beans or legumes are high-quality sources of protein. Within the fruit and vegetable groups, one serving of a citrus fruit and one serving of a vitamin A–rich food, such as deep yellow or dark-green fruits and vegetables, is needed daily.

At the second appointment, the relationship of diet to the health of the oral tissues and evaluation of the patient's diet can be discussed. This will take about 30 to 45 minutes. Nontechnical terms should be used when teaching patients about the diet–oral health relationship. Two concepts are to be stressed. First, the epithelial cells in the mouth have a rapid turnover. Second, the health of the mandible and maxilla depends on a constant supply of calcium and vitamin D. Lack of calcium may accelerate bone resorption. The patient's own radiograph can be used to illustrate the amount of bone remaining in the mandible. This usually is enlightening for patients because they have probably never considered the systemic role of nutrients in maintaining the oral tissues.

When discussing the quality of the patient's diet, always begin by pointing out positive aspects. Identify which food group quotas are being met. If the diet is generally poor, focus on one or two of the most critical deficiencies. Low-calorie, fruit, vegetable, or dairy food intakes, or excessive use of fat-soluble vitamin supplements would be of primary concern. Do not overwhelm patients with information or alarm them by presenting a long list of dietary weaknesses. Remember that older patients with dentures often are particularly sensitive to possible threats to their health and may therefore easily feel disconcerted. If serious dietary problems are detected, referral to a physician or registered dietitian is advisable.

Nutrition goals for the denture-wearing patient are to eat a variety of foods, including protein sources, dairy foods, fruits, vegetable, grains and cereals, and to limit salt, fat, and sugar intake (Box 6-2). Lack of diet diversity, that is, omitting one or more food groups from the daily diet, has been associated with greater risk of death over time.

DEPARTMENT OF PROSTHODONTICS
NUTRITION HISTORY

Name: _____   Date: _____

Age: _____   Height: _____   Weight: _____   Desirable Weight: _____

Food Habits:

1. Do you consider your appetite to be: Good _____   Fair _____   Poor: _____
2. How many meals do you eat each day?   _____
    When are your meals eaten?   _____
    Where are most meals eaten?   _____
3. Do you eat alone?   _____,   with family _____,   with friends _____
4. Do you usually snack between meals?   Every day _____   Seldom _____   Never _____
    What time of day?   _____   Common Snacks: _____
5. How often do you use gum, mints, cough drops?   _____
    What kind?   _____
6. How much sugar do you add to coffee or tea?   _____
    What other beverages do you consume between meals?   _____
7. Are you on a special diet?   Yes _____   No _____
If yes, what kind?   _____
Who recommended the diet?   _____
8. Are there any foods you cannot eat?   Yes _____   No _____
List: _____
9. What kinds of medication, food supplements, or vitamin-mineral pills do you use, if any?
(   )   Medications: _____

(   )   Vitamins, minerals, other supplements: _____

(   )   Antacids, laxatives, others: _____
10. Does your mouth get dry?   Yes _____   No _____   When? _____
What do you eat or drink to moisten your mouth?   _____
11. Do you have difficulty chewing or swallowing?   Yes _____   No _____   Describe: _____
_____
12. How often do you use cigarettes, pipe tobacco, or chewing tobacco?   _____
11. How often do you use wine, beer, whiskey?   Never _____   Daily _____   Weekly _____

Figure 6-2   A nutrition history questionnaire that could be completed by the patient at the time the health history is obtained.

Using the Food Guide Pyramid as a visual tool, the dentist can suggest desirable, nutrient-dense foods to improve the diet, but patients must establish their own dietary goals. Ask patients to describe what foods they could add or substitute in their diet to improve the nutritional balance. Small changes that are possible within the patient's budget and changes that respect food preferences are more likely to be accepted. Adding one glass of milk or orange juice will make a significant contribution to nutrient intake. When it is determined what food changes can be made to improve the patient's diet, the dentist or hygienist can prepare a diet prescription for the patient to take home. The results of the diet assessment and the diet prescription also should be recorded in the patient's dental chart so

DIET EVALUATION SUMMARY

Food groups	Portion size/serving	1st day	2nd day	3rd day	4th day	5th day	Recommended 5-day total	5-day total	Difference
Milk group (milk, cheese) 3-4 servings/day	1 1/2 cups ice cream 1 cup milk, yogurt 1 1/2 oz cheddar cheese 2 oz process cheese						5* 0+		
Meat group (meat, fish, poultry, egg, dried peas, or beans) 2-3 servings/day	2-3 oz cooked lean meat, fish, poultry 2 eggs 4 Tbsp peanut butter 1 cup cooked dry beans or lentils						10		
Fruit group 2-4 servings/day	1 orange 1/2 med grapefruit 3/4 cup fruit juice						5		
	1 med apple, pear, banana 1/2 cup cooked fruit						5		
Vegetable group 3-6 servings/day	1/2 cup cooked dark green, orange, or yellow vegetable						5		
	1/2 cup cooked peas, beans, corn, potatoes 1 cup lettuce						10		
Bread/cereal group 3-5 servings/day	1 pancake, 1 tortilla 1 slice bread, 1/2 bagel 1 oz dry cereal 1/2 cup cooked cereal, rice, noodles, macaroni						30		

*Adults 20-50 yrs   +Adults >50 yrs

Figure 6-3 Form used for evaluating a 5-day food diary submitted by the patient. The average number of servings per day of each food group is compared with the recommended daily intake.

that all members of the dental team can reinforce the dentist's goals.

Compliance with dietary advice is more likely if follow-up is provided. Patients need a trial period to try new foods and eating patterns. Dietary progress should be discussed at future appointments. Roadblocks to modifying a patient's diet should be identified and addressed. Progress may be slow, but modest dietary changes should be praised. Small steps are more likely to result in per-

manent dietary improvement. With continued guidance and encouragement from the dental team, patients are more apt to make permanent changes in their food patterns. In fact, such nutrition care should be an integral part of the overall prosthodontic treatment.

For socially isolated or disabled older adults, there are community-based nutrition programs including food stamps, home-delivered meals, and communal meal programs served in local senior centers, churches, or community centers. Nutrition education, as well as food, is provided. These nutrition services can have a significant impact on nutrient intake and nutritional status of participating older adults. Dental providers can refer patients to these programs.

DIETARY MANAGEMENT WHEN TEETH ARE EXTRACTED

Patients who are candidates for implants or immediate dentures may require several tooth extractions. The patient who is well nourished will experience more rapid tissue healing and will be at lower risk of infection after surgery. If a patient appears poorly nourished (low body weight, weak, disoriented cognition, unexplained skin lesions, glossitis, cheilosis), surgery should be delayed until the individual's body health improves.

Smokers, alcohol abusers, patients with uncontrolled diabetes, and patients with untreated hypertension are at greater risk of having complications after surgery. The smoker and drinker should be advised to abstain or limit their habits for a few weeks before and 1 month after surgery. Consultation

with the physician of the diabetic or hypertensive patient will aid the dentist in determining if the patient is stable enough to undergo the surgical procedure. The adequacy of a patient's diet can be ascertained with the steps just described. To support body functioning and to improve the outcome of surgery, malnourished patients should be instructed to consume high-calorie, high-protein foods before surgery. Milk-based cooked cereals and soups, canned fruits, mashed vegetables, yogurt, ice cream, cottage cheese, ground meat, and eggs are easy for patients with chewing difficulties to eat. A multivitamin containing 100% of the daily value can be prescribed for the high-risk patient.

A generous supply of essential nutrients in the body is basic to tissue healing. It has been clearly shown that when the immune system is depressed, the risk of infection after surgery is greater. Protein, vitamins A and C, folic acid, pyridoxine, vitamin B_{12}, iron, and zinc must be available to body cells for the support of phagocytic activity, cell-mediated immunity, collagen synthesis, and regeneration of epithelial cells. The amount of protein and calories required by the postoperative patient will depend on the amount of metabolic stress experienced during surgery. For the first 24 hours after extractions, the patient should be counseled to consume nutrient-dense liquids. A blender is useful in making cream soups, milkshakes, fruit drinks, or instant breakfast drinks with whole milk or milk with 2% fat. A high-protein milk can be made by adding one cup of dry milk powder to one quart of fluid whole milk. This fortified milk can be used for cooking, for adding to beverages, or for drinking by itself. By using this milk, the patient can boost calories, protein, vitamins, and minerals without increasing serving size. However, milk is a poor source of vitamin C, an essential nutrient for collagen synthesis, so citrus fruit juices or another source of ascorbic acid must be included in the diet. Small, frequent meals throughout the day (every 2 hours) may be required to obtain adequate calories. This is not a desirable time for an adult to try to lose weight.

People's tolerance for solid foods after surgery varies greatly. If blood clot formation is satisfactory, the patient should be encouraged to progress to soft foods by the third day. A variety of soft foods (e.g., cereals, canned fruits, soft-cooked vegetables, cottage cheese, casseroles, chopped meats, and puddings) can be recommended. Without some counseling by the dentist, patients may slow their recovery by limiting themselves to juices, soft drinks, coffee, and tea.

For patients who cannot meet all of their nutritional needs with table foods, commercially produced liquid dietary supplements are available. These products, high in calories and protein and fortified with vitamins and minerals, can be recommended as between-meal snacks. There are milk-based products, and for the lactose-intolerant patient there are soy-based formulas. An 8-oz can provides about 240 to 360 kcal and 10 to 15 g of protein. The use of a high-calorie liquid supplement has been shown to help maintain protein stores and body weight after oral surgery. A less costly alternative is instant breakfasts that have a powdered-milk base.

SUMMARY

Denture wearers are particularly vulnerable to compromised nutritional health. The dentist who is aware of nutritional risk factors can identify patients in need of nutritional guidance. Nutritional deficiencies may result from a combination of low calorie intake, poor chewing efficiency, the presence of chronic disease, economic hardship, and psychological problems. The ability of the oral tissues to withstand the stress of dentures is greater if the patient is well nourished. Dietary guidance is an integral part of treatment for the denture-wearing patient.

Early in treatment, the dentist can assess the general adequacy of the diet and address major deficiencies or refer the patient for care. A patient with dentures will probably not make sweeping dietary changes but will add nutritionally important foods if the need is clearly explained. If the dentally impaired patients are counseled to eat more slowly and chew longer, they can enjoy a wide variety of foods with texture. Foods that require chewing stimulate salivation; saliva lubricates the oral tissues and increases denture comfort. The patient must participate in developing nutrition goals and receive continued encouragement if dietary improvement is to occur.

Bibliography

Ang-Lee MK, Moss J, Yuan CS: Herbal medicines and perioperative care, *JAMA* 286:208-216, 2001.

Brodeur JM, Laurin D, Vallee R et al: Patient intake and gastrointestinal disorders related to masticatory performance in the edentulous elderly, *J Prosthet Dent* 70:468-473, 1993.

Davis DM, Fiske J, Scott B et al: The emotional effects of tooth loss: a preliminary quantitative study, *Br Dent J* 188:503-506, 2000.

Dawson-Hughes B, Jaques P, Shipp C: Dietary calcium intake and bone loss from the spine in healthy postmenopausal women, *Am J Clin Nutr* 46:685-687, 1987.

Duffy VB, Cain WS, Ferris AM: Measurement of sensitivity to olfactory flavor: application in a study of aging and dentures, *Chem Senses* 24:671-677, 1999.

Dwyer JT: Screening older Americans' nutritional health—current practices future possibilities, Washington, DC, 1991, Nutrition Screening Initiative.

Eller WC, Haugen RK: Food asphyxiation—restaurant rescue, *N Engl J Med* 289:81-82, 1973.

Ettinger RL: Changing dietary patterns with changing dentition: how people cope? *Spec Care Dent* 18:33-39, 1998.

Gunne HJ, Wall AK: The effect of new complete dentures on mastication and dietary intake, *Acta Odontol Scand* 43:257-268, 1985.

Herod E: The use of milk as a saliva substitute, *J Public Health Dent* 54:184-189, 1994.

Institute of Medicine: Food and Nutrition Board Dietary reference intakes for calcium, phosphorus, magnesium, vitamin D and fluoride, Washington, DC, 1997, National Academy Press.

Jeffcoat MK, Chestnut CH: Systemic osteoporosis and oral bone loss: evidence shows increased risk factors, *J Am Dent Assoc* 124:49-56, 1993.

Joshipura KJ, Willett WC, Douglass CW: The impact of edentulousness on food and nutrient intake, *J Am Dent Assoc* 127:459-467, 1996.

Kapur KK, Soman SD: Masticatory performance and efficiency in denture wearers, *J Prosthet Dent* 14:687-694, 1964.

Krall EA, Dawson-Hughes B, Papas AS et al: Tooth loss and skeletal bone density in healthy menopausal women, *Osteoporos Int* 4:104-109, 1994.

Krall EA, Hayes C, Garcia R: How dentition status and masticatory function affect nutrient intake, *J Am Dent Assoc* 129:1261-1269, 1998.

Kribbs PJ: Comparison of mandibular bone in normal and osteoporotic women, *J Prosthet Dent* 63:218-222, 1990.

Laurin D, Brodeur JM, Bourdages J, et al: Fibre intake in elderly individuals with poor masticatory performance, *J Canadian Dent Assoc* 60:443-449, 1994.

Marshall TA, Warren JJ, Hand JS, et al: Oral health nutrient intakes and dietary quality in the very old, *J Am Dent Assoc* 133: 1369-1379, 2002.

Mojon P, Budtz-Jorgensen E, Rapin CH: Relationship between oral health and nutrition in very old people, *Age Ageing* 28:463-468, 1999.

Moynihan P, Bradbury J: Compromised dental function and nutrition, *Nutrition* 17:177-178, 2001.

Natow AB, Heslin J: Counseling and compliance. In *Nutritional care of the older adult,* New York, 1986, Macmillan Publishing, pp 65-76.

Palmer CA: Nutrition in oral health. In Papas AS, Niessen LC, Chauncey HH, editors: *Geriatric dentistry: aging and oral health,* St Louis, 1991, Mosby, pp 264-281.

Papas AS, Joshi A, Giunta JL et al: Relationship among education, dentate status and diet in adults, *Spec Care Dent* 18: 26-32, 1998.

Papas AS, Palmer CA, Rounds MC et al: Longitudinal relationship between nutrition and oral health, *Ann NY Acad Sci* 560:124-142, 1989.

Papas AS, Palmer, CA, Rounds MC et al: The effects of denture status on nutrition, *Spec Care Dent* 18:17-25, 1998.

Position of the American Dietetic Association: Food fortification and dietary supplements, *J Am Diet Assoc* 101:115-125, 2001.

Sandström B, Lindquist LW: The effect of different prosthetic restorations on the dietary selection in edentulous patients, *Acta Odontol Scand* 45:423-428, 1987.

Sheiham A, Steele JG, Marcenes W et al: The relationship among dental status, nutrient intake, and nutritional status in older people, *J Dent Res* 80:408-413, 2001.

Shinkai RSA, Hatch JP, Sakai S et al: Oral function and diet quality in a community-based sample, *J Dent Res* 80: 1625-1630, 2001.

Slagter AP, Olthoff LW, Bosman F et al: Masticatory ability, denture quality and oral conditions in edentulous subjects, *J Prosthet Dent* 68:299-307, 1992.

Sullivan DH, Martin W, Flaxman N et al: Oral health problems and involuntary weight loss in a population of frail elderly, *J Am Geriatr Soc* 41:725-731, 1993.

Touger-Decker R, Scafer M, Flinton R et al: Effect of tooth loss and dentures on diet habits, *J Prosthet* Dent 75:831-837, 1996.

Truhar MR: Saliva . . . in health . . . in sickness . . . in aging, *Adult Oral Health* 2:1-11, 1995.

Walls AWG, Steele JG, Sheiham A et al: Oral health and nutrition in older people, *J Public Health Dent* 60:304-307, 2000.

Wayler AH, Chauncey HH: Impact of complete dentures and impaired dentition on masticatory performance and food choice in healthy aging men, *J Prosthet Dent* 49:427-433, 1983.)

PREPARING THE PATIENT FOR COMPLETE DENTURE TREATMENT

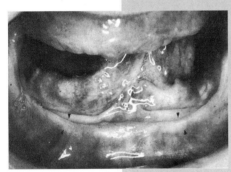

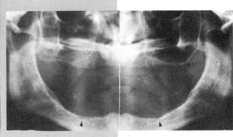

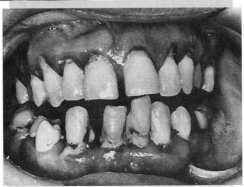

Diagnosis and Treatment Planning for Edentulous or Potentially Edentulous Patients

Douglas V. Chaytor

DIAGNOSIS

Diagnosis for prosthodontic care requires the use of general diagnostic skills and accumulated knowledge from other aspects of dentistry and its supporting science. In this chapter emphasis is placed on diagnostic procedures and findings that are particularly relevant to edentulous and nearly edentulous patients.

Familiarity with the Patient

The patient who is seeking prosthodontic care is prepared by past experiences, good or bad. If the patient has a treatment history in the present practice, both dentist and patient have the advantages of prior knowledge. The dentist also has the potential disadvantage of proceeding on assumptions. Both new and returning patients need their complete medical history taken or reviewed and need to undergo thorough examinations.

Principles of Perception

Visual perception will be the primary mode of data gathering in the examination. A variety of theories of visual perception have been advanced, but it is perhaps easiest to think of its simplest components as seeing with the eyes and interpreting with the brain. Typical of the tasks identified in this process are detection, discrimination, recognition, identification, and judgment. It is not difficult to extend these tasks to the other senses, such as touch and hearing. If the tasks are interpreted in a little more detail, then *detection* is merely noticing something

(i.e., determining its presence). *Discrimination* requires distinguishing that which has been noticed from something else. *Recognition* requires deciding whether this, or at least something similar, has been perceived on some previous occasion. *Identification* moves the process into specificity; what has been observed can now be communicated. *Judgment* allows something that has been observed to be placed within a spectrum of knowledge. In everyday life, these tasks usually proceed automatically, and certainly no attempt is made to fully perceive all aspects of the environment. In diagnosis, there is a professional responsibility to omit nothing of consequence. A consistent, methodical approach to examining patients is required.

The Setting

Health questionnaires and identification data can be gathered in the reception area. The dentist's review and clarification of the responses on the questionnaire, as well as the examination of the patient, are appropriately carried out in the private operatory. The operatory should be comfortably equipped, tastefully decorated, and well lit. It should be free of distractions and provide patients with the sense of security and privacy that will allow them to communicate honestly and completely.

Problem Identification

Diagnosis, in its broadest sense, is an evaluation of existing conditions. More specifically, diagnosing involves identifying, and making judgments about, departures from a healthy state. These departures might simply be thought of as problems. The detection of these problems is the essential first step, but the dentist's perception of them must move through the perceptual tasks to judgment. The latter tasks may not be accomplished until after the examination. The dentist may have to use additional resources to determine the exact nature of a problem and whether it requires treatment. Most important, the dentist cannot act on observations that have not been made. It is dangerous and inappropriate to substitute assumptions for observations. The importance of a thorough examination with accurately recorded observations cannot be overemphasized.

Prognosis and Treatment Planning

Although logic suggests the tidy sequence of data gathering, interpretation into a diagnosis, then treatment planning, the experienced clinician will be thinking ahead during the data gathering and its interpretation. The consequences of both treatment and no treatment will be borne in mind with particular reference to how such action might change the prognosis. The objective of the process is the development of a treatment plan that specifically addresses the diagnosed needs of the patient and accommodates treatment as it progresses.

CONTRIBUTING HISTORY: THE PATIENT'S STORY

Placing a patient's prosthodontic needs in the broader contexts of general health, socioeconomic status, lifestyle, and dental expectations will allow the dentist to deliver treatment specifically appropriate for that patient.

Social Information

A necessary first step for all patients is the establishment of their identity. Information received in referral letters, by receptionists over telephones, or even on forms completed by the patient should be confirmed. The staff can check administrative information such as telephone numbers and addresses. The dentist should address the patient by name and confirm more personal information such as date of birth. Reviewing already completed

forms provides some opportunities for opening conversation and directly, or indirectly, confirming the contained information. A question about hours of work might well prompt a patient who has given an occupation of "school board employee" to say, "I work in the cafeteria, so I am off at 2:30." Now the dentist not only knows when the patient might be available for appointments but also knows that the patient works in a high-risk area for frequent eating.

Knowledge of patients' social settings can help the dentist understand patients' expectations and the evolution of their dental status. Family and social circle norms influence people. There are still sectors of society that are not distressed by tooth loss or by the prospect of wearing complete dentures. Other patients come from unfortunate circumstances where care has been inadequate, but given the resources, they would have done better. Most people have close friends or relatives whose judgment they value. It is helpful to have patients identify these people during the examination and, if possible, gain some insight into their views.

An exploration of a patient's habits will help identify those who might have contributed to their present condition and those who will help ensure success or failure for the treatment to be supplied. The potential for modification or reinforcement of habits should be noted for inclusion in the treatment plan. The dentist will like to know a patient's oral and denture hygiene procedures. The dentist can also find out some of the patient's less favorable habits by explaining their significance for treatment. Smoking is an example. A patient who has not been convinced of the long-term detrimental effects of smoking might respond when learning of its detrimental effects on wound healing and the durability of tissue conditioners.

Patient expectations are founded in the realities and perceptions of the past and influenced by knowledge and emotions of the present but are validated only in the unknowns of the future. Prosthodontics is the most creative segment of dentistry. Its intelligent use of modern techniques and materials justifies raising the expectations of patients with poor dental histories and inadequate knowledge of dentistry today. These patients can be great practice builders when treatment exceeds their expectations. Other people have expectations that far exceed the possibilities for treatment by even the most skilled professionals. If the dentist does not identify this discrepancy between expectations and reality before treatment is started, success will probably elude both dentist and patient. Educating patients is part of the dentist's responsibility for providing dental care. Diagnosing the need for education is as important as diagnosing the need for prostheses.

Medical Status

As health care professionals, dentists are responsible for the well-being of patients under their care. They are not entitled to "just make a denture." They must be aware of each patient's general health, especially conditions that might influence the choice of treatment or that can be aggravated by something that might be done for the patient. Dentists should collect this information early in the diagnostic appointment because of its potential to influence everything else that is done. Early collection of these data also allows the dentist to proceed with diagnostic procedures without having to give undue emphasis to findings by asking related health questions during the visual examination. Minor preprosthetic oral surgery is a frequent requirement and can be presented to the patient in a nonthreatening manner. The patient's perception may be skeptical, however, if at the same time the dentist has to ask about bleeding history or drug allergies.

The exploration of a patient's medical history is a written and verbal art. A well-designed health questionnaire provides clues for more detailed examination by the dentist. The primary objective is the identification of conditions or incidents that have implications for current treatment. Other information assists the dentist in understanding the patient's current condition and in developing a prognosis. It also serves as a context for counseling.

A patient's present conditions are most likely to require accommodation if they physically disadvantage the patient, require medication, or have the potential for causing unfavorable reactions to treatment. Physical incapacity is not always visible. Inquiry may reveal back problems that prevent the patient from tolerating long appointments.

Determination of vital signs will sometimes allow the dentist to find deviations from the norm and in turn advise the patient to seek the services of a physician. It also provides a reference for the patient's record that can be used for comparison should a medical emergency occur during treatment.

Knowledge of all medications that a patient is taking is important to avoid any conflict in therapy. Such conflicts can range from interference with effectiveness of a medication to the precipitation of a medical emergency. Incidents of this nature resulting from failure to elicit a medication history from a patient or from a failure to determine the significance and possible interactions of the medications cannot be justified.

Mental Health

Patients seeking prosthodontic care arrive with an accumulation of experiences and resulting attitudes. These may range from optimism through resignation to despair. All may be set against a background of psychoses or neuroses. When taking the patient's medical history and discussing conditions with the patient, the dentist must seek an understanding of the patient's mental health, particularly attitudes toward receiving new dentures. Much of this can be revealed through discussion of the reason for lost teeth, the importance of any remaining teeth, and the patient's experiences with dentistry, especially experience with any previously worn prostheses. Danger lurks at both ends of the positive-negative spectrum. The overly optimistic patient may have unrealistically high expectations for success with all aspects of the dentures, such as esthetics and masticatory ability. At the other end of the spectrum is the patient who has agreed to treatment only to please someone else, such as a spouse. In all instances, the dentist must seek to improve patient understanding and strive to adjust expectations to reality.

Psychological inventories have been used to assess the personality characteristics of patients who have difficulty wearing dentures. Such studies have shown that many of these patients have high scores on indices of neuroticism. Neurosis is regarded as a chronic anxiety state at the physiological level and is known to affect the performance of tasks requiring neuromuscular coordination. Both learning and skilled performance show optimal relationships with moderate levels of anxiety, whereas levels of anxiety that are too high or too low appear to be incapacitating. Although this suggests that only the most anxious patients should have trouble with their dentures, clinical experience suggests that such a conclusion may be narrow and restrictive. On the other hand, cheerful extroverts are rarely found in the ranks of patients who have difficulty with dentures and who complain unceasingly, although no causative factors can be found for their problems.

Dental Health

Success or failure in the provision of prosthodontic care is frequently the direct result of how adequately the patient's dental history has been gathered and analyzed. Through the telling of their stories and responses to purposeful questions, patients will often provide the essence of a diagnosis of their dental health and needs.

An understanding of the etiology of tooth loss by a patient will help a dentist estimate the patient's appreciation of dentistry and contribute to the prognosis for prosthodontic success. Although patients can change their attitudes and habits, it is reasonable to be suspicious that patients who have lost teeth in an accident might be much more unhappy about their edentulous state than patients who lost teeth as a consequence of decay resulting from neglect. Similarly, the expectations for the amount of alveolar bone remaining would be greater for the patient with a history of rapid tooth loss from decay than for the patient with a long history of progressive periodontal disease.

Patients' expectations will be strongly influenced by their denture experiences. Those experiences may be the source of both good and bad habits. Aside from biological compatibility and mechanical precision, success in prosthodontic treatment is largely dependent on matching patient expectations to the treatment provided. Although it is important to strive to raise the quality of care to match the highest of patient expectations, it also is appropriate to lower the patient's expectations through education about denture wearing.

Considerable information can be gained from observations of dentures being used by patients or saved from previous treatment. The warning to

beware of patients who have a "bag of dentures" is widely known. The more appropriate warning is grounded in diagnosis: the dentist should refrain from treating such a patient unless it is possible to determine ways in which new prostheses can be made significantly better than previous attempts.

Compromising Factors

Treatment planning is defined later in this chapter as a process of matching treatment options with a patient's specific needs as determined by careful diagnosis. Part of that detailed diagnosis must include identification of any factors that have the potential to prevent the delivery of a desirable treatment. Detailed and analytical examination for these factors allows the dentist to move from general knowledge to specific knowledge of the patient being examined. Some factors that should be examined are anatomical, physiological, pathological, psychological, esthetic, and financial.

The examination of the patient's anatomy focuses on the head and neck, with emphasis on the denture-supporting structures for the patient seeking prosthodontic care. However, the patient's general appearance should be observed for characteristics such as asymmetries, irregular gait, and physical defects. Facial asymmetries, disparities in jaw size and concentricity, interarch space, ridge shape, sulcus depth, and muscle attachments are examples of anatomical variations that can require preprosthetic correction or special accommodation in a treatment plan.

Normal physiological functioning contributes to denture success. For example, the successful use of dentures requires adequate neuromuscular control. Deficiencies must therefore be noted and compensatory measures planned. The quality and quantity of saliva are also factors in a patient's toleration of dentures. Thick, ropey saliva tends to dislodge dentures, and thin saliva or low salivary flows tend to provide an insufficient film for retention of dentures or lubrication of the mucosa. Although these factors are unlikely to be modified for prosthodontic purposes, an explanation of their effects can help patients understand related problems and thereby increase their willingness to accept the associated limitations on treatment success.

Perhaps the most obvious, and certainly the most common, objective of diagnosis is the identification of pathoses. Classically, treatment first addresses the elimination of pain and infection. Neoplasms and other active problems also have to be identified for appropriate treatment. Decisions have to be made about inactive problems such as noninfected retained roots. Aside from any immediate harm, consideration must be given to the potential for posttreatment complications. Some potential complications can be sufficiently addressed by simply informing the patient about them. Some problems relate frequently to denture wearing. These include hyperplasia of the denture-bearing area and tissues adjacent to denture flanges, which frequently occurs in the area of the rugae of the palate. This reactive tissue is cauliflower-like in appearance. The inflammation often is the result of a superimposed infection with *Candida albicans*. Concomitant infections at the commissures of the lips appear in many patients. Hyperplastic tissue also occurs at the borders of ill-fitting dentures and was formerly known as *epulis Fissuratum* because of its characteristic form and location. Dysplasia of the ridge crest makes an unstable denture support.

All patients will be psychologically prepared for treatment. The problem for the dentist is to determine if that preparation is positive or negative. Some people will be approaching treatment with enthusiastic optimism; others will be merely resigned to it as a necessity. Some will be cooperative and happy to participate in the decision making and continuing care. Others will want to defer to the dentist and avoid accepting responsibility for their own well-being. With reasonable care and effort in patient management, most patients can be successfully treated. There are people who have real psychological problems that require professional help. Some of these problems can find focus in dental needs. The dentist should not assume the role of the psychologist or psychiatrist. Consultations should be sought with appropriate professionals. Because of the sensitive nature of this type of referral, it usually is best to start with the patient's physician. If patients reveal that they are already in the care of a psychologist or psychiatrist, a direct consultation is in order. Danger lies more in treating the undiagnosed patient than in the patient undergoing therapy.

Desire for an esthetic appearance is a major motivating factor for patients seeking new dentures. Society places considerable emphasis on physical appearance. Advertising uses the "perfect smile" extensively. Preventive measures have helped increasing numbers of people to preserve natural teeth into old age. Improvements have enabled dentistry to provide lifelike prosthetic replacements for natural teeth. All these factors have raised patient expectations. Success in treatment requires matching these expectations or modifying them to meet the reality of current prosthodontic care. It is therefore important for the diagnosis to address patient expectations for esthetic aspects of treatment. The consequences of responding to these expectations also must be considered. The extraction of a few less-than-perfect teeth that retained a removable partial denture satisfactorily can produce a very difficult, and indeed unsatisfactory, complete denture situation. An obvious example of this occurs in a patient who has a Class II jaw relationship requiring a maxillary complete denture to replace a maxillary removable partial denture, but has remaining overerupted teeth in the anterior mandible. Although the mandibular teeth can adequately retain a mandibular removable partial denture, the esthetic requirements for vertical and horizontal overlaps of the anterior teeth make the development of a stable occlusion very difficult.

Both the dentist and patient have reasons to consider the financial implications of treatment plans. The best treatment plans are useless if the patient cannot afford the treatment. The diagnosis must therefore determine the significance of problems and the priority of the need for treatment to permit the development of a treatment plan that addresses the patient's needs in keeping with an ability to pay. The diagnostic findings must be evaluated to allow consideration of interim care, deferred treatment, and alternative treatment.

DATA COLLECTION AND RECORDING

Accurate diagnosis depends on the collection of accurate data. The means of collection and the form of the data will vary. To be useful, data must be stored in a readily retrievable format. They must be respected for their contribution to the diagnosis. They must be kept confidential as a fundamental principle of dentist/patient relations. Office staff must be made aware of these principles. They should know that no patient information should be shared with others, neither through conversation nor through careless exposure on computer screens or written records that can be viewed by other patients.

Record keeping is rapidly moving to computers instead of the traditional paper chart. Computer-based record keeping offers some definite advantages in formatting, manipulation, and data retrieval. Unfortunately, some programs can limit natural expression and thereby present a risk of limiting the scope and depth of information gathered. It is not the role of this text to debate the merits and technology of computerization. The following discussion of gathering and recording information will not be specific to either format.

Questions

The gathering of information starts with the first contact about, or with, the patient. The information may come in a referral letter or a telephone call from the patient or another dentist. Whatever the source, the record keeping should begin with this contact.

A registration form facilitates the capturing of basic information such as the patient's name, address, and telephone number. The name and address of the patient's physician, insurance information, referral source, and any other information that might need frequent or quick access also can be recorded here. Gathering information with health questionnaires has several advantages, but they should not be used alone. Their main advantages are consistency of predetermined questions and ease of patient response. They therefore provide a quick overview for the dentist. Staff should be advised to try to detect people who might have reading problems arising from lack of education, learning disabilities, or language problems because the patient's first language is different from the language used in the questionnaire. For most people, a verbal administration of the questionnaire will overcome the problem, but for some people the help of family, a friend, or an interpreter may be required. However completion of the questionnaire is achieved, the dentist should review it and discuss it with the patient. Because the responses provide only an overview derived from standardized questions, the dentist must explore any suspicious or incomplete responses in more detail. Direct conversation with people will probably be more revealing than written communication. This is partly due to its spontaneity and interactive nature. It also overcomes a natural reluctance by some people to put candid or confidential information in writing. The referring person is the first source of information. If this is another dentist, something of the patient's attitudes or behavior might be revealed. If the referring person is a family member or friend, it is wise to be more cautious in the questioning. However, that person might reveal something of the new patient's hopes and fears and, specifically, the reason for the referral. Given a chance, most patients will tell their own story. Indeed, most patients will have at least a lay idea of their diagnosis and a possible treatment plan. The dentist will learn this through careful listening. An interpretation of this information will assist the dentist in determining what the patients' dental awareness is and how much education will be required to help patients understand their problems and what dentistry can do for them. Patients must be assisted in this process by addressing them at their level of understanding, avoiding unnecessary dental jargon or an approach that might inhibit the conversation. Some patients are reluctant to reveal information in their health or social histories that they feel is not pertinent to dentistry. A simple explanation of dentistry's responsibility for the health of the whole patient as dental treatment might affect it, or might be influenced by it, usually will help.

Records

Whether patients have been edentulous for long or short periods, or are about to be rendered edentulous, it is important to review information about their progression from a full complement of natural teeth to their present state. The primary purpose of this review is to enable the dentist to base restoration on original information and avoid replication of errors in existing prostheses. Some historical records will be available for most patients. The continuity of records is one advantage a patient gains from remaining in one practice. Referring, or previous, dentists usually will be helpful in supplying information. Information normally found in dental charts should be reviewed to provide background for current conditions and treatment needs. Charts should at least provide a chronology of previous treatment. They should also contain some preextraction information such as tooth shade and vertical dimension of occlusion. They also can provide previous health history and an indication of patient compliance with previously prescribed routines such as home care or recall appointments.

Although radiographs reduce the three-dimensional oral structures to two-dimensional shadow pictures, somewhat enlarged and perhaps distorted, they do provide very useful information. They can, for example, contribute an indication of the relative sizes and arrangement of teeth. Old radiographs might reveal how cysts or neoplasms influenced the tooth arrangement. The most valuable records to examine are casts because they provide true three-dimensional information on tooth size and arrangement. Articulator mounted casts also reveal jaw relationships and interarch tooth relationships. Examination of old prostheses, coupled with discussion with the patient, can reveal much about what the patient likes and dislikes and can or cannot tolerate. It is important to note characteristics such as the arch form of the teeth relative to the arch form of the residual alveolar ridge, the orientation of the occlusal plane, the relationship of anterior teeth to the lips, denture base extensions, the thickness and contours of the flanges, and any wear patterns.

Systematically taken preextraction photographs can be useful for determining tooth arrangement. Measurements of teeth also can be made from them. Observations on face form and jaw relations also can be made. Frequently, patients can supply nonstandardized photographs that reveal much of the same information. Age is not a serious factor in selecting teeth from preextraction information. The presence of natural teeth is important even if the patient's mouth is closed. When asking patients for such pictures, it helps to explain how they will be used (i.e., for background information and not necessarily as a blueprint for new dentures).

Visual Observations

Our primary data-gathering sense is vision. In daily life, vision is taken for granted and used unconsciously. In a dental examination, it must be used consciously. Conditions should be designed for optimal effectiveness. Adequate lighting is essential for making correct visual observations. Both quality and quantity are important. Dentists routinely use task lighting to supplement ambient room light. To avoid eye strain, the gradient between the two must not be too great. The ambient light should be diffuse to prevent the production of high-contrast shadows. The task lighting should not produce glare. Visual acuity diminishes with age, and higher levels of lighting are required. Color balance is important for not only shade selection but also for the correct evaluation of soft tissue.

Observing the patient should begin extraorally. There is much to be learned from watching the patient entering the operatory and sitting in the dental chair. Are the patient's movements sprightly or impaired? Does the patient use a walking cane or tend to rest on furniture? Is there pallor or flushing of the face? Does the patient appear to be short of breath? Are there any signs of injury or impairment? Is the patient wearing eyeglasses? Is the patient wearing a hearing aid? Do the patient's hands appear arthritic? Are there facial asymmetries? Are circumoral tissues adequately supported?

After history taking and extraoral observations, the dentist begins the intraoral examination. The surface quality and contours of the soft and hard tissues are the objects of a careful visual examination of the mouth. The dentist should adopt a routine order for this examination to avoid omissions. Patients frequently will direct a dentist to their chief complaint. This can distract the dentist from a comprehensive evaluation. It is wise to explain to patients what the value of the complete examination is and how this allows for setting the chief complaint in the context of the patient's oral and general health.

Often, aids to vision are helpful. The mouth mirror has been the symbol of dentistry's diagnostic responsibilities for many years. It allows for comfortable viewing angles. It also enables the dentist to direct light to structures and recesses of interest.

Magnification is a simple aid to vision. A hand-held lens will serve in some instances, but many dentists find loupes convenient for most tasks. Beyond magnification, loupes can improve the viewing distance and, with more sophisticated optics, can adjust the viewing angle. The latter features enable the dentist to work using less stressful posture than might be possible with unaided vision.

Still photography can be an aid in diagnosis and treatment planning primarily by allowing the dentist to have recorded images available for study during the development of a treatment plan.

Intraoral videography is promoted as a means for patient education. Its well-lit, magnified image displayed on a monitor also provides the dentist with an excellent image for immediate viewing or for storage and retrieval. The stored images supplement other records for a variety of uses from patient education to legal defenses. The ability to view such rich visual information when developing a treatment plan is a major asset.

Digitization of images makes computer-assisted vision possible. Although video images can be converted for this purpose, still digital photography has developed to a practical state.

Radiography

The transition from emulsion-based film radiography to photostimuable phosphor-based films, CCD (charge couple device) and CMOS (complementary metal oxide semiconductor) image sensing, is well underway. This transition is reducing patient exposure to radiation; is eliminating image inconsistencies related to concentrations, depletion, and temperature of chemicals; and also is eliminating chemical disposal as a problem. Experienced dentists will find that displayed digital images differ in appearance from conventional radiographs viewed with transmitted light on a viewbox. Direct viewing of the small film image gives the perception of precision in the image that may appear to be lacking in the enlarged digital image displayed on a monitor. The apparent lack of precision is a function of magnification and the resolution of the digital image. Any digital image can be enhanced to bring out specific features.

Radiographs are important aids in the evaluation of submucosal conditions in patients seeking prosthodontic care. The presence of abnormalities in edentulous jaws, or in the edentulous segments of partially edentulous jaws, may be unsuspected because of the absence of clinical signs or symptoms. Abnormalities do occur and can be seen on radiographic examination. These may be foreign bodies; retained tooth roots; unerupted teeth; or various pathoses of developmental, inflammatory, or neoplastic origin. Radiographs aid in determining the depth of periodontal pockets. They provide information about the bone surrounding the apices of pulpless teeth. They can show the amount of bone lost around the remaining teeth and in the edentulous regions (Figure 7-1). They also can show the relative thickness of the submucosa covering the bone in edentulous regions, the location of the mandibular canal, and the mental foramina in relation to the basal seat for dentures. They can give an indication of the quality of the bone that supports the teeth and will support the dentures. Unfortunately, this information is not always reliable because of variations in radiographic techniques, exposure times, and developing procedures. However, the denser (radiopaque) the bone appears to be, the better the bony foundation. Sharp spicules of bone on ridge crests and spiny ridges also are apparent on dental radiographs. These conditions may affect decisions about the types of impressions and denture-base design that should be used.

Extraoral radiographs can provide a general survey of a patient's denture foundation and surrounding structures. Panoramic dental radiography is readily available for the convenient examination of dentulous and edentulous patients. The dentist must be aware that such radiographs incorporate inaccuracies resulting from the tomographic principles of this type of radiograph. Modern machines have adjustments to compensate for some of these problems, but they do not produce precisely accurate pictures of the anatomical structures. Magnification of structures is common with this technique and is of the order of 25%. Because the machines are programmed to capture a predetermined "slice" of anatomy, structures outside that slice can be missed.

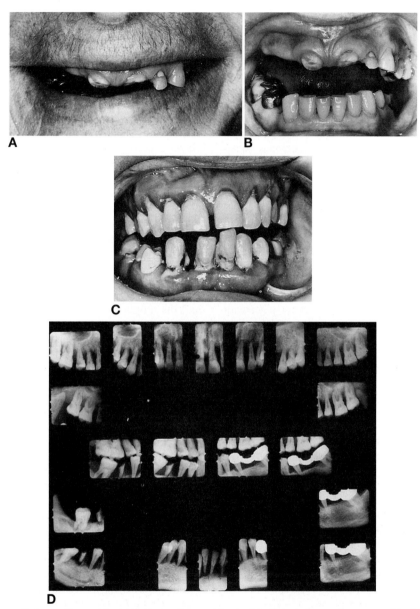

Figure 7-1   Radiographic evidence can be combined with clinical observations to enable the dentist to prescribe optimal treatment. The patient in *A* and *B* and the one in *C* are partially edentulous, and each requested complete denture treatment. In *A* and *B*, clinical and radiographic examinations indicate that all the teeth can be retained and a maxillary removable partial overdenture can be prescribed, rather than a complete denture. In *C* and *D*, a minimum of two bilaterally located and suitable abutments to support an overdenture is not present. This patient was therefore treated with immediate dentures because of the untreatable periodontal disease present.

This can happen most easily for small structures such as ectopic root tips. Knowledge of the location of anatomical structures, as they are normally projected on panoramic radiographs, is an essential prerequisite for reading panoramic radiographs. Suspicious areas should be examined in more detail with intraoral radiographic techniques. Special film holders and central ray aiming aids are available for making some radiographs. Cephalometric and temporomandibular joint (TMJ) radiography are examples. Some large-format views, such as the lateral jaw projection, can be obtained by having the patient hold a cassette loaded with film against the face while exposure is made with the regular chairside dental x-ray machine.

Intraoral radiography is the most frequently used format in dentistry, with the periapical approach considered essential for caries detection and the evaluation of periodontal support. Although periapical radiography is convenient, it also has diagnostic advantages. The small film size allows placement close to the structures of interest, resulting in less magnification than panoramic radiography. Similarly, the small films can be kept flat and thus avoid distortion of the image. Although these features suggest the value of this format when teeth are present, this format should not be overlooked in edentulous patients. Maxillary tuberosities, for example, often are not clearly seen in panoramic radiographs but can be clearly seen in profile on periapical films. In fact, this format should be used to further explore any suspicious areas not clearly seen on large-format films. Although the word *film* has been used here, the same comments will apply to this format when recorded by means of direct digital radiography. Occlusal format films are designed to be held on the occlusal surface of the teeth and exposed appropriately from above or below the jaws to provide a view of a whole arch. Like the periapical approach, it captures all structures in the path of radiation. The profile it provides is particularly helpful for diagnosing apparent expansion of the bone buccally or lingually, such as may occur with cysts or retained roots.

Palpation

Although it is important to use all senses in diagnosis, touch is probably second only to vision in importance. For submucosal structures, it competes with, or perhaps more correctly, complements, radiography. A sensitive finger will detect abnormalities such as displaceable structures, discontinuities, and enlargements of structures. It will reveal textural differences and unusual contours. A light touch should be used for most of the examination, but patient response to pressure also is helpful. Certain areas, such as sharp residual alveolar ridges and mylohyoid ridges, typically are tender. Before patients are palpated, they should be told to expect pressure. They should be assisted in distinguishing the normal sensation of pressure from pain and tenderness. Tenderness or pain, in apparently normal areas, may indicate underlying pathoses and should be investigated radiographically.

Dentists should follow a routine pattern of intraoral palpation to avoid omissions. Typically, one might start with lips and cheeks, moving to the denture-supporting areas, the floor of the mouth, and the tongue. Aside from noting the features of each area, it is important to also note asymmetries with the contralateral structures.

Both primary and secondary denture support areas should be palpated. The sides of residual alveolar ridges should be palpated in addition to the ridge crest. Irregularities and patient reactions should be noted. The contents of the floor of the mouth are best palpated with one finger from one hand inside the mouth and two fingers of the other hand applied extraorally. The outside fingers prevent the displacement of the structures during palpation by the intraoral finger. The patency of Wharton's duct and the production of saliva by the submandibular gland should be demonstrated by watching for the expression of saliva from the duct orifice as the gland and duct are gently squeezed. Palpation of the tongue is essential for a thorough examination and should be done in sequence with the visual examination. The patient is asked to protrude the tongue onto gauze. Aided by the gauze, the dentist can hold the tongue while using a mirror to examine it. Palpation of the tongue should be done both left to right and right to left. Obviously, this must be done quickly. The targeted areas are the lateral borders and the region of the vallate papillae. The dentist will use extraoral palpation to corroborate intraoral findings and explore other structures such as the TMJ and associated muscles. It has been said that the exposed head and neck are areas of responsibility for dentists. This may not be a view shared by patients if they are unaware of the need to look for structures such as lymph nodes in the neck. Extraoral palpation requires explanation to the patient to avoid misunderstanding of the dentist's purpose.

Measurement

Classification of some structures as large or small, and sulci or fossae as deep and wide, or shallow and narrow, is adequate for a general appraisal of a patient's anatomy. However, some structures and spaces require more precise recording. Students new to the field of prosthodontics will find measuring helpful in developing their abilities to estimate size. Recorded measurements often are helpful in the laboratory for fabrication of prostheses. They also allow the dentist to verify the attainment of some treatment objectives. Later they serve as references for reevaluation of prostheses during recall examinations.

The most fundamental extraoral measurement is the vertical dimension of occlusion. A little more difficult to establish, but also important, is the vertical dimension of rest. Techniques for making these measurements often suggest making arbitrary marks on the nose and chin for reference. However, such references disappear at the end of the appointment. Anatomical references such as menton and the columella of the nose remain with the patient and therefore allow repeated comparative measurements at future appointments. The anatomical references used should be noted in the patient's chart. Consistency of technique by the dentist will foster reliability of these repeated measurements. Other extraoral measurements relate to specific procedures such as tooth selection. For example, the patient's true interpupillary distance can be compared with the interpupillary distance on a photograph of the patient; a ratio can be calculated and then used to calculate a replacement tooth size from the patient's tooth size measured on the photograph.

A periodontal probe or dividers and a ruler or Boley gauge can be used to make intraoral measurements. Size is a factor to be considered in mon-itoring any traumatic lesion or other lesions of the mucosa. Measurements also are helpful in designing prostheses or items used in their construction such as impression trays. In the latter instance, measurements of sulcular depth can be transferred to casts to indicate the height of tray flanges required. Of course, some measurements of intraoral structures can be made more easily on the diagnostic casts, for example, the size of remaining teeth.

Diagnostic Casts

Diagnostic casts are at least a convenience and, in most instances, a necessity. They allow for an evaluation of anatomy and relationships in the absence of the patient. The mounting of casts on an articulator allows for a dynamic evaluation of the interarch relations. A facebow can be used to conveniently relate the casts to an approximate hinge axis. Eccentric records can be made to set the condylar guidances. The mounted casts can be surveyed and analyzed at the dentist's convenience. The casts may reveal new information or confirm that which has already been observed intraorally. The dentist will be looking at arch size and symmetry, interarch space, arch concentricity, anteroposterior jaw relationship, and lateral jaw relationships, especially posteriorly where an occlusal crossbite might be indicated. The dentist also will be looking for signs of underlying abnormalities. Measurement and a determination of relationships to other structures will assist in making decisions on preprosthetic surgery. Undercuts may be observed unaided, or their significance can be determined more precisely with the aid of a dental surveyor. Even soft tissue disease may be more obvious on a cast than intraorally when saliva and color may obscure it. The rugae provide an example. Displacement from the pressure of an old denture can be more obvious on a dry cast than in the mouth.

SPECIFIC OBSERVATIONS

Experienced dentists use the full spectrum of data-gathering techniques and aids in accomplishing a compilation of complete information to use in developing a diagnosis for a patient. Regardless of how the information is obtained, the objective is the gathering of specific information from specific observations.

Existing Dentures

The patient's existing dentures should be examined carefully. The objectives of this examination are to determine exactly the quality of the dentures and how that relates to the experiences cited earlier by the patient and to determine the potential for improvement. If the dentist cannot identify specific attributes of the dentures that can be improved to alleviate specific problems, embarking on the making of new dentures is tantamount to embarking on a sailing voyage without a navigation chart. The same rocks and shoals that spoiled the last voyage are probably going to produce failure again. Base, framework, and tooth material can be determined by visual inspection or light scratching with a metal instrument. Transmitted light will reveal the retentive pins of porcelain teeth. Set against the age of the denture and the material of the opposing occlusion, some estimates of patient use and abuse of the prostheses can be made. For example, porcelain teeth are more wear resistant than acrylic resin teeth; thus the resin teeth will show more wear than porcelain teeth over the same period of use. However, porcelain teeth are more brittle; they will likely be chipped if the patient has not been careful, especially when cleaning them. Chipping also may be the result of lack of harmony in the occlusion. An evaluation of the fit of a denture will determine how well it is adapted to the denture-bearing area, how well the flanges fill the sulci, how correct the border extensions are, and where the posterior palatal seal is located. Dentures with flanges that are deficient in extent or thickness fail to achieve their potential for support, stability, and retention. A variety of proprietary products can be applied to the tissue surface of the denture before seating that will reveal the distribution of tissue contact. These products include pressure-indicating pastes and special formulations of silicone impression materials. A thin mix of irreversible hydrocolloid impression material also works. A clue to poor denture-base fit is the finding of plaque on selected sites of the tissue surface of the denture. The tissue surface of the labial flange is a typical location.

The most important observation that must be made of the occlusion is whether the occlusion is in harmony with the patient's jaw relations. Large discrepancies will be immediately obvious if the patient is guided into centric relation and the occlusion is observed as the patient brings the teeth together and subsequently is guided into eccentric contacts. Small discrepancies may only be suggested by tooth wear patterns. The level and orientation of the occlusal plane must be assessed—so must the tooth-to-tooth and tooth-to-ridge relationships. The length of the plane relative to the size and shape of the denture-bearing area also must be assessed. Denture teeth set over the slope of the mandibular ridge as it approaches the retromolar pad are recognized as a source of denture instability. Tissue trauma and a patient's inability to successfully use dentures can frequently be traced to errors in occlusion.

An evaluation of the esthetics of existing dentures should be approached first from the perspective of the knowledge and professional judgment of the dentist. Second, there must be an evaluation in the light of information about the patient's natural teeth. The third phase of the evaluation must take into consideration the patient's views. These perspectives must all be reconciled to achieve success in the making of new prostheses. A patient will sometimes be satisfied with esthetically inappropriate dentures because of conditioning through long-term use. These patients often are reluctant to have significant changes made because they would be noticeable to other people. Patients who desire change must have their expectations clarified because these expectations may not correspond with the dentist's intentions or abilities. The esthetic appropriateness of a patient's existing dentures and the possibilities for improvement can be determined by comparing the observed and contemplated characteristics with the recommendations made later in this book for selecting and arranging prosthetic teeth.

Soft Tissue Health

Complete dentures are entirely dependent for support on soft tissue (mucoperiosteum) and underlying hard tissue (bone). The health and quality of those tissues are therefore very important determi-

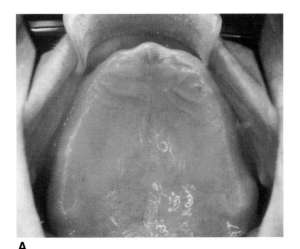

A

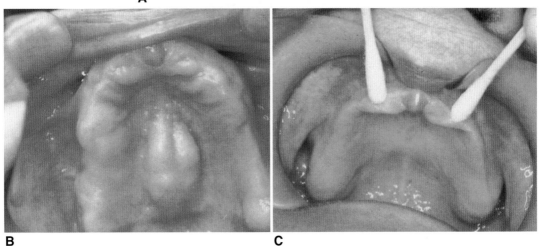

B   **C**

Plate 7-1   An extensive range of morphological tissue health variables must be diagnosed before treatment planning is finished and complete denture fabrication is started. Six different edentulous maxillae underscore some of the frequently encountered variables. **A,** This residual ridge shows minimal resorption and is covered by firm, healthy, soft tissues. Hamular notches are well defined, and no tissue adhesions are present. This maxillary basal seat area offers an excellent morphological prognosis. **B,** This residual ridge, though substantial, is irregular, with bony undercuts and small exostoses present. The left tuberosity is pendulous and mobile, and a large torus is present. A denture can be built on these foundations, but surgical considerations also should be addressed to optimize the basal seat area. **C,** Anterior localized ridge resorption has occurred and been replaced by hyperplastic tissue. This tissue is usually exised before impression making. When a patient's health precludes this option, a modified impression technique is employed.

Continued

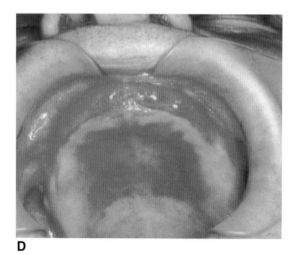

D

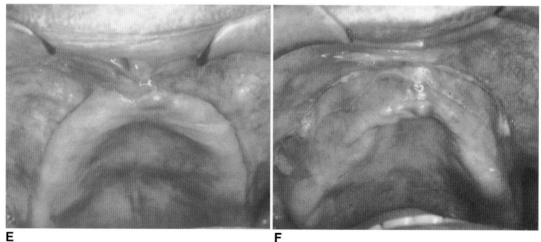

E   F

Plate 7-1 *cont'd* **D,** Home care and a regular recall program were not instituted for this patient. Consequently, the basal seat area became inflamed, and an epulis resulted. Tissue rest, massage, and the prescription of a treatment liner should precede a surgical assessment in this patient. **E,** Advanced residual ridge resorption is evident, with low mobile peripheral tissue attachments and obliteration of the hamular notches. As a result, compromise in both peripheral and posterior palatal seals will negate a favorable prognosis for a retentive and stable denture. **F,** A morphological picture similar to the one in **E** has been rectified by a preprosthetic sulcus deepening with skin graft placement. This prescription used to be frequently used in the mandible but has been virtually eclipsed by implant treatment.

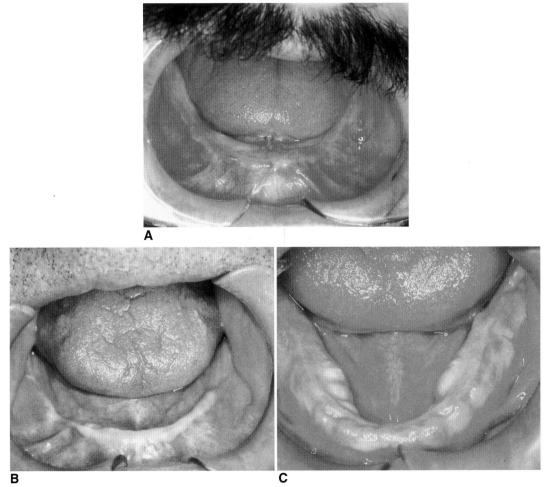

Plate 7-2 Six diverse edentulous mandibular morphologic outcomes. **A,** A firm, broad, and well developed ridge accompanied by a favorable tongue size and position suggests a good prognosis. **B** and **C,** Alveolar ridge undercuts are present, though ridge size differs substantially. Surgical removal of the undercuts can be readily avoided by prudent relief of the denture base. However, tender areas over the exostoses and/or the tori in **C** may have to be treated surgically to ensure a comfortable prosthetic experience.

Continued

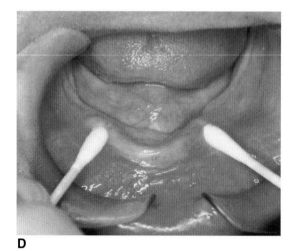

D

E   **F**

Plate 7-2 *cont'd* **D** to **F,** Hyperplastic replacement of the entire residual ridge does not usually provide a firm denture-bearing area. However, surgical excision may result in a significantly reduced basal area, as in **E.** Extension of the denture's posterior lingual flanges usually will allow for a stable denture in **E.** This objective may not be fulfilled in **F** because of the unfavorably high attachment of the floor of the mouth. Also notice the virtual continuity of mobile mucosa in the floor of the mouth and the labial/buccal vestibule. They are separated by a thin, mobile, fibrous band. From a morphologic point of view, this does not provide a favorable prognosis. Preprosthetic surgery for placement of osseointegrated implants is likely to be needed in these situations.

nants of success in the wearing of complete dentures (see Plates 7-1 and 7-2). The dentures are surrounded by the cheeks and lips, which are covered by lining mucosa. This mucosa moves in intimate contact with the dentures during functioning of the related facial and masticatory muscles. The lining mucosa of the lips and cheeks and floor of the mouth is relatively thin and easily traumatized. It is also the site of a variety of pathoses. The lingual and palatal surfaces of the dentures are in intimate contact with the tongue and its specialized mucosa. The specialized mucosa covering the tongue is sometimes said to be a "window" on systemic disorders. All these tissues must be examined in detail for individual anatomy and for abnormalities, irregularities, and pathoses. The term *masticatory mucosa* has been applied to the mucosa covering the residual alveolar ridges and palate. It usually is attached to the underlying periosteum. When it is not attached, denture instability can be a problem. The area of attachment diminishes with ridge resorption. The mandibular ridge is more susceptible to this problem. A total loss of attachment is often first seen above the mandibular symphysis. This loss can be demonstrated by pulling the lower lip and watching the floor of the mouth move.

Diagnosis of abnormalities of the mucosa requires the recall of the normal appearance. Shape, color, and texture are significant characteristics. Some variations occur frequently with no significance and are therefore accepted as normal. These include Fordyce's granules in the buccal fat pads and varicosities in the floor of the mouth of elderly patients. Initially, knowledge of normal appearance is learned from anatomy texts and the study of surface anatomy. However, the required mental picture becomes well developed only through careful examination of many healthy mouths. General knowledge of the anatomy of the mouth provides a background for the examining dentist to focus on the specific details of the anatomy of each patient. The simple questions of presence or absence of the normal structures must be followed by determinations of the detailed characteristics of the structures. The hard palate is examined for its shape, its height, its width, and the quality of the mucosa and submucosa covering it. Does it have a high vault that will resist lateral displacement of a denture? Is the hard palate wide as

to supply denture support and surface area for retention? The soft palate accommodates the posterior palatal seal and distal border of a complete denture and is included in the discussion of border tissues. The cheeks are examined primarily to determine if they are pathoses free. If traumatic lesions are found, their relationship to existing dentures must be determined. The general contour of the cheeks should be noted. Are they full, filling the buccal spaces, which indicates a need for concave buccal contours on the dentures? Does the full shape result from underlying fat (e.g., retained juvenile buccal fat pads) or from well-exercised masseter muscles such as is seen in gum chewers? The latter must be accommodated in the buccal flange contours through the impression making.

The tongue is an important factor in denture success or failure. The size and activity are the main concerns. The tongue will expand into edentulous spaces. The introduction of a new denture will then be met with dislodging competition from the tongue. An edentulous patient who has not been wearing a mandibular denture often will use the tongue as an antagonist for the maxillary arch in mastication. In these situations, the tongue can become enlarged and very strong. Examination of the floor of the mouth includes examination of deep structures. The surface contours are important but can change as a result of underlying activity. Contraction of the mylohyoid muscles will raise the floor of the mouth. This will dislodge a complete denture made from an impression that did not record the floor of the mouth with the mylohyoid muscle in a contracted state. The visual examination requires that the depths of mucosal folds be exposed to be sure hidden lesions are not missed. The patency of the submandibular ducts should be checked. Bidigital palpation should express saliva from the duct. This technique helps identify abnormalities such as sialoliths in the submandibular duct, fibrosed glands, and enlarged lymph nodes. Many types of pathological lesions can be found in and around the oral cavity, including lesions of the mucous membrane and tissues under it. They may be in the bone or glandular tissue; on the soft palate, hard palate, lips, cheeks, tongue, or floor of the mouth; or in the throat. Like mechanical cuts and abrasions, pathological lesions should be diagnosed and treated before impressions are made.

Among the more common lesions found in the mouth of edentulous patients are pseudoepitheliomatous hyperplasia, papillary hyperplasia, aphthous ulcers, lichen planus, hyperkeratosis, leukoplakia, and epulis fissuratum (hyperplasia). Other lesions may be more serious; for example, lumps and ulcers can be evidence of malignancies. These may be found anywhere in the oral cavity. If they are not detected, serious consequences can result for the patient and for the dentist. If suspicious lesions are found, adequate steps must be taken to determine their precise nature. These include biopsy and referral for further tests. Oral malignancies are most common in people who are old enough to need complete dentures, but they may occur in people of all ages. The obligations of dentists for maintaining health do not end when the teeth are gone. Instead, they become more important. Patients must be questioned about their knowledge of any suspicious findings. Questioning should start with the patient's awareness of the abnormality and progress through symptoms, duration, and any home remedies that might have been applied. The patient's perception of whether a lesion is healing or spreading is important.

The color of the mucosa will reveal much about its health. The differences in appearance between a healthy, pink mucosa and red, inflamed tissue will be apparent. The cause of any inflammation must be determined. Is it the result of trauma from an old denture? Is it a manifestation of infection? Abrasions, cuts, or other sore spots may be found in any location under the basal seats of the existing dentures or at the borders. They may be the result of overextended or even underextended borders. Malocclusion is also a major source of tissue trauma. Sharp or overextended denture borders will produce red lines of inflammation or ulcerations. Evidence of cheek biting will appear at the level of the occlusal plane. It often will be white scar tissue indicating a mucosa that has been traumatized and is now healing. Sometimes soreness results from something as simple as a berry seed getting under the denture. At the time of the examination, the causes should be determined to allow correction before impressions are made. Although infections may arise from a variety of sources, fungal infections are common in edentulous patients. Concomitant inflammation of the corners of the

mouth should raise suspicions of *C. albicans* infection. A cytosmear may be made easily and examined for pseudohyphae. Smears also may be cultured to confirm the clinical diagnosis.

Hyperplasia of the tissue associated with ill-fitting dentures is a common finding. Hyperplastic tissue will be found in relation to edentulous ridges and border tissues, as a reaction either to trauma or to the resorption of supporting bone. When bone resorbs, it leaves a void in the denture foundation as defined by the existing denture. This space often will remain at least partially filled with hyperplastic tissue. This condition seems to appear more frequently in the maxillary arch. On the mandible, it is seen most frequently in the anterior region when the posterior regions are relatively stable but the dentures were not relined in more recent anterior extraction sites. Occlusal trauma from decreased vertical dimension of the jaws and posterior tooth wear is concentrated in the anterior regions and contributes to this problem. Border tissues chronically traumatized by overextended flanges, or by flanges of dentures that have settled as result of lost ridge support, often will produce a reactive hyperplasia that has commonly been referred to as *epulis fissuratum*. Similarly, tissue will proliferate inside a loose-fitting flange. The labial surface of the maxillary residual alveolar ridge is a common site. Papillary hyperplasia is cauliflower-like in appearance and tends to occur on the anterior of the palate, in the area of the rugae, of long-term denture wearers. Often this tissue is inflamed and is then referred to as *inflammatory papillary hyperplasia*. The deep crevices of papillary hyperplasia are prone to infection. The infection frequently is found to be *C. albicans*. Obviously, infection must be treated before new dentures are made, but recurrence is likely unless the hyperplastic tissue is removed.

Excess fibrous tissue commonly occurs under very normal-appearing mucosa. Although it is sometimes quite firm, it does not provide sound denture support. This is in part due to its uneven distribution. The maxillary tuberosities, if fibrous, may not only provide poor denture support but may also be so large as to interfere with the correct placement of the occlusal plane. If they are mobile, they will diminish the stability of the denture. The anterior region of the maxillary residual alveolar ridge also may be fibrous, but usually it is flabby if bone resorption has occurred and the denture has not been relined to compensate for the loss. A ridge supporting a complete denture opposed by only anterior teeth in the mandible seems to be especially prone to this type of deterioration. Resorption of the mandibular residual alveolar ridge sometimes leaves a tight band of fibrous tissue above the ridge crest. This too is nonsupportive for a complete denture and is difficult to record accurately in an impression because of its displaceability.

Hard Tissue Health

Teeth   All teeth should be examined and evaluated carefully. The loss of all remaining teeth can be a terrible psychological shock to patients, even though some of them may not admit it. Consequently, the dentist should be empathetic to patients who must lose their teeth. Every possibility for saving them should be explored. When patients recognize that the dentist does not want them to lose their teeth, a necessary feeling of confidence can be developed. Even patients who say that they cannot wait to get rid of their teeth so that they will not have to see dentists anymore usually do not really want to lose their teeth. Often they are only trying to prepare their defenses against future difficulties they do not understand. If the dentist removes teeth without adequate reason, physical, mental, and even legal problems may arise. The answer as far as the dentist is concerned is simple: get all the facts and consider all possibilities before making the decision to remove the remaining teeth. Many diagnostic factors are involved. To ignore or fail to recognize any of them can lead to incorrect decisions. Valid reasons for extractions may include one or more of the following conditions:

1. Advanced periodontal disease with severe bone loss around the teeth
2. Severely broken-down crowns (subgingival) that cannot be adequately restored
3. Fractured roots
4. Periapical or periodontal abscesses that cannot be successfully treated
5. Unfavorably tipped or inclined teeth that pose problems for their use as abutments for fixed or removable prostheses
6. Extruded or tipped teeth that interfere with the proper location of the occlusal plane

The number and location of remaining teeth must be carefully noted. Perception sometimes fulfills expectations, as was mentioned earlier. Drifted teeth can masquerade as missing neighbors. Each tooth should be identified and notations should be made of drifted or malaligned teeth. The coronal structure of remaining teeth should be examined for the quality of both the natural components and any restorations. The fracture or ditching of restorations, the extent of caries, and the presence of cracks, especially vertical cracks extending into the root, should be determined. The questions to be answered include the following: Is this tooth satisfactory to survive on its own? Can it support a removable partial denture? Can it be restored? Can it be used as an overdenture abutment? Periodontal support is another major factor in the decision to preserve teeth or render a patient edentulous. If significant periodontal disease is found, its extent and the prognosis for treatment become factors in deciding on retention or extraction of the affected teeth.

Bone   Bone is the firm, yet physiologically dynamic, support for teeth and prostheses. Its external form and internal structure are influenced by systemic and local factors. Even though whole bones are permeated with other structures such as blood vessels, bone tissue is primarily a collagenous protein matrix impregnated with mineral salts. Its stability is dependent on good nutrition and hormone balance. A thorough discussion of bone diseases of systemic origin is beyond the scope of this book, but the dentist must be alert to their negative influence on the success of prosthodontic treatment. Patients may reveal these diseases in their health histories. Alternatively, they may be unaware of the problem yet exhibit symptoms on examination. Commonly identified metabolic bone diseases are osteosclerosis, osteomalacia, and osteoporosis. *Osteosclerosis* refers to increased amounts of calcified bone. It can be associated with metastatic tumors or hypoparathyroidism. A deficiency in the amount of minerals relative to the amount of matrix is referred to as *osteomalacia*. *Osteoporosis* is a decrease in bone mass but with a normal ratio of minerals and matrix. Adult women, especially after menopause, are particularly inclined to have osteoporosis. Local bone disease and anatomy can be significant factors in prosthodontic care. Retained roots of teeth, abscesses, cysts, and neoplasms have to be identified and differentially diagnosed. Appropriate treatment must then be planned. Some retained roots will be partially resorbed and difficult to distinguish from surrounding bone. Attempts to remove these surgically often are frustrating and only partially successful. If such roots are asymptomatic and apparently covered completely in bone, they are usually best left undisturbed. The patient should be made aware of their presence and the rationale for leaving them. Roots covered only by mucosa and roots with clearly defined periodontal ligaments, associated cysts, or abscesses should be removed. Neoplasms require complete diagnosis and treatment.

The anatomy of structures particularly related to the provision of prosthodontic treatment is described and illustrated in later chapters. Diagnosis in preparation for new dentures requires a detailed examination of the specific anatomy of the individual patient. Many variations will be found. Some will present no special problems. Others will require accommodation in impression making. Still others will require surgical correction. Sharp and spiny residual alveolar ridge crests can be products of preextraction bone destruction, trauma during extractions, or postextraction resorption. Crestal bone irregularities and increasing radiolucency toward the ridge crest suggest this in radiographs showing the ridge in profile. Palpation usually will reveal the sensitivity of the mucoperiosteum over the crest. Because of the sensitivity, spiny ridge crests cannot contribute much to the support of a denture. Surgical reduction is tempting and sometimes indicated, but the reduction in ridge height adversely affects the stability of a denture. The ridges can sometimes be kept for their contribution to stability if they are relieved of direct pressure by using a selective pressure impression technique that gains support for the denture from other areas. Severe resorption will expose the mental foramina on the crest of the mandibular residual alveolar ridge. This may be seen radiographically. The exposed mental nerve is sensitive to pressure. The patient wearing dentures may report a sporadic shooting pain in the distribution area of nerve.

Palpation will produce the same pain. Relief of the denture to bridge over the nerve must be provided but is not completely effective because conventional complete dentures move in function. Stabilization of dentures with implants has overcome this problem. The location and size of the mandibular canal usually are important only if surgery, such as the placement of implants, is contemplated. Enlarged maxillary sinuses preclude, or at least complicate, reduction of maxillary residual alveolar ridge height such as might be needed to allow correct orientation of the occlusal plane. Placement of implants in the region of the maxillary sinuses will usually require the grafting of bone to the inner wall of the sinus by a procedure generally referred to as a *sinus lift*.

Tori are benign bony enlargements found in some patients at the midline of the hard palate or on the lingual aspect of the mandible in the premolar region. They vary in size. Small ones may be accommodated by relief of the denture base. Others are so large that their interference with denture design warrants their surgical removal. Tori are covered with a thin mucoperiosteum; consequently, they are very hard and sensitive to pressure. A torus in the midline of the maxillary arch, torus palatinus, may appear to be nothing more than a prominent midline suture but may be so large that it fills the palate to the level of the occlusal plane. Generally, surgical removal of a torus palatinus should be avoided, but if the torus is so large that it extends beyond the vibrating line and over part of the soft palate, it should be removed or reduced in size. When the torus extends very far back, it can interfere with the development of a posterior palatal seal (see Figure 8-9). Mandibular tori occur singly or in rows just above the floor of the mouth. It often is difficult to provide adequate denture relief for them because it would break the border seal of the denture. If adequate accommodation through relief cannot be anticipated, surgical removal is indicated. Because a torus has a thin covering of cortical bone, the interior cancellous bone will be exposed by surgery. The formation of a new cortical plate takes 2 to 6 months.

Bony undercuts can be found on maxillary and mandibular residual alveolar ridges. They are significant only if the denture base cannot be manipulated into place over them. This usually requires opposing undercuts. A typical example is a railway track–like mandibular residual alveolar ridge with lingual and buccal undercuts. Another typical example is seen when buccal undercuts appear at the distal of the maxillary right and left residual ridges. Although some of these undercuts result from true exostoses, many, such as the maxillary example, arise from inadequate management of the alveolar bone at the time of extractions. Forceps extraction of teeth usually spreads the alveolus. The buccal and lingual plates require repositioning after this occurs; otherwise, the socket will fill with new bone supporting the cortical plates in a splayed relationship.

Biomechanical Considerations

A number of biomechanical factors influence the choice of methods to be used and the difficulties that will be encountered in providing complete denture service. These factors must be recognized even though sometimes not much can be done to eliminate the problems or their causes. Instead, it is sometimes necessary to alter the technical procedures to minimize the adverse effects of the unfavorable conditions.

Jaw Relations Unobtrusive observation usually will provide the first indication of the patient's jaw relations. A later chapter deals with the determination of jaw relations during treatment. Some of these approaches can be applied at the diagnostic appointment. The vertical dimensions of the face at rest and occlusion, as well as the anteroposterior jaw relations, must be estimated during diagnosis to permit provision for their acceptance or correction being included in the treatment plan.

The available amount of support for complete dentures is directly related to the size of the mandible and the maxillae. Although dentists are expected to strive for accuracy in all aspects of denture construction for all patients, it is obvious that errors in patients with small arches can take on more significance than would be the case for patients with large arches. This will be true from impression making to finalization of the occlusal scheme and denture bases. The arch form as it appears from an occlusal viewpoint should be noted. This information is used in several steps of denture construction

(e.g., stock tray selection for preliminary impressions). In the absence of precise information, arch form can be used as a factor in tooth selection. It also may assist in decisions on the arrangement of teeth. If the arches are asymmetric, problems of tooth arrangement and occlusion may occur. Harmony in size and form between maxillary and mandibular jaws allows for the most desirable tooth arrangements and occlusion. However, some patients have large maxillary jaws and small mandibular jaws, or the opposite disharmony. These conditions arise from genetic factors and from imbalance in growth and development. When the natural teeth were present, these patients would have had severe malocclusions, unless they had been treated with orthodontics. The replacement of teeth for people who had a Class II or Class III malocclusion presents some special problems. Generally, the artificial teeth should occupy the same positions as the natural teeth. This requires the occlusion to be planned in relation to the disharmony. The modifications from an ideal occlusion to a crossbite occlusion or one with an excessive horizontal overlap of the upper teeth over the lower teeth will require time to develop. These difficulties should be recognized and anticipated when the diagnosis is made. The cross-sectional contour of a residual alveolar ridge has an important influence on the selection of an impression procedure. Resorption of a residual ridge after the removal of teeth radically changes its cross-sectional form. When the teeth are first removed, the ridge is broad at its occlusal surface, but as resorption occurs, the residual ridge becomes progressively narrower and shorter. The ideal ridge has a broad top and parallel sides. As the ridge becomes narrower, it becomes sharper and consequently is unable to withstand as much occlusal pressure as a broader ridge. Ridge relations change as shrinkage occurs. Therefore the amount of resorption that has occurred after teeth have been lost affects the relationship between the maxillary and mandibular support areas. The bone of the maxillae resorbs primarily from the occlusal surface and from the buccal and labial surfaces. Thus the maxillary residual ridge loses height, and the maxillary arch becomes narrower from side to side and shorter anteroposteriorly. The mandibular ridge resorbs primarily from the occlusal surface. Because the mandible is wider at its inferior border than at the residual alveolar ridge in the posterior part of the mouth, resorption, in effect, moves the left and right ridges progressively farther apart. The mandibular arch appears to become wider, while the maxillary arch becomes narrower. The cross-section shrinkage in the molar region is downward and outward. The cross-section shrinkage in the anterior region at first is downward and backward. Then, as shrinkage continues, the anterior part of the basal seat for the mandibular denture moves forward. These changes must be noted at the time of the examination to plan for the resultant problems of leverage, occlusion, and tooth position for esthetics.

Denture stability is enhanced by parallelism of the primary denture-bearing areas. When natural teeth contact in centric occlusion, the surfaces of the maxillary and mandibular arches are, in effect, parallel. This is a very stable relationship. Even though denture teeth will be set to contact evenly in centric occlusion, the surface of the arches that support the dentures may be resorbed out of parallelism. This diminishes the stability of the dentures. This problem must be noted at examination for consideration in denture design. For example, implant-supported dentures are especially helpful in this situation. To determine this relationship, the patient should be coached to position the jaws at the vertical dimension of occlusion and hold the position while the examining dentist parts the lips with fingers and mouth mirror to observe the ridges. The relationship also will be obvious on mounted diagnostic casts. Mounted diagnostic casts also will reveal the amount of interarch space. This is important information because a lack of space can lead to denture failure from improperly positioned teeth. Excessive space usually is related to severe ridge resorption. The resulting instability also limits denture success. Even when severe ridge resorption indicates excessive interarch space in the anterior of the mouth, the posterior should be examined to determine if there is sufficient space. If some teeth are present, they must not interfere with the placement of the occlusal plane. Extraction may be indicated if a tooth is so extruded that its occlusal surface is above the desired occlusal plane, unless it can be shortened sufficiently to be on the same plane with the other teeth in that dental arch.

If the maxillary tuberosities are so large that they will prevent the correct location of the occlusal plane or require the omission of some teeth or prevent the correct distal extensions of the denture bases, they could be surgically reduced. The fact that a patient may have been wearing dentures does not rule out these difficulties. Denture-base wear on old dentures over the retromolar pads and the maxillary tuberosities suggests an interarch space deficiency. Radiographs will show whether large tuberosities are bone or an overgrowth of fibrous connective tissue. Where possible, the reduction should be limited to the fibrous tissue. The resulting closed soft tissue wound heals quickly and predictably. Should bone have to be removed, remodeling is initiated, making the result less predictable and prolonging the healing. Sometimes space can be gained by dissecting out nonessential contents from large retromolar pads.

Border Tissues Retention of a complete denture is partially dependent on an effective border seal. The seal is created by closely adapting the denture to its surrounding tissues. Therefore the tissues that will surround the denture flanges and the spaces that will accommodate them should be examined thoroughly. Noting their specific anatomical characteristics and dimensions during the diagnosis will help in designing the denture, in determining the size and shape of a custom tray, and in evaluating of the impressions.

The labial sulci anterior to the buccal frenula are often obliterated by the lips resting against the residual alveolar ridges. With severe ridge resorption, the lingual boundary is undefined. An estimate of the depth and labiolingual width of each sulcus will help by setting an objective for impression making and ultimately for the height and thickness of the labial flanges. The goal is to provide a denture flange that correctly supports, but does not distort, the lips while also creating a border-sealing contact with the boundary tissues without impingement. Essentially the same can be said of the buccal sulci, which are located distal to the buccal frenula. However, some related structures must be examined for their influence on the space. Lateral jaw movement will advance the coronoid process of the mandible toward the maxillary tuberosity. In so doing, it may obliterate the sulcus, indicating that a very thin denture flange will be needed. This diminished space will have to be recorded during impression making. The masseter muscle, when contracting, can act through the buccinator muscle and impinge on the buccal sulcus. This effect usually is much more pronounced in the mandibular buccal sulcus. The external oblique line of the mandible defines the lateral boundary of the buccal shelf and frequently defines the buccal boundary of the mandibular buccal sulcus. However, sometimes the tissues of the cheek are easily displaced and will allow a wider mandibular buccal flange.

The alveolingual sulcus lies between the tongue and the residual alveolar ridge and body of the mandible. The mylohyoid muscle underlying its floor modifies its depth and shape during function. The sulcus should therefore be observed during movements of the tongue. Having the patient lick the lower lip from side to side with the tip of the tongue can raise the floor of this sulcus to a reasonable level. The retromylohyoid fossa is the pouch forming the posterior terminus of the alveolingual sulcus on each side. The few mylohyoid muscle fibers found here are usually weak and displaceable. However, the posterior wall of the fossa is the retromylohyoid curtain, which contains the superior constrictor of the pharynx. Contraction of this muscle will alter the shape of the fossa; so too will protrusion of the tongue. An estimate of usable space must be made. Having the patient place the tongue tip in the opposite buccal sulcus usually will demonstrate the usable space. It may be necessary to use a mouth mirror to control the tongue to permit observation.

The anatomy of the soft palate usually will determine the location of the distal border of the maxillary complete denture and its posterior palatal seal. A soft palate that turns down abruptly limits the distal extension of the denture. A palate that slopes down gradually allows more discretion in locating the denture border. The vibrating line is used as a guide to this location. It is the area of transition from immovable palatal tissue to the movable soft palate. Observation of the palate with the mouth open and the patient attempting to say the letter "k" usually will reveal the vibrating line and the extent of palatal movement. The depth to which the tissue anterior to the vibrating line can be

displaced will determine the depth of the posterior palatal seal. The hamular notches, which appear between the maxillary tuberosities and the hamular processes of the medial pterygoid plates, should be demonstrated. Even though these bone boundaries are covered by soft tissue, they usually can be palpated. Between them, the soft tissue is quite displaceable, thus affording a location for the posterior palatal seal of the maxillary denture. However, the pterygomandibular raphe originates in this area; it must not be encroached upon by the denture. The various sulci are traversed by frenula. Some contain muscles. Others are moved by neighboring muscles. If they are displaced by the denture base, the denture will be dislodged when the muscles contract. If the notches made in the denture base to accommodate the frenula are too large, a seal will not be achieved, and air will leak in and break the potential vacuum that helps retain the denture. The potential for these problems must be estimated at the diagnosis. If it is determined that their location, size, or activity will adversely affect denture retention, surgical repositioning or removal should be considered. Each labial and buccal frenulum must be examined to make specific determinations. The lingual frenulum also must be examined, but surgical correction often has to involve the floor of the mouth, making it uncomfortable for the patient and hence less desirable. An important consideration is interaction between the lingual frenulum and the mandibular labial frenulum. If there is insufficient attached mucosa on the ridge between the frenula to prevent movement of one causing movement in the other, the area of attachment must be improved surgically. Otherwise, the mandibular denture will be unstable because its mucosal support is unstable.

Saliva Saliva often does not receive the attention it deserves. Both the flow rate and the viscosity are important to denture success. Normal resting salivary flow is about 1 ml/min. A flow of medium viscosity at this rate lubricates the mucosa and assists retention of complete dentures. Many factors can affect the flow rate, but aging is no longer considered to be a primary factor in diminished flow. Many patients of denture-wearing age, however, take medications that can reduce salivary flow. Patients who have received radiation therapy in the region of the salivary glands usually have glandular tissue destruction with resulting reduction in salivary flow. In the absence of a history of radiation or antisialagogue drugs to explain diminished flows, further investigation is warranted. The glands themselves may be diseased or ducts can be blocked, although the latter would usually produce acute distress. Often the palatal glands are destroyed in patients who have worn a complete maxillary denture for many years. The cause is really pressure atrophy resulting from lost residual alveolar ridge support of the denture.

Muscular Development

The oral cavity is surrounded by muscles. Jaw and soft tissue movements are the products of muscle activity. If the muscles are strong and their activity well coordinated, they will help the patient use a correctly designed denture. Conversely, poor denture design, weak muscles, and poor muscle coordination all detract from denture stability and retention.

Muscle Tonus The tone of the facial tissues is critical to several steps of denture construction. Tissue tone that is either too strong or too weak is unfavorable. As a result, completing clinical procedures may require more than the usual amount of time. If the muscles are too tense, cheek and lip manipulations will be difficult; if too slack, the lips and cheeks may be displaced easily by impression materials. Patients may take more time than usual to learn to use the dentures. Optimal functioning of the postural and facial expression muscles requires correct support from the natural teeth and ridges or from correctly designed and built prostheses.

Neuromuscular Coordination Good muscular control and coordination are essential to the effective use of complete dentures. They also are helpful in denture construction. For example, when tongue movements are used for border molding the lingual flanges of a mandibular impression, the timing, direction, and amount of movement are critical to the success of the molding. Similarly, coordination of jaw movements is important during denture construction and use.

A patient lacking ability to move the mandible to the right place at the right time reveals the poten-

tial for problems in making jaw relation records before they are attempted. To make an observation of muscular control, the dentist can ask the patient to open the mouth about halfway and move the lower jaw from left to right, then to put the tongue into the right cheek and into the left cheek, to stick it out, and to put it up and back inside the mouth. The ability, or lack of ability, to do these movements on demand will be apparent. The treatment schedule can be modified accordingly. If the dentist feels the problems are significant, the patient can be asked to practice jaw movements at home. Emphasis can be placed on deliberate border movements ending in centric relation. Practicing in front of a mirror will allow the patient to visually coordinate the movements.

Patients with one or more of the following symptoms usually are considered to have a temporomandibular disorder (TMD). The symptoms include (1) pain and tenderness in the muscles of mastication and the TMJs, (2) sounds during condylar movements, and (3) limitations of mandibular movement. Quite logically, the TMJs should be healthy before new dentures are made.

Unhealthy TMJs complicate the registration of jaw relation records. If it is to be a functional position, centric relation depends on the structural and functional harmony of osseous structures, the intraarticular tissue, and the capsular ligaments. If these specifications cannot be fulfilled, the patient will not be able to position the mandible in a correct centric relation or, for that matter, provide the dentist with a repeatable one; thus the importance of the routine evaluation of a patient's temporomandibular function as an integral part of complete denture treatment. The diagnosis and management of TMDs were addressed in detail in Chapter 5.

Tongue Apart from the example of tongue movement coordination during impression making previously mentioned, tongue position and coordination are significant in complete denture functioning. A retruded tongue position deprives the patient of a border seal of the lingual flange in the sublingual crescent and also may produce dislodging forces on the distal regions of the lingual flanges. Normally, the tongue should be expected to rest in a relaxed position on the lingual flanges, which, if properly contoured, will allow the tongue to help retain the denture. A tongue thrust tends to dislodge a lower complete denture by raising the floor of the mouth and, in so doing, lifting the lingual flanges and by exerting pressure on the anterior teeth. Attempts at retraining may not be very successful but will at least make patients aware of the problem and help them to understand the adverse effects.

Dentists should have a basic knowledge of speech, particularly its articulatory component. Articulation is the modification of speech sounds by structures of the throat, mouth, and nose. Fortunately, the neuromuscular activity that produces speech can adapt to, or accommodate, some structural change. The relationship of the positions teeth, lips, and tongue have to each other in the articulation of speech is discussed later (see Chapter 19). An assessment must be made during diagnosis to identify existing problems and determine the potential for improvement.

A patient's protective gag reflex can compromise dental treatment. A thorough history and oral examination will reveal the presence of an overly active reflex early in the patient/dentist relationship. The dentist can then assess the possible cause of the problem as being attributable to iatrogenic factors, organic disturbances, anatomical anomalies, biomechanical inadequacies of existing prostheses, or psychological factors. Effective management of gagging tends to be based on experience and anecdote, with combinations of distraction techniques, prosthodontic management, and medication. Usually, counseling, reassurance, and kind handling of the patient prove to be useful therapeutic adjuncts. However, patients whose gagging cannot be controlled by counseling or distractions may need the services of a psychologist.

Cheeks and Lips The external form of the cheeks and lips is dependent on their internal structure and their underlying support. This support may be natural teeth and ridges or denture teeth and bases. The muscles in the cheeks and lips have a critical function in successful use of dentures. The denture flanges must be properly shaped to aid in maintaining the dentures in place without conscious effort by the patient. This involves the development of the correct arch form and tooth positions, as well as the shape of the polished surfaces and the

thickness of the denture borders. The amount of denture space must be considered carefully if a fixed implant-supported prosthesis is planned because it does not usually provide a tissue-supporting base.

Patients with very thick cheeks may present technical problems during some clinical steps. Thick cheeks often do not allow easy manipulation for border molding of impression materials. Various characteristics of the lips not only are significant for denture retention but also are prominent in considerations of esthetics and phonetics. Fortunately, phonetics involving the lips does not tend to pose many independent problems when esthetic requirements are satisfied. If the tissue around the mouth has wrinkles and the rest of the face does not, lack of lip support can be suspected and significant improvement can be expected. A rolled-in vermilion border is evidence of inadequate lip support and historically has characterized denture wearing. If the problem appears to be anterior teeth set too far lingually or palatally, the lack of support can be tested by adding wax to the labial surfaces. If the addition of wax improves the appearance of the lip, plans can be made to bring the new teeth further forward and thus provide the necessary support to help eliminate the wrinkles. If the wrinkles, especially the vertical lines in the lower half of the lip, are long-standing, they will not disappear at once, and patients should be warned about this. Questions about the prominence of the natural upper anterior teeth may reveal that the residual alveolar ridge was reduced when the teeth were removed "to get rid of the buck teeth I never liked." Attempts to reduce the horizontal overlap of anterior teeth by setting the teeth back "under the ridge" and through surgery usually lead to a lack of lip support that produces vertical lines as tissue tone deteriorates later in life. Patients should be told that for a short time their mouths might appear to them to be too full because of the sudden change. The danger insofar as the dentist is concerned is that too much support for the lips might be provided in an attempt to eliminate the vertical lines in the upper lip. The apparent fullness of the lip is directly related to the support it gets from the bone or denture base and the teeth behind it. Lip fullness should not be confused with lip thickness, which involves the intrinsic structure of the lip. A denture with an excessively thick labial flange may make the lip appear to be too full rather than displaced. Excessively thick denture bases also can make the lip appear thick or short. An obliterated philtrum or mentolabial fold suggests excessive support. The problem with lip fullness is in the patient's reaction to changes. If the existing dentures have the teeth set too far palatally, the patient may feel that the new and corrected tooth arrangement makes the lip too full. Extra time will be needed at the try-in of the wax dentures.

Patients with thin lips present special problems. Any slight change in the labiolingual tooth position makes an immediate change in the lip contour. This can be so critical that even overlapping of teeth may distort the surface of the lip. Both the arch form and the individual tooth positions are involved. Thick lips give the dentist a little more opportunity for variations in the arch form and individual tooth arrangement before the changes are obvious in the lip contour.

The evaluation of anterior tooth position is complicated by short or incompetent lips. The patient may ask for a less-than-natural show of teeth. Long lips tend to hide the teeth, thus presenting the dentist with a temptation to set the teeth too long to make them visible. Awareness of these problems can help the dentist overcome them. A patient with a short upper lip may expose all the upper anterior teeth when properly set and much of the labial flange of the denture base as well.

INTERPRETING DIAGNOSTIC FINDINGS

After all the intraoral and general physical and dental conditions have been recorded and radiographs, casts, and other visual aids are at hand, they can be interpreted, and the treatment plan can be developed. This includes which teeth are to be saved and how, which teeth are to be extracted, the tooth-removal sequence, the type and extent of oral surgery that might be required, and the type of prosthesis that is indicated. Should it be an overdenture, an immediate overdenture, a conventional immediate complete denture, or an interim immediate denture, or even a transitional denture? Is it the unusual situation where all the teeth should be removed and a waiting period allowed so that the tissues can heal somewhat before new dentures are

made? Is the ultimate goal an implant supported prosthesis?

Obvious, Congruent, or Incongruent?

Some diagnostic findings have obvious significance and suggest treatment that is just as obvious. The incidence of this will increase as a dentist becomes more experienced in treating edentulous and partially edentulous patients. These apparently easy decisions become the basis for developing a treatment plan. However, such a treatment plan should be looked on as a hypothesis in need of testing. The testing may lead to modifications. The first test of the obvious is to determine if such findings are consistent with other findings that have been made. Is there congruency between the disease that appears to be present and the probable etiology? Incongruity of information gathered about a patient signals the need for further investigation.

Summary

A diagnosis must be based on adequate information and must account for the findings from the history and examination. Where findings cannot be accounted for, further investigation may be incorporated into the treatment plan, provided such action would not be injurious to the patient. A summary of the points addressed in developing a thorough diagnosis can serve as a primer on determining patient problems (Box 7-1).

TREATMENT PLANNING

Treatment planning is the process of matching possible treatment options with patient needs and systematically arranging the treatment in order of priority but in keeping with a logical or technically necessary sequence. The process requires a broad knowledge of treatment possibilities and detailed knowledge of patient needs determined by a careful diagnosis. A dentist approaching treatment planning with a deficiency in either of these categories of knowledge places the patient in jeopardy of receiving inadequate or inappropriate treatment. The dentist also must resist the natural tendency to include in a treatment plan only that treatment that the dentist feels competent to deliver. Patients requiring treatment beyond

---

Box 7-1

A Primer on Determining Patient Problems

History: The Patient's Story
Social
Medical
Mental
Dental
Compromising factors
Specific Observations
Existing dentures
   Materials
   Fit
   Occlusion
   Esthetics
Soft and hard tissue health
   Lining and specialized mucosa
   Mucoperiosteum
   Teeth
   Bone
Biomechanical considerations
   Denture support
   Interarch relations
   Border seal areas
Muscular development
   Muscle tonus
   Neuromuscular coordination
   Cheeks and lips

---

the competency of the treatment planner should be referred to more competent colleagues or specialists. When presented with adequate explanations, patients appreciate referrals as expressions of the dentist acting in the patients' best interests. Failure to make such referrals is unethical and can lead to litigation. The consequences of both treatment and no treatment must be considered. Treatment planning must have a parallel process of developing a prognosis. Treatment planning is driven by the diagnosis but must take other factors such as a prognosis, patient health, and attitudes into account.

WHY TREATMENT PLAN

A treatment plan is required to specifically state the treatment that will address a particular patient's needs (Figure 7-2). That treatment will be stated in a logical sequence and will include adjunctive care. Its detail and clarity will permit estimates of operatory time and laboratory time, as well as associated fees. Failure to have such a plan makes informed consent by the patient impossible. Proceeding without informed consent exposes the dentist to problems ranging from loss of patient confidence to difficulty with fee collection or even to litigation. Inadequate plans also make it difficult or impossible for staff to do their part in maintaining a smooth delivery of patient care.

Treatment Planning Is Problem Solving

Problem-solving techniques usually involve careful analysis of a problem, breaking it into components where possible, then generating and weighing a list of possible component solutions to ultimately construct a comprehensive solution. The problems are not solved until the solutions are implemented. Untried solutions might reasonably be thought of as hypotheses in need of testing. Dental treatment planning might be thought of in the same manner. The first step is a careful analysis of the diagnostic findings, paying particular attention to specific components (see Box 7-1). With knowledge of these needs, the second step involves developing a list of possible means of addressing them (Box 7-2). Although this may be a mental exercise, there are times when a written list assists thinking. The integration of these component solutions into a comprehensive treatment plan requires an estimation of the impact of the components on each other.

The Matching Process

The information that should be gathered on individual patients and the techniques for gathering it are discussed earlier in this chapter. The details of the specific observations determine the details of the treatment required (Figure 7-3). A decision to supply a set of complete dentures to an edentulous patient does not require very sophisticated thinking. Left at that level, the results might be equally unsophisticated. Truly professional care requires the dentist to consider all information gathered and appropriately address it in the treatment plan.

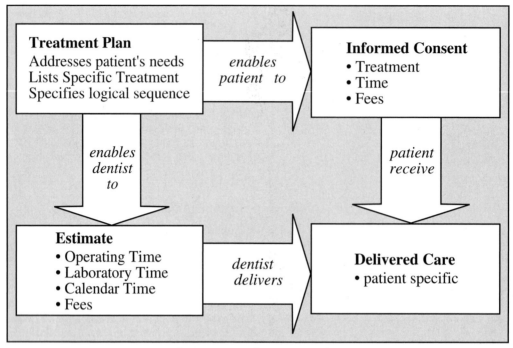

Figure 7-2 Why treatment plan.

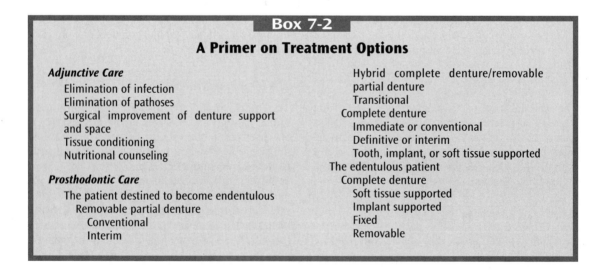

Box 7-2

A Primer on Treatment Options

Adjunctive Care

Elimination of infection

Elimination of pathoses

Surgical improvement of denture support and space

Tissue conditioning

Nutritional counseling

Prosthodontic Care

The patient destined to become endentulous

Removable partial denture

Conventional

Interim

Hybrid complete denture/removable partial denture

Transitional

Complete denture

Immediate or conventional

Definitive or interim

Tooth, implant, or soft tissue supported

The edentulous patient

Complete denture

Soft tissue supported

Implant supported

Fixed

Removable

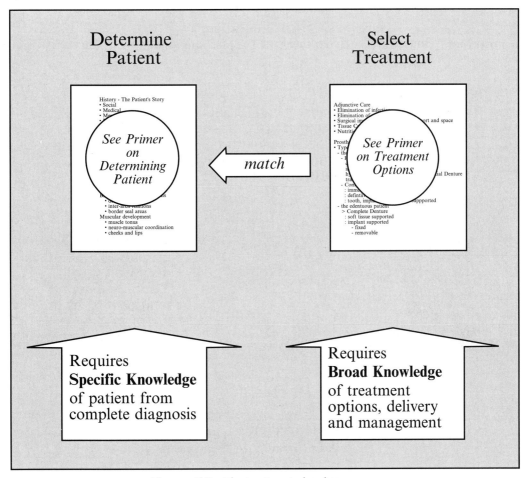

Figure 7-3 The treatment planning process.

There are many occasions when the patient will benefit from preparatory care such as the treatment of candidiasis, the repositioning of frenula, and the reduction of fibrous maxillary tuberosities. The presence of active periodontal disease may make prediction of the form of the postextraction ridge impossible and thereby suggest the use of an interim immediate denture for the patient who is about to have remaining teeth extracted. A history of denture dissatisfaction, the financial means to afford quality care, and findings of a deficient, denture-supporting foundation but adequate bone suggest the patient would ben-

efit from implant-supported prostheses. Design, fabrication, and delivery of prostheses as the focus of prosthodontic care are discussed later in this book. The dentist must customize the care for each patient.

The information accumulated from the diagnosis must be systematically analyzed to identify each patient's problems and to determine their related needs. A problem list for a patient might include (1) large areas of edentulous residual alveolar ridges and (2) three remaining teeth that can be restored only with the aid of endodontic and periodontal treatment. When a patient is

---

Patient Education:
an initial and continuing activity integral to, and supportive of, a treatment plan

Purposes
- inform the patient of their dental health and its significance.
- give the patient understanding of significance of edentulism.
- match the patient's expectation with reality of treatment potential.
- explain nature, use, and shortcomings of prostheses.
- identify alternative treatments and their consequences.

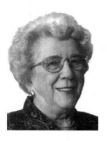

Will help patient understand
- diagnostic procedures
- diagnostic results
- treatment plan
- treatment to be provided
- use of prostheses
- continuing care
- fees

Should facilitate
- acceptance of treatment
- acceptance of fees
- continuing care

Figure 7-4 Patient education.

unhappy with his or her appearance and expresses a desire for replacement of missing teeth, the dentist might be tempted to decide the patient needs extensive endodontic, periodontic, and prosthodontic treatment to address all problems. However, if the patient has limited financial resources, he or she is more likely to translate the problems into a need for extractions and complete dentures. Agreement must be reached on the needs and the treatment options to be applied. This may require modifications in a treatment plan as first conceived by a dentist. One might think of this process as transforming a dentist-oriented treatment plan to patient-oriented treatment plan in light of a variety of influencing factors such as accessibility and finances. However, the modifications should not be such that they would jeopardize the health of the patient.

Patient Preparation

All patients seeking dental services do so with some degree of understanding and experience. The extent of the experience and the validity of the understanding will vary greatly. This diversity must be recognized by the dentist and addressed in the treatment plan and its presentation. Respecting the patient's uniqueness, the dentist must use the treatment plan as an educational tool to raise the patient's level of understanding of dentistry and their understanding of how the proposed treatment will meet their individual needs identified through diagnosis. Patient education is an essential element in patient care that should start with the initial contact with the patient (Figure 7-4).

SUMMARY

The treatment plan developed for a patient should reflect the dentist's best efforts at interpreting the diagnostic findings and addressing the patient's needs in keeping with their appreciation for dentistry and their ability to accept the proposed treatment. The presentation of a treatment plan to a patient is an offer to contract with a patient for the provision of treatment. It is therefore helpful to the patient, and prudent for the dentist, to supply a written summary of the treatment plan and patient obligations associated with its acceptance. Licensing boards and insurance companies report that the underlying reason for complaints by patients can frequently be traced to dentists' inadequate communication with patients, especially concerning an explanation of treatment and fees. The treatment plan therefore not only provides direction for the dentist but also contributes a measure of protection by aiding the patient in understanding the care that will be provided and the obligations that go with it. It is well to remember that good treatment plans are conducive to good care and to mutual understanding between dentists and patients.

Bibliography

Barsh LI: *Dental treatment planning for the adult patient*, Philadelphia, 1981, WB Saunders.

Bohay NB, Stephens RG, Kogan, SL : A study of the impact of screening or selective radiography on the treatment and postdelivery outcome for edentulous patients, *Oral Surg Oral Med Oral Pathol Oral Radiol Endod* 86:353-359, 1998.

Coleman GC, Nelson JF: *Principles of oral diagnosis*, St Louis, 1993, Mosby–Year Book.

Ganong WF: *Review of medical physiology*, ed 16, Norwalk, Conn, 1993, Appleton and Lange.

Goaz PW, White SC: *Oral radiology: principles and interpretation*, ed 3, St Louis, 1994, Mosby–Year Book.

Hall WB, Robert WE, LaBarre EE: *Decision making in dental treatment planning*, St Louis, 1994, Mosby–Year Book.

Ivanhoe JR, Cibirka RM< Parr GR: Treating the modern denture patient: A review of the literature, *J Prosthet Dent* 88: 631-635, 2002.

Little JW: *Dental management of the medically compromised patient*, ed 5, St Louis, 1997, Mosby–Year Book.

McCord JF, Grant AA: Identification of complete denture problems: a summary, *Br Dent J* 189:128-134, 2000.

Miles DA, Razamus TF, Van Dis ML: *Basic principles of oral and maxillofacial radiology*, Philadelphia, 1992, WB Saunders.

Morris RB: *Principles of dental treatment planning*, Philadelphia, 1983, Lea & Febiger.

Owall B, Kayser AF, Carlsson GE: *Prosthodontics: principle and management strategies*, London, 1996, Mosby–Wolfe.

Papas AS, Niessen IC, Chauncey HH: *Geriatric dentistry: aging and oral health*, St Louis, 1991, Mosby–Year Book.

United States Pharmacopeial Convention: *Drug information for the health care professional*, ed 6, Rockville, Md, 1996, The United States Pharmacopeial Convention, Inc.

Wood NK, Goaz PW: *Differential diagnosis of oral and maxillofacial lesions*, ed 5, St Louis, 1997, Mosby–Year Book.

CHAPTER 8

Preprosthetic Surgery: Improving the Patients' Denture-Bearing Areas and Ridge Relations

George A. Zarb, S. Ross Bryant

The vast majority of patients for whom complete denture therapy is prescribed have already been wearing dentures. As suggested earlier, there is a risk in patients wearing dentures for prolonged periods. This risk, or *biological price*, manifests itself in a number of adverse changes in the dentures' foundations. Consequently, several conditions in the edentulous mouth should be corrected or treated before the construction of complete dentures. Often, patients are unaware that tissues in the mouth have been damaged or deformed by the presence of old prostheses. Other oral conditions may have developed that must be managed to increase the chances for success of the new dentures. The patient must be made cognizant of these problems, and a logical explanation by the dentist, supplemented with radiographs and, where required, diagnostic casts, usually will convince the patient of the necessity for the suggested treatment.

Treatment methods to improve the patient's denture foundation and ridge relations are usually either nonsurgical or surgical in nature, but can be a combination of both methods.

NONSURGICAL METHODS

Nonsurgical methods of edentulous mouth preparation include the following methods.

Rest for the Denture-Supporting Tissues

Rest for the denture-supporting tissues can be achieved by removal of the dentures from the mouth for an extended period or the use of temporary soft liners inside the old dentures. Both proce-dures allow deformed tissue of the residual ridges to return to normal form (Figures 8-1 and 8-2). Clinical reports and experience also support the merits of regular finger or toothbrush massage of denture-bearing mucosa, especially of those areas that appear edematous and enlarged.

It has been demonstrated that tissue abuse caused by improper occlusion can be made to disappear by (1) withholding the faulty dentures from the patient, (2) adjusting/correcting the occlusion and refitting the denture by means of a tissue conditioner, or (3) substituting properly made dentures. When the latter is undertaken, it is necessary to allow the soft tissues to recover by removing the dentures for 48 to 72 hours before impressions are made for the construction of new dentures. However, it generally is not feasible to withhold a patient's dentures for an extended period while the tissues are recovering. Therefore temporary soft liners have been developed as tissue treatment or conditioning materials. The softness of these materials is maintained for several days while the tissues recover. Tissue conditioners consist of a polymer powder and an aromatic ester-ethanol mixture (see Chapter 12). They have been widely used in dentistry for years and provide the dentist with an expanded scope for short-term resolution of patient problems.

The major uses of these tissue-conditioning materials are tissue treatment, liners for surgical splints, trial denture-base stabilizers, and optimal arch form or neutral zone determinants. Clinical experience indicates that soft liners also can be used as functional impression materials when relining or refitting complete dentures (see Chapter 24).

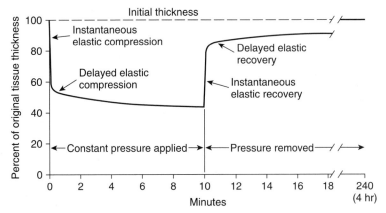

Figure 8-1   Typical behavior of tissue under a constant pressure load for 10 minutes. Notice the 90% recovery within 8 minutes after removal of the pressure. Total recovery requires 4 hours. (From Kydd WL, Daly CH, and Wheeler JB: *Int Dent J* 21:430-441, 1971.)

It is well recognized that denture-bearing tissues demonstrate microscopic evidence of inflammation, even if they appear clinically normal. Consequently, tissue rest for at least 24 hours and preferably the use of tissue conditioners are essential preliminaries to each prosthetic appointment. Tissues recover rapidly when the dentures are not worn or when treatment liners are used. The method of achieving optimal health of the denture-bearing tissues is not as important as the result (the tissues being made healthy). Many dentures fail because the impressions or registrations of the relations are made when the tissues are distorted by the old dentures. The same error is frequently committed when dentures are relined without adequate denture-bearing tissue rest or tissue treatment.

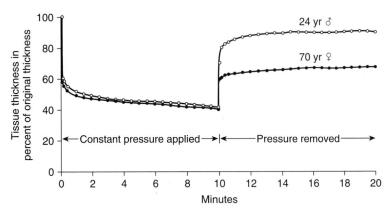

Figure 8-2   Comparison of responses to tissue loading and removal of the load in an elderly adult and a young adult. The compression curve is essentially the same. However, the removal of load shows definite differences in rate of recovery. The load was 11 g/mm^2. (From Kydd WL, Daly CH, and Wheeler JB: *Int Dent J* 21:430-441, 1971.)

Occlusal Correction of the Old Prostheses

An attempt should first be made to restore an optimal vertical dimension of occlusion to the dentures presently worn by the patient with an interim resilient lining material. This step enables the dentist to prognosticate the amount of vertical facial support that the patient can tolerate, and it allows the presumably deformed tissues to recover. The decision to create room inside the denture depends on its fit and the condition of the tissues. The tissue treatment material also permits some movement of the denture base, so its position becomes compatible with the existing occlusion, apart from allowing the displaced tissues to recover their original form. Consequently, ridge relations are improved, and this improvement facilitates the dentist's eventual relation registration procedures.*

It also may be necessary to correct the extent of tissue coverage by the old denture base so all usable supporting tissue is included in the treatment. This correction can easily be achieved by use of one of the resin border-molding materials combined with a tissue conditioner.

Good Nutrition

A good nutritional program must be emphasized for each edentulous patient. This program is especially important for the geriatric patient whose metabolic and masticatory efficiency may be compromised (see Chapter 6).

Conditioning of the Patient's Musculature

The use of jaw exercises can permit relaxation of the muscles of mastication and strengthen their coordination and help prepare the patient psychologically for the prosthetic service. If at the initial appointment the dentist observes that the patient responds with difficulty to instructions for relaxation and coordinated mandibular movement, a program of mandibular exercises may be prescribed. Clinical experience indicates that such a program may be beneficial and the subsequent registration of jaw relations facilitated.

---

*This will in turn facilitate an occlusal adjustment that can be accomplished intraorally or extraorally (with an articulator).

SURGICAL METHODS

Frequently, certain conditions of the denture-bearing tissues require edentulous patients to be treated surgically. These conditions are the result of unfavorable morphological variations of the denture-bearing area or, more commonly, result from long-term wear of ill-fitting dentures. The objectives of prescribing a preprosthetic surgical procedure are listed in Box 8-1. It must be emphasized that these interventions are infrequently mandatory undertakings. It is often far easier to make alterations in the prosthetic techniques and materials used than to subject the patient to a surgical intervention. The key consideration is whether a good prosthodontic prognosis will result from the surgical outcome. In fact, it is only the provision of dental implants that has been shown to have the best prognosis for morphological problems associated with maladaptive denture-wearing behavior.

Correction of Conditions That Preclude Optimal Prosthetic Function

Hyperplastic Ridge, Epulis Fissuratum, and Papillomatosis The premise underscoring surgical intervention is that mobile tissues (e.g., a

---

Box 8-1

Objectives of Preprosthodontic Surgical Prescriptions

1. Correcting conditions that preclude optimal prosthetic function
   Localized or generalized hyperplastic replacement of resorbed ridges
   Epulis fissuratum
   Papillomatosis
   Unfavorably located frenular attachments
   Pendulous maxillary tuberosities
   Bony prominences, undercuts, and ridges
   Discrepancies in jaw size relationships
   Pressure on mental foramen
2. Enlargement of denture-bearing area(s)
   Vestibuloplasty
   Ridge augmentation
3. Provision for placing tooth root analogues by means of osseointegrated dental implants

hyperplastic ridge), tissues that interfere with optimal seating of the denture-localized enlargement of peripheral tissues (an epulis), or tissues that readily harbor microorganisms (a papillomatosis) are not conducive to firm, healthy foundations for complete dentures. Whenever possible, these tissues should be rested, massaged, or treated with an antifungal agent before their surgical excision. If the patient's health or a personal choice precludes surgical intervention, the impression technique and design of the denture base have to be modified to accommodate the mobile tissue and minimize its distortion.

Frenular Attachments and Pendulous Maxillary Tuberosities   *Frena* are fibrous bands of tissue attached to the bone of the mandible and maxillae and are frequently superficial to muscle attachments. If the frenum is close to the crest of the bony ridge (Figure 8-3), it may be difficult to obtain the

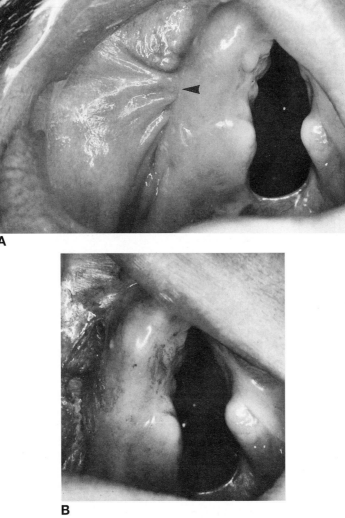

Figure 8-3   Preoperative **(A)** and postoperative **(B)** views of the maxillary buccal frenum *(arrowhead)* in an edentulous patient with an unrepaired palatal cleft. Excision allowed for optimal extension of the denture flange into this area.

ideal extension and border of the flange of the denture. The upper labial frenum in particular may be composed of a strong band of fibrous connective tissue that attaches on the lingual side of the crest of the residual ridge. This tissue should usually be removed surgically. Frena often become prominent as a result of reduction of the residual ridges. If muscle fibers are attached close to the crest of the ridge when frena are removed, the muscles usually are detached and elevated or depressed to expose the amount of desired ridge height. The frenectomy can be carried out before prosthetic treatment is begun, or it can be done at the time of denture insertion when the new denture can act as a surgical template. The former is preferred because the patient will not have to contend with postoperative discomfort along with adjustment to the dentures.

Pendulous fibrous maxillary tuberosities (Figure 8-4) are frequently encountered. They occur unilaterally or bilaterally and may interfere with denture construction by excessive encroachment on

or obliteration of the interarch space. Surgical excision is the treatment of choice (Figure 8-5), but occasionally maxillary bone must be removed. Care must be used to avoid opening into the maxillary sinus. In those instances in which the sinus dips down into a pneumatized and elongated tuberosity, it may be possible to collapse the sinus floor upward without danger of opening into it. This technique also is used when a bony undercut exists on the buccal side of the tuberosity and the sinus has pneumatized into the undercut (Figure 8-6).

Bony prominences, undercuts, spiny ridges, and mandibular tori may have to be removed to avoid painful denture flange impingement and to achieve a border seal beyond them against the floor of the mouth (Figure 8-7). They frequently occur so close to the floor of the mouth that a border seal cannot be made. On the other hand, maxillary tori are rarely removed. Satisfactory dentures can be made over most of them by careful relief of the palatal denture base material. The following are indications for the removal of maxillary tori:

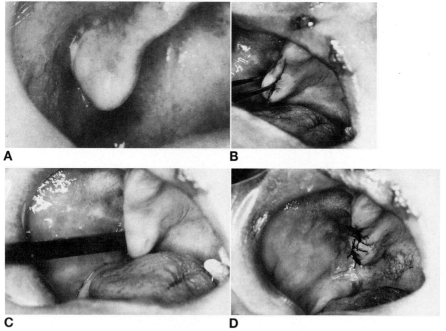

Figure 8-4   **A,** A pendulous, fibrous, mobile right maxillary tuberosity that is easily displaced. **B,** Two elliptic incisions undermine the mass (**C**) and allow for approximation of the mucosal surfaces (**D**) over a firm, bony base.

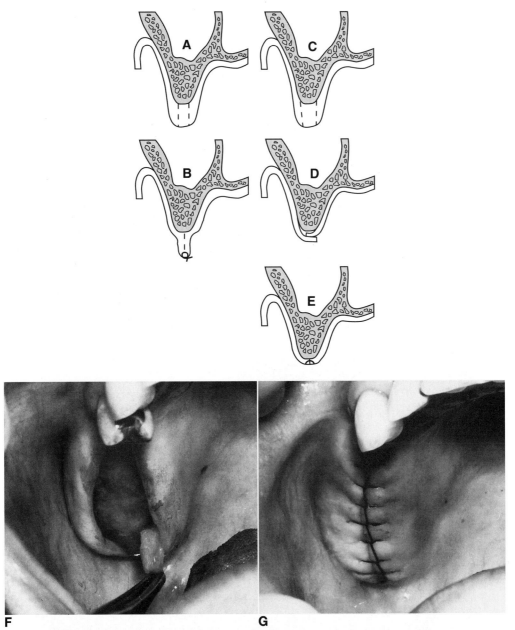

Figure 8-5 Procedure for reducing the vertical height of a maxillary tuberosity.
A, Incisions are made in the fibrous tuberosity. **B,** A wedge of fibrous tissue is removed. The tuberosity is less bulky but is still as vertically long as before. **C,** Incisions made just under the mucosa permit removal of all unwanted fibrous connective tissue. **D** and **E,** Thin mucosal flaps are fitted, trimmed, and sutured. This technique decreases vertical length of the tuberosity. **F** and **G** are clinical views of **C** and **E.**

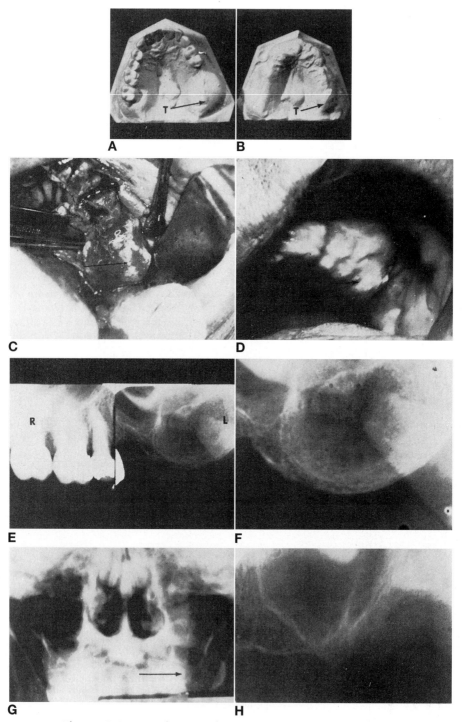

Figure 8-6   Legend on opposite page.

Figure 8-6 Reduction of a huge pneumatized tuberosity *(T)*. **A,** Preoperative diagnostic cast. **B,** Cast made 2 years after surgery. **C,** Clinical view of the enlarged and exposed bony tuberosity. **D,** The tuberosity 2 years after surgery. **E,** Dental radiographs of the patient's right and left maxillary molar regions. **F,** Radiograph of the enlarged pneumatized tuberosity. **G,** Radiograph shows the buccal undercut of a pneumatized sinus *(arrow)*. **H,** Another radiograph, 2 years after surgery.

1. An extremely large torus that fills the palatal vault and prevents the formation of an adequately extended and stable maxillary denture (Figure 8-8)
2. An undercut torus that traps food debris, causing a chronic inflammatory condition; surgical excision is necessary to create optimal oral hygiene
3. A torus that extends past the junction of the hard and soft palates and prevents the development of an adequate posterior palatal seal (Figure 8-9)
4. A torus that causes the patient concern

Exostoses may occur on both jaws but are more frequent on the buccal sides of the posterior maxillary segments (Figures 8-10 and 8-11). They may create discomfort if covered by a denture and usually are excised. It must be emphasized that routine excision of all mandibular exostoses is rarely recommended (see Figure 8-10, *B*). Frequently, the denture can be easily relieved to accommodate the exostoses, or a permanent soft liner can be used.

Sometimes the genial tubercles are extremely prominent as a result of advanced ridge reduction in the anterior part of the body of the mandible (Figure 8-12). If the activity of the genioglossus muscle has a tendency to displace the lower denture or if the tubercle cannot tolerate the pressure or contact of the denture flange in this area, the genial tubercle is removed and the genioglossus muscle detached. If it is clinically necessary to deepen the alveololingual sulcus in this area, the genioglossus muscle is sutured to the geniohyoid muscle below it (see Figure 8-12).

Residual alveolar ridge undercuts (Figure 8-13) are rarely excised as a routine part of improving a patient's denture foundations. Usually, a path of insertion and withdrawal of the prosthesis can be determined together with careful adjustment of a denture flange, which enables the dentist to use the undercuts for extra stability. Diagnostic casts can be surveyed as a guide in the assessment of the minimal amount of tissue to be removed. Considerable evidence exists that residual ridge surgery causes excessive bone reduction. However, the dentist may comfortably choose to remove a severe undercut that occurs opposite the lingual side of mandibular second and third molars and is tender to palpitation (Figure 8-14). Such an undercut is caused by a sharp mylohyoid ridge that (usually) is covered by very thin mucosa. When painless undercuts occur in this area, they can help achieve added stability for the denture (Figure 8-15). The path of insertion in such a situation is altered to allow for distal placement of the lingual flanges with a downward and forward final seating movement. Alternatively, one undercut area can be relieved in the denture to permit engagement of the remaining undercut area for retentive purposes.

Discrepancies in Jaw Size Impressive advances in surgical techniques of mandibular and maxillary osteotomy have enabled the oral and maxillofacial surgeon to create optimal jaw relations for patients who have discrepancies in jaw size. The patient with prognathism frequently places considerable stress and unfavorable leverages on the maxillary basal seat under a complete denture. This may cause excessive reduction of the maxillary residual ridge. Such a condition is even more conspicuous when some mandibular teeth are still present. A mandibular osteotomy in these cases can create a more favorable arch alignment and improve the appearance as well (Figure 8-16). However, changes in the soft tissues of the face tend to be accentuated by such a procedure (as shown by the patient in Figure 8-16). Usually, an adjunctive face-lifting procedure in this type of patient produces impressive results. Alternatively, these patients may be considered for implant-supported or retained dentures to address their prosthodontic problems. Such a procedure would less invasive, but its outcome is determined by host bone site and esthetic considerations.

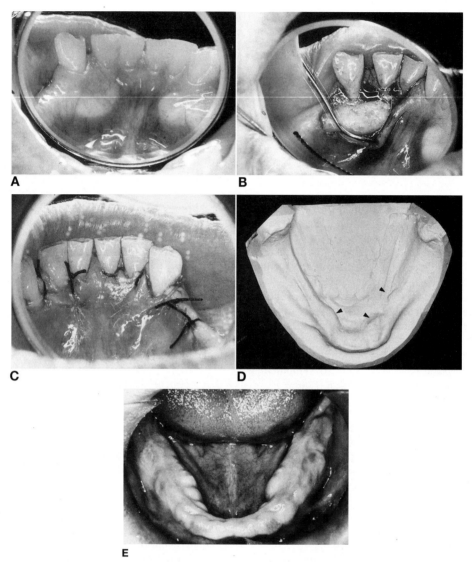

Figure 8-7   Conspicuous mandibular tori (**A**) are surgically exposed (**B**). A mucoperiosteal flap (**C**) is replaced and sutured interdentally. **D,** Prominent mandibular tori on an edentulous cast *(arrowheads)*. **E,** Intraoral view of the tori that must be excised before denture construction.

Pressure on the Mental Foramen   If bone resorption in the mandible has been extreme, the mental foramen may open near or directly at the crest of the residual bony process (Figure 8-17). When this happens, the bony margins of the mental foramen usually are more dense and resistant to resorption than the bone anterior or posterior to the foramen is. This causes the margins of the mental foramen to extend and have very sharp edges 2 to 3 mm higher than the surrounding mandibular bone. Pressure

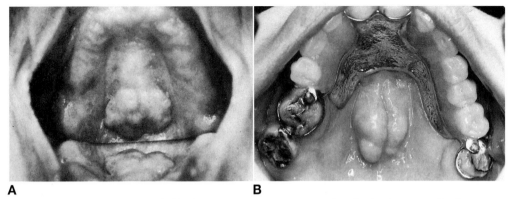

A   **B**

Figure 8-8 The sheer bulk of a torus may prevent conventional palatal coverage by the denture base (**A**). This situation can be ameliorated in a partially edentulous mouth by modification of the design of major connectors (**B**), or (less frequently) the torus may be considered for surgical removal.

from the denture against the mental nerve exiting the foramen and over this sharp bony edge will cause pain. Also, pressure against the sharp bone will cause pain because the oral mucosa is pinched between the sharp bony margin of the mental foramen and the denture. The most suitable way of managing this is to alter the denture so pressure does not exist. However, in rare instances it may be necessary to trim the bone to relieve the mental nerve of pressure. Pressure on the mental nerve is reduced by increasing the opening of the mental foramen downward toward the

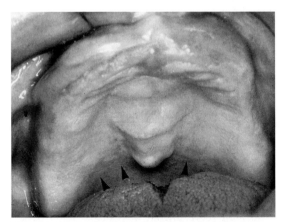

Figure 8-9 A large maxillary torus that extends distally past the proposed posterior palatal seal area.

inferior border of the body of the mandible. Such a change permits the mental nerve to exit the bone at a point lower than it had previously, thereby taking pressure off the nerve.

Occasionally, the anterior part of the residual ridges becomes so resorbed that it is extremely thin labiolingually, and it may have a sharp knife-edge with small spicules of bone protruding from it (Figure 8-18). Careful denture relief in these areas frequently overcomes this problem. If, however, constant irritation develops as a result of the soft tissue being pinched between the denture and the bone, the spicules and the knife-edged ridge must be surgically reduced.

A lack of parallelism between the maxillary and mandibular ridges can be encountered and, on occasion, may require surgical correction. This lack of parallelism may be caused by an absence of trimming of the tuberosity and ridge behind the last maxillary tooth when it is removed or may be the result of jaw defects, unequal ridge reduction, or abnormalities of growth and development. Most clinicians favor parallel ridges for their denture foundations because the resultant forces generated are directed in a way that tends to seat the denture rather than dislodge it. Also, the height of the occlusal plane of the upper denture can be elevated posteriorly to improve the denture esthetically.

Virtually all the surgical procedures described necessitate the use of a surgical template effect. The

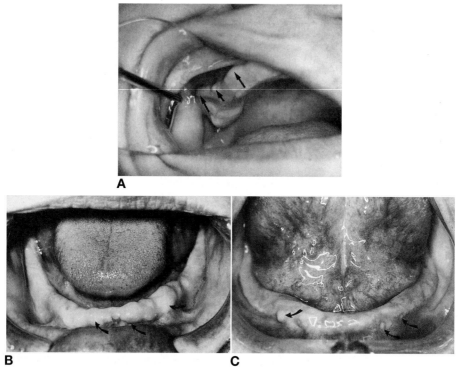

Figure 8-10   Bony exostoses *(arrows)* on the right buccal aspect of the maxillary residual ridge **(A)** and on the labial and buccal aspects of the anterior mandibular ridge **(B** and **C).**

patient's old dentures can usually be modified and lined with a tissue conditioner to function as such. The use of a soft-lined prosthesis protects the operated area from trauma and enables the patient to continue wearing the dentures. All the surgical interventions mentioned in this chapter must be considered in the context that there are potential effects on residual ridge resorption and that extensive surgical preparation of the edentulous mouth is rarely necessary. In fact, clinical experience indicates that careful prosthetic technique and design can frequently preclude a surgical intervention. The obvious exception to this observation is the use of implants, which have significantly improved treatment outcomes for patients with maladaptive denture experience.

Enlargement of Denture-Bearing Areas

The surgical techniques of vestibuloplasty and ridge augmentation have been largely eclipsed by

osseointegrated implant modalities. However, some explanatory observations about the rationale are relevant.

Vestibuloplasty   The reduction of alveolar ridge size is frequently accompanied by an apparent encroachment of muscle attachments on the crest of the ridge. These so-called high (mandibular) or low (maxillary) attachments serve to reduce the available denture-bearing area and to undermine denture stability. The anterior part of the body of the mandible is the site most frequently involved: the labial sulcus is virtually obliterated, and the mentalis muscle attachments appear to "migrate" to the crest of the residual ridge (Figure 8-19). This usually results in the dentist's arranging the teeth in a position more lingual than the position of the former anterior teeth. Such lingual crowding may not be tolerated by the patient, and when the absent sulcus is accompanied by little or no attached

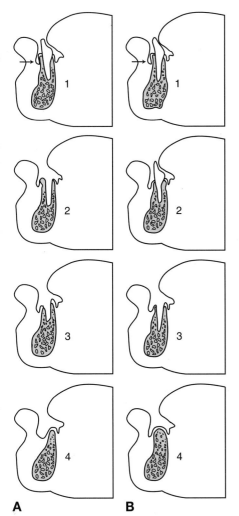

A   **B**

Figure 8-11 Incorrect (**A**) and correct (**B**) methods for trimming an exostosis of the crest of the alveolar process labial to the mandibular incisors. The exostosis should be removed before the incisor teeth are removed. (In **A** an undesirable loss of bone occurs if a labial undercut is trimmed after the tooth is removed. *1*, Tooth in position [notice the labial bony prominence]; *2*, the removed tooth leaves an undercut; *3*, removal of the undercut shortens the labial plate of bone; *4*, the end result is a lingually placed sharp residual ridge. The correct method [**B**] is to remove a labial undercut before the teeth are removed. This conserves bone and leaves a larger and more desirable residual ridge. *1*, Tooth in position, with a labial bony prominence; *2*, the bony prominence is removed, but the height of bone is retained; *3*, tooth removed; *4*, the resulting residual ridge is favorable.)

alveolar mucosa in this area, it is virtually impossible for a lower denture to be retained. Myoplasty accompanied by sulcus deepening has been proposed in an attempt to improve denture retention. With this operation the oral surgeon detaches the origin of muscles on either the labial or the lingual, or both, sides of the edentulous residual ridges. This allows for an increase in the vertical extensions of the denture flanges. When horizontal bony shelving is present in the mentalis muscle region, the surgical procedure is less successful, and its relative efficacy is attributable to the modification of the powerful mentalis muscle's activity. The risk of altered lower lip and chin sensation may also result from such mandibular intervention.

Over the years close cooperation between the two involved disciplines has resulted in a clearer understanding of what the surgical intervention should achieve. A wide and deep sulcus is not essential for success (Figure 8-20, *A* and *B*), and the vestibuloplasty can be restricted to the interpremolar region because the buccinator muscles are not the major cause of the problem (see Figure 8-19, *D* and *E*). Displacement of the mentalis muscle and adjacent muscle slips allow for the production of a looser lower lip, along with a low wound margin down in the sulcus and an increase in both stability and depth of the labial flange. The situation varies in the maxillae, where a muscle comparable to the action of the mentalis in its unstabilizing potential is not encountered. A broader vestibuloplasty is indicated here.

Although a lingual vestibuloplasty can provide for a major denture dimensional increase, the procedure is traumatic, particularly in frail and elderly patients; therefore the procedure is only very infrequently recommended. The long-standing clinical impression that free-skin grafts lose resiliency and develop nuisance crinkling has been confirmed in several reports. Skin grafts tend to result in a noticeable increase in parakeratosis, with subsequent clinical sogginess. Furthermore, they seem to exhibit poor cohesion and adhesion qualities with acrylic resin when compared with mucosa. Whenever possible, mucosal grafts are preferred.

The use of customized acrylic resin templates or the modified previous denture to support vestibuloplasty in the mandible is essential. These templates are usually fastened to the mandible with circummandibular wires for 1 week or longer. Carefully

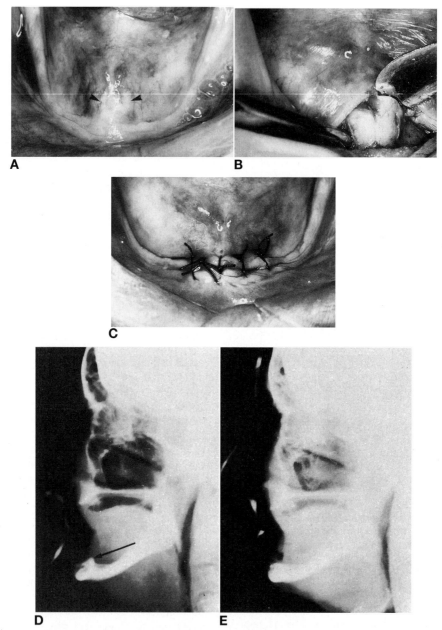

Figure 8-12   A prominent and painful superior genial tubercle (**A,** *arrowheads*) is surgically exposed (**B**) and excised (**C**). Cephalometric radiographs (**D** and **E**) show the thinness of the mandible. In **D,** notice that the superior genial tubercle *(arrow)* is higher than the crest of the bony ridge. Notice also the extreme interarch distance at the rest position. **E,** After the tubercle had been removed.

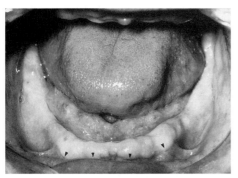

Figure 8-13 Anterior mandibular alveolar ridge undercuts *(arrowheads)* are rarely excised.

designed splints will reduce inflammation, reduce postoperative scarring, and maintain muscles in the desired position, thereby improving the result. The effect of mandibular vestibule-extension surgery on muscle activity and prosthesis retention has been investigated. The electromyographic activity of the mentalis and inferior orbicularis muscles was shown to undergo only slight changes despite the mentalis muscle's being severed completely from its origin in the mandible. The presumed cause of this minor change was that the mentalis muscle was given a new origin in the lower lip, with mainly the same activity pattern. However, a variable change in the apparent prominence of the chin can result. The altered appearance has been described as a "witch's chin."

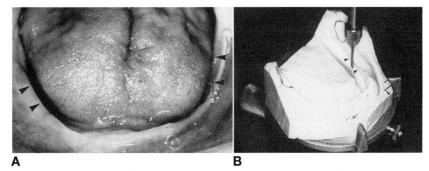

A   **B**

Figure 8-14 Undercuts frequently occur on the lingual of the mandibular second and third molars. Occasionally, they are very tender, and a sharp mylohyoid ridge of bone must be excised (**A,** *arrowheads*). **B,** A surveyor is used to emphasize the undercut that such a ridge can create.

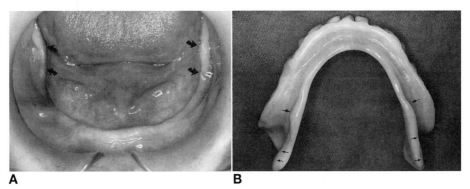

A   **B**

Figure 8-15 Posterior mandibular lingual undercuts (**A,** *arrows*), occur frequently and can be used to enhance mandibular denture stability (**B**) via selective reduction of the acrylic resin flange(s).

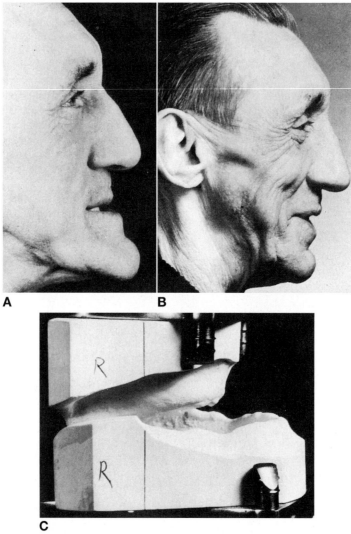

Figure 8-16 Preoperative (**A**) and postoperative (**B**) views of a man who underwent mandibular osteotomy. **C,** The preoperative diagnostic cast.

Continued

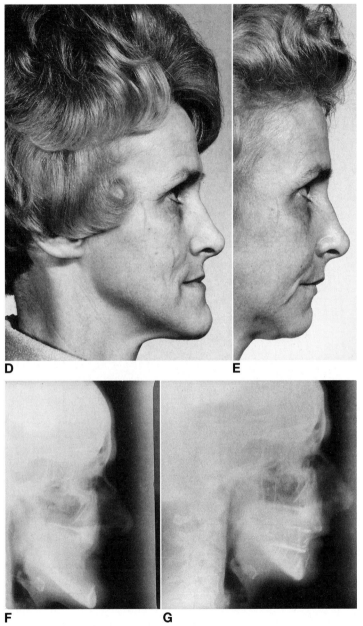

Figure 8-16 *cont'd* Preoperative **(D)** and postoperative **(E)** profiles and cephalometric views **(F, G)** of a woman treated in a similar manner. (Courtesy Dr. P. Symlski.)

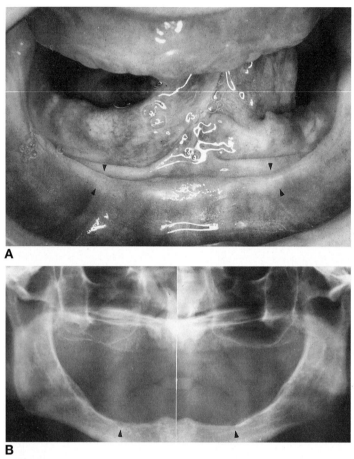

Figure 8-17 Intraoral **(A)** and radiographic **(B)** views of an edentulous mandible with superficially placed mental foramina *(arrowheads),* resulting from extensive residual ridge reduction. The foramina usually are quite palpable in such situations.

Another result of excessive alveolar bone loss or reduction is obliteration of the hamular notch. This "anatomical cul-de-sac," with its potential for displacement, makes it an important part of the posterior palatal seal of the maxillary denture. Its absence can severely undermine retention of the denture, and a small, localized deepening of the sulcus in this area may be attempted. The patient's old denture or a surgical template is used after the surgery to help retain the patency of the newly formed, yet small sulcus, or notch.

Ridge Augmentation For many years oral and maxillofacial surgeons have attempted to restore advanced jaw residual ridge resorption by placing onlay bone grafts from an iliac or rib source above or below the mandible. Unfortunately, follow-up reports suggest that the result generally leaves much to be desired with respect to predictable recovery of ridge height and minimal morbidity as a treatment outcome. Considerable caution is recommended with these procedures because they are a formidable undertaking, particularly for elderly patients. Nevertheless, current surgical reports suggest promise for combining grafts with implants to rectify serious residual ridge resorption problems, particularly in the maxilla.

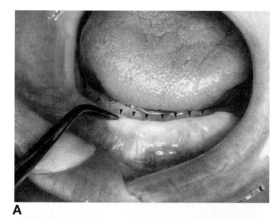

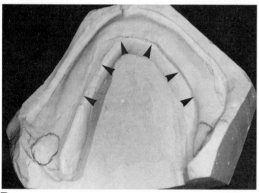

Figure 8-18   **A,** The slender knife-edge mandibular alveolar ridge is covered by a thin and nonresilient mucosa. **B,** The working cast clearly demonstrates the knife-edged character of the ridge *(arrowheads).*

Replacement of Tooth Roots with Osseointegrated Dental Implants

Whenever complete dentures are prescribed, the optimization of a denture-bearing area is a logical and compelling objective. For some patients this demands a preprosthetic surgical prescription. Two decades of studies about treatment outcome with osseointegration have provided irrefutable evidence to support this type of preprosthetic surgery. This scientific advance has ushered in a new era of efficacy and effectiveness in preprosthetic surgery. The denture-bearing area is no longer the prime or exclusive source of support, and the focus has now shifted to an endosseous one. Different numbers of implants are prescribed for different prosthesis designs, such as an electively fixed prosthesis, which is entirely implant borne (Figure 8-21), or an overdenture, which relies both on implant and residual ridge support (Figure 8-22). Implant management of edentulous jaws is described in Part 4.

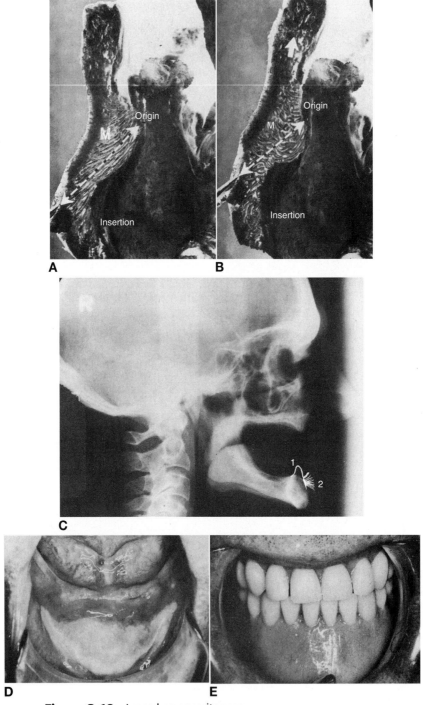

Figure 8-19   Legend on opposite page.

Figure 8-19   Sagittal sections through the lower lip and anterior part of the mandible (**A** and **B**) show the space available for a labial flange and the effect of the mentalis muscle *(M)* on this space. The muscle originates on the bone and inserts into the skin. Contraction of the muscle lifts the lip and reduces the space available for the flange of a denture. A lateral cephalogram (**C**) shows the contour of the residual alveolar ridge immediately after tooth extraction *(1)* and at the origin of the mentalis muscle (simulated at *2*). When *1* resorbs to its present level, the relative locale of origin of this muscle now obliterates the labial sulcus. **D** and **E,** A mandibular vestibuloplasty provides for dramatic increase in the labial flange extension.

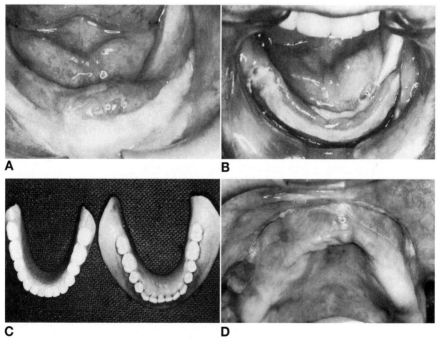

Figure 8-20   Deepened facial mandibular (**A** and **B**) and maxillary vestibules (**C**) with skin grafts in place. Note that current procedures do not aim at achieving such a wide area of operation and restrict the intersection to interforamina site in the mandible. Mandibular dentures before and after sulcus deepening are compared (**D**).

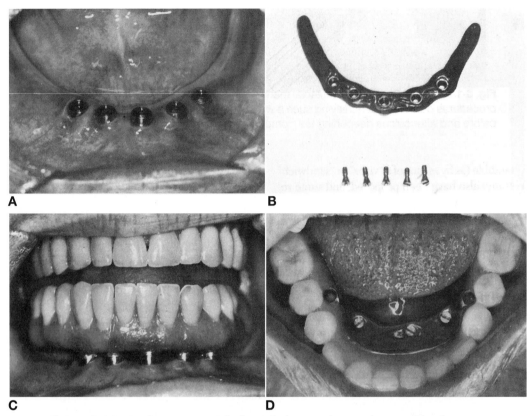

Figure 8-21   **A,** After two preprosthetic surgical stages, the osseointegrated implants are used as abutments for an electively removable fixed prosthesis. Prosthetic cylinders are matched to the implants and joined together by means of a wax scaffolding **(B),** which is cast to provide support for the final prosthesis **(C and D).** Notice that access to the retaining screws allows for ready removal of the prosthesis and that the gingival surface design allows for hygiene maintenance as with standard fixed prostheses.

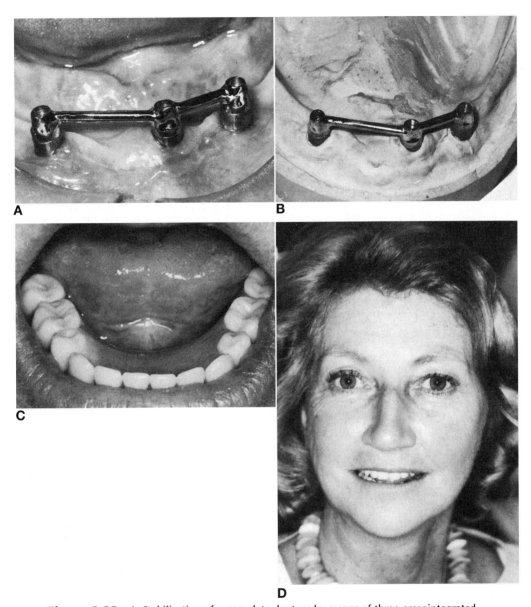

Figure 8-22 **A,** Stabilization of a complete denture by means of three osseointegrated implants joined together with a cast gold bar (**B**). Clip attachments inside the mandibular prosthesis ensure retention and stability without compromising the esthetic result (**C** and **D**). The quality of a patient's prosthetic experience can be greatly enhanced by prescribing this cost-effective method.

Bibliography

Björlin G, Palmquist J, Ahlgren J: Muscle activity and denture retention after vestibular extension surgery, *Odontol Rev* 18:179-190, 1967.

Cawood JI, Howell RA: A classification of the edentulous jaws, *Int J Oral Maxillofac Surg* 17:232-236, 1988.

de Koomen HA, Stoelinga PJW, Tideman H et al: Interposed bone-graft augmentation of the atrophic mandible, *J Maxillofac Surg* 7:129, 1979.

Harrison A: Temporary lining materials: a review of their uses, *Br Dent J* 151(12):419-422, 1981.

Hillerup S: Preprosthetic mandibular vestibuloplasty with split-skin graft: a two-year follow-up study, *Int J Oral Maxillofac Surg* 16:270-278, 1987.

Hillerup S, Hjørting-Hansen E, Eriksen E et al : Influence of skin graft pathology on residual ridge reduction after mandibular vestibuloplasty: a 5-year clinical and radiological follow-up study, *Int J Oral Maxillofac Surg* 19:212-215, 1990.

Hjørting-Hansen E, Adawy AM, Hillerup S: Mandibular vestibulolingual sulcoplasty with free skin graft: a five-year clinical follow-up study, *J Oral Maxillofac Surg* 41: 173-176, 1983.

Hopkins R: *A colour atlas of preprosthetic oral surgery,* London, 1987, Wolfe Medical Publications.

Lytle RB: Complete denture construction based on a study of the deformation of the underlying soft tissues, *J Prosthet Dent* 9:539-551, 1959.

Møller JF, Jolst O: A histologic follow-up study of free autogenous skin grafts to the alveolar ridge in humans, *Int J Oral Surg* 1:283, 1972.

Quayle AA: The atrophic mandible: aspects of technique in lower labial sulcoplasty, *Br J Oral Surg* 16:169-178, 1979.

Taylor RL: A chronological review of the changing concepts related to modifications, treatment, preservation, and augmentation of the complete denture basal seat, *Aust Prosthodont Soc Bull* 16:17-39, 1986.

Weingart D, Strub JR, Schilli W: Mandibular ridge augmentation with autogenous bone grafting and immediate implants: a 3-year longitudinal study (abstract), Abstracts from the fifth International Congress of Preprosthetic Surgery, Vienna, 1993.

Wowern N. Bone mineral contents of mandibles: normal reference values—rate of age-related bone loss, *Calcif Tissue Int* 43:193-198, 1988.

CHAPTER 9

Immediate Dentures

Nancy S. Arbree

An immediate denture is "a complete denture or removable partial denture fabricated for placement immediately after the removal of natural teeth" (according to the *Glossary of Prosthodontic Terms,* Academy of Prosthodontics, 1999). An immediate denture can also be an overdenture. One of the first references to immediate dentures in the literature was that of Richardson in 1860 (Seals, 1999).

Immediate dentures are more challenging to make than routine complete dentures for both the dentist and the patient. Because a try-in is not possible beforehand, the patient may not be completely comfortable with the resulting appearance and fit on the day the immediate denture is inserted. The dentist must explain and the patient must fully understand the limitations of the procedure before beginning treatment.

Immediate dentures may be either single immediate dentures or upper and lower immediate dentures in the same patient. The latter should be made together to ensure optimal esthetics and occlusal relationships.

DEFINITIONS IN CURRENT PRACTICE

Currently, there are two popular types of immediate dentures:

1. *Conventional (or classic) immediate denture (CID):* After this immediate denture is placed and after healing is completed, the denture is refitted or relined to serve as the long-term prosthesis.
2. *Interim (or transitional or nontraditional) immediate denture (IID):* After this immediate denture is made and after healing is com-

pleted, a second, new complete denture is fabricated as the long-term prosthesis. The *Glossary of Prosthodontics Terms* defines interim prosthesis as a prosthesis designed to enhance esthetics, stabilization and/or function for a limited period of time, after which it is replaced by a definitive prosthesis (Academy of Prosthondontics, 1999). Practically speaking, the CID is usually selected when only anterior teeth remain or if the patient is willing to have the posterior teeth extracted before immediate denture procedures begin. The IID is used most often when anterior and posterior teeth remain until the day of extraction and placement of the immediate denture.

An abbreviated type of IID has been called the "jiffy" denture (Raczka and Esposito, 1995). It is similar to the IID because it is replaced by a second complete denture after healing. Some dentists use it when the immediate denture needs to be fabricated *very quickly* (in one day or session) because of extenuating emergency circumstances or medical indications. It differs from the IID in that the denture "teeth" are usually made with tooth-colored, autopolymerizing acrylic resin (Hay, 1998; Raczka and Esposito, 1995; Seals, Kuebker, and Stewart, 1996; Pence, Lee, and Baum, 1992; Rayson and Wesley, 1970) or portions of the patient's preexisting fixed or removable partial denture(s) (Cohen and Mullick, 1994; Zalkind and Hochman, 1997). These tooth/prosthesis components are converted with the use of irreversible hydrocolloid impressions, stone casts, and either autopolymerizing or light-cured, tooth-colored and pink resins (Khan and Haeberle, 1992) into an IID.

The low cost and efficiency with which these jiffy dentures can be made allow their fabrication in extreme circumstances. Refer to the literature references for the precise techniques for these IIDs. They are not described here because they do not usually use conventional denture teeth and processing techniques. The main disadvantage of "jiffy dentures" is that the materials used are not as long lasting (e.g., in wear and color stability) as conventional denture teeth and processed bases.

ADVANTAGES AND DISADVANTAGES FOR ALL TYPES OF IMMEDIATE DENTURES

Advantages

1. The primary advantage of an immediate denture is the maintenance of a patient's appearance because there is no edentulous period.
2. Circumoral support, muscle tone, vertical dimension of occlusion, jaw relationship, and face height can be maintained. The tongue will not spread out as a result of tooth loss.
3. Less postoperative pain is likely to be encountered because the extraction sites are protected. Some authors have discussed whether immediate dentures reduce residual ridge resorption (Heartwell, 1965; Johnson, 1966; Kelly, 1958; Campbell, 1960; Carlsson, 1967).
4. It is easier to duplicate (if desired) the natural tooth shape and position, plus arch form and width. If desired, the horizontal and vertical positions of the anterior teeth can be more accurately replicated.
5. The patient is likely to adapt more easily to dentures at the same time that recovery from surgery is progressing. Speech and mastication are rarely compromised, and nutrition can be maintained.
6. The availability of tissue-conditioning material allows for considerable versatility in the correction and refinement of the denture's fitting surface, both at the insertion stage and at subsequent appointments.

7. Overall, the patient's psychological and social well-being is preserved. The most compelling reasons for the immediate denture prescription are that a patient does not have to go without teeth and that there is no interruption of a normal lifestyle of smiling, talking, eating, and socializing. The reasons are supported by a study (Jonkman, Van Waas, and Kalk, 1995), which found that 1 year after denture placement, a majority (76% to 79%) of patients with immediate dentures (when compared with two groups of control subjects, one who had immediate overdentures and one who had tooth-attachment overdentures) could eat properly and had easily adapted to wearing the denture. No difference in denture satisfaction, comfort, chewing ability, esthetics, and general satisfaction was found among the three groups.

Disadvantages

Immediate dentures are a more challenging modality than complete dentures because the presence of teeth makes impressions and maxillomandibular positions more difficult to record.

Specific disadvantages include the following:

1. The anterior ridge undercut (often severe) that is caused by the presence of the remaining teeth may interfere with the impression procedures and therefore preclude also accurately capturing a posteriorly located undercut, which is important for retention.
2. The presence of different numbers of remaining teeth in various locations (anteriorly, posteriorly, or both) frequently leads to recording incorrectly the centric relation position or planning improperly the appropriate vertical dimension of occlusion. An occlusal adjustment, or even selective pretreatment extractions, may be needed to make accurate records at the proper vertical dimension of occlusion.
3. The inability to accomplish a denture tooth try-in in advance on extractions precludes knowing what the denture will actually look like on the day of insertion. Careful planning, operator experience,

attention to details of the technique, and explanation to the patient best address this inherent problem.

4. Because this is a more difficult and demanding procedure, more chair time, additional appointments, and therefore increased costs are unavoidable.

5. Functional activities (e.g., speech and mastication) are likely to be impaired. However, this is a temporary inconvenience.

Additional Comparative Advantages and Disadvantages

The CID and the IID have advantages and disadvantages when the two techniques are compared with each other. Many of these are described in Table 9-1. Advantages are as follows:

1. The CID will usually have better initial retention and stability because fewer teeth are usually extracted on the day of placement.

2. The CID has an easier surgical session on the second surgical (denture placement) date.

3. The overall cost of the CID is less.

4. The IID technique results in two dentures, which is advantageous for some patients.

5. The IID has only one surgical visit.

6. The IID procedure takes less overall time, from the dentist's meeting the patient to placing the denture.

7. Patient with IIDs can use all their teeth or wear their existing removable partial denture(s) up until the day of extraction.

8. The IID lends itself better to complex treatment plans, especially in a patient who needs an upper immediate denture opposing a lower transitional removable partial denture.

9. The IID is better for less experienced practitioners because a second denture can correct any imperfections.

The following are disadvantages:

1. The CID technique results in only one denture.

2. The CID technique requires two surgical visits.

3. The CID technique includes a period of posterior partial edentulism, which impairs mastication and compromises esthetics.

4. The CID takes longer to fabricate, especially in complex treatment plans.

5. The single surgical visit for the IID is more involved and lengthy than for a CID.

6. The retention and stability of the IID is less at insertion. However, modern tissue conditioning techniques negate this disadvantage.

CONTRAINDICATIONS

A few patients are not good candidates for immediate dentures. They include (1) patients who are in poor general health or who are poor surgical risks (e.g., postirradiation of the head and neck regions, systemic conditions that affect healing or blood clotting, cardiac or endocrine gland disturbances, and psychological disorders) and (2) patients who are identified as uncooperative because they cannot understand and appreciate the scope, demands, and limitations to the course of immediate denture treatment.

On occasion, patients will not object to going without teeth during the healing period. This is especially true if these patients have extensive tooth loss (or teeth decoronated by decay) already. For these patients, immediate extractions followed by conventional complete denture treatment are simpler and less expensive.

DIAGNOSIS, TREATMENT PLANNING, AND PROGNOSIS

Which Type of Immediate Denture Should Be Prescribed?

Scrupulous treatment planning and patient education, plus meticulous clinical performance aided by the careful use of tissue conditioners, will virtually ensure a predictable treatment outcome for most CIDs (see candidate for upper and lower immediate dentures in Figure 9-1). With well-planned monitoring and modifications, these dentures can become the definitive prostheses for long-term wear. Such results can be achieved routinely. In some cases, the presence of numerous posterior teeth and the need for other hard and soft tissue related procedures can complicate treatment. In some patients, the sequelae of advanced periodontal disease, including aberrant occlusal relationships, might require a "staged" surgical approach to the final objective of a definitive prosthesis. Extracting the posterior teeth and performing other necessary procedures first in these patients can lead to predictable results for the CID.

However for other patients, the idea of a period without posterior teeth is impossible to imagine. The IID essentially reconciles these considerations: (1) expediency for the patient where smile, occupation, and preference demand a full display of teeth at all times and (2) recognition of the educated guesswork necessitated by this type of service. The proviso (agreed to by both patient and dentist) is

that if the esthetic and occlusal outcome is not satisfactory, a new definitive prosthesis will be made. In this manner, a patient can be reassured while the dentist acknowledges the inherent risks in this type of service.

More and more patients are opting for the convenience of the IID choice. If the dentist performs the technique meticulously and the patient is cooperative, the resulting IID can be very successful. The second denture procedures allow optimization of the end result.

The final decision as to which type of immediate denture best suits the treatment needs and social history of the patient can be confusing. Table 9-1 summarizes a comparison of the CID and IID for assistance during preliminary patient discussions and at the final treatment-planning visit.

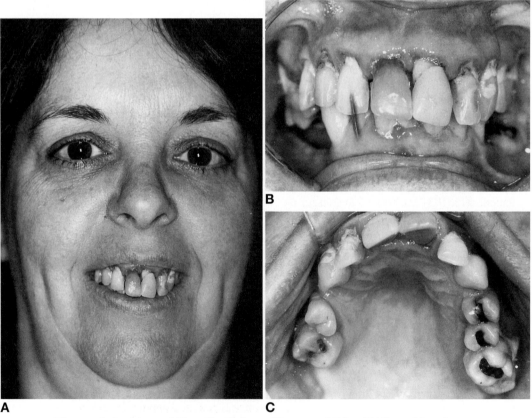

A **C**

Figure 9-1 Advanced (Class III—McGarry, Nimmo, and Skiba, 2002) candidate for immediate denture treatment. **A,** Natural tooth display. **B,** Teeth in centric occlusion. **C,** Maxillary occlusal view. *Continued*

Explanation to the Patient

A careful explanation to the patient of the limitations of immediate denture service should always be given. It is helpful to have a list including all possible difficulties (Box 9-1). Practitioners should also include an informed consent with wording specific to the nature of the immediate denture (Box 9-2). At this stage of diagnosis and treatment planning, patients should be provided with written information (to take home) concerning dentures,

immediate dentures, or both so that they have time to ask questions at a subsequent visit when treatment procedures begin.

Oral Examination

The usual full mouth series of radiographs should be taken. The dental and medical history of the patient should be reviewed. A head and neck examination is performed. During the normal

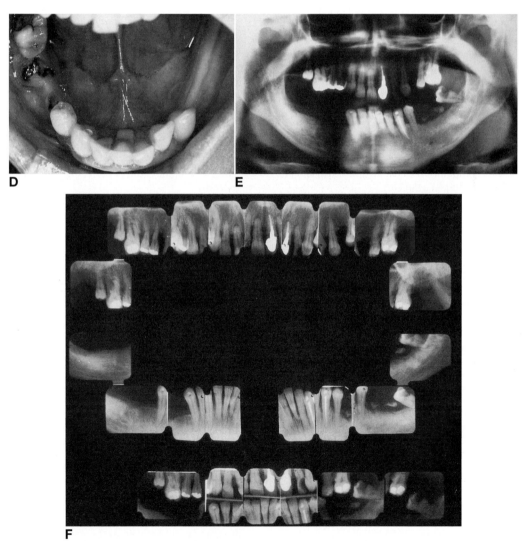

Figure 9-1 *cont'd* **D,** Mandibular occlusal view. Panoramic (**E**) and full mouth (**F**).

Table 9-1
Comparative Indications for the Conventional (or Classic) Immediate Denture versus the Interim (or Transitional or Nontraditional) Denture

Conventional Immediate Denture (CID)	Interim Immediate Denture (IID)
Intended as definitive or long-term prosthesis	Transitional or short-term prosthesis
After healing is complete, it is relined	After healing, a second denture is made; the IID is kept as a spare denture and may be relined for use as a spare
At the patient's initial presentation, usually only anterior teeth (plus possibly premolars) are remaining	At initial presentation, usually both anterior and posterior teeth are remaining
Usually has good retention and stability at placement, which is possible to maintain during healing	Usually has only fair retention and stability at insertion, which must be improved by provisional relines (tissue conditioning) during healing
The overall cost of CID treatment is less than IID treatment because it is the cost of the CID plus a reline	The overall cost of IID treatment is greater than CID treatment because it includes the cost of the interim denture and a second denture
Treatment process takes longer than the IID because there is a delay of 3-4 weeks for the posterior teeth extraction areas to heal partially before making the final impression.	Treatment process takes less time than the CID as denture fabrication procedures can begin right away
Generally indicated when only anterior teeth are present or few posterior teeth remain *that do not support an existing removable partial denture*	Generally indicated when there are multiple anterior and posterior teeth remaining or full arch extractions and/or these teeth support a removable partial denture that the patient desires to retain until insertion
Generally indicated when patient can function without posterior teeth for approximately 3 months (3-4 weeks posterior area healing time plus 2 months to fabricate and place the CID)	Generally indicated when the patient cannot or will not go without posterior teeth or an existing removable partial denture because of esthetic or functional concerns
At placement of the CID, usually only anterior teeth are extracted (possibly also one premolar on each side that had been retained to preserve the vertical dimension of occlusion)	At placement of the IID, usually both anterior and posterior teeth are extracted
Indicated when two extraction visits are feasible	Indicated when only one surgical visit is preferable (e.g., to meet "one hospital surgical visit" insurance benefits or when the patient's medical condition warrants) only one surgical and/or hospital visit.
Esthetics of the CID cannot be changed	The second denture procedure after the IID allows an alteration of esthetics and any other factors if indicated.
At the end of the treatment, the patient has one denture.	At the end of the treatment, the patient has a spare denture to use in case of extenuating circumstances
If all posterior teeth are initially removed, the vertical dimension of occlusion is not preserved; opposing premolars can be maintained for this purpose	Because posterior teeth need not be removed before fabrication of the IID, the vertical dimension of occlusion may be preserved
Contraindicated for a patient who has a complex treatment plan (e.g., periodontal therapy, crowns, fixed partial dentures and removable partial dentures in the opposing arch) or for changes in the vertical dimension of occlusion	Indicated when the patient will become edentulous in one arch and become partially edentulous in the opposing arch for the first time or complex procedures are needed (such as crowns, fixed partial dentures, and removable partial dentures) or changes in the vertical dimension of or changes in the vertical dimension of occlusion; an upper IID against a transitional lower partial denture can be made; then any periodontal procedures, crowns, and fixed partial dentures can be done during the initial healing stage
Not useful for converting existing prostheses such as removable partial dentures	Can be useful in converting existing prostheses to an IID

Box 9-1

Explanation to the Patient Concerning Immediate Dentures

1. They do not fit as well as complete dentures. They may need temporary linings with tissue conditioners and may require the use of denture adhesives.
2. They will cause discomfort. The pain of the extractions, in addition to the sore spots caused by the immediate denture, will make the first week or two after insertion difficult.
3. It will be difficult to eat and speak initially, almost like learning to eat and speak all over again.
4. The esthetics may be unpredictable. Without an anterior try-in, the appearance of the immediate denture may be different from what you or the dentist expected.
5. Many other denture factors are unpredictable such as the gagging tendency, increased saliva-

tion, different chewing sounds, and facial contour.
6. It may be difficult or impossible to insert the immediate denture on the first day. Every effort will be made to do so. If it is not possible, it will be inserted or remade as quickly as possible.
7. Immediate dentures must be worn for the first 24 hours without being removed by the patient. If they are removed, they may not be able to be reinserted for 3 to 4 days. The dentist will remove them at the 24-hour visit.
8. Because supporting tissue changes are unpredictable, immediate dentures may loosen up during the first 1 to 2 years. The patient is responsible for all fees involved in refitting or relining the dentures.

---

intraoral examination, the dentist should include and record periodontal probings, a full charting of all the teeth, and a note of need for frenum release, tori reduction or any other hard and soft tissue surgery, if necessary. When possible, teeth should be selected for retention as overdenture abutments. A careful evaluation and palpation of the potential denture-supporting tissues and the posterior palatal seal area should be carried out. The patient should be classified according to the partially edentulous classification system of the American College of Prosthodontists (McGarry, Nimmo, and Skiba, 2002) or another system. This aids in the determination of prognosis.

The shade and mold of the existing teeth should be determined. A gingival shade should be taken with denture-base shade tabs. Patients should be asked if they like their current shade and tooth position and what changes they would make if any. This discussion should include deciding whether to preserve diastemata, rotations, and overlapping of teeth for a more natural transition and a more natural-looking denture. This initial esthetic dialogue will streamline the final tooth selection process at a later visit. It also is best to include photographs as part of the permanent record, including full-size face and profile, lips

closed and smiling, and an intraoral view of the teeth in maximum occlusion.

Time should be spent evaluating the lip support, philtrum shape, position of high lip line, low lip line, and amount of tooth exposure in function while the patient is both silent and talking. Notation of the following factors will help in later visits:

1. The patient's existing midline and need for modification of its position (existing teeth may have drifted, especially if a nearby tooth has been lost for some time)
2. The patient's existing vertical dimension of occlusion and amount of interocclusal distance (freeway space) and the need for conforming to or changing it, according to whether the patient's existing maximum occlusal position coincides with the planned centric relation position for the immediate dentures and how difficult it is to manipulate or achieve that position for recording
3. The present amount of horizontal and vertical overlap of anterior teeth
4. An estimate of the Angle's classification of occlusion for the patient
5. Display of posterior tooth in the buccal corridor

Box 9-2

Example of Informed Consent for Immediate Dentures

An immediate denture is a denture that is inserted immediately on extraction of your remaining teeth. The fit, appearance, or comfort of such dentures is very difficult to predict. There is no way that teeth can be fitted in advance to show you what the denture will look like, how well you will be able to bite and chew, and how they will fit.

Immediate dentures often require tissue conditioning or temporary liners during the healing phase as the natural process of gum and bone shrinking takes place. After several months, the immediate denture will need a definitive reline or a new denture. The costs of these liners, relines, or the new denture are not included in the fee for the immediate denture. The fee for each of these services has been discussed with you.

Every effort will be made to duplicate or improve on the position of your natural teeth, but if the immediate denture is not quite what you expected, you may *have* to have a second denture made, even if a reline was what was originally planned.

Examination of Existing Prosthesis

Any existing prostheses should be examined for shade, mold, tooth position, lip support, and smile line. The shade of the denture base should also be noted.

Tooth Modification

Many immediate dentures will require modification of opposing teeth to correct the occlusal plane or to eliminate prematurities in centric relation. Occlusal plane adjustment is necessary because the factors that necessitate tooth extraction (e.g., extensive caries, periodontal disease, and extrusion or drifting) often are associated with occlusal discrepancies (Figure 9-2). These can affect the correct registration of centric relation, especially when they interfere with guiding the patient into the centric relation

position. They can also interfere with the proper determination of the occlusal vertical dimension. These tooth modifications should be made to the patient in advance of the final impressions.

At times it is determined that the analysis of the occlusion and the plane of occlusion is best made by performing a diagnostic mounting of the preliminary casts (impression technique for these is described later) to carefully evaluate the planned changes. The esthetic dialogue initiated at the oral examination visit can be recorded and marked on the mounted diagnostic casts. These casts are also used to plan and mark the occlusal tooth modifications that will need to be done at the final impression visit later (Figure 9-3). These preliminary casts also serve as a preextraction record.

Prognosis

All of the foregoing features will allow the dentist to determine a prognosis for the immediate denture. The professional fee should be quoted only after this thorough examination. At this point, there will be a good indication of the best type of immediate denture for the patient, the anticipated difficulties (e.g., inability to achieve a reliable centric relation position), esthetic demands on the part of the patient, a compromised residual ridge for denture support, systemic diseases and medications that may affect denture success, sensitive tissues or sharp, bony prominences that may necessitate more sore spot adjustment, and other concerns. The American College of Prosthodontics Classification for Partially Edentulous Patients (McGarry, Nimmo, Skiba et al., 2002) should be noted; it is helpful to both the dentist and the patient to use this system to understand the nature of the patient's diagnosis and prognosis. It also serves as a basis to refer to specialists (prosthodontists) when indicated. Once the patient understands and accepts the diagnosis, treatment plan, and prognosis, treatment can begin.

Referrals/Adjunctive Care

If other dentists are to be involved in the patient's treatment, referrals for required consultations are requested at this time. When required, a surgical consultation should occur early in the treatment to establish good communication

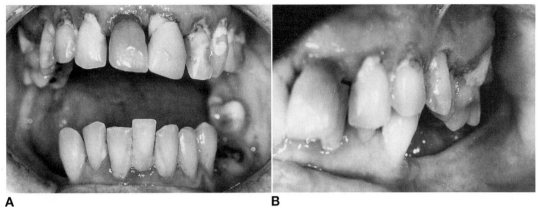

Figure 9-2 **A,** The lower anterior teeth requiring modification to correct them to an even plane of occlusion. **B,** Note the supereruption of the upper right molar (mirror view), which must be corrected in the final planned prosthesis

among the patient, practitioner, and the surgeon. Common preprosthetic surgical procedures are considered (Terry and Hillenbrand, 1994). A written referral with a copy of the radiographs should be sent to the surgeon in advance. Requests for surgery, where *not* to do surgery (e.g., when bone trimming is not needed or when saving teeth for overdenture abutments), and future surgical considerations (e.g., dental implants) are also identified.

This surgical consultation visit will further reassure the patient as to events that will occur on the surgical date(s). If the patient desires any type of sedation anesthesia, the details of this can be worked out in advance. The surgeon and the practitioner should communicate after the consultation so that they can arrange a mutually convenient surgical date and so that the practitioner can receive input and suggestions from the surgeon's examination of the patient.

An endodontic consultation concerning any treatment needed for planned overdenture abutments should be done, if necessary. The endodontic treatment can start at any time. Periodontal consultations should also be scheduled for any remaining teeth in the opposing arch or overdenture abutments as needed. It is usually preferable to do any needed periodontal therapy *after* the placement of the immediate denture. Clinical experience indicates that the removal of periodontally compromised adjacent teeth frequently improves and even reduces the periodontal treatment that may be required for the remaining teeth.

Oral Prophylaxis

The patient should have a general scaling of the teeth to minimize calculus deposits. This will reduce the postoperative edema and chance of infection.

Other Treatment Needs

Often, patients with single immediate dentures also require restorations, crowns, or removable partial dentures. Restorations are usually performed coincident with the immediate denture procedures.

For the patient with a single CID, restorations and crowns can be completed during the 3 to 4 weeks of healing after the first surgical visit and also coincident with the immediate denture procedures. For the patient with a single IID, restorations, crowns, and the definitive removable partial dentures procedures for the opposing arch are done after placement of the IID. The only exception to this is if a transitional removable partial denture is planned for the opposing arch; this is fabricated coincident with the immediate denture procedures.

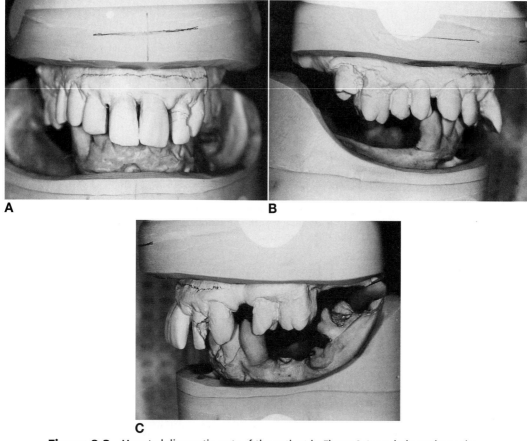

Figure 9-3   Mounted diagnostic casts of the patient in Figure 9-1 can help evaluate the plane of occlusion, extruded teeth, diastemata, and rotated teeth. They can be marked for smile line, midline, posterior limit, and planes of occlusion such as interpupillary and ala-tragus. They serve as a permanent preextraction record. **A,** Front view with marks for midline, interpupillary line, and smile line. **B,** Right lateral view with ala-tragus line. **C,** Left lateral view.

CLINICAL AND LABORATORY PROCEDURES

The procedures for fabrication of immediate dentures are similar to those for making complete dentures, with some modifications. If overdenture abutments are planned, endodontic treatment is preferably completed coincident with the immediate denture procedures. The abutments can be morphologically modified when the denture is ready to be inserted. Final preparation of overden-

ture abutments and placement of any copings or attachments should be done after the immediate denture is inserted and the patients' ridge healing is complete.

First Extraction/Surgical Visit

If a clinical decision is made to undertake preliminary extractions (CID technique), the patient should have the identified (usually posterior) teeth removed as soon as possible. Opposing premolars may be retained to preserve the vertical dimension of occlusion, although canines or other anterior teeth may provide the required so-called centric or vertical stops. Any other required hard and soft tissue operation is also usually done at this first surgical visit. Examples include tori reduction, tuberosity reduction, and frenectomy.

These posterior extraction and other operated-on areas are allowed to heal for a short time, usually only 3 to 4 weeks, before the preliminary impressions are made. If any posterior teeth are proposed as overdenture abutments, and if the patient does not object, the endodontic treatment can be done earlier and these teeth reduced before the impression appointment.

Preliminary Impressions and Diagnostic Casts

Impressions are made in irreversible hydrocolloid (alginate) in stock metal or plastic trays. The tray should be selected based on its ability to reach all peripheral tissue borders and posterior extensions, such as the retromolar pad on the mandibular arch and the posterior limit (hamular notches and post-dam area) on the maxillary arch. Periphery (rope) wax is adapted to the borders of the tray to reach toward the vestibule and into the often-extensive undercuts accentuated by the presence of teeth. The palatal surface of the upper tray needs to have wax added to reach the palatal tissues (Figure 9-4). Location of the posterior limit can be marked in the patient's mouth with an indelible stick. This often will transfer to the impression surface, or it can be drawn (copied from the mouth) on the impression later before pouring.

The wax may show through these initial impressions, but this will not significantly alter the cast accuracy because of the softness of the wax. The impressions should be free of voids and should record the full extensions planned for the denture prosthesis. These impressions are poured in stone and are used to make custom trays for the final impressions. If an IID is planned, these preliminary impressions and casts will contain all of the remaining teeth (Figure 9-5, *A* and *B*, and Figure 9-6, *A* and *B*). If a CID is planned, these will contain only anterior teeth (Figure 9-5, *C* and *D*, and Figure 9-6, *C* and *D*).

Loose Teeth

Several authors have made suggestions for protecting loose teeth from extractions during preliminary or final impression procedures for immediate dentures. Loose teeth can be blocked out by adding periphery wax at the cervical areas, by generously applying a lubricating medium to the teeth, by placing copper bands over the loose teeth (Soni, 1999), by placing a vacuum-formed plastic over the teeth (Vellis, Wright, Evans et al., 2001), or by placing holes in the tray and using an amalgam condenser to release the tray over loose teeth (Goldstein, 1992).

Custom Trays, Final Impressions, and Final Casts

Many successful tray types and impression techniques for immediate dentures are described in the dental literature. There are two basic ways to fabricate the final impression tray, depending on the location of the remaining teeth and operator preference. Both are successful as long as they are done properly.

Type One: Single Full Arch Custom Impression Tray   The type one method more closely resembles a routine custom impression tray for removable partial dentures. It can be used in the CID technique. It is the *only* tray that can be used for the IID technique. This type of tray is effective when only anterior teeth are remaining or when anterior *and* posterior teeth are remaining.

The process for tray fabrication is as follows:

1. The areas of the casts with remaining teeth are blocked out with two sheet wax thicknesses as for a fixed partial denture custom impression tray; undercuts in the edentulous areas are blocked out as for a complete denture custom tray. In the IID technique, both anterior and posterior teeth areas are blocked out with two thicknesses of wax (Figure 9-7, *A* and *B*). In the CID technique, only anterior teeth are blocked out in this manner.
2. A stop effect is established by providing holes through the wax anteriorly (CID and IID) or posteriorly (IID only) on one or two teeth and posteriorly in the tuberosity or posterior palatal seal areas (CID and IID).

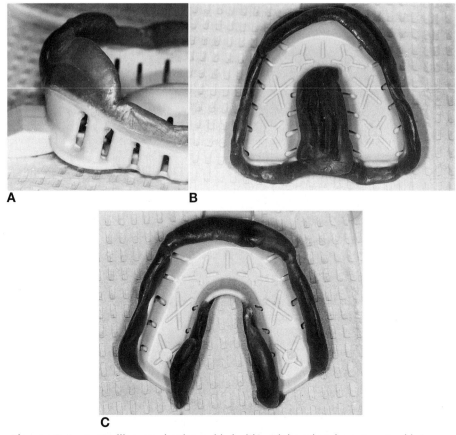

Figure 9-4 **A,** Maxillary tray border molded with periphery (rope) wax to extend into undercuts and onto the vestibular roll area and palatal area (**B**). **C,** Mandibular tray similarly prepared.

3. The tray is outlined to be 2 to 3 mm short of the vestibular roll and to extend and include the posterior limit (posterior palatal seal and hamular notch area).

4. Autopolymerizing acrylic resin or light-cured resin is adapted over the cast, into the stops, and to the planned outline. A handle is added to the anterior palate or to the mid-palate. The latter is regarded as advantageous because if the anterior handle is too long, it may interfere with proper anterior vestibule border molding. A sketch of the cross section of a full arch tray for a CID is shown in Figure 9-8. The full arch tray for an IID would be similar except that it would have teeth under the posterior section as well as under the anterior section. The tray is allowed to polymerize (Figure 9-9).

5. As with the usual technique in complete dentures (see Chapters 13 and 14), the tray is polished, tried in, and relieved. Border molding is accomplished, the appropriate adhesive added, and a final impression is made in any preferred elastomeric material (irreversible hydrocolloid, polysulfide rubber base, polyvinyl silicone, or polyether) (Figure 9-10).

Type Two: Two-Tray or Sectional Custom Impression Tray The type two method is used only when the posterior teeth have been removed (CID). It cannot be used in the IID technique because usually

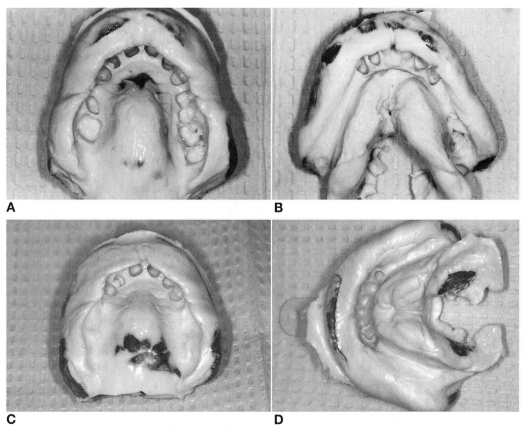

Figure 9-5 Maxillary (**A**) and mandibular (**B**) preliminary impressions for the IID technique and maxillary (**C**) and mandibular (**D**) preliminary impressions for the CID technique. *CID,* Conventional immediate denture; *IID,* interim immediate denture.

there are posterior teeth present. It involves fabricating two trays on the same cast—one in the posterior, which is made like a complete denture tray, and one in the anterior (backless tray). Some operators eliminate the anterior tray.

1. Outline the borders of the tray(s) again to be 2 to 3 mm short of the vestibule but covering the posterior limit and/or the retromolar pads.
2. Use melted wax to block out tissue undercuts, interdental spaces, and undercuts around the anterior teeth. *Note:* A double sheet of wax is not used because intimate adaptation of the tray is desired.
3. Adapt autopolymerizing acrylic resin or light-cured resin to the posterior edentu-

lous areas. This section or posterior tray should cover the lingual surfaces of the teeth (only) and extend up beyond the incisal edges of the teeth to include a handle (Figure 9-11).
4. For the anterior section or tray, there are varying techniques: one is to adapt a custom tray, and another is to cut and modify a plastic stock tray (Figure 9-12). Alternately, some operators prefer to *not* use a tray. Instead, they adapt plaster impression material or a heavy mix of an elastomeric impression material directly in the mouth. The anterior section/impression material must cover the labial surfaces of the teeth and the vestibule. All variations can be used successfully.

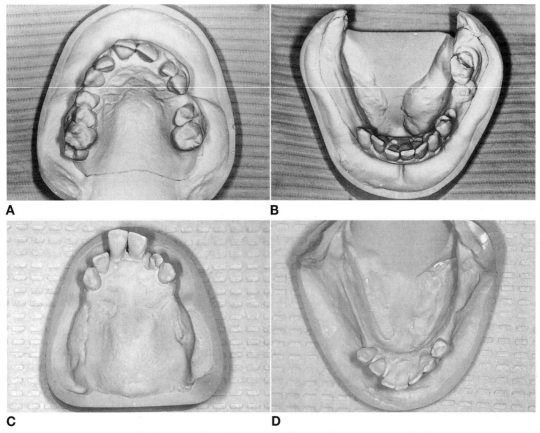

A   B

C   D

Figure 9-6   Preliminary maxillary (**A**) and mandibular (**B**) casts for IID technique. Preliminary maxillary (**C**) and mandibular (**D**) casts for the CID technique. *CID*, Conventional immediate denture; *IID*, interim immediate denture.

5. The posterior sectional tray is tried in, relieved as with a complete denture tray, border molded, and adhesive applied; then the posterior impression is made in any impression material desired (zinc oxide–eugenol paste, polysulfide rubber base, polyvinyl silicones, polyether) (Figure 9-13). This material does not have to be elastomeric because it will not lock into tooth undercuts because it includes only the lingual areas of the teeth and the posterior ridge. If severe posterior ridge undercuts are present, an elastomeric material should be used.

6. The posterior impression is removed and inspected. Excess material is removed,

and it is replaced in the mouth. The anterior section of the impression is made to it by one of the variations described in step 4. Figure 9-14 shows the sectional custom tray technique for a patient with a CID.

7. The most important consideration in the sectional tray technique is the careful, proper reassembly of the two separate components of the impression. Care must be taken not to distort this assembly during removal from the mouth and during the pouring of the impression. The method of boxing the impression with a mixture of plaster and pumice is suggested as least likely to cause distortion (Figure 9-15). The final casts are trimmed (Figure 9-16).

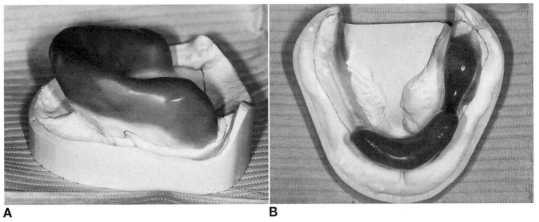

A   **B**

Figure 9-7 Wax block-out of maxillary (**A**) and mandibular (**B**) casts for an interim immediate denture (IID).

Another tray variation is the maxillary Campagna tray (Campagna, 1968). It looks like a full arch tray with a hole cut out where the remaining anterior teeth are (CID technique). A stock tray is used over the full arch tray to capture the anterior teeth in the impression.

Note: At the final impression visit (preferable) or at the jaw relation record visit, the teeth selected earlier for the patient should be shown to the patient for his or her approval. A change can be made at this time if necessary.

Location of Posterior Limit and Jaw Relation Records

The procedures for locating the posterior limit and jaw relation records are identical to those for complete dentures (see Chapter 15). If there are enough anterior and posterior teeth remaining (in some patients with IIDs), there may not be a need for a record base and occlusion rim. If not (as in some patients with IIDs and all patients with CIDs),

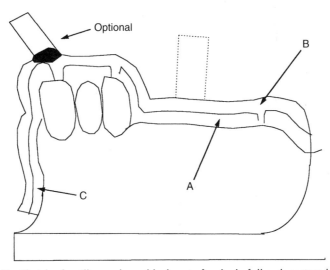

Figure 9-8 Sketch of outline and wax block-out of a single full arch custom impression tray for a conventional immediate denture (CID). **A,** Wax for spacer. **B,** Stop. **C,** Wax block-out.

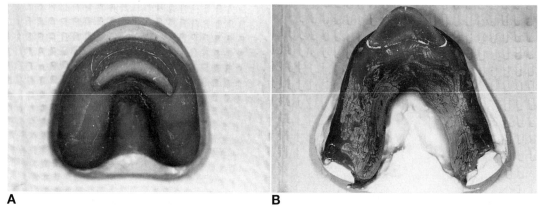

A   **B**

Figure 9-9   Maxillary (**A**) and mandibular (**B**) full arch custom impression trays. This view would look the same for either a CID or an IID. In the IID, teeth would also be present under the posterior sections. *CID*, Conventional immediate denture; *IID*, interim immediate denture.

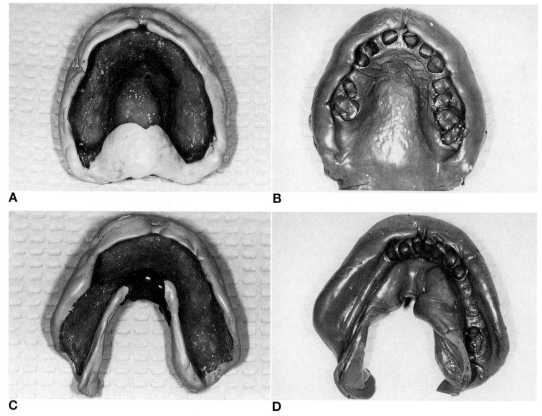

A   **B**

C   **D**

Figure 9-10   Border molding (**A**) and final impressions (**B**) for maxillary (**C**) and mandibular (**D**) immediate dentures (IID) in full arch custom impression trays. In the CID technique, posterior teeth would not usually be present in the full arch final impression. *CID*, Conventional immediate denture; *IID*, interim immediate denture.

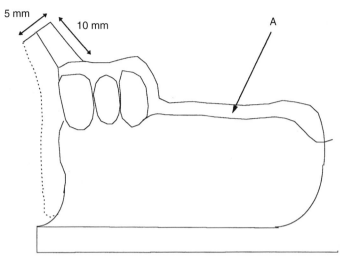

Figure 9-11 Sketch of the two-tray or sectional custom impression tray method, which can be used only when there are no posterior teeth present (CID). *A,* Posterior tray; *dotted line,* anterior tray/impression material; *CID,* conventional immediate denture.

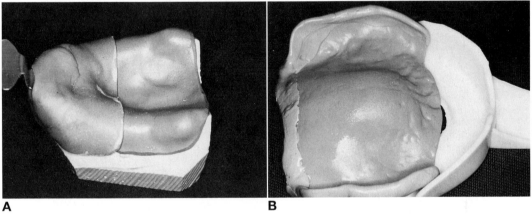

Figure 9-12 Sectional tray techniques use a posterior custom impression tray, which can be covered by an anterior custom impression tray (**A**) or a stock tray (**B**). (Courtesy Dr. Arnold Rosen.)

record bases and occlusion rims are made on the master casts.

1. Undercut areas around teeth and on edentulous areas are blocked out with wax, and autopolymerizing acrylic resin or light-cured resin is adapted to the edentulous areas of the cast as for complete dentures. Wax occlusion rims are added to the proper height and width. The remaining teeth and anatomical landmarks, such as the retromolar pad, can serve as a guide to the height of the rim (Figure 9-17). It is important that these record bases be stable and strong enough to record jaw relations.

2. The record bases and occlusion rims are tried in for patient comfort. They are removed. The posterior limit is marked as discussed in Chapter 15 and transferred to the upper record base and then to the cast. Alternatively, if a

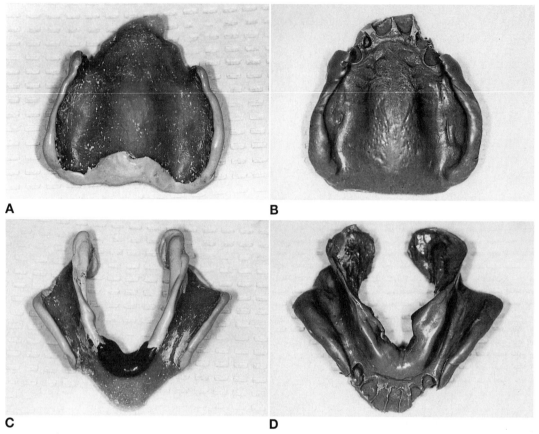

Figure 9-13 The posterior component of the sectional impression technique (conventional immediate denture [CID]). Maxillary posterior section is border molded (**A**), and the final impression is made (**B**). **C,** Mandibular border molding. **D,** Impression.

record base was unnecessary, this transfer also can occur "by eye."

3. An evaluation of the patient's existing vertical dimension of occlusion is accomplished, determining if it should be retained. On occasion, the operator may wish to restore it by opening because the patient's uneven tooth loss, loosening of the remaining teeth, and tooth wear created overclosure. At times, the vertical dimension of occlusion will have to be closed because drifting and extrusion of the patient's teeth opened it.

The latter can be accomplished by grinding the natural or stone teeth on the master cast.

4. The occlusion rims (and teeth if necessary) are trimmed to the desired vertical dimension of occlusion. A face-bow transfer and a recording of centric relation are made (see Chapter 16).

5. The casts are mounted on the articulator (Figure 9-18).

6. Protrusive relation records are made, if desired, to transfer to the articulator in order to set the condylar guidance.

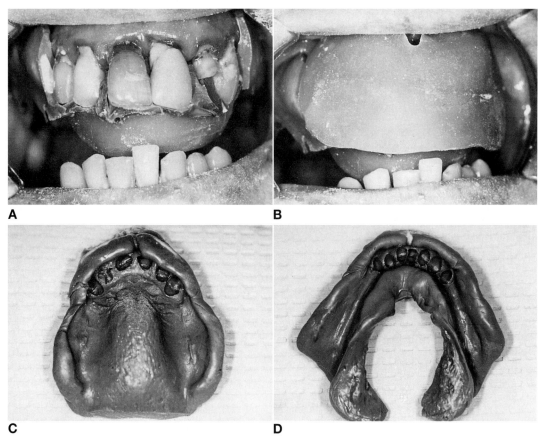

A   **B**

C   **D**

Figure 9-14   The anterior component of the sectional impression technique and reassembly with posterior section (conventional immediate denture [CID]). **A,** Maxillary posterior impression reseated in the mouth. **B,** Try-in of the anterior section of maxillary tray. **C,** Sectional maxillary final impression removed (by unhinging) together and reassembled. **D,** Mandibular completed final sectional impression.

Setting the Denture Teeth/Verifying Jaw Relations and the Patient Try-in Appointment

The articulated casts are used for setting any anterior/posterior teeth that are missing so that a try-in can be accomplished with the patient. A try-in is not always possible (e.g., when all teeth in the arch are present as in some patients with IIDs), but the mounting should still be confirmed at a patient visit. In Figure 9-19, the posterior teeth are missing (CID) so that a try-in is possible.

1. Set the posterior teeth as described in Chapter 17. Set the teeth in tight centric occlusion.

2. The trial denture bases are tried in the mouth and used to verify vertical dimension of occlusion and centric relation as with complete dentures. If necessary, the lower cast is remounted with a new centric relation record until the articulator mounting and the patient's centric relation coincide. Teeth are reset to any new mounting and tried in again. For patients where a try-in is not possible, a verifying centric relation record should be taken to confirm the jaw relationship.

3. Now it is important to take time with the patient to record landmarks on the casts and to confirm the patient's esthetic desires. Much of what follows has already been done as a preliminary

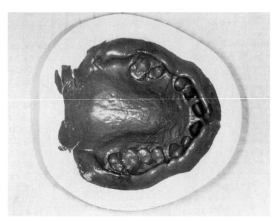

Figure 9-15 Plaster and pumice (50:50) mix for boxing is the method least likely to cause distortion of sectional impressions. Boxing wax is applied to this to complete the boxing before pouring the impression.

measure at the diagnostic or diagnostic mounting phase. If available, the mounted diagnostic casts should accompany this visit to serve as a reference.

a. The midline or newly selected midline is recorded on the base area of the master casts. The middle of the face is usually the best choice for the midline, but this should be confirmed with the patient. It should be pointed out to the patient if the selected midline does or does not coincide with the middle of the philtrum or the midline of the lower teeth. Some patients will prefer that it does.

b. The anterior plane of occlusion (using the interpupillary line as a guide) is determined and marked on the base of the cast. The remaining canines may not be coincident with this plane. Two teeth should be found that are parallel to the desired anterior plane of occlusion. If posterior teeth are still present at this stage, they may be extruded, which would distort the desired occlusal plane. Intraoral landmarks that correspond to the ala-tragus plane should be located and noted. These can be used as an aid to draw an ala-tragus line on the base of the cast. If posterior teeth are missing at this stage, it is easy to establish and record the ala-tragus line with the posterior tooth set up.

c. The high lip line should be determined. A discussion can then occur with the patient as to the display of tooth/gingiva that will be attempted or the need for a localized anterior alveolectomy if too much tooth/gingiva display is anticipated (see patient in Figure 9-1, *A*). Also note and show the patient the posterior tooth display in the buccal corridor. Make sure the patient sees and approves this.

d. A discussion of placement of diastemata, rotated teeth, notches, and other natural arrangements should occur so that the patient is actively involved in the esthetic decisions. Some patients want perfect-looking teeth because they never had them, whereas other patients will prefer a more natural arrangement. They may not want friends and colleagues to know that any change has occurred.

e. Note the existing anterior vertical and horizontal overlap. Often, in patients in whom drifting and excursion have occurred, this will be severe. Most patients will want to duplicate the position of their natural teeth, but some do have rather unesthetic arrangements, the result of advanced periodontal disease and drifting of teeth.

   Determine how much vertical overlap needs to be maintained for esthetics and phonetics. Deep vertical overlaps are detrimental to denture stability. If it is excessive, discuss with the patient the possibility of denture retentive loss during excursions. Using a posterior anatomical tooth or increasing the horizontal overlap to minimize the incisal guidance may be able to help here.

   If horizontal overlap is excessive, determine if maxillary anterior teeth need to be placed farther back into the mouth to eliminate an unesthetic position or if the horizontal overlap needs to be preserved for lip support and phonetics. Lower anterior denture teeth can be tipped forward to eliminate some of the excess horizontal overlap. Discuss with the patient the fact that anterior teeth in dentures do not have centric relation contact; this will be especially true if the horizontal overlap is excessive. Make notes

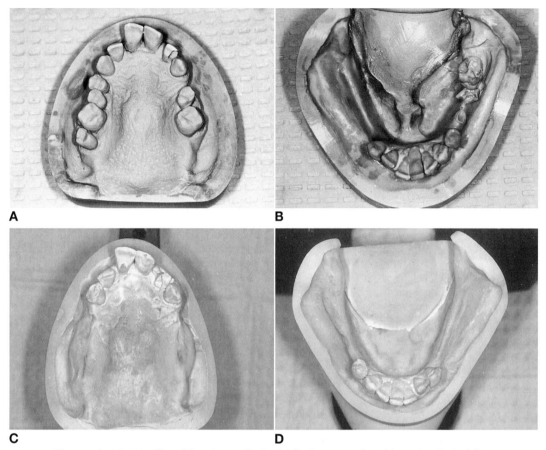

Figure 9-16 Maxillary **(A)** and mandibular **(B)** final casts produced from the single full arch custom impression tray method shown in Figure 9-10, for interim immediate dentures (IIDs). The final casts for a maxillary **(C)** and mandibular **(D)** conventional immediate denture (CID) are also shown.

and mark the casts with planned changes after receiving the patient's approval.

4. Reevaluate any further tooth modifications for a smooth occlusal plane or for better centric relation.

5. The casts are marked with all the information just listed and with information gathered during the initial oral examination. This should include pocket depths, free gingival margins, a line marking the interproximal of each tooth, and a drawing of where the new tooth position should be. One should duplicate these markings on the diagnostic casts for a back-up reference. The

tooth selection is confirmed with the patient (Figure 9-20).

6. A discussion of the surgical and denture placement protocol should occur to prepare the patient further and to answer any questions that the patient may have had after reading the written instructions given earlier. It is always wise to mention to the patient that circumoral tissues will become edematous and discolored in the few days or even weeks after insertion. Once the inflammatory response is resolved, the patient will still experience a local sense of upper lip puffiness, due to the presence of a flange, which

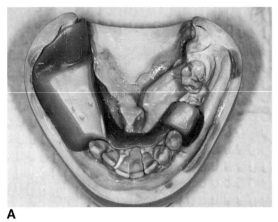

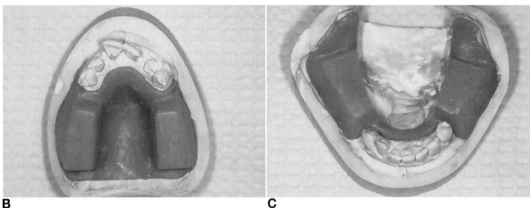

Figure 9-17 **A,** Mandibular record base with occlusion rim for an IID that uses the remaining teeth and halfway up the height of the retromolar pad as a guide to location of the posterior plane of occlusion. Maxillary **(B)** and mandibular **(C)** final casts and record bases for conventional immediate dentures (CIDs).

is necessary for denture retention. This can be thinned after sore spots are eliminated, and the patient should be reassured that the full upper lip sensation is usually temporary until the soft tissues adapt.

7. If a change in the vertical dimension of occlusion is desired, and indeed feasible, the denture teeth are reset or modified to the preferred vertical dimension of occlusion.

Setting the Anterior Teeth: Laboratory Phase

Setting anterior teeth for immediate dentures differs from that for complete dentures. An *alternative* or *"every other"* tooth setup is suggested even if duplicating the exact position of the remaining tooth is not the goal. Some authors have suggested the removal of all the teeth at this stage and then a setting of the denture teeth with the desired tooth arrangement irrespective of where the natural teeth were. However, this method eliminates much valuable information provided by the remaining teeth. The following tooth set-up technique is suggested:

1. Mark with an "X" (overdenture abutments can be marked with an "O") and remove with a saw or cutting disk every other anterior tooth (in the case of IIDs, every other posterior tooth as well) from the cast,

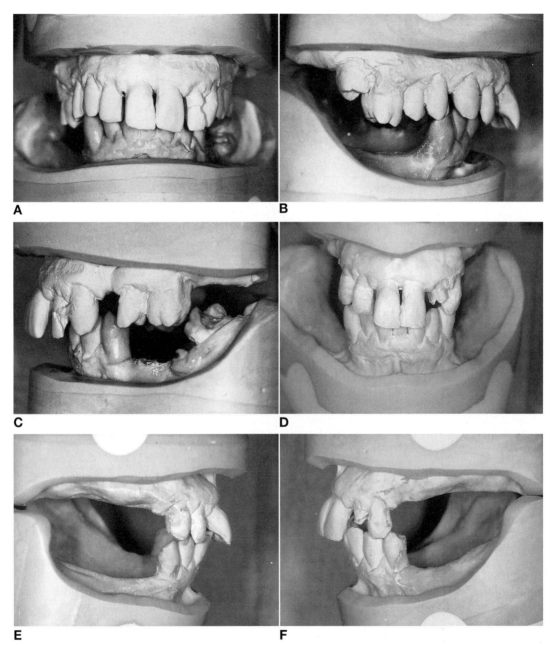

Figure 9-18 **A,** Mounted casts for immediate upper and lower dentures (IID). Right lateral view (**B**) and left lateral view (**C**). For upper and lower CIDs, **D,** Frontal view. **E,** Right lateral view. **F,** Left lateral view. *CID,* Conventional immediate denture; *IID,* interim immediate denture.

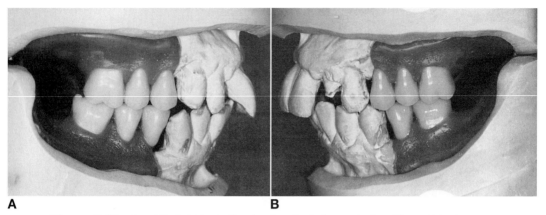

Figure 9-19 **A** and **B,** Posterior tooth setup for a try-in for conventional immediate dentures (CIDs).

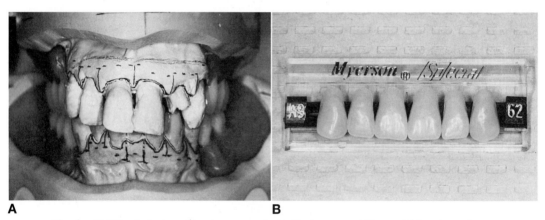

Figure 9-20 **A,** Casts and land areas marked with the new midline, anterior plane of occlusion (interpupillary), high lip line, gingival margins, interproximals, and pocket depths. **B,** Tooth selection is confirmed with the patient.

leaving at least one canine, central incisor, and lateral incisor. Trim the extraction site on the cast with a carbide bur (wide, fluted ones designed for stone trimming are best) as if the tooth had been removed and a small clot had formed in the site. In other words, the resulting area should be concave and not convex (Figure 9-21). Be conservative in this trimming (Jerbi, 1966), using the pocket depths as guides. The facial (only) portion of the extraction site can be further trimmed conservatively to the pocket depth line with a bur or a knife blade. The lingual or palatal tissues should not be trimmed because they

will not collapse to the pocket depth after extraction.

Overdenture abutments are trimmed to a dome shape to approximately 3 mm above the free gingival margin or slightly higher than the final form (1 to 2 mm above the gingival margin) planned. In the foregoing description, it is assumed that little or no bone will be removed during the extraction. If an anterior alveolectomy is needed, the casts should be trimmed according to esthetic requirements and as dictated by careful radiographic scrutiny and surgical operator input. The maximum

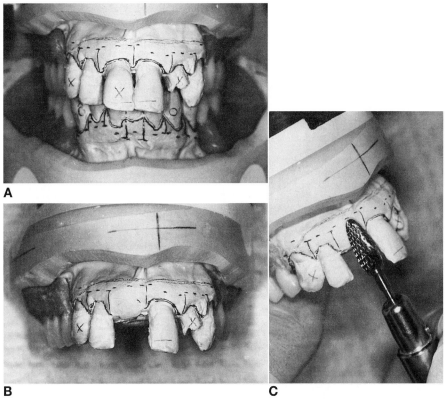

Figure 9-21 **A,** Use an "X" to mark an alternate tooth for removal, an "O" to mark an overdenture abutment, lines to mark interproximals, lines to mark the free gingival margin, and a line on the tooth to mark any planned raised position. **B,** The extraction site is trimmed conservatively. **C,** The extraction site should be convex (not concave). Note the midline and interpupillary line, which has been transferred to the base of the cast.

amount of trimming possible is usually about halfway between the buccal and the palatal gingival margins. Final smoothing of the cast must be completed at the wax boil-out stage, often by the dental technician. The prescription to the technician should note that this trimming should be conservative and serve only to smooth sharp edges and blend in the trimmed areas.

2. Set every other tooth in the maxilla first and then the mandible, referring to the notes and marks made at the try-in visit. The goal is an optimal esthetic result.
3. Then remove the remaining teeth and com-
plete the entire setup. Bring posterior teeth forward, close diastemata if desired, and finalize the setup for a balanced occlusion as needed (Figure 9-22). A Boley gauge or visualization can be used to compare the preexisting distance between the canines on the preextraction diagnostic cast and the new tooth arrangement (Figure 9-23).
4. An extra visit to recall the patient for a look at the final wax-up is a good idea at this time. This serves to reassure some apprehensive patients and may even provide them an opportunity to introduce minor artistic refinements in the setup.

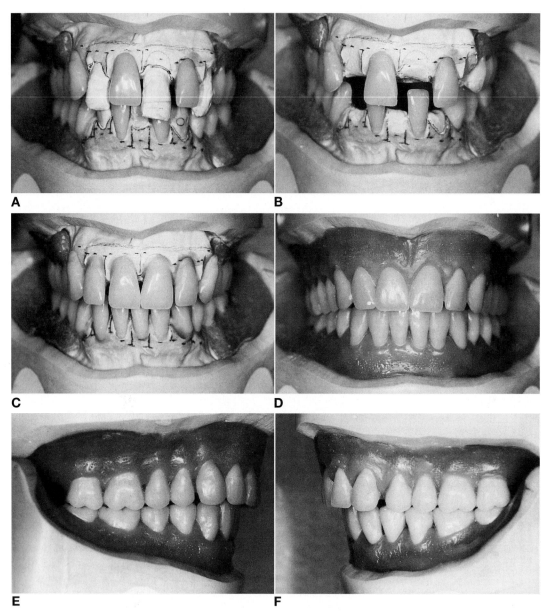

Figure 9-22 **A,** Every other tooth is set on the maxillary and the mandibular casts. **B,** The remaining teeth are removed. **C** to **F,** The setup is completed and waxed-up.

Wax Contouring, Flasking, and Boil-Out

1. The wax contour is similar to that for complete dentures, although the immediate denture may be thinner, especially in the anterior. Make sure that wax is added to provide a thickness of

material for strength during future deflasking. Also, when denture insertion is first attempted, it will undoubtedly bind on undercut areas. Thickness of the acrylic resin is needed to provide room to trim from the inside to relieve the sore spot or to seat the denture.

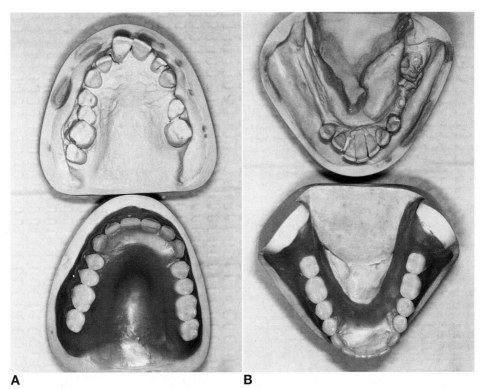

A   **B**

Figure 9-23 The preextraction casts and the final immediate denture wax-up can be compared. **A,** Maxillary. **B,** Mandibular.

2. A remount cast to preserve the face-bow should be done for later patient remounting 2 to 4 weeks after delivery.
3. The casts are flasked in the usual manner for complete dentures. At boil-out, the cast should be smoothed with a knife to a harmonious rounded contour (Figure 9-24). Custom characterization of the denture bases also is possible at this time.

Surgical Templates

A surgical template is a thin, transparent form duplicating the tissue surface of an immediate denture and is used as a guide for surgically shaping the alveolar process (Farmer, 1983). It is a prescription for the surgical procedure and is essential when any amount of bone trimming is necessary.

This template is fabricated (usually by the dental technician) by the following procedure:

1. Make an irreversible hydrocolloid (alginate) impression of the edentulous ridge after the cast has been trimmed at boil-out.
2. Pour the impression in stone.
3. Make a clear resin template on this duplicate cast by any of these four methods:
   a. Vacuum form method (a hole is placed in the center of the cast and a clear sheet is vacuumed onto the cast)
   b. Sprinkle-on technique (a clear acrylic [orthodontic] resin is used)
   c. Process template in clear acrylic resin (created by waxing up, flasking, and heat processing [Figure 9-25])
   d. Fabricate the template in light-cured, clear material

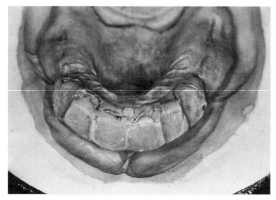

Figure 9-24 At boil-out, a knife is used to smooth the extraction sites to a harmonious rounded contour.

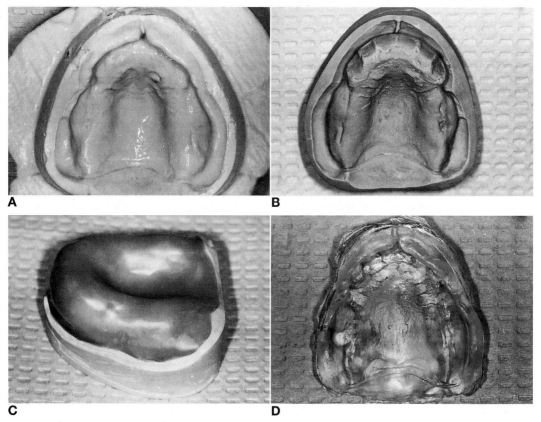

Figure 9-25 A surgical template is made at boil-out from the master cast **(A)** by making an irreversible hydrocolloid (alginate) impression. **B,** This is poured in stone. **C,** A wax-up is done. **D,** This can be processed in clear acrylic resin.

Processing and Finishing

1. The immediate dentures are processed and finished in the usual manner of complete dentures. If desired, a laboratory remount can be accomplished before removing the dentures from their casts and finishing. Keep the undercut areas of the denture slightly thick at this point to allow for insertion over undercuts. Using an upward/backward path of insertion of the immediate denture at placement may allow insertion without trimming; regardless, these areas can be thinned later before sending the patient home.

2. It is best to keep all posterior undercuts at this point because often they do not need reduction but can be well managed by selecting an alternate path of insertion and withdrawal of the denture combined with judicious trimming of the width of the inside of the resin flange in these areas at the placement visit. Any bumps inside the immediate denture resulting from over-trimming of the cast should be reduced to allow for a convex ridge healing. These procedures are duplicated on the surgical template.

3. Both the immediate denture and the surgical template should be placed in a chemical sterilizing solution in a bag for delivery.

Surgery and Immediate Denture Insertion

1. The patient can see the practitioner first for reduction of any overdenture abutments (Figure 9-26) or sectioning of any preexisting fixed partial dentures. The dentist performing the operation then extracts the remaining teeth, taking care to preserve the labial plate of bone. Usually, no bone trimming is done.

2. The surgical template is used as a guide to ensure that the prescribed bone trimming is done adequately. The template should fit and be in contact with all tissue surfaces. Inadequately trimmed areas planned for bone reduction will blanch from the pressure and be seen through the clear template.

The template is removed and the bone or soft tissue trimmed until the template seats uniformly and completely. This indicates that the denture will seat as it was originally intended, to ensure proper occlusion and minimally induced discomfort.

3. Sutures are placed where necessary (Figure 9-27). (With simple extractions, none are preferred.)

4. If the overdenture abutments must be reduced after the extractions, the extraction sockets can be protected during preparation by covering them with Burlew foil.

5. Usually, the dentist or surgeon places the denture so that it seats well with good firm bilateral occlusion and no gross deflective contacts. Pressure areas inside the denture (indicated by rocking) can be located with pressure-indicating paste and trimmed. If the occlusion is not correct, the denture should be rechecked for seating, particularly distally, the so-called denture heel areas, which are checked for interference. When occlusal prematurities are verified, a quick occlusal correction is done to allow simultaneous bilateral contact (Figure 9-28). Further refinement of the occlusion usually is done at a later date. The frena should be checked for proper relief.

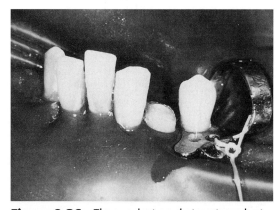

Figure 9-26 The overdenture abutments are best reduced by the application of a rubber dam to prevent amputated crowns from entering the throat or airway.

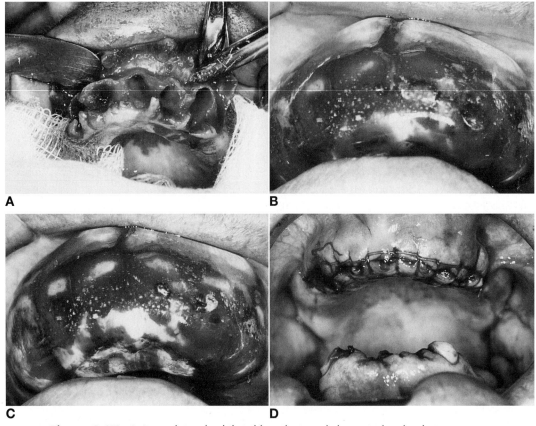

Figure 9-27 **A,** It was determined that this patient needed an anterior alveolectomy. **B,** The seated stent will show blanched areas where bone has not been trimmed adequately. **C,** After proper bone trimming, the template will seat uniformly. **D,** Sutures can then be placed.

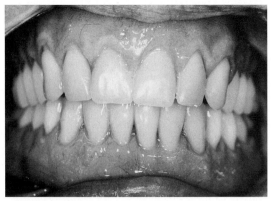

Figure 9-28 At placement, good bilateral contacts should be present.

6. On occasion, the denture will be found to be inadequately retentive. This is frequently the case when both anterior and posterior teeth were extracted. A tissue-conditioning liner can be placed at this stage, but the material should not be allowed to get into the extraction sites. Burlew foil can be used to cover the extraction sites for this procedure. Carefully check the extraction sites before dismissing the patient. Also trim any bumps or projections of tissue conditioning material inside the denture with a rounded hot instrument. If this is overlooked, normal socket healing will be compromised, and the ridge will heal with small concavities overlying the

extraction sites. A knuckle-shaped residual ridge will result.

Some authors (Woloch, 1998) recommend that instead of extracting the remaining anterior teeth, decoronation (with pulpectomy as indicated) of the crowns should be done instead. The advantages cited are better visualization (less blood), shorter placement visit, no need for surgeon on the day of placement, minimal pain and swelling, and ease of distinguishing sore spots at adjustment visits (versus pain from extraction sites). The roots are removed after several days through 2 to 3 weeks. Disadvantages are that there is no tissue collapse that can be planned when setting denture teeth and extraction might be more difficult in some instances without the clinical crown. Contraindications include acutely infected teeth and severe bilateral undercuts.

Postoperative Care and Patient Instructions

First 24 Hours The patient should avoid rinsing, avoid drinking hot liquids or alcohol, and not remove the immediate denture(s) during the first 24 hours. Because inflammation, swelling, and discoloration are likely to occur, their partial control can be helped with ice packs (20 minutes on, 20 minutes off) on the first day. Because of swelling, premature removal of the immediate denture could make its reinsertion impossible for 3 to 4 days or until reduction of swelling. In addition, if swelling occurs and the denture can be reinserted, the amount of sore spots created will be increased. The patient should be reminded that the pain from the trauma of extraction would not be eliminated by removal of the dentures from the mouth. Analgesic medications are prescribed as required (Holt, 1986).

Patients should be alerted to expect minimal blood on their pillow during the first night, but troublesome hemorrhaging is rare because the denture acts as a bandage. The diet for the first 24 hours should be liquid or soft, if tolerated.

The following should occur at the 24-hour visit (Figure 9-29):

1. Ask patients where they feel sore. Warn them that you are going to remove the den-

ture and that this will cause some discomfort. Have some dilute mouthwash ready for the patient to rinse with. Remove the denture and wash it.
2. Quickly check the tissues for sore spots related to the denture; these will appear as strawberry-red spots. Usually, these areas include canine eminences, lateral to tuberosities; posterior limit areas; and retromylohyoid undercuts as well as any other undercut ridge areas.
3. These areas may be related to the denture bases visually or with the adjunctive use of pressure indicator paste. The corresponding areas are relieved in the acrylic resin. The denture should be kept out of the mouth only for a very short time.
4. Adjust any gross occlusal discrepancy in centric relation or excursions.
5. Reevaluate the denture for retention. Place a tissue conditioner if denture retention is unsatisfactory.

First Postoperative Week Counsel the patient to continue to wear the immediate denture at night for 7 days after extraction or until swelling reduction. This ensures that a recurrence of nocturnal swelling will not preclude reinserting the denture in the morning. Starting immediately after the 24-hour visit, the patient should be shown how to remove the denture after eating to clean it and to rinse the mouth at least three to four times daily to keep the extraction sites clean. The denture should then be quickly reinserted and worn continuously. After 1 week, sutures can be removed (Figure 9-30), and the patient can begin removing the denture at night.

Further Follow-up Care

During the first month after insertion, the patient is seen on request or else weekly as required for sore spot adjustments. Denture adhesives can be used during this period as an aid if retention is lost between visits. After 2 weeks, remount casts are poured, the maxillary denture is related to its semiadjustable articulator using the remount matrix made before flasking, a centric relation

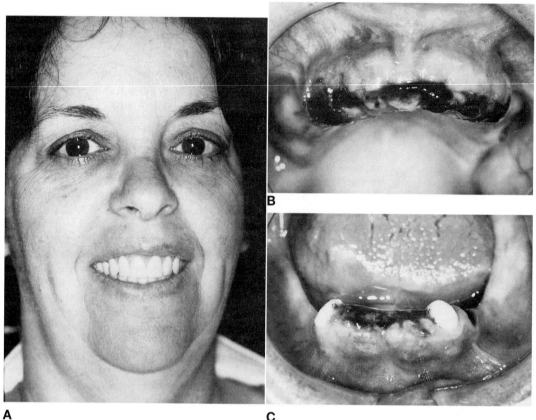

A   B   C

Figure 9-29   The patient (**A**) and the maxillary (**B**) and mandibular (**C**) arches 24 hours after extraction. Sore spots are evident on the mandibular anterior buccal ridge.

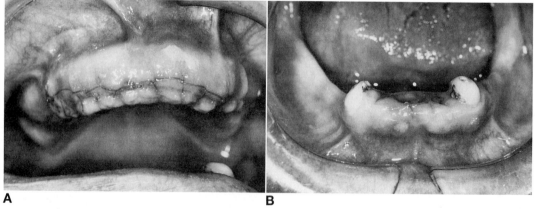

A   B

Figure 9-30   Patient's healing after 1 week in the maxillary (**A**) and mandibular (**B**) arch.

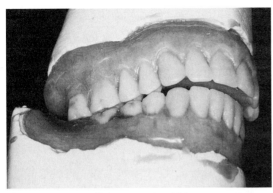

Figure 9-31   All dentures should be remounted after delivery. Remounting the immediate denture should occur after swelling has subsided, between week 1 and week 2 postoperatively.

record is used to remount the mandibular denture, and refinement of the occlusion is performed (Figure 9-31).

If the opposing arch is not a denture, a cast of the opposing restored or unrestored arch is made in an irreversible hydrocolloid (alginate) impression and related to the immediate denture on the articulator in a manner similar to the one just described.

Subsequent Service for the Patient with an Immediate Denture

After the sore spots are eliminated and the tissues have healed, a recall program for changing the tissue-conditioner liner is organized. Ridge resorption is fastest during the first 3 months (Tallgren, Lang, and Walker, 1980). The frequency of changing these liners varies from patient to patient and is influenced by denture hygiene frequency and methods, diet, and smoking habits. New light-cured soft liners may last longer in some patients. The major determinants of the frequency of changing temporary liners are the rate and amount of ensuing bone resorption and the ability of the patient to keep the liner clean.

Research shows that complete socket calcification is complete at 8 to 12 months after tooth extraction and that bone volume of the ridge is reduced 20% to 30% during the first 12 months. The resorp-

tion in the lower ridge is about twice that for the upper ridge (Tallgren, Lang, and Walker, 1980) Practically speaking, patients with CIDs frequently prefer to have a definitive reline (laboratory acrylic or chair side acrylic or light-cured resin) done within the first 3 to 6 months. This is acceptable, but patients should be told that their denture-supporting area will continue to remodel and that further relines will probably be necessary (at an additional fee for service). Regular visits and adjustments are needed throughout the first year (Tallgren, Lang, and Walker, 1980).

Patients with IIDs can have their second denture started within 3 to 6 months if desired. Again, this second denture may need a reline (laboratory acrylic or chair side acrylic or light-cured resin) after tissues complete their full healing. The advantage here is that the IID can be worn as a spare if a laboratory reline is selected for the second denture.

Change in Plans

Infrequently, imperfect results demand that the patient with a CID become the patient with the IID by default, or after the fact. This may be due to processing errors or unmet expectations for the CID. In such situations, a new second denture (instead of a reline of the CID) is fabricated. Because of this possibility, all patients with CIDs should be informed that there is always the remote chance that the CID could turn out to be an IID and a second denture may need to be made. The fee structure would be adjusted because clearly, a second denture is more expensive than a reline.

In a similar manner, a planned IID can turn out to be the final prosthesis (as in the CID). When all goes well, the dentist and the patient may be so pleased with the interim denture that it is relined as the final denture.

Overdenture Tooth Attachments, Implants, or Implant Attachments

When patients with immediate overdentures have an indication for an overdenture attachment, it should be accomplished after healing and before the definitive prosthesis so that attachment components can be processed into the second denture or reline (Figure 9-32).

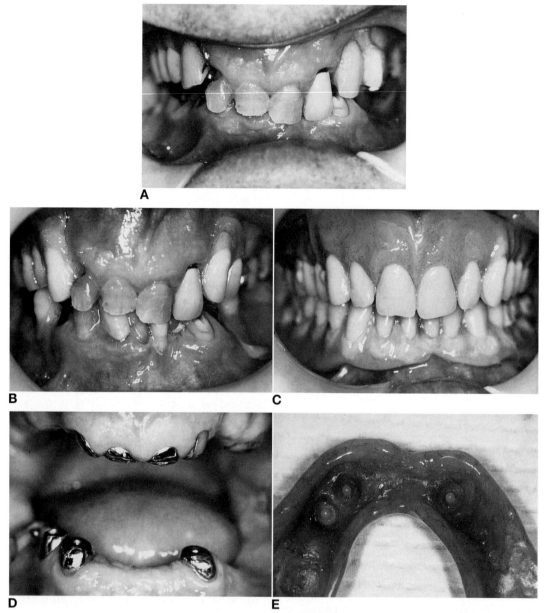

Figure 9-32 **A,** Patient for whom immediate overdentures with lower attachments are planned if the retention of the lower overdenture is not as expected. **B,** Denture try-in at correct vertical dimension of occlusion. **C,** Placement of immediate upper and lower overdentures. **D,** Zest Anchor attachments are done after healing and before reline or second denture **(E)** so that attachment components can be processed into the definitive prosthesis. (**D,** Zest Anchor, Inc, Irvine, Calif.)

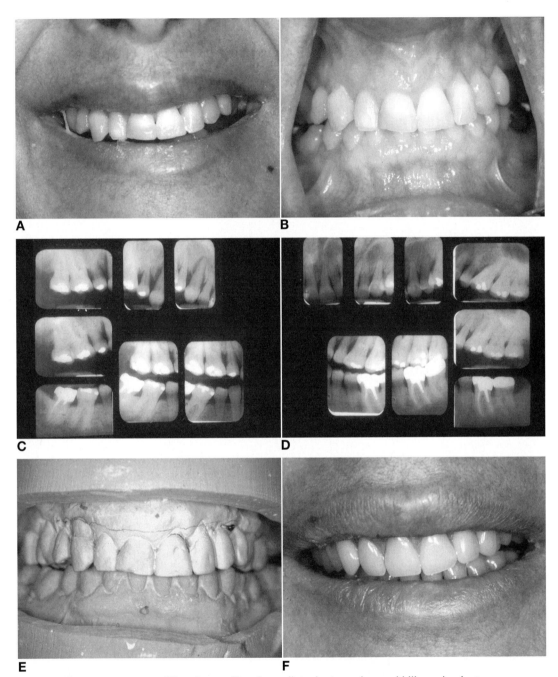

Figure 9-33 Candidate for maxillary immediate denture who would like an implant retained overdenture as her final treatment outcome. **A,** Patient's smile with her remaining teeth. **B,** Teeth in occlusion. **C** and **D,** Preoperative radiographs. **E,** Final mounted interim denture maxillary cast against opposing arch. Denture tooth position planning must occur at this stage for the eventual placement of the four implants and bar assembly. **F,** Placement of the interim denture (IID). *Continued*

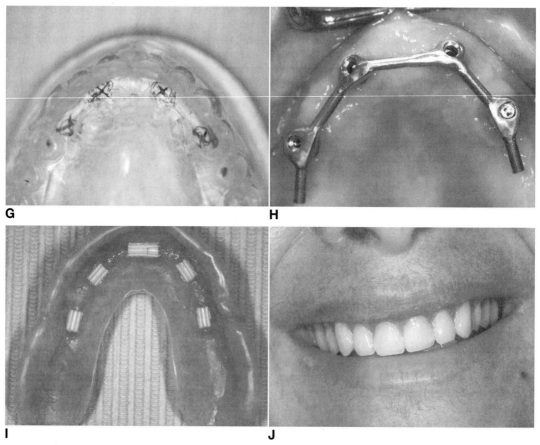

Figure 9-33 *cont'd* **G,** A clear resin duplicate of the interim denture serves as a surgical template. Its placement on the preliminary cast helps to plan the best implant/bar assembly location. **H,** After implant placement and healing, try-in of final implant bar assembly. **I,** Final implant attachment overdenture. **J,** Patient's smile with (second) implant overdenture. If planned well, the patient's interim denture can also be relined to "fit" the bar assembly.

If the patient's treatment plan includes implants, such as an implant retained overdenture, the implants can be placed and allowed to heal under the immediate denture. Care should be taken to avoid wearing the prosthesis for the determined time after implant surgery (usually 1 to 2 weeks). The immediate denture can be reinserted after relieving and tissue-conditioning procedures.

After implant uncovering, the immediate denture is relieved to accommodate the healing abutments and serve as the prosthesis until replacement by the implement prosthesis. Figure 9-33 shows an immediate denture patient who illustrates this sequence of events.

SUMMARY

Immediate dentures fulfill an important role in today's treatment modalities by providing the patients with esthetics, function, and psychological support after extractions and during the healing phase. The technique is more demanding than regular complete dentures for both the patient and the dentist. If the patient is well prepared and the appropriate type of immediate denture is selected (conventional or interim), the resulting prosthesis can be a success.

ACKNOWLEDGMENTS

Gratitude is expressed to Dr. Arnold Rosen for his slides in Figure 9-12, Dr. Victor Fong for his treatment/laboratory procedure shown in his patient throughout the chapter, and Mr. David Baptiste for his tinting and processing of the photographed dentures.

References

Academy of Prosthodontics Editorial Staff. The glossary of prosthodontic terms: seventh edition, *J Prosthet Dent* 81:76, 78, 1999.

Campagna SJ: An impression technique for immediate dentures, *J Prosthet Dent* 20:198-202, 1968.

Campbell RL: A comparative study of the resorption of the alveolar ridges in denture wearers and non-denture wearers, *J Amer Dental Ass* 60: 146-148, 1960.

Carlsson GE, Bergman B, Hedegard B: Changes in contour of the maxillary alveolar process under immediate dentures: a longitudinal clinical and x-ray cephalometric study covering 5 years, *Acta Odontol Scand* 25: 45-75, 1967.

Cohen BD, Mullick SC: Conversion of a fixed/removable partial denture into an immediate provisional complete denture, *J N J Dent Assoc* 65:19-21, 1994.

Farmer JB: Surgical template fabrication for immediate dentures, *J Prosthet Dent* 49:579-580, 1983.

Goldstein GR: An alternative immediate complete denture impression technique, *J Prosthet Dent* 67:892-893, 1992.

Hay CD: Direct provisional immediate denture is comfortable transition, *J Indiana Dent Assoc* 77:14, 1998.

Heartwell CM and Salisbury FW: Immediate dentures: an evaluation, *J Prosthet Dent* 15(4): 616-618, 1965.

Holt RA Jr: Instructions for patients who receive immediate dentures, *J Am Dent Assoc* 112:645-646, 1986.

Jerbi FC: Trimming the cast in the construction of immediate dentures, *J Prosthet Dent* 16(6): 1048-1051, 1966.

Jonkman RE, Van Waas M, Kalk W: Satisfaction with complete immediate dentures and complete immediate overdentures: a 1-year survey, *J Oral Rehabil* 22:791-796, 1995.

Kelly EK, Sievers RF: The influence of immediate dentures on tissue heating and alveolar ridge form, *J Prosthet Dent* 9(5): 739-742, 1958.

Khan Z, Haeberle CB: One appointment construction of an immediate transitional complete denture using visible light-cured resin, *J Prosthet Dent* 68:500-502, 1992.

McGarry TJ, Nimmo A, Skiba, JF et al: Classification system for partial edentulism, *J Prosthodont* 11:181-193, 2002.

Payne SH: A transitional denture, *J Prosthet Dent* 14: 221-2241964.

Pence B Sr, Lee MW, Baum L: Transitional dentures: a better immediate prosthesis leads to successful restoration, *General Dentistry* 40:319-23, 1992.

Raczka TC, Esposito SJ: The "jiffy" denture: a simple solution to a sometimes difficult problem, *Compendium of Continuing Education in Dentistry* 16: 914, 1995.

Rayson JH, Wesley RC: An intermediate denture technique, *J Prosthet Dent* 23:456-463, 1970.

Seals RR Jr, Kuebker WA, Stewart KL: Immediate complete dentures, *Dent Clin North Am* 40:151, 1996.

Soni A: Use of loose fitting copper bands over extremely mobile teeth while making impressions for immediate dentures, *J Prosthet Dent* 81:638-639, 1999.

Tallgren A, Lang BR, Walker GF et al: Roentgen cephalometric analysis of ridge resorption and changes in jaw and occlusal relationships in immediate complete denture wearers, *J Oral Rehabil* 7:92, 1980.

Terry BC, Hillenbrand DG: Minor preprosthetic surgical procedures, *Dent Clin North Am* 38:193-216, 1994 (review).

Vellis PA, Wright RF, Evans JH et al. Prosthodontic management of periodontally compromised patient, *N Y State Dent J* 67:16-20, 2001.

Woloch MM: Nontraumatic immediate complete denture placement: a clinical report, *J Prosthet Dent* 80:391-393, 1998.

Zalkind M, Hochman N: Converting a fixed partial denture to an interim complete denture: esthetic and functional considerations, *Quintessence Int* 28:121-125, 1997.

CHAPTER 10

Overdentures

George A. Zarb, Rhonda F. Jacob, John P. Zarb

Dentists have long recognized the difference that the presence of teeth makes to preservation of alveolar ridge integrity (Figure 10-1). It appears that the presence of a healthy periodontal ligament maintains alveolar ridge morphology, whereas a diseased periodontal ligament, or its absence, is associated with variable but inevitable time-dependent reduction in residual ridge dimensions (see Chapter 2). In the past the extraction of entire dentitions with complete denture replacements used to be promoted as an inexpensive and permanent solution for oral health care. The legacy of this approach has become a major oral morphological problem: advanced residual ridge resorption (RRR). Ongoing and frequently rapid reduction in edentulous ridge size appears to be multifactorial and is imperfectly understood. However, clinical experience and compellingly documented research have underscored the merits of retaining natural teeth to serve as abutments under complete dentures or else under extensive or distal extension areas of removable partial dentures. The premise is that occlusal forces of a functional and parafunctional nature that exert an adverse influence on denture-supporting tissues need to be attenuated or reduced and that attempts to clinically address this problem are an important part of the RRR paradigm that the dentist can control. Thus we have the technique of designing overdentures, which also have been described as hybrid dentures, or teeth-supported or assisted complete dentures. The retained teeth abutments may be few or numerous, coronally modified or restored, and frequently endodontically prepared. The objective is to distribute stress concentration between retained teeth abutments and denture-supporting tissues (Figure 10-2).

The overdenture technique was originally introduced to reconcile a need for maximum support in morphologically compromised dental arches with a desire to improve equally compromised esthetic appearance resulting from undersupported circumoral tissues. Consequently, patients with congenital anomalies such as cleft palates or those with sequelae of maxillofacial trauma were the usual candidates for the service (Figure 10-3). Eventually, the merits and ingenuity of the technique encouraged dentists to prescribe it for patients who had worn dentitions or anomalies that included missing teeth and when unfavorable jaw size or position could not be rectified by orthognathic surgery (Figures 10-4 and 10-5). Above all, the technique was incorporated into the management of patients with partial or terminal dentitions, especially when complete dentures seemed a likely therapeutic option. In fact, in today's dental practices, it is most unlikely that immediate dentures are ever prescribed without diligent efforts made to retain abutment teeth (even if provisionally) for an immediate overdenture service (see Chapter 9).

Most prosthodontic educators and researchers now recognize that the technique helps reduce the impact of some of complete denture-wearing consequences: RRR, loss of occlusal stability, undermined esthetic appearance, and compromised masticatory function. The technique has also been regarded as a gentler transition to the completely edentulous state.

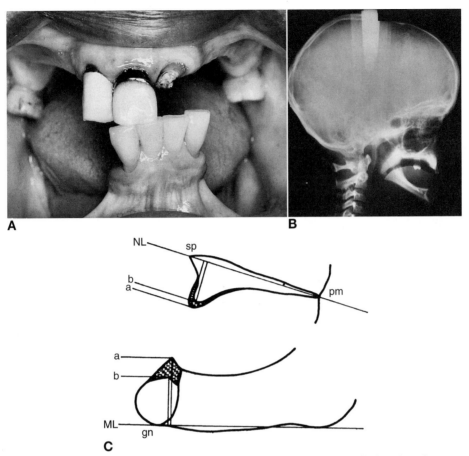

Figure 10-1   A, Dramatic residual ridge reduction (RRR) of the mandibular edentulous segments contrasts sharply with integrity of the alveolar ridge where the incisors are present. **B,** Virtual absence of the upper and lower alveolar ridges in the mandible of a 13-year-old boy whose dentition was congenitally absent. **C,** Measurements of ridge reduction/resorption. The anterior height of the upper and lower alveolar ridges at two stages of observation (*a* and *b*). The difference (*a* and *b*) represents reduction of the ridges between observations. Shaded area denotes the resorption. (**C,** Modified from Tallgren A: *J Prosthet Dent* 27:120-132, 1972.)

Van Waas et al. (1993) randomly assigned 74 subjects to immediate complete dentures versus immediate complete overdenture prostheses supported on two mandibular canines. They evaluated the loss of bone in the canine area using cephalometric radiographs. The authors reported a reduction of 0.9 mm in the overdenture group and 1.8 mm in the denture group; in the molar area the loss of bone was 0.7 mm and 1.9 mm, respectively, with all measurements being statistically signifi-

cant. The clinical retention of bone surrounding the abutments has been clinically observed by most clinicians using this technique.

ADVANTAGES AND DISADVANTAGES

Demonstrated, cited advantages of overdentures include the following: (1) There is maintenance of more residual ridge integrity than if an "unsupported" denture is worn. This results from presumed

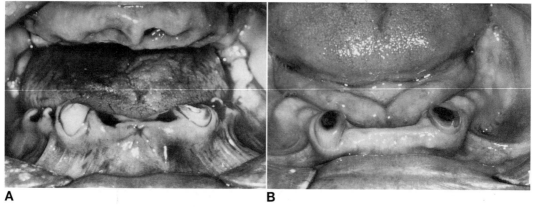

A **B**

Figure 10-2 The entire notion of the classic overdenture technique is depicted in **A** and **B**. Two mandibular canines are morphologically altered after root canal therapy and extraction of adjacent teeth that demonstrated advanced periodontal disease. Their retention and use as overdenture abutments ensure dentogingival support for the complete denture and an expected reduction in residual ridge resorption (RRR) at least around and between the abutments. Overdenture treatment planning reconciles clinical decisions regarding number and location of potential abutments, their restorative and endodontic status, and their use for retention and support. A management strategy for their continued health status is also a required consideration.

improved occlusal stress distribution. (2) Denture stability and even retention (particularly in the mandible) may be enhanced. (3) Patients' subjective perceptions regarding a retained "natural feeling" tend to be positive ones. This may translate into better occlusal awareness, biting force, and consequent neuromuscular control than if the abutments in the overdenture were absent. (4) The technique is a viable and simple alternative to complete denture therapy, and it is frequently self-reported as providing immense psychological support for patients. (5) Its application is virtually unlimited and depends on the dentist's judgment and skill and, above all, on the patient's motivation to maintain an impeccable oral environment (Figure 10-6). There are also disadvantages to the technique, and it is prudent to regard it as a likely provisional one. The likely time-dependent transition to complete denture treatment is largely related to the patient's oral hygiene commitment and the nature of the selected abutments. It must be emphasized that the covered teeth abutments' environment is not conducive to maintaining a plaque-free milieu with its serious risk of adverse sequelae. Furthermore, the age-related inability to apply a scrupulous hygiene

protocol and the presence of refractory periodontal disease are serious deterrents to successful teeth retention outcomes. Thus many clinicians frequently cite significant occurrence of caries and periodontal disease around abutments. Caries can, of course, develop rapidly, with different degrees of susceptibility recorded, particularly among older persons. However, some studies have also emphasized the feasibility of controlling carious lesions through nutritional counseling, sustained program of oral hygiene, and regular fluoride applications.

The prevention of gingival and periodontal disease is a very compelling concern because it remains the patient's responsibility, and scrupulous hygiene accompanied by biannual professional monitoring is mandatory to ensure continued abutment-supporting tissues' health. This entails a rigid and frequent recall appointment protocol with its implied additional expense, and it is one that is increased in the context of endodontic and frequent restorative requirements. Furthermore, available interarch space is sometimes judged inadequate on technical convenience grounds, and extensive abutment or design modifications will be required to

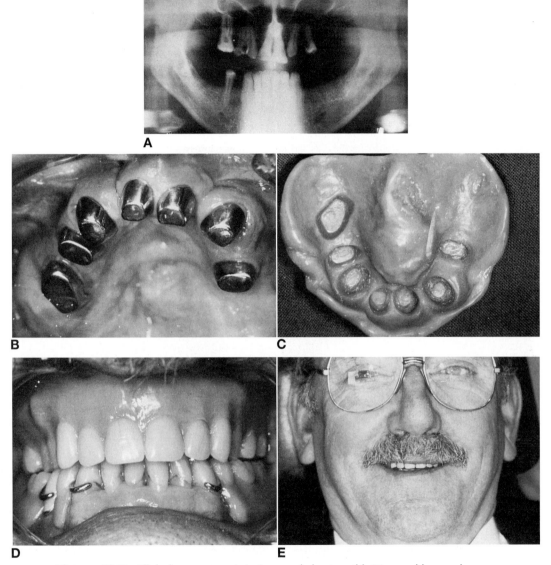

Figure 10-3 Clinical management strategy carried out on this 54-year-old man whose congenital anomaly was surgically repaired in his youth (**A** to **E**). Note that congenitally impaired horizontal and vertical dimensions of the facial profile were esthetically corrected with an overdenture.

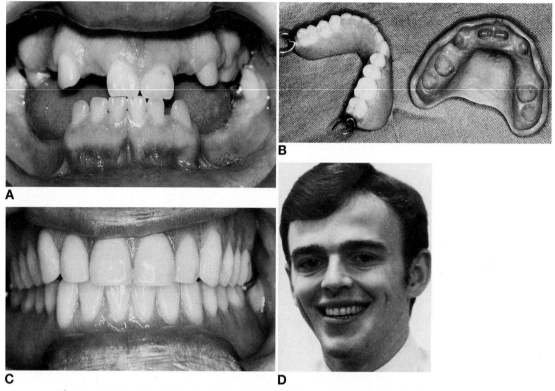

Figure 10-4 **A** to **D,** Congenitally missing teeth have undermined both the appearance and the functional efficiency of this patient. A maxillary overdenture resolved the problem and created a normal appearance. Note that minimal horizontal labiofacial support was required here.

expedite treatment. Potential weakness in the acrylic resin denture base also will need to be determined, and extra laboratory steps such as a cast metal superstructure fabrication can lead to additional expenses.

The increased costs associated with the technique are, however, justified because overdentures *are* a superior health service compared to the standard complete denture.

INDICATIONS AND TREATMENT PLANNING

The versatility of the overdenture service is demonstrated in Figures 10-2 to 10-8. These patient examples were selected to emphasize the range of treatment possibilities. Above all, they

underscore the logic of including the method as an integral part of every dentist's treatment-planning repertoire. In general, there are two major groups of patients who benefit from the technique. Group 1 comprises patients with a few remaining teeth that may be healthy or with reversible periodontal disease, that are coronally intact, or that are malpositioned or morphologically compromised. These teeth can be modified for use as abutments. Treatment here is conceptually and technically straightforward with minimal preprosthodontic intervention needed. Analysis of articulated diagnostic casts, full-mouth radiographs, and overall patient concerns will enable the dentist to determine potential abutment teeth's restorative and endodontic requirements (if any) in the context of

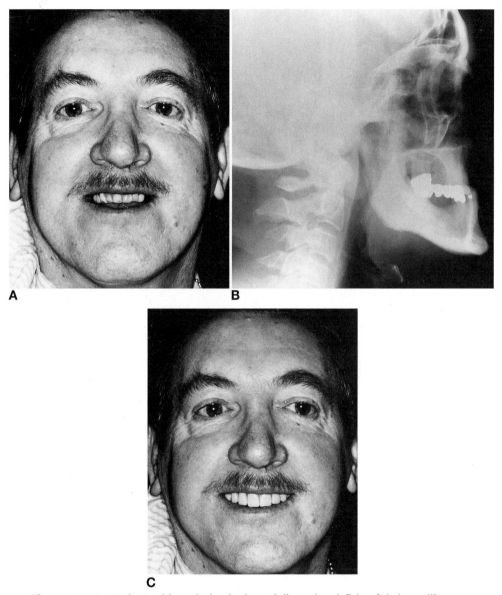

Figure 10-5 Patients with vertical or horizontal dimension deficits of their maxillary arches can be managed prosthodontically by overlaying their maxillary dentition. This approach permits improved horizontal facial support and increased vertical dimension of occlusion. **A, B, D,** and **E,** Pretreatment views of a patient whose complaint of compromised masticatory function and poor esthetic appearance was attributable to a discrepancy in facial development. **C** and **F,** Post-treatment results were achieved without surgical orthognathic interventions. *Continued*

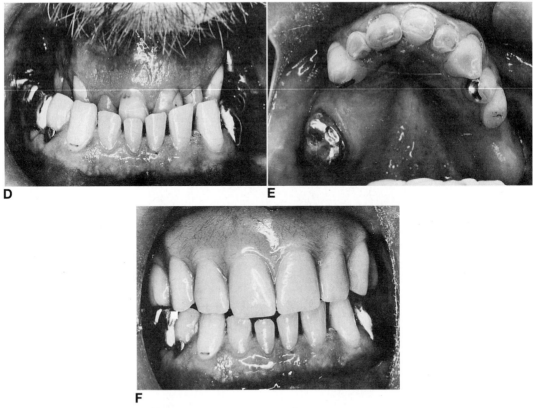

Figure 10-5 *cont'd*

the proposed overdenture's design. Particular consideration should be given to those patients in whom the overdenture will oppose a natural or restored natural dentition (see Chapter 21). The presence of overdentured abutments in an otherwise edentulous arch will reduce the considerable risk inherent in the stresses associated with an unbalanced hammer and anvil effect simulated by single complete denture therapy (see Chapter 2).

Group 2 comprises patients who received a diagnosis of so-called mutilated or severely compromised dentitions. These patients appear to be heading in an edentulous direction, and their treatment is defined by the complexity, expense, and time implications of the intervention. Selected extractions will need to be carried out, keeping in mind that retention of teeth with good alveolar support will preserve bone at the selected sites. Conversely, retention of periodontally compromised teeth can only risk further depletion of

bone levels if such teeth are retained—thus the need for their early extraction. Such an initiative could also serve to improve the periodontal status of the adjacent retained teeth.

SELECTION OF ABUTMENT TEETH

Specific critical factors that influence the selection of abutment teeth include periodontal status, mobility, location, and endodontic and prosthodontic considerations, with costs an ever-present and often overriding consideration. The treatment plan is defined by the number and required interventions on the retained teeth, as well as the following:

1. Periodontal and mobility status: An abutment root or tooth must be chosen that is surrounded by healthy periodontal tissues. The tissues may already be healthy or

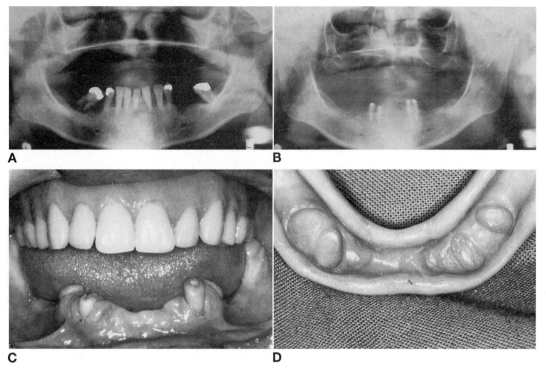

Figure 10-6 This example of mandibular overdenture treatment in a 45-year-old woman with periodontal disease underscores the simplicity of the technique as well as its advantages and disadvantages. The panoramic views in **A** and **B** are separated by an interval of 7 years. Although such radiographic precision is not scientifically quantifiable, it still suggests an impressive retardation in residual ridge resorption (RRR). **C,** The prepared root surfaces were left "bare," but no caries activity or increased periodontal disease progress was noted. Clearly, the patient's home maintenance program, which included fluoride gel use, has yielded a very good treatment outcome (**D**). The status of the prosthesis has been well monitored.

rendered so by appropriate periodontal therapy (see Figures 10-6 and 10-7). Compromised teeth with a good treatment prognosis are popularly regarded as suitable candidates, even when horizontal bone loss is present. Conversely, significant vertical bone loss, particularly if accompanied by type 2 or 3 mobility, generally precludes a tooth's selection. Slight tooth mobility per se is not a contraindication because a favorable change in the crown-root ratio may ameliorate this sign. A circumferential band of attached gingiva, albeit a narrow one, is regarded as a mandatory requirement for abutment selection.

2. Abutment location: Because the anterior mandibular alveolar ridge appears to be most vulnerable to time-dependent RRR, canines or premolars are regarded as the best overdenture abutments to reduce adverse forces at this site. This conviction applies to the maxilla as well, although incisors are also frequently used. The latter is particularly desirable if the mandibular arch is intact or is a naturally restored one. Clinical experience supports the recommendation of at least one tooth per quadrant. If this recommendation is exceeded, retained teeth should preferably not be adjacent ones, or there should be several millimeters of space between the reduced tooth forms.

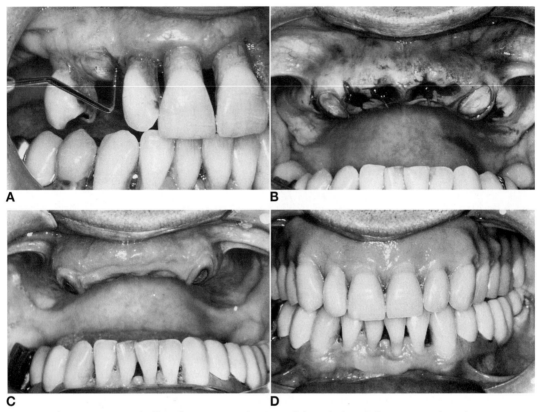

Figure 10-7   **A** and **B,** The presence of severe adult periodontal disease necessitated extraction of selected teeth and subgingival root planing of retained overdenture abutments. **C** and **D,** Endodontic treatment and alloy restorations ensured 6 years of excellent prosthodontic rehabilitation. With ongoing clinical monitoring and good home care, we anticipate a good prognosis for this patient's treatment outcome.

This will minimize the risks of compromise in soft tissue health. Some authors have expressed serious concerns about preserving or restoring balance of forces between the opposing arches. This notion underscores the importance of the dentist's reconciliation of the number and location of retained abutments in either arch and the status of the opposing one. Ultimately, this must be assessed in the context of the status of the mandibular "hammer" and maxillary "anvil" concept discussed earlier. Considerations for selecting maxillary overdenture abutments are summed up in Table 10-1.

3. Endodontic and prosthodontic status: Anterior single-rooted teeth are easier and less expensive to manage endodontically. Whenever pulpal recession to the extent of calcification has occurred, endodontic treatment usually can be avoided. The clinical crowns can be modified for technical convenience and treated with sealant restorations or fluoride applications. In recent years the use of cast copings has been largely eclipsed by composite and alloy restorations, with or without adjunctive retention.

Various methods and devices have been proposed for preparing abutment teeth to receive an over-

Table 10-1
Considerations in Selection of Maxillary Teeth as Overdenture Abutments

Maxillary Teeth	Advantages	Disadvantages
Central incisors	Ideal location, provide protection of the premaxilla	Proximity and alveolar prominence may complicate utilization
Lateral incisors	Widely separated, facilitating plaque control Tissue undercuts do not pose a problem Path of placement/removal is not compromised Ability to create a flange/peripheral seal	Diminished root surface area
Canines	Longest root of the anterior teeth	Diverging facial tissue undercuts Overcontoured flanges Excessive lip support Potentially uncomfortable placement/removal of prosthesis Complicates placement of prosthetic teeth Internal relief to accommodate canines may weaken, create a food trap, compromise the peripheral seal

From Nelson DR, von Gonten AS: Biomechanical and esthetic considerations for maxillary anterior overdenture abutment selection, *J Prosthet Dent* 72:133-136, 1994.

denture. It is our impression that the essential feature in this technique is not the type of attachment used per se but the following basic principles:

1. Maximum reduction of the coronal portion of the tooth should be accomplished. A better crown-to-root ratio is established, and minimal interference will be encountered with the placement of artificial teeth. The routine use of endodontic therapy increases the coronal reduction that can be achieved. Patients with advanced pulpal recession, usually combined with extensive tooth wear, can undergo coronal reduction without the need for endodontic treatment (see Figure 10-8). A clinical decision to leave the prepared abutment tooth "bare" or "unprotected" versus "to protect" it with a coping has fiscal and design implications. Frequently, a devitalized and broken-down tooth can be restored with an alloy or a composite, reshaped, and polished with fine sandpaper disks. In most situations, a bare tooth root preparation can provide adequate

long-term service for both immediate and replacement overdentures and is the selection of choice. This preparation is made when time is needed to evaluate the status of selected abutment teeth and when a patient's (usually an elderly one's) general health precludes several dental appointments. It is also the least expensive option, and a coping's presumed protective qualities can probably be exceeded with fluoride gel application, maintenance of an excellent level of oral hygiene, the use of chlorhexidine mouthwashes, and appropriate adjunctive restorative therapy. Study results are ambiguous at this time as to whether alloy, resin composite, glass ionomer, or resin-modified glass ionomer materials are the recommended material for filling endodontic openings. All these materials have produced clinical successes. Fluoride release of glass ionomers has not been compellingly evaluated in an overdenture population, and use of this material should not preclude additional daily fluoride regimens. Success of any of the materials requires routine follow-up to

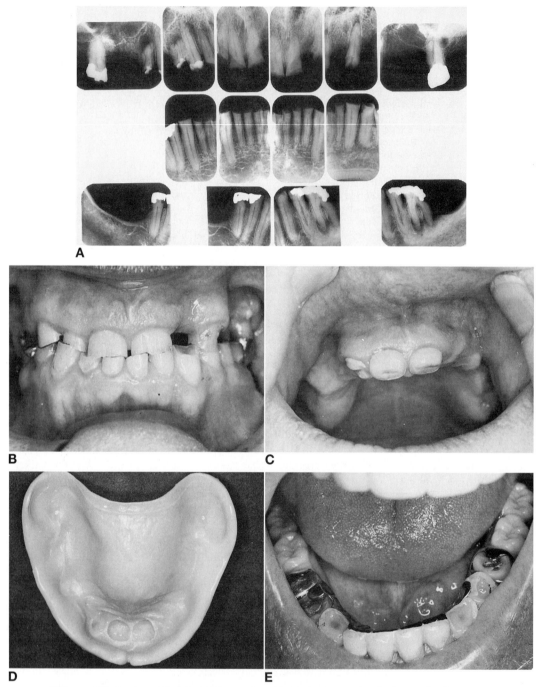

Figure 10-8 A and B, Advanced, symptomatic teeth wear and pulpal recession in a patient whose dentition showed considerable morphological changes and neglect. C and D, Three maxillary anterior teeth were retained, and an overdenture was constructed (E). Some of the badly worn anterior mandibular teeth were reduced/reshaped, polished, and partially "restored" with a cast removable partial denture of the overlay type.

evaluate the integrity of the restoration, and moreover, to evaluate home care of the abutment. The clinician is encouraged to continually evaluate current dental literature on this topic of dental materials for abutment restoration.

2. The need for a gold coping or a crown-and-sleeve coping retainer depends on several factors. Occasionally, a gold coping is necessary and can be prepared with or without a post or retentive pins, depending on the amount of tooth structure remaining above the gingival attachment. Often the coping preparation can extend into the endodontic preparation to gain increased surface area. The gold coping (Figure 10-9)

does involve an additional expense, but some patients are uncomfortable with the sight of discolored and "unprotected" roots in their mouth. The patient's susceptibility to caries must also be considered because provision of a coping does not guarantee reduced caries activity. Tooth preparation is similar to that for a complete gold crown, with or without additional pin retention, and it includes a combination of shoulder and chamfered gingival margins as dictated by the amount of residual tooth structure. It must be emphasized that the main objective in preparing and restoring overdenture abutments is to prolong the useful life span of the retained abutments and the preservation

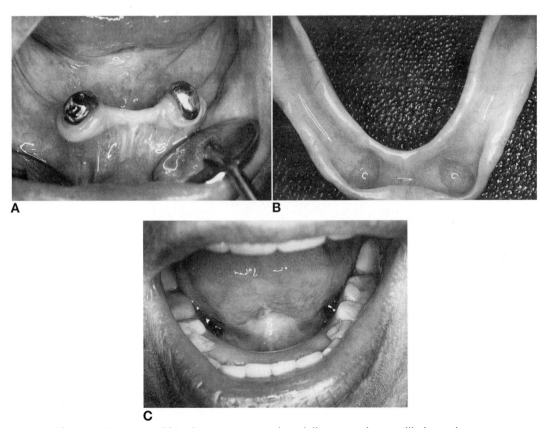

A   **B**   **C**

Figure 10-9 **A,** Gold copings to protect and partially restore the mandibular canines. **B,** An overdenture has been modified out in these areas to conform to the abutment contours. **C,** The cosmetic merits of the complete denture are in no way compromised.

of alveolar bone; it is not necessarily to introduce a technique for more retentive dentures. Consequently, a simple, short, convex abutment preparation (with or without a casting) appears to be the optimal root surface preparation.

3. Provision of some sort of attachment mechanism on a cast coping also is popular (Figure 10-10). This is an extension of the precision-retained abutment concept used in removable partial dentures and modified for use with overdenture abutments. It is a technically ingenious idea and offers a diversity of techniques, for example, intracoronal and extracoronal attachments, chairside attachments, or indirect attachments with cast copings. Several of these attachments are available in resilient and nonresilient designs. The notion of underscoring the use of such attachments shifts the overdenture design from stability and retardation of RRR concerns to major emphasis on prosthesis retention. Apart from the increased expense, the risks are increased technical demands and difficulties, particularly when repairs are required, oral hygiene maintenance requirements may be more demanding, and esthetic plus interarch

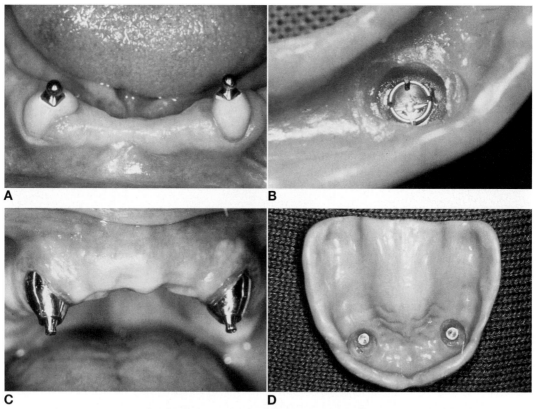

Figure 10-10 Although attachments in general may not be needed, they can improve support, stability, and retention of the overdenture. Some clinical examples are shown. **A** and **B,** The Dalbo Rotex chairside attachment system: male portion cemented in the abutment teeth and female housing embedded in the acrylic of the overdenture. **C** and **D,** The Ceka-Revax attachment system: the male stud-type attachment is soldered to a coping. Fixation is achieved by the female housing embedded in the (maxillary) overdenture.

space concerns are usually more severe. Nonetheless, attachment systems expand the scope of the overdenture technique in selected specific situations in which retention concerns dominate in the context of available design considerations.

Gold copings and telescopic crowns are a method of improving overdenture retention. These may be conical crowns with a friction adaptation at the marginal area of the abutment or milled crowns with larger surface area for frictional retention. Frictional retention is more commonly used in exclusively tooth-supported overdentures that are not supported by soft tissue. In overdenture situations where the prosthesis also rests on resilient edentulous ridges, the copings and telescopic crowns are usually designed with a relief area of 0.3 to 0.5 mm, allowing tissue-ward movement and lateral movements. Retention is obtained by other devices. The remainder of the edentulous ridge is covered by acrylic resin bases. The telescopic crowns resemble porcelain crowns, and they are incorporated in the overdenture. Wenz et al. (2001) have described these methods with both (1) complete tooth-supported and (2) tooth- and tissue-supported dentures. Tooth- and tissue-supported dentures had an average of three or fewer abutments. The total of both groups in the Wenz study was 125 subjects with 460 abutments. A total of only 16 subjects lost 38 abutments, and the probability of keeping all abutments was similar in both groups, with 84% (95% confidence interval [CI], 67-94) at 5 years and 66% (95% CI, 38-84) at 10 years. We stress that these abutments should be in very good health when considered for this restoration technique.

LOSS OF ABUTMENT TEETH

Several studies have reported loss of abutment teeth during varying observational follow-up periods. After 5 to 6 years, about 10% of abutment teeth supporting overdentures were lost. The most frequent causes were periodontal disease (about 70%), caries (about 25%), and endodontic complications (about 5%). Many of the long-term clinical studies of overdenture populations have been fraught with logistical problems of poor clinical follow-up and poor patient compliance in home care. Therefore their projection of abutment loss is a suspect point estimate, but one that can be explained through little fault of the investigators or clinicians. This patient population is usually older, with other health problems, social problems of finances and transportation, and an overall lack of perceived dental need. Many authors reported that although yearly or biannual examinations were planned, after a few years, more than 25% of populations ceased evaluations or were sporadic in attendance. The level of compliance with home care was also sporadic and at times nonexistent because this was a patient population that likely had long-standing habits leading to a terminal dentition that culminated in the overdenture treatment plan. What is compelling in this population is the possible vulnerability of the abutments, and it is clear that the success of overdenture treatment demands effective prevention of caries and periodontal disease. Regular follow-up visits are essential, and oral health maintenance measures are periodically reviewed and revised as necessary.

Ideally the patient must be well motivated to maintain the hygienic phase of periodontal care. It has been amply demonstrated that inadequate oral hygiene is a major contributor to abutment loss. Given the fact that this population may lack dexterity and motivation for adequate hygiene, one might consider the many mechanical toothbrushes that are available. Lack of patient compliance and predicted lack of motivation should not exclude a patient from overdenture therapy. Griess, Reilmann, and Chanavaz (1998) described mentally challenged subjects who maintained 81% of three-teeth telescopic overdentures at 8 years. Unfortunately actual "loss of dentures" was more a problem then loss of abutments. One-tooth mandibular overdentures were not as well tolerated, and patients often discarded these dentures.

Long-term monitoring of patients with overdentures reveals the occasional need for removal of one or more abutment teeth. This must be expected, and the cause is usually a periodontal abscess. Removal of the affected tooth, with appropriate filling in of the contacting site in the overdenture, can be done readily and inexpensively, without loss of the prosthesis. Caries accounts for the remainder of maintenance issues and abutment loss. Fluoride gel is prescribed for daily application to the inside of the overdenture to bring the fluoride into intimate contact with the natural tooth structure. It is understood that the effectiveness of fluoride on root and dentinal surfaces has not been as well defined as fluoride remineralization and incorporation in enamel. Studies of root surface caries in patients exposed to lifelong fluoridated water supply reveal a decrease in caries activity. Its use has been prescribed for patients with overdentures and seems to decrease caries activity. As in enamel, the greater the fluoride concentration, the greater the efficiency of the fluoride.

An in vitro evaluation was performed by Ettinger et al. (1997) to simulate overdenture abutment root surface caries, and the depth of remineralization bands were evaluated with polarized light microscopy. Fluoride preparations were 5000-ppm acidulated phosphate fluoride (pH 5.6), 5000-ppm neutral sodium fluoride, and 1000-ppm neutral sodium fluoride, with a distilled water control. Over 18 days the extracted teeth with exposed root surfaces were repeatedly placed in fluoride for 4 minutes, then in a demineralizing solution for 6 hours, and then in a remineralizing solution for 17 hours. The lesions in the 5000-ppm preparation had statistically shallower lesions. All groups except the control group exhibited remineralization bands. Reduction of demineralization was found to have a dose response in favor of the greater 5000 ppm. These findings are consistent with in vivo fluoridated dentifrice studies on root surface caries.

Given these findings, one should consider the preparations with greater fluoride concentrations. There are also dentifices with 5000-ppm fluoride that can be prescribed. The role of preparation pH is also being questioned in root surface caries models. The thought that the tissues may be severely irritated by the daily use of fluorides with low pH is an unlikely scenario because patients undergoing irradiation have been using daily stannous fluoride preparations (pH 4.0) in tray applicators for 10 minutes daily for many years without noticeable tissue irritation or patient complaints. In addition, stannous fluoride (SnF_2) preparations have been shown to inhibit plaque formation and periodontal microorganisms in multiple periodontal studies. If patients complain about tissue irritations, neutral preparations can be considered. The clinician should continue to evaluate the commercially fluoride preparations and the fluoride literature as it relates to root surface caries and overdenture abutments.

CLINICAL PROCEDURES

The procedures will vary depending on whether a tooth-supported complete denture is being constructed or a tooth-supported immediate-insertion complete denture is planned (see Chapter 9).

Tooth-Supported Complete Denture

The important principles of complete denture construction must be respected and when required, matched to the technical and laboratory dictates of selected attachment type. These principles are identical to those described in subsequent chapters, and they should be meticulously observed.

One frequently encountered problem of tooth-supported complete denture service is the tendency for an unfavorable gingival response around the abutment teeth (Figure 10-11). The following may cause gingival irritation: (1) movement of the denture base (more apparent in mandibular dentures), with the development of a loading factor

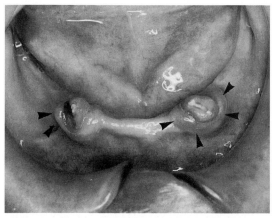

Figure 10-11 Gingivitis *(arrowheads)* around the abutments of an overdenture caused by inadequate hygiene measures of the patient. If untreated, the condition may precipitate a series of adverse changes and actually progress to periodontal disease.

at the gingival margins; (2) poor oral hygiene with failure to remove plaque or to pay sufficient attention to tissue rest and periodic recall assessments; and (3) excess space in the prosthesis around the gingival margins of the abutment teeth, which leads to the development of a "dead space" (a potential source of inflammation and tissue hypertrophy).

Clinical experience suggests that a slight space around the gingival margin is essential to avoid overloading this particularly vulnerable site, especially with mandibular dentures because they appear to become dislodged more easily than maxillary dentures. On the other hand, a dead space may lead to a combined hypertrophic/hyperplastic response of the gingival margin similar to that elicited by a relief chamber in a complete maxillary denture. One way to avoid this is to hollow out an area in the resin overdenture over the abutment site and line it with a tissue conditioner at the time of denture placement. The resiliency of the liner, combined with its need for frequent replacement, can create an optimal schedule for recall appointments. However, there also may be subsequent deterioration of the material and, with it, the risk of gingival tissue damage. Our preference therefore is to use an autopolymerizing hard acrylic resin to reline the abutment area at delivery of the prosthesis.

Tooth-Supported Immediate-Insertion Complete Denture

The procedures for immediate tooth-supported complete dentures are identical to those described in Chapter 9, except that the coronal reduction of the selected abutment teeth is done at the time the remaining teeth are extracted. The teeth to be retained are prepared on the master cast to the approximate shape of the pending abutment, and the remaining teeth are trimmed from the cast in the usual manner. The processed immediate denture thus demonstrates depressions on its impression surface that will conform to the teeth that are being retained. The endodontic treatment is completed during one or more appointments before the immediate denture insertion or just before the combined surgical-prosthetic appointment. Some dentists prefer the latter because removal of the

tooth crown facilitates the endodontic procedures. Immediate denture insertion and follow-up are carried out in the usual manner (see Chapter 9). The need for refining the impression surface of the denture in the operated on and abutment sites, by the addition of a treatment resin, is essential because rapid tissue changes are to be anticipated. When healing has occurred and tissues and remodeling bone have achieved a stable contour, additional coping preparation may be necessary with refitting of the prosthesis in this area.

TREATMENT OUTCOME STUDIES

The desire to prolong the useful life of at least a few of our patients' teeth led to a dramatic surge of interest in the overdenture concept. Several reports endorsing the technique have been published and many anecdotal claims made, but until recently there has been a lack of well-documented, long-term clinical follow-up of these patients. Current research appears to endorse the claim that overdentures are an effective alternative to conventional complete denture therapy, and their use in routine practice continues to be endorsed. However, the very nature of overdenture design and its relationship to plaque must always be kept in mind if this treatment modality is to fulfill its potential. Furthermore, the impressive and virtually morbidity-free outcomes reported in implant-supported overdenture studies are now beginning to eclipse the traditional role of teeth-supported overdentures.

SUMMARY

Relatively short-term favorable outcomes with the overdenture technique are well demonstrated and endorse routine prescription of the technique. Furthermore, the recent introduction of the osseointegration technique created the possibility of converting patients with maladaptive complete dentures into ones with adaptive overdentures when implants are used to stabilize "offending" prostheses. As a result, the twin techniques (traditional complete denture fabrication with natural teeth abutments or with implants) now offer dentists and patients a new standard of prosthodontic therapy (see Part 4).

References

Becker CM, Kaldahl WB: An overdenture technique designed to protect the remaining periodontium, *Int J Periodont Restor Dent* 4:28-41, 1984.

Budt-Jörgensen E: Prognosis of overdenture abutments in elderly patients with controlled oral hygiene: a 5 year study, *J Oral Rehabil* 22:3-8, 1995.

Derkson GD, MacEntee MM: Effect of 0.4% stannous fluoride gel on the gingival health of overdenture abutments, *J Prosth Dent* 48:23-26, 1982.

Ettinger RL, Jakobsen J: Caries: a problem in an overdenture population, *Community Dent Oral Epidemiol* 18:42-45, 1990.

Ettinger RL, Krell K: Endodontic problems in an overdenture population, *J Prosthet Dent* 59:459-462, 1988.

Ettinger RL, Olson RJ, Wefel JS et al: In vitro evaluation of topical fluorides for overdenture abutments, *J Prosthent Dent* 78:309-314, 1997.

Ettinger RL, Taylor TD, Scandrett FR: Treatment needs of overdenture patients in a longitudinal study: five-year results, *J Prosthet Dent* 52:532-537, 1984.

Geertman ME, Slagter AP, Van Waas MAJ et al: Comminution of food with mandibular implant-retained overdentures, *J Dent Res* 73:1858-1864, 1994.

Gotfredsen K: ITI-implants with overdentures: a prevention of bone loss in edentulous mandibles? *Int J Oral Maxillofac Implant* 5:135-139, 1990.

Griess M, Reilmann B, Chanavaz M: The multi-modal prosthetic treatment of mentally handicapped patients-necessity and challenge, *Eur J Prosthodont Rest Dent* 6:115-120, 1998.

Hussey DL, Linden GL: The efficacy of overdentures in clinical practice, *Br Dent J* 161:104-107, 1986.

Jensen ME, Kohout F: The effect of a fluoridated dentifrice on root and coronal caries in an older adult population, *J Amer Dent Assoc* 117:829-832, 1988

Johnson GK, Sivers JE: Periodontal considerations for overdentures, *J Am Dent Assoc* 114:468-471, 1987.

Kalk W, Käyser AF, Witter DJ: Needs for tooth replacement, *Int Dent J* 43:41-49, 1993.

Keltjens HMAM, Creugers TJ, Mulder J et al: Survival and retreatment need of abutment teeth in patients with overdentures: a retrospective study, *Community Dent Oral Epidemiol* 22:453-455, 1994.

Keltjens HMAM, Creugers TJ, Schaeken MJ et al: Effects of chlorhexidine-containing gel and varnish on abutment teeth in patients with overdentures, *J Dent Res* 71:1582-1586, 1992.

Keltjens HMAN, Creugers TJ, van't Hof MA et al: A 4-year clinical study on amalgam, resin composite and resin-modified glass ionomer cement restoration in overdenture abutments, *J Dent* 27:551-555, 1999.

Keltjens HMAM, Schaeken MJM, Van der Hoeven JS et al: Caries control in overdenture patients: 18-month evaluation on fluoride and chlorhexidine therapies, *Caries Res* 24:371-375, 1990.

Keltjens HMAM, Schaeken MJM, Van der Hoeven JS et al: Effects of chlorhexidine gel on periodontal health of abutment teeth in patients with overdentures, *Clin Oral Implants Resh* 2:71-74, 1991.

Lauciello FR, Ciancio SG: Overdenture therapy: a longitudinal report, *Int J Periodont Restor Dent* 5:62-71, 1985.

Mericske-Stern EA, Mericske-Stern R: Overdenture abutments and reduced periodontium in elderly patients: a retrospective study, *Schweig Monatssche Zahnmed* 103:1245-1251, 1993.

Mushimoto E: The role in masseter muscle activities of functionally elicited periodontal afferents from abutment teeth under overdentures, *J Oral Rehabil* 8:441-455, 1981.

Shaw MJ: Attachment retained overdentures: a report on their maintenance requirements, *J Oral Rehabil* 11:373-379, 1984.

Toolson LB, Smith DE: A five-year longitudinal study of patients treated with overdentures, *J Prosthet Dent* 49:749-756, 1983.

Toolson LB, Taylor TD: A 10-year study of a longitudinal recall of overdenture patients, *J Prosthet Dent* 62:179-181, 1989.

Van Waas MAJ, Jonkman REG, Kalk W et al: Differences two years after tooth extraction in mandibular bone reduction in patients treated with immediate overdentures or with immediate complete dentures, *J Dent Res* 72:1001-1004, 1993.

Van Waas MAJ, Kalk W, van Zetten BL et al: Treatment results with immediate overdentures: an evaluation of 4.5 years, *J Prosthet Dent* 76:153-157, 1996

Wenz HJ, Hertrampf K et al: Clinical longevity of removable partial dentures retained by telescopic crowns: outcome of the double crown with clearance fit, *Int J Prosthodont* 14:207-213, 2001.

Zarb GA, Schmitt A: The edentulous predicament, II: longitudinal effectiveness of implant supported overdentures, *J Am Dent Assoc* 127:59-65, 1996.

CHAPTER 11

Building Rapport: The Art of Communication in the Management of the Edentulous Predicament

Howard M. Landesman

There is an overwhelming amount of research data to confirm the enormous success achieved through incorporating implants for managing the edentulous predicament. Accordingly, it is easy to conclude that it is no longer necessary for the practitioner to spend countless hours with patients discussing how to adapt to a removable prosthesis.

The dentist can assume that the objectives of therapy for the edentulous patient—retention, stability, support, and esthetics—can be satisfied by the use of implants. In fact, those dentists who throughout their professional career declined to accept edentulous patients now use implants to achieve the same optimal result in much the same manner as restoring a partially edentulous space with a fixed prosthesis. It is a "dream come true" for the technically oriented dental professional. Is it therefore possible for the practitioner to declare victory in his or her need to communicate with patients, and can effective communication skills be minimized?

This author wishes to convey to the reader that communication is more than transmitting information. Communication is essential because it is an act of sharing. It is a participation in a relationship that involves a deep understanding of the patient. It includes an ability to listen, empathize, and ultimately establish a trusting doctor/patient relationship.

Dentists are taught to be masters in technical skills and to provide quick solutions to problems. However, many problems require "patience with patients" through effective communication techniques and listening to the needs of those who seek dental help. The purpose of this chapter is to sensitize the practicing dentist to the importance of the doctor/patient relationship by building rapport through effective communication skills.

In his acceptance speech for the Nobel Prize for literature, John Steinbeck noted that ". . . they are offered for increased and continuing knowledge of man and of his world—for understanding and communication. . . ." Steinbeck was, of course, referring to categories of the Nobel Prize; however, even a cursory reading reveals that his words are equally true of his art with its offering of human diversity. Communication and understanding are not the sole purview of the literary artist, however, but are necessary components of all human life from the individual to the familial, social, and professional.

For health care professionals, in particular, such skills are as essential as impeccable clinical technique because communication and understanding are tools of healing. Despite ever-increasing evidence that effective communicative skills are essential to the practice of even the most science-based and technical-helping professions, communication is often underemphasized in the curricula of medical, dental, and other health care colleges. This scarcity is no doubt attributable to the monumental proportions of biological and physical sciences to be absorbed from a weighty curriculum and the equally daunting task of acquiring and honing clinical skills to competency within a prescribed time frame. The unfortunate, but avoidable, result is too often uncomfortable and unproductive confrontations with those "problem patients" encountered by adept practitioners.

This chapter does not aspire to offer a crash course in effective communication. Rather it is designed to give an overview of the subject colored by the precepts of humanistic psychology. The aim is to evoke within the thoughtful clinician an appreciation of and interest in communicative skills by offering an elemental framework from which to practice, with the hope of inspiring further inquiry. To these ends, it addresses the following questions: (1) What is communication? (2) Why is it important? (3) What are the techniques of effective communication? and (4) What is the special significance of doctor/patient communication?

WHAT IS COMMUNICATION?

Scope

In the beginning was the word: the Latin *communicare*, which means to share, impart, and partake. The 1989 edition of the Oxford English Dictionary cites 10 definitions for the English verb *communicate* and 12 for the noun *communication*. These meanings are layered, like an onion, with, for example, high-tech informatics outermost and spiritual communion at the core. The multiplicity implies an organic universality.

Communication is ubiquitous—the thread that weaves an individual pattern into the universal web. In the arts, for example, a poet perceives the wind communicating with trees, and a deaf composer hears a symphony performed by the orchestra within his mind. In science, the biologist knows that the waters lead salmon to the spawning ground by means of subtle chemical messages and that migrating birds navigate by electromagnetic broadcasts from the Earth's poles. In quantum physics, an observer measuring a particle's position or momentum is aware that the very act of observation will influence the outcome. This interaction between subject and object implies something communicated; there is an informational transaction between bird and earth, between physicist and subatomic particle.

Among the multitude of communicators, human beings are by far the most complex, the most prolific, and the most likely to be misunderstood. Humankind alone consciously experiences the misunderstanding and separation, the alienation and longing, identified and defined by the existentialists. Martin Buber wrote the following: "Man wishes to be confirmed in his being by man and wishes to have presence in the being of the other . . . secretly and bashfully he watches for a Yes which allows him to be and which can come to him only from one human person to another."

Human beings are separated from other terrestrial species by consciousness, reflectiveness, and the ability to create and communicate through the medium of language. As Buber suggests, they are dependent on quality interactions with others for spiritual, mental, emotional, and physical well-being, for integration and affirmation. Communication is the medium through which individuals are able to transform a sense of alienation into the sense of self, of community, and of union.

The existential plea continues to be addressed by theologians and philosophers, by social scientists and psychologists, striving to create new paradigms rooted in a holistic view of the human being. Those helping professions oriented predominately by bioscience (medicine and dentistry, for example) are responding by incorporating new themes such as the "person centeredness" advocated by the humanistic psychologist Carl Rogers.

The scope of communication extends from the individual to society. If (1) the well-being of the person is related to the quality of his or her communication and (2) society is composed of persons, then (3) a measure of that society's health is the quality of its communications.

A Model of Communication

Communication among human beings is a transactional process used to impart or share ideas and other information. Its most commonly recognized vehicle is language.

If evolutionary theory is accepted, it becomes reasonable to suppose that since appearing on the planet, the genus *Homo* struggled to convey meaning to fellow primates through symbolic gestures, grunts, and other sounds that eventually led to assigning common significance to specific vocal symbols and language. By the time animals and crops were domesticated, in 9000 BCE, spoken language was the norm. Written language appeared in 3100 BCE in the form of pictographs, and the

Phoenicians invented alphabetical script about 1200 BCE.

Until the nineteenth century, Western culture subscribed to the notion that language was a gift from God and that human behavior was divinely directed. Consequently, any inquiry into communication or the other social sciences was based on religious dogma. In the twentieth century, speech communication studies were instituted because of an interest in politics and persuasion during World War II, not surprisingly because propaganda is an important weapon of war.

From the social unrest of the late twentieth century and with the emergence and increasing influence of humanistic psychology, interest in communication expanded to include the dynamics of the transaction among individual human beings. Results of current studies continue to reveal new information.

Figure 11-1 offers an animated model of communication, which consists of nouns and verbs, things and actions. The nouns are (1) participants, (2) messages, (3) channels or vehicles, (4) noise, and (5) environments. The verbs or actions are (1) encoding, (2) sending, (3) receiving, (4) decoding, and (5) responding.

Let us examine the model using the example of a man and a woman conversing. In this sample, the initiating participant or sender, the woman, experiences thoughts, feelings, or other mental images she wishes to convey to the man, or receiver. Before this intent can be actualized, the internal images must be translated or encoded into language. Although this process involves complex neurological activity, it usually occurs without effort or awareness. When, however, the woman pauses before speaking to seek a word appropriate to the internal experience she wishes to share, she is afforded an opportunity to become aware of the act of encoding.

Encoded, the message is sent, traveling by way of the selected channel or vehicle to the receiver. In the example dialogue, the channel is vocalized language. Other examples of channels include telephoning, writing a letter, or typing an e-mail message.

The man receives the message through the auditory sense. Neurons in his brain engage in translating the words into thoughts or other personally meaningful internal experience; he decodes the message. Even as the decoding process occurs, the man assumes the role of sender, responding to his

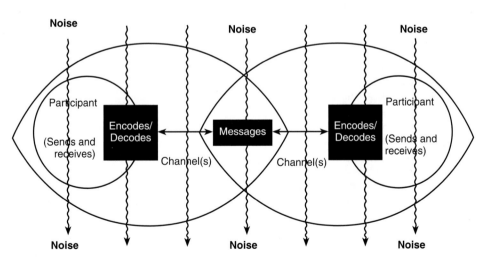

Figure 11-1   Communication is a continuous, irreversible, transactive process involving participants who occupy different but overlapping environments and are simultaneously senders and receivers of messages, many of which are distorted by external, physiological, and psychological noise. (From Adler RB, Towne N: *Looking out/looking in,* ed 5, New York, 1987, Holt, Rinehart and Winston.)

interpretation of the message and sending intentional or unintentional signals or verbal feedback or nonverbal messages to the woman, who becomes the receiver, then the sender as she responds. Participants send and receive messages simultaneously.

The purpose of the dialogue is to exchange information that is understood. Consequently, the outcome of successful communication is a consonance of the mental images of each participant. All communicative efforts do not succeed because this congruence is dependent on the participants' ability to express and interpret accurately.

These capabilities are affected by the two factors known to social scientists as *environment* and *noise*. Environment is twofold: in addition to the physical locale, it encompasses the internal environment or personal history each participant brings to the dialogue. As Figure 11-1 illustrates, internal environments overlap, but only to the extent that the participants' experience and knowledge are shared. If the English-speaking woman says "fork," the English-speaking man receives the correct mental image. If one or the other understands only French, the message is aborted by conflicting internal environments.

The major portion of each internal environment is not common to both participants. Differences in age, life experience, socioeconomic status, and interests, among many others, create varied internal environments that affect accurate communication. In the sample scenario, the quality and content of the interaction will be affected if the woman's internal environment is that of a chief executive officer of a major corporation and the man works as a day laborer. What if he is fascinated by baseball and she is uninterested in it, or she is an 80-year-old grandmother and he is a 40-year-old bachelor?

The second factor affecting the success of communication, noise, also has two aspects: the external and internal. The effects of external noise are obvious. Loud music, for example, hinders the communicants' ability to hear and, consequently, the quality of their vocal interaction.

Less obvious, internal noise is attributed to physiological and psychological factors. The former affects reception and stems from the participant's physiological condition (e.g., is he ill? is she hearing impaired?). The latter includes elements such as a participant's preoccupation, emotional state, and defensiveness. In short, anything happening in a participant's consciousness that distorts attention or distracts it from the communicative process is psychological noise and impinges on both the accuracy of expression and of reception. Adler and Towne define this transactional model of communication as "a continuous, irreversible, transactive process involving participants who occupy different but overlapping environments and are simultaneously senders and receivers of messages, many of which are distorted by external, physiological, and psychological noise."

WHY IS COMMUNICATION IMPORTANT?

"Man is the talking animal." Speech and gesture saturate every facet of human existence. Why are the only animals that obviously and continuously engage in symbol making so occupied with this complex activity? Since the first tribal group agreed that certain noises would represent specified external objects or internal states of being, *Homo sapiens* have used language as a tool for fulfilling needs.

Abraham Maslow set forth a hierarchical taxonomy of human needs: (1) life, (2) safety, (3) belongingness and affection, (4) respect and self-respect, and (5) self-actualization or the realization of individual potential. On the most basic level (need for life), the ability to communicate, to share sensory impressions, played a substantive role in the success of the species by expanding the limits of individual perception to include sensory data from others' nervous systems and by supporting the cooperative activity necessary to survival. People warned one another of danger by shouting words that meant "watch out"; they shared and passed to their progeny stores of knowledge to facilitate life. Part of a tribal repertoire that was shared by symbols included information such as what plants to eat or make soap or baskets from and what dangerous animals or places to avoid. Through verbal and nonverbal exchanges with immediate family, shamans, and chiefs, people learned and fulfilled needs for safety, inclusion, affection, and esteem. Because the basic needs (integral to all human beings since the origin of the species) have been satisfied over millennia through personal interaction with the external environment, human beings are dependent on their habitat and social structure—the components of this environment.

In contemporary Western society, practically speaking, communication continues to serve humanity by permitting people to tell the dentist which tooth hurts, to order a favorite meal, and to ask directions from a passerby. Psychologically, our interactions with others mold the sense of identity and the concept of self. Personal value and worth are equated by inclusion in the group, by esteem, and by recognition. People influence their social environment by conveying needs and desires that can then be fulfilled and, conversely, by responding to needs communicated by others.

Ultimately, as these basic, species-wide requirements are met, the need at the apex of the hierarchy enters awareness. Once thirst is quenched, hunger is sated, and the person is snug in the esteem of a group, there is an opportunity for the person to listen and respond to the unique aspects of the individual psyche. This urge to seek self-actualization is nourished by interaction with the internal environment and is characterized by personal uniqueness and independence. It reveals who we are and what we can offer to others. Thus symbol making can free the individual from total dependence on, and consequent attention to, the supporting external environment and allow the spontaneity, creativity, and holistic sense of belonging within the cosmos that distinguishes self-actualization.

The importance of communication lies in its functions. It is the nexus between human beings and the universal context, the external and internal environments that nourish. It enabled the cave dweller to thrive and proliferate; it makes possible the sophisticated business of contemporary life practically, socially, professionally, and spiritually.

WHAT ARE THE ELEMENTS OF EFFECTIVE COMMUNICATION?

Social science describes myriad elements that overlap psychological principles and combine to influence this art. These factors include dissonant and confirming relational climates, defensiveness, selective perception, social intelligence, self-image, genuineness, and empathy. An in-depth examination of the many psychosocial dynamics acting on the exchange of information among people is not possible within the confines of one chapter. Therefore this discussion is limited to an examination of some of the skills used by high-level communicators. Because communication is an art, the maestro becomes proficient in specific techniques that include self-awareness, genuineness, attending behavior, listening, empathy, self-disclosure, and deep understanding.

Self-awareness is the cornerstone of effective communicative skill. Abraham Maslow described the self as " . . . a kind of intrinsic nature which is very subtle, which is not necessarily conscious, which has to be sought for, and which has to be uncovered and then built upon, actualized, taught, educated." Carl Jung went so far as to suggest that full understanding of human nature may not be possible without a similarly intelligent species for comparison.

Human beings are singular among animals because their inner natures and consequent behaviors are not obviously and completely dictated by instinct. Other animals express their biological natures confidently without thought or attention. All cats, for example, hunt, groom themselves, and sleep copiously; they announce "catness" effortlessly and unconsciously. On the other hand, what defines humanity is an elusive and complex question. Knowing oneself is not an easy task.

Maslow postulates a three-faceted human nature: instincts common to the species; individual uniqueness; and a higher, spiritual or actualized self. To achieve the full, meaningful expression and understanding necessary for expert communication, one needs to be in touch with these three aspects and to be tuned in to the feelings, self-concept, ideas, attitudes, and values that make up the inner environment.

Because feelings are basic to all facets of the self and are not always articulated with ease, they can serve as a model for this discussion. Social roles and taboos, perceived risks, and difficulty of expression combine to suppress the sharing of emotions. Cultural admonitions such as "anger is bad" lead to misunderstanding and even fear of feelings. Unexpressed emotions are likely to be ignored and may ultimately be relegated to the realm of the unconscious. The inaccurate and often negative mythology surrounding the acceptance and expression of emotion can close the door on self-awareness. For example, people often believe that their feelings come from others. "You make me happy" or "You make me angry" are common expressions. However, emotions, which are based on thoughts in response to situations and circumstances, are generated from within. We are responsible for how we feel. Replacing "you" statements with "I" statements, such as "I feel happy (angry) when you call," conveys the notion of responsibility and defuses the threatening implication of emotional control from without and resultant dependency. In addition, "I" statements reduce the risk that the receiver will react defensively.

Another common myth is the belief that being aware of a feeling or expressing it is synonymous with acting on it. Acknowledging anger does not commit one to yelling and throwing things. Rather than a call to immediate action, a feeling is a message from the inner self, an invitation to self-awareness. How or if to act on it is subject to the discretion of the individual relative to the situation.

Awareness of physical reactions, followed by introspection, assists in recognizing and defining feelings. Strong emotions elicit rapid heartbeat, perspiring, and a shaky sensation—signs of both fear and anticipation. Subtle feelings are most frequently felt in the solar plexus or heart. A flutter or a pang here is a feeling message. Another way to tune in on feelings is to monitor inner dialogue. What are you saying to yourself: that you are worthy and capable? Feedback fr om others can also bring emotions and other unknown aspects of self into awareness and clarity. Genuineness, a quality of self-awareness, is expressed when communication accurately portrays inner experience. Sir Francis Bacon stated the essence of genuineness when he wrote, "Be so true to thyself as thou be not false to others." Communicators who display genuineness inspire trust by exhibiting specific behaviors. They are free from playing roles; that is to say, they do not disguise themselves or play games to manipulate others. They are aware and accepting of personal strengths and weaknesses; they tend not to react defensively; and they are open and consistent in thought, feeling, and behavior.

Attending behavior means paying attention to or being with another and communicating this nonverbally with physical proximity; relaxed, open posture; turning toward the partner; and eye contact. It includes sensitive interpretation of nonverbal messages. Attending behavior speaks of affection, respect, and esteem.

Listening, which is closely related to attending skills, is not merely hearing the other's words while waiting impatiently for a turn to talk. Effective listening means being committed to understanding another. It also requires attention to, and accurate decoding of, both verbal and nonverbal messages. Nonverbal language (proxemics, kinesics, and paralanguage) conveys feelings and attitudes. Proxemics is the study of the space between communicators; kinesics concerns postures and facial expressions; and paralanguage is the use of sounds other than words, such as pause, pitch, and intonation. Accurate decoding of nonverbal language requires understanding that its messages are ambiguous and sensitivity to their meaning within the context of the situation. Listening is essential for empathetic responding.

Empathy is the ability to see a situation from another's frame of reference and to understand and appreciate someone else's feelings, perceptions, or attitudes. It does not necessarily connote agreement but does relay respect or the belief that the other is a worthwhile and capable individual. It functions to promote and communicate understanding, laying the groundwork for trust. It is a difficult skill because personal feelings and attitudes must be exchanged for openness and acceptance.

Self-disclosure broadens the base of understanding and increases rapport. Persons reveal themselves continuously through nonverbal behavior, but people frequently feel that self-disclosure means confessing faults and weaknesses. It is more accurately a sharing of experience and resulting feelings within the context of an interaction. Self-disclosure promotes trust in a relationship and encourages others to respond in kind.

Deep understanding combines the skills of attending, listening, and empathy to perceive and communicate information about another that may be unknown or unclear to that person. For instance, if a friend shows a pattern of self-criticism, one could intuit a lack of self-esteem. If the hunch is accurate, expressing it appropriately to the friend can stimulate insight. Deep understanding lets people know how others perceive them, which aids self-awareness. To be effective, one must understand it as intuition and express observations tentatively as a personal perception, rather than as absolutes or judgments.

Self-awareness, genuineness, attending behavior, listening, empathy, self-disclosure, deep understanding, and other techniques used by high-level communicators are underscored by the principles of concrete expression, discipline, and person centeredness.

Concrete expression adds clarity and captures the meaning of experience. It is characterized by describing perceptions, rather than stating inferences. For instance, to say, "I see you are angry," is inferred from perceived behavior. Instead, saying, "Your face is red, jaw clenched, and you're yelling. It looks like you're angry," is concrete. Such statements check accuracy with a summation or question that encourages the other to clarify, refute, or acknowledge the truth of the observation.

Discipline implies that a communicator possesses a wide variety of communicative behaviors and the social intelligence to know which is most appropriate in a particular situation. A skilled communicator does not articulate emotions indiscriminately, but expresses those feelings and thoughts that suit the occasion and individuals involved. Discipline tempers self-disclosure and reduces risks involved in talking about feelings. A quality of discrimination, it boosts courage and confidence.

Person centeredness is an attitude that unites the attributes of communication in a matrix of respect and esteem. Based on acceptance, it is feeling that others are of value and worthy of attention by virtue of their humanness, and it fuels the communicator's skills.

SPECIAL SIGNIFICANCE OF DOCTOR/PATIENT COMMUNICATION

Dentists are in significant agreement that success or failure in fabricating dentures is not exclusively predicated on a patient's residual form, but on the patient's attitude toward the prosthesis as well. It has been noted that the body schema (the psychological image of the physical self) is heavily invested with emotional meaning. Significant changes in body image result in varying degrees of emotional instability that affect adaptive competence. Given time, most people can absorb the trauma involved in body changes and develop new adaptations to changed circumstance. Although it appears that most patients adapt to the denture-wearing experience, many do not. They comprise a group of people who are more emotionally fragile and who find that they cannot adjust to the physical change or else cannot cope with the tissues' complex adverse response to prostheses. The loss of teeth in both general patient groups, morphologically or emotionally maladaptive, is an obstacle they cannot surmount despite provision of excellent prosthetic replacements.

There are many critical elements to consider in managing the adaptive and maladaptive patients with dentures. The two most important are the behavior of the doctor and the iatrosedative interview, both of which involve a skillful handling of verbal and nonverbal communication.

THE DOCTOR'S BEHAVIOR

For the emotionally maladaptive patient with dentures, the sense of loss and the prospect of a life of discomfort and discontent are powerful feelings that may create a sense of hopelessness. The doctor, on whom the patient is dependent to make a significant change in his or her life, becomes an important figure. The patient must have an alliance with the doctor to cross over to adaptability. Consequently, there are strong feelings associated with such a doctor. They will be powerfully positive or negative, depending on the doctor's behavior and attitude. Those feelings will become "incorporated" into the denture. If the patient distrusts and resents that behavior and attitude, the resulting denture will be "contaminated" by those feelings. The consequence is rejection of the denture as well as the doctor. On the other hand, if the doctor creates a warm, trusting relationship, the goodwill becomes embedded in the denture, resulting in patient acceptance of it along with acceptance of the doctor. Trust and a warm relationship will override the mechanical and psychological factors that ordinarily create a maladaptive response to the prosthesis. The first few minutes of an interaction are critical in creating trust. A warm relationship should be generated at the greeting before the initial interview starts. This is accomplished by empathetic nonverbal and verbal communications, a skill some doctors have intuitively and others have acquired in learning the role of a doctor and dedicating themselves to mastering it.

Bowlby's research suggested that attachment behavior is among the instinctive responses that appear at birth. This response is biologically preset and therefore not dependent on prior learning. Attachment behavior is defined as "seeking and maintaining proximity to another individual." Attachment behavior is one set of instinctive responses that operates in the service of species survival. For the remainder of one's life, seeking and maintaining proximity to another individual will be a matter of central importance to existence.

All relationships of consequence include attachment behavior and trust if they are to effectively survive. When patients require the help of care providers (such as a dentist or physician) to care for their most prized possession (effective physical functioning), attachment and trust needs are activated. The way in which the clinician recognizes and responds to such needs can make a crucial difference in outcome.

A patient may view a prosthesis prescription with some degree of alarm. Others regard the prescription as the ultimate disaster because previous experiences have indicated a maladaptive response. This can be the case even when an initial prosthetic experience is an adaptive one, only to undergo a prognostic change as a result of a continuum of adverse morphological sequelae. Hopefully, latent attachment behaviors are stimulated as the patient looks for a caretaker who is confident, caring, sensitive, and supportive. The dentist who can satisfy these attachment behaviors is likely to have a considerable advantage in preparing a denture that is acceptable to the patient, both physically and emotionally.

THE IATROSEDATIVE INTERVIEW

The iatrosedative interview is designed to help dentists mobilize their resources so that they operate in the most efficient way to create the climate of involvement and trust indispensable to altering maladaptiveness.

The iatrosedative model is a systematic, pragmatic, "cherished" interaction used to reduce or eliminate most of the dental fears encountered in practice. The definition of iatrosedation is "making calm by the doctor's behavior." The word is a combination of *iatro* (doctor) and *sedation* (the act of making calm). The goal of iatrosedation is to create a relearning experience wherein the feelings originally learned will be unlearned and a new set of feelings generated as a consequence of the interaction between the doctor and the patient. The iatrosedative interview is composed of four parts: (1) recognizing and acknowledging the problem, (2) exploring and identifying the problem, (3) interpreting and explaining the problem, and (4) offering a solution to the problem.

RECOGNIZING AND ACKNOWLEDGING THE PROBLEM

The following example started as an open-ended initial interview. The patient immediately indicated that emotional factors were an important component of her request for a new denture. The doctor recognized this and acknowledged it by shifting into an iatrosedative interview. Had the doctor responded to the patient's opening statement by asking, "Well, what's the problem with your denture?" this would indicate nonacknowledgment and the desire to move the interview into the technical-anatomical arena.

Example

A 57-year-old woman has an appointment to see a dentist concerning her inability to adapt to dentures. Other than this information, he knows virtually nothing about this patient. When he enters the operatory, his first impression is of an attractive, petite woman who seems younger than her stated age. She is seated, her face is expressionless, and the doctor infers that she is anxious or depressed. He begins with a greeting and some brief pleasantries, the continues:

Doctor: What kind of difficulties are you having?

This type of opening permits the patient to tell her story in the way she wishes. An open-ended question often elicits the patient's dominant concern.

Patient: I am awfully unhappy. (Pauses.)

Doctor: Unhappy?

The patient chooses to convey her emotional uneasiness as a primary complaint. The doctor repeats the significant word, indicating to the patient that he wishes to hear more. This also conveys to the patient his willingness to consider psychological factors as well as physical ones. This is a first step toward developing a strong working relationship.

Patient: I have grown into an old woman long before my time. The day they removed my teeth, I felt I had aged 20 years.

The patient is defining one potentially major factor in her maladaptive response to dentures. There may be others, but she has provided the doctor with an important diagnostic clue.

Doctor: That feeling must be quite distressing. However, you do not give the appearance of an old woman.

The doctor again recognizes the emotional issues and indicates his acknowledgment by providing some support in making a realistic appraisal of her appearance. To go beyond this limited observation may make the patient feel that the doctor is trying to make her feel better but is in reality insincere. He will continue to explore the emotional factors.

Exploring the Problem

Patient: Yes, everyone tells me that, but that's not how I feel.

(She smiles for the first time.) And that is what counts. The doctor's observation has been validated, but she emphasizes that the only thing that matters is how she feels. Again, she underscores the importance of her inner state. The smile signals that her earlier tension is probably receding, and the doctor's style of communication is beginning to have an effect.

Doctor: I agree with you. In the end, it is only how we feel that really matters. (He waits to see if the patient will respond to this remark. She does not.) Aside from the fact that the loss of teeth and

the denture makes you feel like an old woman, how are you having difficulty with the denture?

The doctor agrees with this very realistic assessment by the patient, that is, the nature of one's feelings. No matter how fine the prosthesis, all is for naught if the patient feels miserable. He pauses to see whether the patient wants to add anything more to this point. If she does not, he now shifts his focus from the generalized emotional state to ask what specific complaints there are. This will lead shortly to an interruption to evaluate the oral condition and the dentures.

Patient: I find it very uncomfortable. It slips. I have a burning sensation. My food seems tasteless. But I wear the denture all the time despite the discomfort because I'm shocked by how I look without it.

She mentions physical difficulties but indicates that the discomfort is overridden by the dread of appearing aged. Even when she is talking about physical factors, the pull is always back to emotional distress.

Doctor: I see. Your emotional discomfort is even greater than your physical discomfort. But can you give me more details about the physical difficulties?

The doctor makes explicit what is implicit in the patient's observations. This is another way of indicating to the patient that she has been heard and understood. Because the doctor needs more information about physical difficulties, he shifts back to this area.

Patient: The denture seems to move in my mouth. When I chew, it seems to slip from side to side. The only time it doesn't is if I eat soft foods. But my gums seem to be sore all the time. Seems like a burning sensation. Spicy foods make it much worse. I have given up all alcohol because it now seems to burn my mouth.

The physical symptoms that accompany the emotional ones have now been clarified. In a brief period of time, the doctor has acquired some knowledge of the patient's emotional and physical symptoms. This seems an appropriate time to gather information about previous attempts to fabricate dentures.

Doctor: As I understand it, you've had several other dentures made.

Patient: Yes, none of them worked. Dr. L did two, and Dr. Y did the other two. Each one didn't work, and I don't know why. To be honest, I really don't know why I came to see you. If two perfectly competent specialists could not make one denture that I could wear comfortably, I really don't know what I could expect from you.

During the early part of the interview the patient appeared tense and anxious. Her emotional state has shifted to a more aggressive position in which the edge of sarcasm and challenge can be detected in both the tone of her voice and her words. The doctor has two possible responses. The first is to simply ask her why she requested a consultation despite her pessimism. A second possibility is to pick up on her thinly veiled anger. For the moment, the doctor chooses the first maneuver. However, he will keep in mind the anger and the challenge for another point in the interview.

Patient: Well, I haven't given up. Somehow I have the feeling that someone must have the answer to my problem. (Long pause.) You can help.

Her pessimism is not total, but the doctor must be cautious. What happened with the previous "very competent dentists" who she says failed, could also be the fate of this doctor.

Doctor: You are not very happy with the previous dentists you went to?

As noted earlier, her manner indicated anger at the previous practitioners. Is there something of consequence he can learn from her past encounters? The dentist puts the question directly to the patient in looking for the doctor-behavior link to maladaptiveness.

Patient: Each one was quite confident that he could make a denture that I would be happy with. I remember telling them that I hated wearing a denture, but they just said that they could make one that would fit.

The statement is at the crux of the matter because the previous dentists and this patient were talking at different levels. In each instance, the dentist was focused on fit, but she was talking about emotional fit.

Doctor: You were talking about your emotional distress mostly.

The doctor explicitly interprets what the patient has been telling him. At this point, he realizes that if there is any chance of success, he must hear both levels and set up a treatment plan that incorporates both aspects.

Patient: Exactly. I must say, doctor, I am somewhat encouraged because you seem to appreciate what I'm going through.

This is a positive movement in cementing a relationship. The doctor is now fully aware that attention to the psychological factors will be important because emotional concerns will always be present. This is an appropriate time to interrupt the interview and examine the dentures in the mouth to determine whether the burning and soreness of the tissues are related to any pathosis such as lesions or inflammation; whether there are any problems with inadequate ridges; and whether the denture is well fabricated. If all of these factors are within a satisfactory range, the question of nonacceptance maladaptiveness arises. (The oral examination revealed that the patient was wearing mandibular and maxillary dentures. The ridges were more than adequate in size and shape, and the dentures were well fabricated and adapted. No lesions were visible, and the mucosa was free of inflammation. The tentative diagnosis was "maladaptive Class II, unable to adapt psychologically and physically.")

Part of the exploration of the problem was stated in the previous portion of the interview. Some of the feelings were revealed, and the previous doctors' behaviors seemed to have been limited to technical aspects of the problem. It is probable that some of the patient's hostility may be related to these experiences. Further exploration is necessary to determine whether previous learning has conditioned the patient and, if so, how the recommendation of total tooth loss and complete dentures affected her. In addition, what were her feelings when the teeth were extracted and the dentures placed?

Doctor: You mentioned that you hate wearing dentures. Before we talk more about that, I'd like to ask if your parents or grandparents had dentures.

Patient: Yes, my mother did, and she suffered so with them. I remember as a child that she was unable to wear them and had several sets made. She was unable to eat with them, and I was frightened because I thought that this might happen to me. I am so much like my mother.

Doctor: That must have been terrifying to you as a child. Did you ever get used to the idea?

The doctor makes an understanding statement and follows it with a facilitative question to get more information about her feelings.

Patient: No, no, I never did. I've never forgotten the first time I saw my mother with her dentures out. Her face fell in—it was so shrunken that I panicked. And when the doctor told me that I had to have my teeth pulled, that horrible image flashed through my mind.

Doctor: Did you tell the doctor how you felt?

Patient: Yes, I did, but he didn't seem to care too much and repeatedly said that I should get used to it and get along just fine.

Doctor: How did that make you feel?

Patient: It made me angry and frightened me even more than I was.

This example represented the most common basis for maladaptiveness as a result of depression and anxiety related to toothlessness and dentures. Whatever feelings are expressed—the depression and fears of aging, loss of body integrity, femininity, masculinity, youthfulness, or beauty—may be the core around which the explanatory and interpretive segment of the interview will be built. The responses to the questions about the feelings associated with the doctors' behaviors will provide insight as to the probable effect on adaptiveness and also will be used in the explanatory interpretive phase of the interview.

INTERPRETING AND EXPLAINING THE PROBLEM

There is more than one way to use the information garnered by the exploration of the feelings and events preceding and following the advents of tooth loss and replacement by artificial substitutes. The doctor's style will determine this. The iatrosedative model is a vehicle to create mutual involvement by a combination of expressions of feelings of confidence and trust by both parties, the inclusion of the patient as participating in achieving success, and the use of the acquired information to suggest that feelings may affect success or failure in adapting to dentures. The sincerity of the tone the doctor brings to the situation probably will have a profound effect on the patient.

Doctor: I feel that you have suffered a great deal at the loss of your teeth. It was a terrible blow, and it seems as if you have never really gotten over it. You were frightened as a child when your mother lost her beautiful teeth and her face sunk in, making her look very old suddenly. You learned to fear dentures because of this, and because of this fear, you fought to avoid losing your teeth. Unfortunately, you did lose them. The dentures are a constant reminder of that loss, and your feelings may have an effect on your being able to accept them. You may have learned to fear having dentures because of your mother's unhappy experience. This may have set the stage for your not being able to accept dentures for yourself. Furthermore, the condition, or quantity and quality of your denture-supporting tissues, may not be optimal for an adaptive denture experience. A thorough examination will enable me to determine whether adjunctive methods of denture support, such as implants, may be required in your particular case. What do you think? Does this make sense to you?

Patient: Yes, that sounds possible. (The examination is carried out.)

Doctor: I want you to know your feelings can change, and with that change we can expect you to be able to wear the dentures with comfort. Your gums, although tender, are healthy. They are not infected, but the stress of your unhappiness with the dentures can and does affect the way your gums tolerate the pressure of the dentures. With your new dentures and a new set of feelings, it is likely that you will not have the soreness you have now. Let's talk about what we can do.

OFFERING A SOLUTION TO THE PROBLEM

Doctor: We will work together in making new dentures, and I am quite confident that, as we work things out together, your feelings about yourself and your dentures will change so that you will be able to live with them comfortably. It is going to take time to fabricate well-fitting dentures for you. It may take as long as 3 to 4 months.

Patient: Doctor, why so long?

Doctor: It takes time to make dentures that are well fitting, dentures that you will be able to function with properly, and I want you to know that the day I place the dentures in your mouth is in essence the first day of treatment. From that time on, I will be available to help make you comfortable.

Patient: I really appreciate that, doctor. The other doctors were so impatient with me and didn't seem to realize that I was suffering so much emotionally. I feel hopeful and would like us to start.

The patient is grateful that the dentist is willing to spend the necessary time to make a good set of dentures. The great advantage is that the patient will get involved with the dentist as the helping, understanding, and supportive figure, realizing that the dentist is extremely concerned about her long-term well-being. She also realizes that this dentist is maintaining an open-door policy. This continues the building process toward an ever-more-positive trusting relationship.

Doctor: Good. I am glad you feel optimistic about our working together. Let's set up an appointment to start treatment. I would like you to bring some photographs of you when you had your natural (own) teeth. They will be of great help to both of us in determining what your teeth looked like before and also help us in determining how to arrange the new teeth.

Patient: I'll start looking for them. I think I have wedding pictures when I had a big smile on my face.

The patient is now involved in the fabrication of the new dentures, which adds another increment of relationship building. If, after a considerable amount of treatment, it becomes apparent that the patient's adaptive ability is not increasing sufficiently, it would be in her best interest and the dentist's to address the issue. The timing is important here. This is a difficult issue. Most patients reject the initial recommendation of dealing directly with the emotional aspects of the problem. Nevertheless, with an understanding approach, coupled with a strong relationship, such as exists with this patient, an initial rejection may change to acceptance.

Doctor: I am very concerned about our progress at this point. We have done everything that we can together, and things are not going as well for you as they should. My experience has been that most patients would be able to manage these dentures. I am quite confident that the stress you have undergone in losing your teeth and struggling with the dentures is still affecting you. Therefore I think we should bring someone in to help us with those stress factors.

Patient: No, I don't think I want to do this. I don't think I am emotionally disturbed.

Doctor: I did not mean to imply that you were an emotionally disturbed individual. We all have specific areas in our lives that are upsetting, and for many people, accepting dentures is very difficult. I need to discuss this with you at this point because without solving this emotional aspect, we chance failure again, and you may be spending time, effort, and money unnecessarily. What I would like you to do is think about it because I sincerely believe it would be in your best interest. Perhaps share these thoughts with someone who is particularly close to you and whose opinion you value. Call me next week, and let us discuss this over the phone. One last point: next week you may still be opposed to my suggestion; however, in 4 or 6 months you may feel differently about it and want to explore my suggestion further. If that happens, feel free to call me, and I'll be happy to help you in any way I can.

There are a small percentage of patients who cannot adapt because they need their symptoms. Patients maintain symptoms for a variety of reasons. The symptoms may represent a way of rationalizing other problems and manipulating people, and they may be an exhibitionistic attempt to draw sympathy from other people. These symptoms may be absolutely necessary to maintain a precarious psychological equilibrium. If the patient cannot relinquish such symptoms, the dentist will fail.

SUMMARY

Some patients are maladaptive because morphological or neuromuscular deficits preclude successful wearing of dentures. Other patients are emotionally maladaptive. For these patients, effective verbal and nonverbal communication is significant in maximizing an effective doctor/patient relationship and minimizing the maladaptive response. Often, patients who seek technical advice relative to a prosthesis are seeking emotional solutions.

If the patient is maladaptive, the dentist cannot conclude that the patient is "neurotic" and beyond the dentist's capacity to help. The dentist who shuts off the patient's desire to share his or her feelings about wearing a denture is putting obstacles in the path to achieving a successful outcome. It is not the denture that is the problem; it is the patient's feelings about that particular denture.

A major aspect of the solution is the dentist's ability to first listen and gather information and then communicate effectively. In general, dentists are excellent communicators in the areas of physical and anatomical problems, but reticent when the issues are emotional.

The iatrosedative interview is an effective method of communication to help patients who are unable to adapt to dentures. It creates an indispensable trusting relationship in the process of determining the factors responsible for the problem and offers a solution.

It is worth reiterating that dentists become masters in technical skills and very adept at providing quick solutions to problems. However, many practice problems require significant commitment to "patience with patients." Effective techniques of communication remain an indispensable determinant of favorable management outcomes.

ACKNOWLEDGMENTS

The author is indebted to Dr. Nathan Friedman, who coauthored previous manuscripts that influenced this chapter's preparation. The significant assistance received from Ms. Virginia S. Watson also is gratefully acknowledged.

Bibliography

Adler RB, Towne N: *Looking out/looking in,* ed 5, New York, 1987, Holt, Rinehart and Winston.

Bowlby J: *Attachment and loss, vol 1,* p 194, New York, 1979, Basic Books.

Capra F: *The Tao of physics,* New York, 1984, Bantam Books.

Cassell EJ: *Talking with patients, vol 1, The theory of doctor-patient communication,* Cambridge, Mass, 1985, The MIT Press.

Covici P, editor: *The portable Steinbeck,* New York, 1971, The Viking Press.

Davis AJ: *Listening and responding,* St Louis, 1984, Mosby–Year Book.

Egbert L, Battit G, Turndoff H, et al: Value of the preoperative visit by an anesthetist, *JAMA* 195:553, 1963.

Friedman N: Iatrosedation: the treatment of fear in the dental patient, *J Dent Educ* 47:91-95, 1983.

Friedman N, Landesman HM, Wexler M: The influence of fear, anxiety, and depression on the patient's adaptive response to complete dentures, Part I. *J Prosthet Dent* 58:687-689, 1987; Part II. *J Prosthet Dent* 59:169-173, 1988.

Hayakawa SI: *Language in thought and action,* New York, 1972, Harcourt Brace Jovanovich.

Hirsch B, Levin B, Tiber N: The effect of patient involvement and esthetic preference on denture acceptance, *J Prosthet Dent* 28:127-132, 1972.

Kelly EW Jr: *Effective interpersonal communication: a manual for skill development,* Washington, DC, 1979, University Press of America.

Kirschenbaum H, Henderson VL: *Carl Rogers: dialoges,* Boston, 1989, Houghton Mifflin.

Lefer L, Pleasure MA, Rosenthal L: A psychiatric approach to the denture patient, *J Psychosom Res* 6:199-207, 1962.

Maslow AH: *Toward a psychology of being,* New York, 1968, D Van Nostrand.

The Oxford dictionary of quotations, ed 3, Oxford, 1980, Oxford University Press.

Pitts WC: Difficult denture patients: observation and hypothesis, *J Prosthet Dent* 53:532-534, 1985.

Rogers C: *A way of being,* Boston, 1980, Houghton Mifflin.

Welch ID, Tate GA, Richards F, editors: *Humanistic psychology: a source book,* Buffalo, NY, 1978, Prometheus Books.

Zunin L: *Contact: the first four minutes,* p 194, New York, 1979, Basic Books.

CHAPTER 12

Materials Prescribed in the Management of Edentulous Patients

Randa R. Diwan

The selection of materials is based on a reconciliation of their biocompatibility, optimum physical and mechanical properties and, where indicated, their superior esthetic qualities. A fundamental knowledge of the properties, as well as the limitations of dental materials is crucial, so that dentists can carefully manipulate those materials to the best benefit of the patient. This is further underscored by the fact that none of the materials used in dentistry or medicine are totally inert. Biodegradation of materials in the oral environment has been frequently related to chemical or mechanical factors prevailing in the oral cavity such as bacteria, saliva, and other oral fluids.

The aim of this chapter is to present a synthesis of key information regarding biomaterials prescribed in the management of the edentulous patient. It is organized in five sections: denture base materials, denture teeth materials, lining materials, denture cleansers, and cast metal alloys.

Fulfilling the requirements listed in Box 12-1 may be a challenge for dental practitioners, considering the number of new materials available on the dental market, often with unproven claims of superiority in biocompatibility, physical, and mechanical properties. The clinical efficiency of all prosthodontic materials should essentially be based on long-term, large-scale clinical trials, as well as strict adherence to internationally recognized specifications and standards that gauge the quality and properties of those materials to ensure maximum safety, durability, and effectiveness.

DENTURE BASE MATERIALS

Over the years a variety of materials have been used for the fabrication of denture bases. The most commonly used materials are polymers such as polymethylmethacrylate (PMMA) or acrylic resins. Popularity of PMMA accrues from the fact that the material exhibits favorable working characteristics, has acceptable physical mechanical and esthetic properties, and is easy to fabricate with inexpensive equipment. However, as with all other known denture base materials, acrylic resin has its inherent limitations and does not fulfill all the requirements of a hypothetically ideal denture base material (Box 12-2).

The polymerization process of PMMA involves the conversion of low molecular weight monomers to high molecular weight polymers. Denture base resins are formed by a process of additional polymerization through the release of free radicals. The reaction passes through three stages, namely, activation and initiation, propagation, and finally, termination. An initiator like benzyl peroxide yields free radicals, which sets off the chain reaction. Activation of the initiator can be achieved through the application of heat (heat-activated or cured PMMA), chemicals, such as tertiary amines (chemically activated PMMA), or by other sources of energy, such as visible light-activated (VLC) urethane dimethacrylate, or through electromagnetic radiation such as in the case of microwave-activated resins.

Copolymers are formed when monomers of two or more compatible types are joined. The vast

---

Box 12-1

General Requirements of Biomaterials for Edentulous Patients

1. The material must be biocompatible:
   No harmful effects on the oral tissues
   Nontoxic, nonirritant
   Nonallergenic, noncarcinogenic
2. The material must fulfill clinical objectives:
   Optimum physical and mechanical properties:
   Adequate hardness, rigidity, strength
   High abrasion resistance
   Adequate thermal properties
   Adequate viscoelastic properties
   Chemical nondegradability
   Superior esthetic properties
   High cleansability
   Easy to fabricate and manipulate
   Readily available and economical to use
   Permits easy and inexpensive maintenance
   such as repairs and additions

Box 12-2

Requirements of an Ideal Denture Base

Biocompatible (nontoxic, nonirritant)
Adequate physical and mechanical properties:
   High flexural and impact strength
   High modulus of elasticity for better rigidity
   Long fatigue life
   High abrasion resistance
   High craze resistance
   High creep resistance
   High thermal conductivity
   Low density
   Low solubility and sorption of oral fluids
   Softening temperature higher than that of
      oral fluids and food
   Dimensionally stable and accurate
Superior esthetics and color stability
Radiopacity
Good adhesion with denture teeth and liners
Ease of fabrication with minimum expenses
Easily repaired if fractured
Readily cleansable

---

majority of today's dentures are made of heat-activated PMMA and copolymers, such as rubber reinforced PMMA. The latter is a high-impact acrylic resin, where the PMMA forms graft copolymers with polystyrene-butadiene rubber. The rubber inclusions significantly improve impact strength of the polymerized denture base.

Polymers with chemical bonds between different chains are termed *cross-linked*. This process affects physical properties of the polymer. In the case of PMMA, it increases rigidity as well as craze resistance, which is the tendency of resins to form minute surface cracks, and reduces the resin's solubility in organic solvents. The chemical composition of frequently used denture base resins is listed in Box 12-3.

Box 12-3

Chemical Composition of Denture Base Resins

Heat-Activated PMMA

Powder-liquid system
Powder: prepolymerized spheres of PMMA
   Initiator: benzoyl peroxide (~0.5%)
   Pigments and dyed synthetic fibers
Liquid: methyl methacrylate monomer
   Inhibitor: hydroquinone (traces)
   Cross-linking agent: ethylene glycol dimetha-
      crylate (~10%)
   Activator-NN-dimethyl-p-toluidine[*]

Microwave-Activated PMMA

Powder-liquid system
Similar to heat-activated PMMA: with slight
   modifications to accommodate the microwave activation procedure

Light-Activated Resins (single component, premixed composite sheets and ropes)

Matrix: urethane dimethacrylate, microfine silica
Filler: acrylic resin beads
Photoinitiator: camphoroquine-amine

[*]Only in chemically activated resins.
PMMA, Polymethylmethacrylate.

Technical Considerations and Properties of Denture Base Resins

Heat-Activated PMMA These resins are commonly processed in a brass flask using a compression-molding technique (dough technique). The polymer and monomer are mixed in the proper ratio of 3:1 by volume or 2.5:1 by weight. The mixed material goes through four stages: first, a wet, sandlike stage; second, a tacky fibrous stage as the polymer dissolves in the monomer; third, a smooth, doughlike stage, suitable for packing into a mold; and fourth, a stiff, rubberlike stage. Dough formation is assisted by internal plasticizers chemically attached to the polymer beads that locally softens them and facilitates monomer diffusion.

After wax elimination, the dough is packed in a gypsum mold. The flasks are placed, under pressure, in a time-temperature controlled water bath to initiate polymerization of the resin.

The polymerization reaction is exothermic in nature and should be carefully controlled to avoid a marked increase in temperature, which may exceed the boiling point of unreacted monomer (100.8°C), leading to denture porosity. Gaseous porosity due to rapid heating and monomer evaporation appears as fine, uniform spherical pores, localized more often in the thicker portions of the denture.

Inadequate pressure during flask closure, an insufficient amount of dough present on packing of the mold, or improper mixing of powder/liquid components may also result in denture porosity. The resulting porosity will inevitably compromise the physical properties and denture esthetics and may promote the accumulation of denture deposits, which could adversely affect the health of the denture-supporting tissues.

In general, heat-activated acrylic resins are polymerized by placing the flasks in a constant-temperature water bath at 74°C (165°F) for 8 hours or longer with or without a 2- to 3-hour terminal boil at 100°C. A shorter cycle involves processing the resin at 74°C for approximately 2 hours then boiling at 100°C for 1 hour or longer.

Rapid-cure type resins have been recently introduced in the market. The resins are polymerized by rapidly heating the packed dough in boiling water for 20 minutes. The materials are hybrid acrylics, in which activation of the polymerization reaction is carried out through both chemical and heat activators, allowing rapid polymerization without porosity.

It should be noted, however, that processing at temperatures that are too low or for shorter times increases the residual monomer content in the processed denture base. Excess residual monomer in the polymerized resin base could lead to tissue irritation, sensitivity, or even allergic reactions in some patients. The plasticizing effects of excess monomer could also adversely affect the properties and dimensional stability of the denture. Fortunately, allergies to residual monomer are relatively rare, and most patients are well able to tolerate the 0.2% to 0.5 % of residual monomer that often remains, even in a properly polymerized base.

After the polymerization procedure, the denture flasks are cooled slowly to room temperature to allow adequate release of internal stresses and thus minimize warpage of the bases. Deflasking then follows and should be done carefully to avoid fracture or flexing of the dentures.

The popularity and relative simplicity of the compression molding technique are usually overshadowed by the high-processing stresses that are induced in the resins during polymerization. These stresses result from various factors. First, polymerization shrinkage, which occurs as polymer chains are formed, accounts for a volumetric shrinkage of about 7%. Second, thermal shrinkage follows as the resin cools. In addition, differences in thermal contraction of the resin and gypsum mold collectively yield stresses in the resin. It is tempting to assume that the release of such cumulative stresses may give rise to dimensional changes and inaccuracies in the fit of the denture base. However, these changes have been found to be clinically insignificant in the fit of heat-activated acrylic resin denture bases, and in most instances they do not cause discomfort to the patient. Occlusal errors that are commonly encountered after processing are effectively corrected and the predetermined vertical dimension of occlusion restored through routine laboratory remount procedures.

Denture base resins are also subjected to a variety of stresses during function. Midline fractures of dentures during function have been considered a flexural fatigue failure because of cyclic deformation of the base during function. This is usually more evident in ill-fitting or poorly designed dentures. Impact fracture, on the other hand, may result from accidental dropping of the dentures by the patients. Denture fractures or distortions may be expected considering the far-from-ideal mechanical properties of conventional unmodified heat-activated resins, particularly their inferior tensile, flexural, and impact strength as well as poor fatigue resistance.

Other physical and biological considerations of conventional heat-activated resins include the following points:

1. Denture bases undergo water absorption, mostly through diffusion, which results in linear expansion. The resulting expansion has been found to offset the thermal shrinkage that occurs during polymerization. Similarly, conventional acrylic base resins do dry out, causing shrinkage. Patients are routinely cautioned to store their dentures in water when out of the mouth.

2. Acrylic resin dentures have a low thermal conductivity, portrayed as a substantial decrease of thermal stimulation of the patient's oral tissues under the denture base. This could be a source of inconvenience, particularly to first-time denture wearers.

3. Denture base resins deform under load with time. This viscoelastic property, termed *creep*, is minimized, but not entirely eliminated, especially under high stresses, by the addition of cross-linking agents.

4. One of the main advantages of heat-activated resins is their excellent chemical bond with acrylic resin denture teeth. This is a result of the increased rate of diffusion of monomers into polymers at the high temperatures involved in processing, leading to the formation of chemical welts between the teeth and the bases. On the contrary, adhesion of acrylic polymers to metal and untreated porcelain is weak and can only be effectively accomplished through mechanical retention. Treatment of the ridge lap area of porcelain teeth with organosilane compounds and the use of adhesive primers to chemically bond acrylic resin to metal

alloys has been advocated to overcome this problem.

5. Biocompatibility of acrylic resin in the surrounding oral environment is considered an attribute to the material. However, water absorption of the bases is usually associated with the ability of certain organisms to colonize the fitting surface of the denture (e.g., *Candida albicans)*, particularly in association with poor denture hygiene. Frequent cleansing and soaking the dentures in chemical cleansers is usually sufficient to minimize this problem. The use of chlorhexidine gluconate has been recommended to effectively eliminate *C. albicans*, as well as treating the resin surface with nystatin.

Heat-activated PMMA is less frequently processed using an injection-molding technique. The resin mix is injected into a closed, sprued flask under continuous pressure. The resulting dentures usually demonstrate minimum polymerization shrinkage. Other plastics that are injection molded include polycarbonates, nylon, and polyvinyl acrylics. The latter plastics could be considered in patients with a confirmed allergy to the methacrylate monomer. However, high capital costs and sensitivity of the technique limit its application for denture fabrication.

Chemically Activated Resins

These resins are often referred to as *cold-curing, self-curing,* or *autopolymerizing* resins. As pointed out earlier, the methyl methacrylate monomer contains a chemical initiator, a tertiary amine, which activates the polymerization process without the need of any heat. Chemically activated resins are much less frequently used for denture fabrication as compared with the heat-activated resins. Processing of the resins could be carried out by compression molding in a flask, where initial hardening of the resin occurs within 30 minutes of flask closure. The resins could also be used to produce dentures using a *pour* or *fluid resin technique.* The principal difference in chemical composition of the resins used in this technique is the smaller size of the powder particles necessary to ensure fluidity of the mix.

The pour technique involves pouring the fluid mix into a sprued mold made of a reversible hydrocolloid material (agar agar). The flask is placed under pressure at room temperature or at a slightly higher temperature (45°C). Polymerization is completed in about 30 to 45 minutes. The technique is obviously simpler and cleaner with regard to flasking and deflasking but is prone to problems, such as shifting of denture teeth during pouring of the acrylic into the mold. The use of a hydroflask increases atmospheric pressure around the mold, minimizing air inclusions in the mix, thus yielding a denser resin base.

In comparison with heat-activated resins, chemically activated resins do, in general, have a higher residual monomer content of 3% to 5%. Polymerization in those resins is never as complete as in heat-activated resins. This results in inferior mechanical properties and dramatically compromises biocompatibility of the denture bases. The materials exhibit higher solubility; they have inferior color stability, due to oxidation of the amine accelerator; and creep rates are usually high, especially under increased stresses. However, chemically activated resins, particularly when compression molded, display less shrinkage on polymerization than their heat-activated counterparts, leading to greater dimensional accuracy. This could be attributed to a reduction in the residual stresses induced during the processing cycle.

Microwave-Activated Resins

Microwaves are electromagnetic waves in the megahertz frequency range that have been recently advocated to activate the polymerization process of acrylic resin base. The procedure was greatly simplified in 1983, with the introduction of a special glass fiber–reinforced plastic flask, suitable for use in a microwave oven. The acrylic resin is mixed in the proper powder/liquid ratios, and the composition of the liquid monomer is usually modified to control the boiling of monomer, in a very short curing cycle of about 3 minutes. In this technique heat is rapidly generated within the monomer as a result of numerous rapid intermolecular collisions. As the degree of polymerization increases, monomer content decreases proportionally, and as energy is further absorbed, the remaining monomer

is converted into a polymer. Careful control of the time and wattage of the oven is essential to yield porous-free resins and still ensure complete polymerization. The technique is more time efficient and cleaner than the conventional technique. However, its limitations are related due to its cost-effectiveness for a wide production base, particularly because of high equipment expenses and fragility of the plastic flasks, which are easily prone to damage. Microwave-activated resins have comparable physical and mechanical properties to conventionally heat-activated resins, with claims of even greater dimensional stability. This could be attributed to the excellent temperature control in the resin and equal distribution of temperature throughout the resin and gypsum mold, respectively.

Light-Activated Resin Bases

Light-activated resins, also termed VLC resins, are copolymers of urethane dimethacrylate and an acrylic resin copolymer along with microfine silica fillers. The polymerization process is activated by placing the premixed, moldable resin on the master cast on a rotating table, in a light chamber and exposing it to high intensity visible light of 400 to 500 nm, for an appropriate period of about 10 minutes. In this technique, after an initial cure of the resin base, the teeth are repositioned on the base using a light-cured template, and contouring is carried out, followed by a final cure in the light chamber. The resin is coated with a nonreactive barrier compound to prevent oxygen inhibition of the polymerization process. Light-activated resins contain no methacrylate monomer and could be readily used in monomer-sensitive patients. The produced resin contains high molecular weight oligomers, which results in smaller polymerization shrinkage, reportedly half that of conventional resins. The physical and mechanical properties of the resins compare well with conventional heat-activated resins, particularly in regard to impact strength and hardness. Some studies, however, have reported lower elastic moduli and slightly lower flexural strength for VLC resins, which could increase deformation of the dentures during function. The inferior bond strength of VLC resins to resin denture teeth has been a main concern;

however, significant improvement of this bond has been achieved with the use of bonding agents.

Modified Acrylic Resin Bases

For the prevention of shortcomings in the mechanical properties of conventional heat-activated acrylic resins, modifications have been introduced into the structure of the polymers to improve mechanical properties, such as flexural, tensile, and impact strengths, as well as fatigue resistance. Chemical modifications to produce graft copolymer resins, through the incorporation of a rubber phase, have been attempted. The resulting resin consists of a matrix of PMMA in which is dispersed an interpenetrating network (IPN) of rubber and PMMA. The resins absorb more energy at higher strain rates before fracture occurs, resulting in a significant increase in impact strength. However, this modification has been shown to be accompanied by a reduction in the stiffness or rigidity of the resins.

Rubber reinforcement of PMMA is a successful alternative to conventional resins. However, the high cost of the material restricts its routine use for denture fabrication. Mechanical reinforcement of acrylics has also been attempted through the inclusion of fibers such as glass, carbon, aramid (Kevlar) fibers, nylon and ultra high modulus polyethylene (UHMPE) polymers, as well as metal inserts (wires, plates, fillers). The resulting resins have demonstrated an increase in impact and flexural strength, as well as a significant improvement in fatigue resistance, effectively minimizing denture fractures.

Various problems have been associated with this route of reinforcement of PMMA resins. This includes tissue irritation from protruding glass fibers, poor esthetics associated with dark carbon fibers (black), or straw-colored Kevlar fibers. Other limitations relate to an increase in production time, difficulties in handling, precise orientation, placement, or bonding of the fibers within the resin. In the case of metal inserts, failure due to stress concentration around the embedded inserts has been reported.

The availability and quality of fibers for denture reinforcement are improving very quickly with great promises for better results in the near future. Attempts to improve radiopacity of the denture bases have been carried out to facilitate the detection of fragments of resin bases that may be accidentally ingested or, more seriously, inhaled by the patient. These attempts included the use of metal inserts, radiopaque salts and fillers, and organometallic compounds. Examples are barium sulphate (8% wt), bismuth (10% to 15% concentrations), halogen-containing copolymers, or additives such as 2,3-dibromopropyl methacrylate. Unfortunately, many of those attempts have been accompanied by adverse effects on the esthetics and strength of the denture base resins or, more seriously, cytotoxic effects that may endanger the patient. Table 12-1 provides a summary of commonly used denture base resins, their processing techniques, and properties.

MATERIALS USED IN THE FABRICATION OF PROSTHETIC DENTURE TEETH

Prosthetic or denture teeth are produced in a variety of molds and shades and are available as vacuum-fired porcelain, acrylic resins, modified acrylic, and composite resins. In general, teeth used in the fabrication of dentures should demonstrate optimum physical and mechanical properties to withstand rigorous demands of masticatory functions, such as chewing, biting, shearing, or crushing of food, and simultaneously exhibit superior esthetics, particularly in the anterior region of the mouth (Box 12-4).

Acrylic Resin Teeth

Acrylic resin (PMMA) denture teeth are manufactured either by the compression-molded dough technique or by injection molding. Some teeth contain an IPN. Such resins exhibit low creep and flow rates, and minimum dissolution in solvents, which is an important requirement for resin teeth. Most resin teeth are highly cross-linked in the coronal portion to provide resistance to crazing, but with little or slight cross-linking in the gingival or body portion to improve bond to the denture base. A significant advantage of acrylic resin teeth is that they bond chemically to the denture base, provided

Table 12-1
Processing Techniques and Properties of Denture Base Resins

Denture Base Resin	Processing Technique/ Method of Activation	Advantages	Disadvantages
Conventional heat-activated PMMA	Compression-molded/dough technique Flask and gypsum mold Water bath short or long cycles	Good biocompatibility Low density Good esthetics, color stability, surface finish Insoluble in oral fluids Chemical bond with resin teeth Acceptable dimensional stability Easily repaired/modified Easy to fabricate/low cost	Low thermal conductivity Low impact and flexural strengths Short fatigue life Low abrasion resistance Radiolucent
Heat-activated rubber reinforced PMMA	Compression molded Water bath short or long cycles	High impact strength	Reduced stiffness/rigidity More expensive than conventional PMMA
Heat-activated fiber reinforced PMMA	Compression molded Water bath short or long cycles	High impact and flexural strengths Good fatigue resistance High stiffness	Unesthetic color of Carbon and Kevlar fibers Inferior surface finish Increased production time Difficulty in handling and placement of fibers
Chemically activated PMMA	Compression-molded/dough or pour/fluid resin Agar mold Chemically activated	Dimensionally accurate Pour resins easy to deflask Processing is less time-consuming	High residual monomer content High creep rates Reduced stiffness Lower impact/fatigue strength Color instability High solubility Tooth movement/tooth bond failures in pour resins
Microwave-activated PMMA	Compression molded Fiber reinforced plastic flask Microwave energy in an oven at 500-600 W Curing time as short as 3 minutes	Short processing time Processing technique easy/clean Dimensional accuracy Comparable physical/ mechanical properties to conventionally processed resins	High capital cost Flasks easily fractures/ limited serviceability Porosity if time/temperature of oven not controlled
Light-activated PMMA	No flask required High intensity visible light (wavelength 400-500 nm) In special light chamber Curing time 10 minutes	Simple processing technique Short processing time No methacrylate monomer Low polymerization shrinkage Improved fit Comparable impact strength and hardness to conventionally processed resins	High capital cost Inferior bond to resin denture Decreased elastic teeth modulus Slightly lower flexural strength

PMMA, Polymethylmethacrylate.

that the tooth surface was thoroughly dewaxed. This in turn facilitates grinding of the teeth to accommodate the available interocclusal spaces and allows reshaping of the teeth to fit small spaces for esthetic purposes, without fear of destroying the bond to the base. The use of adhesive promoters such as (4-methacryloxyethyl trimellitic anhydride [4-META]) has been recently advocated to facilitate bonding of highly cross-linked acrylic teeth to resin bases. Adhesive resin cements containing this compound have also been used to facilitate bonding of resin bases to base metal alloys.

The esthetic qualities of acrylic resin teeth have improved significantly over the years, and clinically they are quite acceptable. The teeth are prepared in layers of different shades with lighter shades towards the incisal or occlusal portions, thus increasing their translucency. Both acrylic and porcelain teeth can also be characterized with surface stains to enhance their natural appearance. A specifically great advantage of acrylic resin teeth is the ease of their occlusal reshaping to achieve the desired articulation needed for various occlusal schemes. Resin teeth have high resiliency and are tougher than porcelain teeth, making them less liable to fracture or chipping on impact. Unfortunately, they exhibit inferior abrasion resistance, which could lead to alteration in the vertical

dimension of occlusion, particularly in long-time denture wearers. However, newer, chemically modified acrylic resin teeth are more wear resistant and stain much less than earlier-used resin teeth.

Composite resin teeth have also been introduced as a suitable material for fabrication of denture teeth. They contain microfine filler particles of silica and have demonstrated wear properties that are clinically acceptable. Continued improvements in the polymer structure may facilitate its widespread use by most clinicians in the future.

Porcelain is another material that has been quite popular for fabrication of denture teeth for many years. Porcelain teeth, in general, exhibit superior esthetic qualities, excellent color stability, and high abrasion resistance. They are mechanically attached to resin bases by means of pins or diatoric holes, and this attachment precludes their ability to be ground, or reshaped, to fit limited interarch spaces. Bonding of porcelain teeth to acrylic bases has been recently enhanced by a combination of micromechanical retention and chemical bonding. This is carried out by treating the ridge lap area of the tooth with an etchant such as hydrofluoric acid gel, followed by a silane-coupling agent.

Another limitation of porcelain teeth includes their ability to cause significant wear of opposing enamel and metallic occlusal surfaces. The teeth are quite brittle, can easily crack or chip on impact, and are difficult to grind for occlusal adjustments because they lose their surface glaze and repolishing is quite difficult. Porcelain teeth produce noisy clicking sounds on contact with each other. However, the teeth are not without merits. They are dimensionally stable; are hard, in comparison with the softer acrylic resins; exhibit no permanent deformation under occlusal loading; and are insoluble in oral fluids and in most organic solvents.

In the selection of denture teeth for complete dentures, and considering the recently mentioned properties of the various materials, the dentist should avoid combining posterior resin teeth with porcelain anterior teeth. The significant differences in abrasion resistances in both materials, with acrylic resin wearing more rapidly than porcelain, would potentially create destructive occlusal forces in the anterior region of the mouth. Table 12-2 compares the properties of acrylic and porcelain teeth.

DENTURE-LINING MATERIALS

Denture-lining materials are used to refit the surfaces of complete dentures and to help condition traumatized tissues, providing an interim or permanent cushionlike effect. These materials are generally classified into the following types:

1. Short-term soft liners (tissue conditioners)
2. Long-term soft liners

Soft denture liners are polymers with a glass transition temperature (T_g) that is below that of mouth temperature. The T_g is the temperature at which a polymer ceases to be glossy and brittle and changes to a rubberlike form. The soft resilient nature of these materials inside the mouth provides them with a whole range of diagnostic, adjunctive, and treatment purposes in the management of edentulous patients.

Short-Term Soft Liners (Tissue Conditioners)

These materials are soft, resilient materials commonly used as temporary liners and have been widely used in dentistry to manage a multitude of patient problems and for various clinical applications (Box 12-5).

Tissue conditioners are provided mostly as a powder/liquid system, but preformed sheets of acrylic gels are also available. The powder contains a polymer, a polyethylmethacrylate (PEMA), or its copolymers, and the liquid contains a mixture of ethyl alcohol (solvent) and an aromatic ester (dibutyl phthalate), which acts as a plasticizer that lowers the T_g of the polymer rendering it a soft gel. The gelation of tissue conditioners is a physical process, which is devoid of any chemical reaction or any monomeric substances that could cause tissue irritation. Upon mixing the powder and

Table 12-2
Advantages and Disadvantages of Acrylic Resin and Porcelain Teeth

Property	Acrylic Resin Teeth	Porcelain Teeth
Bond with resin base	Chemical bond	Mechanical via pins or diatoric holes
Mechanical properties	Less brittle than porcelain High resilience and toughness	Very brittle/chipping occurs on impact
Solubility in oral fluids and dimensional changes	Insoluble; some dimensional changes	Insoluble; inert in oral fluids; no dimensional changes
Maintenance of vertical dimension (VDO)	Poor abrasion resistance; wear is significant, wear can result in reduced VDO	Excellent abrasion resistance; hard, wear is insignificant; VDO tends to be maintained
Effect on opposing occlusion	Can oppose natural teeth or metallic occlusal surfaces	Abrades opposing tooth enamel/ metallic surfaces
Tooth contouring/occlusal adjustment/repolishing	Relatively easy	Difficult, may result in loss of surface glaze
Grinding of ridge lap areas	Easy to grind without compromising tooth-resin bond	Difficult to grind; compromises tooth-resin bond; difficult to position or retain in limited interarch spaces
Esthetic properties	Excellent, can be characterized as required	Excellent, can be characterized as required
Clicking sounds	None on contact with opposing teeth	Noisy, clicking occurs with opposing porcelain teeth

Box 12-5

Indications for Short-Term Soft Liners/Tissue Conditioners

1. Treatment and conditioning of abused/irritated denture supporting tissues lining ill-fitting dentures allows the tissues to rest and regain their health prior to impression making for new dentures
2. For provisional adjunctive/diagnostic purposes such as recovery of the vertical dimension of occlusion and correcting occlusion of old prosthesis; also to assess the necessity of using a permanent soft liner for patients with chronic pain or soreness associated with denture wearing
3. Temporary relining of immediate dentures/immediate surgical splints
4. Relining cleft palate speech aids
5. Tissue-conditioning during implant healing
6. Functional impression materials

formulated to remain soft and resilient for longer periods. The mechanism of action of tissue conditioners is related to their specific viscoelastic properties, which is a combination of both viscous fluid and elastic solid behavior. Viscous behavior allows adaptation of the gel to the inflamed/irritated mucosa underlying the denture, which greatly improves the fit of the denture. After an initial easy flow, the gel becomes highly viscous, and its flow thereafter is affected by the magnitude of the load applied on the denture as well as its duration. This consequently affects stress distribution in the mucosa. Concurrently, under cyclic/intermittent loading such as during chewing, the material demonstrates a time-dependent elastic behavior that allows it to recover initial deformation, absorbing impact forces and cushioning the underlying tissues. Thus viscoelastic and elastic properties of tissue conditioners result in an even distribution of load on the underlying mucosa and a cushioning of cyclic forces of mastication. This in turn allows the traumatized mucosa to recover, particularly under an ill-fitting denture.

Short-term soft liners can also be used as functional impression materials. Requirements for this clinical application differ slightly from those required for tissue conditioning.

For traumatized tissues to be effectively conditioned, a tissue conditioner should demonstrate adequate flow and elastic properties. Maintenance of this viscoelastic behavior is the key to its clinical success. A functional impression material, on the other hand, should display good flow but with minimal elastic recovery. The material should flow readily under functional stresses, ensuring continual adaptation to the underlying soft tissues as they are altered under stresses. However, for guaranteed accuracy of the impression, the material must undergo minimum elastic recovery and should exhibit adequate dimensional stability in terms of weight change, water sorption, and solubility. Casts should be poured immediately after removal of the impression from the patient's mouth. Functional impressions are routinely removed from the patient's mouth after a few days. Results of recent studies recommend even shorter periods of 24 hours to obtain optimum results.

Materials that are available as short-term soft liners vary considerably in their compositions and

liquid, the alcohol/plasticizer mix diffuses into the swellable acrylic beads. Gelation involves the entanglement of outer polymer chains of swollen beads, resulting in a tacky set gel with high cohesive properties, which enhances its retention to the fitting surface of the denture. The set gel has viscoelastic and elastic properties that allow it to act as a shock absorber. The temporary nature of tissue conditioners stems from the fact that both the alcohol and the plasticizer leach out and are partially replaced by water. The material thus hardens within a considerably short time, which varies from a few days to a week or two, and gradually loses its proclaimed cushioning effect. In addition, the material becomes increasingly vulnerable to surface deterioration, contamination, and fouling by microorganisms, which in turn can lead to further irritation to the already abused mucosal tissues.

Ideally, for adequate cushioning, a tissue conditioner should be replaced with a fresh mix every 2 to 3 days. This procedure should continue until full recovery of the tissues has occurred. The gelation characteristics and viscoelastic properties of tissue conditioners vary due to differences in their composition and structures, such as powder particle size and ethyl alcohol content. Some materials are properties; some fulfill the requirements of an optimum functional impression material more efficiently than others. The choice of materials should be based on a thorough understanding of their properties in conjunction with their effective clinical applications.

Self-Administered Home Relines

Numerous over-the-counter temporary reline materials are available for patients' use and are marketed as "home relines." The materials allow the patient to adjust the fit of their dentures. They are supplied as preformed thermoplastic pads or in a powder/liquid form and have a similar composition and manipulation as treatment liners. The main limitation and danger of these materials are the high potential for their misuse. Improper adherence to manufacturer's instructions on the proper mixing of the components or long-term use of these liners can lead to trauma, can cause irritation to the underlying tissues, may adversely affect the denture base materials, and may cause occlusal errors. There is a unanimous consensus that patients should be strongly discouraged from using these materials as a substitute for seeking proper professional help.

Long-Term Soft Liners

Long-term/permanent soft liners are mostly used as a therapeutic measure for patients who cannot tolerate the stresses induced by dentures. There is strong theoretical evidence to justify the use of these materials in the management of edentulous patients who suffer from chronic pain, soreness, or discomfort due to prolonged contact between the rigid denture base materials and the underlying tissues. Such as the case in patients with sharp, thin, or heavily resorbed ridges or those with severe bony undercuts. In these situations a viscoelastic soft liner would be a welcome adjunct to compensate for the dramatically depleted mucoperiosteal support. The liner permits wider dispersion of forces and absorption of impact forces that are involved in functional and parafunctional movements.

Materials available as permanent soft liners include plasticized acrylics, silicone rubber, plasticized vinyl polymers and copolymers, hydrophilic polymers, polyphosphazine fluoropolymers, fluoroethylene, and polyvinyl siloxane addition silicones. Currently, the most commonly used materials are plasticized acrylics and silicone rubber, which are either chemically or heat activated. Requirements of an ideal permanent soft liner are presented in Box 12-6.

Plasticized Acrylics

Heat-activated plasticized acrylic liners are supplied as preformed sheets or in a powder/liquid form. The powder consists of a higher methacrylate polymer (PEMA) and benzoyl peroxide as an initiator. The liquid consists of a higher methacrylate monomer (such as ethyl, n-butyl or 2-ethoxyethyl methacrylate) together with a plasticizer, commonly a phthalate ester. The plasticizer lowers the T_g of the resin and acts as a lubricant between the polymer chains, enabling them to deform more easily. The liner is processed in the laboratory, usually at the time of processing a new denture.

Chemically activated acrylic resins are also available as soft liners. Their chemical composition is similar to that of heat-activated resins, but they are polymerized by a peroxide-tertiary amine system. These materials are applied as chairside

---

Box 12-6

Requirements of an Ideal Long-Term Soft Liner

1. Biocompatibility
2. Good dimensional stability
3. Low water sorption and water solubility
4. Good wettability by saliva
5. Permanent softness/compliance/viscoelasticity
6. Adequate abrasion resistance and tear resistance
7. Good bond to the denture base
8. Unaffected by aqueous environment and cleansers, easy to clean
9. Simple to manipulate
10. Color stable and exhibits good esthetics
11. Inhibits colonization of fungi and other microorganisms

relines, and polymerization usually takes a few minutes. However, as with other mouth-cured liners, they can only be used on a temporary basis because of their tendency to foul and debond from the denture within a few weeks, a major drawback that limits their clinical application. The presence of free monomer also results in inferior mechanical properties and reduced biocompatibility.

Silicone Soft Liners

Another commonly used long-term soft liner is silicone rubber. Silicone liners are provided with heat activation or room temperature vulcanization (RTV).

Heat-activated silicone is supplied as a single paste that consists of poly(dimethyl siloxane), a viscous liquid to which silica is added as a filler, and benzoyl peroxide as an initiator. The liner sets by a cross-linking reaction that is catalyzed by heat and the peroxide initiator. It is processed against the acrylic dough of the new denture. The addition of an adhesive usually enhances the bond between the liner and the acrylic resin base.

RTV silicones, on the other hand, use a condensation cross-linking process catalyzed by an organo-tin compound. The materials are supplied as paste and liquid and are also laboratory processed to the fitting surface of the denture base. The fact that these materials achieve a lower degree of cross-linking than their heat-activated counterparts certainly compromises many of their attributes as long-term liners.

Advantages and Disadvantages of Permanent Soft Liners

Despite the vast clinical benefits that have been recognized for plasticized acrylics and silicones as soft liners, both materials exhibit properties that are by far short of fulfilling requirements of an ideal permanent liner. This fact has limited their efficacy and life expectancy, reportedly to a maximum of 1 year of serviceability.

Plasticized acrylic soft liners exhibit good, durable bond strength to the acrylic base, have been shown to exhibit higher tear and abrasion resistance, and can achieve a much better polish than silicones.

However, biodegradation of plasticized acrylics in the oral environment is their main weakness. The plasticizer and other soluble materials in the liner leach out in saliva resulting in a progressive loss of resiliency, diminishing their cushioning effect. The resulting hard, rough surface of the liner then promotes calculus and food accumulation and undergoes fouling with microorganisms, as well as color changes and staining.

The major drawback of silicones as soft liners is their intrinsic inability to bond with the denture base resin, which is more evident around the borders of the denture. High water sorption by the liner accentuates this problem further, detrimentally affecting the adhesion between the liner and resin base. This is a particular problem in RTV silicones, which tend to swell, split, or peel off the denture base. Attempts to enhance the bond with resin bases include adding bonding agents; using special primers applied to the acrylic base, as in the case of RTV silicones; or confining the borders of the liner to end within the denture border, rather than extending it to the periphery of the denture base. However, such a design may be accompanied with the risk of decreasing the shock absorbability of the liner.

Despite their shortcomings, silicone rubbers, particularly those that are heat activated, have a myriad of properties that enhances their clinical preeminence over plasticized acrylics, mostly their high resilience and prolonged elasticity over time, which in turn, enables them to maintain their cushioning effect longer than other soft liners.

Most challenging in the use of long- and short-term soft liners is their tendency to support growth of *C. albicans* and other microorganisms on and within the liners. The porous nature, particularly of silicones, reportedly facilitates water absorption and diffusion of nutrient materials. This is further complicated by the difficulty of cleaning most of these liners with routine mechanical or chemical methods, such as brushing, or hypochlorite and peroxide denture cleansers (Figure 12-1).

Excellent oral and denture hygiene and the use of antimicrobial agents can effectively minimize fungal/microbial colonization of liners. Cleaning of soft liners can be carried out with a soft brush in conjunction with a very mild detergent or nonabrasive dentifrice. Alternatively, the external surface

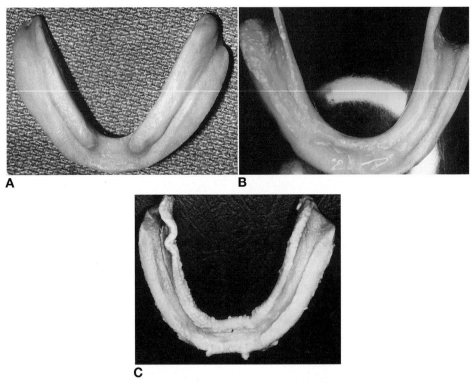

Figure 12-1   **A,** Recently completed resilient liner on a mandibular denture.
B, A 6-month-old resilient liner with foci of yeast colonies already apparent. **C,** A neglected
12-month-old resilient liner with almost total coverage by yeast colonies.

of the denture can be cleaned as described, but the liner itself can be wiped with cotton under cold water. Box 12-7 provides a comparison of properties of plasticized acrylics versus silicone rubber.

Clinical experience indicates almost universal tissue tolerance of soft liners and acceptable patient reactions. However, currently, the materials have to be considered as temporary expedients because none of the advocated permanent soft liners has a life expectancy comparable to that of the resin denture base. Improved strength, permanent resiliency, improved adhesion to the denture bases, the ability to inhibit growth of microorganisms, and chemical stability continue to be the main focus of ongoing research. These attempts include surface coatings of liners with sealants such as fluorinated copolymers and integration with antifungal components. Silicone rubbers, when properly used, may be the most appropriate of the various types available, but they too are only temporary expedients and must be inspected regularly by the dentist and replaced when unsatisfactory. As pointed out earlier, the application of proper cleansers and home care habits has contributed to the use of these materials with significantly beneficial results. It must be emphasized, however, that using these materials does not preclude adherence to the fundamental principles of complete denture construction. Nevertheless, when used intelligently, soft liners are an excellent adjunct in removable prosthodontics.

DENTURE CLEANSERS

Education of patients is crucial to enhance their awareness of both limitations and inherent weak-

---

Box 12-7

A Comparison of the Properties of Plasticized Acrylics versus Silicone Rubber

Plasticized Acrylics

Less resilient
Hardens by time/loss of plasticizer
Good durable bond with denture base
More resistant to growth of *Candida albicans*
Acceptable tear strength
Better abrasion resistance
Reasonable resistance to damage by denture cleanser

Silicone Rubber

Highly resilient
Retains softness and elasticity
Low bond strength to acrylic base, particularly RTV silicones
More susceptible to growth of *C. albicans/* other microorganisms
Low tear strength
Low abrasion resistance
Less resistant to damage by cleansers particularly RTV silicones

RTV, Room temperature vulcanization.

---

nesses in the physical and mechanical properties of the inserted prosthesis. Furthermore, it must be emphasized that improper care of dentures can have serious detrimental effects on the health of the denture-supporting tissues. Most patients are unaware of the risks of microbial plaque accumulations around and under the denture-tissue interfaces and the potential for promoting adverse pathological mucosal reactions such as denture stomatitis and angular cheilitis.

The presence of denture deposits and their rate of accumulation are directly related to the presence of a protein-rich saliva and the microporous nature of the polymeric base, which facilitates microbial plaque formation and ensuing calculus deposition. The organic portion of calculus consists of microproteins that bond the deposits to the denture surface, whereas the inorganic portion mostly contains calcium phosphate and calcium carbonate. Maintenance of adequate denture hygiene, through mechanical or chemical methods, or both, is essential to minimize and preferably eliminate adverse tissue reactions. It must be an integral component of postinsertion patient care.

Denture cleansing materials and techniques include mechanical brushing, the use of chemical cleansers, or both. Commonly available denture cleansing materials include (1) oxygenating cleansers, (2) alkaline hypochlorite solutions, (3) dilute mineral acids, (4) abrasive powders and pastes, and (5) enzyme-containing materials (proteases) (Box 12-8).

Mechanical Techniques

Patients are routinely instructed to clean their dentures by light brushing with a soft denture brush or a multifluted soft nylon brush with rounded ends and soap and water. The mechanical cleaning action of the brush is usually sufficient to remove loosely attached soft food debris, without abrading the denture base and teeth. However, it is ineffective for denture disinfection. The removal of hard calculus deposits, plaque, and stains require more vigorous measures such as the daily use of immersion chemical denture cleansers or brush-on diluted acid cleansers.

The use of hard bristle brushes, forceful brushing, or abrasive dentifrices, such as calcium carbonate or hydrated silica, may cause abrasion of polymeric materials or result in scratches on their surface. The rough, irregular surfaces promote

---

Box 12-8

Requirements of an Ideal Denture Cleanser

1. Nontoxic
2. Easy to remove and harmless to the patient (eyes-skin-clothes) if accidentally spilled or splashed
3. Harmless to the denture base materials and denture teeth as well as soft liners
4. Able to dissolve all the denture deposits such as calculus
5. Exhibits a bacteriocidal and fungicidal effect
6. Long shelf life and inexpensive

accumulation of denture deposits, increase staining and fouling with oral microorganisms, and they dramatically compromise denture esthetics. Pastes with some gentle abrasives (sodium bicarbonate or acrylic resin) may be used. Similarly, patients should be strongly advised against using abrasive household kitchen or bathroom cleansers, such as scouring powder, to clean their dentures.

Chemical Denture Cleansers

The most commonly used commercial chemical denture cleansers use immersion techniques; these include alkaline peroxides and hypochlorites. Advantages of immersion cleansers include full accessibility of the solutions to all areas of the denture, minimum damage from mishandling dentures, minimum abrasion of denture bases and teeth, and use simplicity of the technique.

Oxygenating Cleansers Alkaline peroxides are provided in powder and tablet forms. The material contains alkaline compounds, detergents, sodium perborate, and flavoring agents. When mixed with water, sodium perborate decomposes releasing peroxides, which in turn decomposes releasing oxygen. Cleansing is a result of the oxidizing ability of the peroxide decomposition and from the effervescent action of the evolved oxygen. This effectively breaks down, dissolves, and floats away organic deposits and kills microorganisms. Peroxides are not as effective, though, in removing heavy calculus deposits. Some are not compatible with soft denture liners. Overnight immersion of dentures in an alkaline peroxide solution is a safe, effective method of denture cleaning and sterilization, particularly among geriatric or disabled patients, whose limited manual dexterity may deter them from using mechanical brushing techniques.

Hypochlorite Solutions Diluted household bleaches (sodium hypochlorites) are commonly used as denture cleansers, for removing plaque and light stains, and are capable of killing denture adherent organisms. One technique involves the immersion of the dentures in a solution of one part of 5% sodium hypochlorite in three parts of water (1:3 water) followed by light brushing. Alternatively, the denture is immersed in a solution containing

1 teaspoon of hypochlorite (Clorox) and 2 teaspoons of a glassy phosphate (Calgon) in half a glass of water, to help control calculus and heavy stains.

Alkaline hypochlorites are not recommended for dentures fabricated from cast base metal alloys. The chlorine ions can result in corrosion and darkening of these metals. Concentrated hypochlorite solutions should also not be used because prolonged use may alter the color of the denture base resins. Bleaches may eventually discolor soft denture liners, particularly silicones. The importance of avoiding soaking dentures in hot water should be stressed to the patient to avoid distortion of the denture bases.

Other Techniques/Materials

- Ultrasonic units provide vibrations that can be used to clean dentures. When this technique is used, the denture is placed into a cleaning unit, which is filled with a soaking chemical agent supplied by the manufacturer. The cleansing action of the soaking agent is supplemented by the mechanical debriding action of the ultrasonic vibrations. This in turn creates areas of vacuum next to the denture surface and thus dislodges and dispenses debris. Despite its effectiveness, this technique may not adequately remove plaque on the denture surface. It is mostly available for use in institutions such as nursing homes and hospitals.
- Dilute acids (citric acid, isopropyl alcohol, hydrochloric acid, or plain household vinegar) are available to remove obstinate deposits. The brush-on cleanser is swabbed onto the denture surfaces with a brush. The materials attack the inorganic phosphate portion of denture deposits, thus reducing calculus accumulations. Vinegar can also kill microorganisms but less effectively than bleaching solutions. Brush-on materials must be used cautiously, and the denture must be rinsed thoroughly to avoid contact of the material with the skin and mucosa. Diluted acids may also cause corrosion of some alloys.
- Denture cleansers containing enzymes (mutanese and protease) have been shown to

reduce denture plaque significantly, with a daily 15-minute soak, particularly when combined with mechanical brushing of the dentures.

- Other materials and techniques include the use of silicone polymers. These cleansers provide a protective coating, which interferes with bacterial adherence to the denture surface until their next application. Overnight air-drying and microwave radiation have been also used to disinfect and clean resin bases, mostly in conjunction with mechanical brushing.

Table 12-3 describes disadvantages of the various types of denture cleansers.

CAST METAL ALLOYS AS DENTURES, BASES

Despite the popularity of PMMA as a denture base material, its inherent weaknesses in mechanical properties increases its susceptibility to impact and fatigue failure. Both are considered to be the two main causes of denture fractures. The reinforcement of conventional PMMA resins through the incorporation of rubber inclusions and fibers has significantly enhanced the impact and flexural strengths of the material as well as its fatigue resistance. However, there are various clinical situations where a dentist may select an alternative material. One such situation is where a single maxillary complete denture opposes a full or partial complement of

natural mandibular teeth. An unfavorable/irregular occlusal plane, heavy anterior occlusal contacts, and heavy masticatory forces directed onto a virtually thin palatal resin plate may collectively contribute to denture fracture. In such a situation, the choice of a cast metal base has been recommended as an effective alternative to resin bases.

A variety of metals and metal alloys have been used as complete denture bases. Currently, the materials of choice include cast base metal alloys: cobalt-chromium, nickel-chromium, cobalt chromium nickel, and more recently titanium alloys.

In this technique a relatively thin metal base is cast to contact the denture-bearing mucosa surface, covering the whole palate, providing superior fit and comfort to the patient. Acrylic resin is used to retain the denture teeth and provide buccal/labial flanges that enhance the esthetic quality of the denture. The processed acrylic resin is attached to the cast metal base by a retentive meshwork. The acrylic resin and metal meet at a definite finish line to ensure a strong butt junction. Care must be taken to avoid inadequate shaping of the palatal contours at the finish line or placing the acrylic resin–metal junction too far laterally or medially, which could result in crowding or inadequate contact with the lateral border of the tongue, causing discomfort or altering the patient's phonetics (Figure 12-2).

Cobalt-chromium alloys, often referred to as *stellite alloys,* consist of about 60% cobalt and 25% to 30% chromium, together with minor alloying elements such as manganese and silicone to enhance its fluidity for casting. Other components

Table 12-3
Disadvantages of the Various Types of Denture Cleansers

Cleanser	Main Constituent	Disadvantages
Oxygenating cleansers	Alkaline perborate	Ineffective for removal of heavy calculus deposits; harmful to soft liners
Hypochlorite solutions	Dilute sodium hypochlorite	May bleach denture base resins May discolor soft liners Corrosion of base-metal alloys Unpleasant odor
Dilute acids	Hydrochloric acid Citric acid/isopropyl alcohol	Corrosion of some alloys Unpleasant odor
Denture cleansing powder/paste	Abrasive agents	Abrasion of denture polymeric bases and teeth

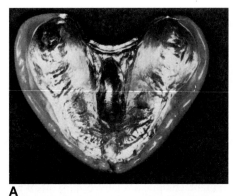

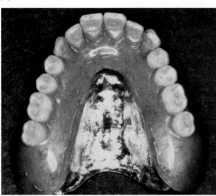

Figure 12-2 Metal bases for complete dentures. **A,** Gold, stellite (cobalt/chromium), or titanium alloy covers the palate and residual ridges with the borders formed in acrylic resin. It should be noted that many dentists prefer to *not* cover the residual ridges with metal so as to facilitate relieving and relining procedures for acrylic resin covered sites in the future. **B,** Also note that the posterior palatal seal area need not be made of metal. Many dentists prefer a "mesh" area here to provide excellent retention for an acrylic posterior palatal seal. The tuberosity regions may need to be entirely covered in metal or a mesh plus acrylic as dictated by the interarch space.

included are aluminum, gallium, copper, iron, and platinum. Molybdenum, tungsten, and carbon are also added as hardening and strengthening elements. The resulting alloys display high strength, hardness, high modulus of elasticity (stiffness), low density, and high corrosion resistance, and they have a substantially lower cost than gold alloys.

Nickel-chromium alloys contain about 70% nickel and a lower content of chromium (16%). The inclusion of beryllium (0.5%) in minor quantities lowers the melting range and enhances fluidity of the alloy. The inclusion of aluminum (2%) leads to the formation of an intermediate (Ni3-Al) compound that increases the strength and hardness of the alloy. Box 12-9 lists the advantages and disadvantages of base metal alloys, as compared to all resin complete denture bases as listed in Table 12-1.

The controversy surrounding the biocompatibility of cobalt- and nickel-containing alloys as potential allergenics and the biological risks of metal ions released in the mouth during corrosion (such as beryllium, a carcinogenic hazard) suggests the merits of another cast base metal, titanium, as an alternative. Superiority of titanium stems from its remarkable biocompatibility and high corrosion resistance. In addition, it exhibits high dimensional stability, low density, and mechanical properties that are comparable to those of cobalt-chromium alloys. The main drawback of titanium as a denture

---

Box 12-9

Advantages and Disadvantages of Base Metal Alloys

Advantages

High thermal conductivity
Increased tissue tolerance
Reduced bulk across the palate creates more tongue space/increased comfort to patient
Dimensional stability/increased accuracy of fit of the denture base
Superior biocompatibility of titanium bases
Stronger bases that withstand high masticatory stresses
Increased weight, enhances stability of a mandibular denture

Disadvantages

Greater technical costs
Difficulty of rebasing and relining metal/currently facilitated with adhesives
Less margin of error permissible in the posterior palate seal area
Increased weight for a maxillary denture

base alloy relates to difficulties in its casting technique. Casting problems of titanium are a result of its relatively low density, high melting point (about 1700° C), high chemical affinity to gases (oxygen, hydrogen, nitrogen), and its reactivity with components of most investment materials. This has led to a variety of problems such as low casting efficiency, casting porosities, difficulty in finishing, soldering, and welding of the metal. Casting titanium is a relatively expensive laboratory technique that requires high-cost equipment.

Recent advances in casting technology and melting techniques, such as electric arc melting and laser welding; in investment materials; and in alloying titanium with other metals to attain lower melting and casting temperatures have greatly facilitated the casting of titanium-based metals and its use in dental laboratories.

SUMMARY

The premise in preparing this review chapter is that dentists should possess sufficient knowledge of the properties of the different prosthodontic materials they deal with so that they can exercise prudent judgment in their selection. This knowledge should be preferably based on evidence-based information plus large scale, long-term clinical trials to ensure treatment efficacy and effectiveness.

Bibliography

Au AR, Lechner SK, Thomas CJ et al: Titanium for removable partial dentures (III): 2-year clinical follow-up in an undergraduate program, *J Oral Rehabil* 27:979-985, 2000.

Blagojevic V, Murphy VM: Microwave polymerization of denture base materials: a comparative study, *J Oral Rehabil* 26:804-808, 1999.

Clarke RL: Glassy polymers. In Braden M, Clarke RL, Nicholson J, Parker S, editors: *Polymeric dental materials*, Verlag Berlin, 1997, Springer.

Combe EC, Burke FJT, Douglas WH: *Dental biomaterials*, Boston, 1999, Kluwer Academic.

Cunningham JL: Shear bond strength of resin teeth to heat-cured and light-cured denture base resins, *J Oral Rehabil* 27:312-316, 2000.

Cunningham JL, Benington IC: An investigation of the variables which may affect the bond between plastic teeth and denture base resins, *J Dent* 27:129-135, 1999.

Da Silva L, Martinez A, Rilo B et al: Titanium for removable denture bases, *J Oral Rehabil* 27:131-135, 2000.

Jagger DC, Harrison A, Jandt KD: The reinforcement of dentures, *J Oral Rehabil* 26:185-194, 1999.

John J, Gangadhar SA, Shah I: Flexural strength of heat-polymerized polymethylmethacrylate denture resin reinforced with glass, aramid or nylon fibres, *J Prosthet Dent* 86: 424-427, 2001.

Kawano F, Ohguri T, Koran A III et al: Influence of lining design of three processed soft denture liners on cushioning effect, *J Oral Rehabil* 26:962-968, 1999.

Koran A III: Prosthetic applications of Polymers. In Craig RG, Powers JM, editors: *Restorative dental materials*, ed 11, St Louis, 2002, Mosby Inc.

Malmström HS, Mehta N, Sanchez R et al: The effect of two different coatings on the surface integrity and softness of a tissue conditioner, *J Prosthet Dent* 87:153-157, 2002.

McCabe JF, Carrick TE, Kamohara H: Adhesive bond strength and compliance for denture soft lining materials, *Biomaterials* 23:1347-1352, 2002.

Murata H, Kawamura M, Hamada T et al: Dimensional stability and weight changes of tissue conditioners, *J Oral Rehabil* 28:918-923, 2001.

O'Brien WJ: *Dental materials and their selection*, ed 3, Chicago, 2002, Quintessence Publishing Co, Inc.

Ödman PA: The effectiveness of an enzyme-containing denture cleanser, *Quintessence Int* 23:187-190, 1992.

Parker S: Soft prosthesis materials. In Braden M, Clarke RL, Nicholson J, Parker S, editors: *Polymeric dental materials*, Verlag Berlin, 1997, Springer.

Phoenix RD: Denture base resins, technical considerations and processing technique. In Anusavice KJ, editor: *Phillips' science of dental materials*, ed 10, Philadelphia, 1996, WB Saunders.

Qudah S, Harrison A, Huggett R: Soft lining materials in prosthetic dentistry: a review, *Int J Prothodont* 3:477-483, 1990.

Shay K: Denture hygiene: a review and update, *J Contemp Dent Pract* 1:28-41, 2000.

Taguchi N, Murata H, Hamada T et al: Effect of viscoelastic properties of resilient denture liners on pressures under dentures, *J Oral Rehabil* 28:1003-1008, 2001.

Takahashi Y, Chai T, Takahashi T et al: The bond strength of denture teeth to denture base resins, *Int J Prosthodont* 13:59-65, 2000.

Takamata T, Setcos JC: Resin denture bases: review of accuracy and methods of polymerization, *Int J Prosthodont* 2: 555-560, 1989.

Tan HK, Woo A, Kim S et al: Effect of denture cleansers, surface finish and temperature on Molloplast B resilient liner, color, hardness and texture, *J Prosthodont* 9:148-155, 2000.

REHABILITATION OF THE EDENTULOUS PATIENT: FABRICATION OF COMPLETE DENTURES

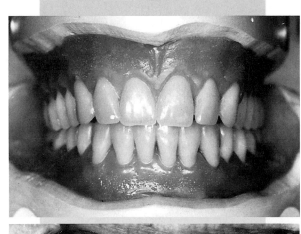

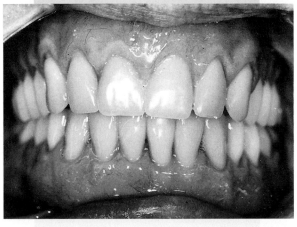

CHAPTER 13

Developing an Analogue/Substitute for the Maxillary Denture-Bearing Area

David M. Davis

If dentures and their supporting tissues are to coexist for a reasonable length of time, the dentist must fully understand the anatomy of the supporting and limiting structures involved, for these are the foundation of the denture-bearing area. The denture base must extend as far as possible without interfering in the health or function of the tissues. It is convenient to regard the impression surface of a denture as comprising two areas: a stress-bearing or supporting area and a peripheral or limiting area. Each of these is discussed separately, but like the sides of a coin they are inseparable.

ANATOMY OF SUPPORTING STRUCTURES

The foundation for dentures is made up of bone of the hard palate and residual ridge, covered by mucous membrane. The denture base rests on the mucous membrane, which serves as a cushion between the base and the supporting bone.

Mucous Membrane

The mucous membrane is composed of mucosa and submucosa. The submucosa is formed by connective tissue that varies in character from dense to loose areolar tissue and also varies considerably in thickness. The submucosa may contain glandular, fat, or muscle cells and transmits the blood and nerve supply to the mucosa. Where the mucous membrane is attached to bone, the attachment occurs between the submucosa and the periosteal covering of the bone.

The mucosa is formed by stratified squamous epithelium, which often is keratinized, and a subjacent narrow layer of connective tissue known as the *lamina propria*. In the edentulous person, the mucosa covering the hard palate and the crest of the residual ridge, including the residual attached gingiva, is classified as masticatory mucosa. It is characterized by a well-defined keratinized layer on its outermost surface that is subject to changes in thickness depending on whether dentures are worn and on the clinical acceptability of the dentures.

Although the importance of the mucosa from a health standpoint cannot be neglected, the thickness and consistency of the submucosa are largely responsible for the support that the mucous membrane affords a denture because in most instances, the submucosa makes up the bulk of the mucous membrane. In a healthy mouth, the submucosa is firmly attached to the periosteum of the underlying supporting bone and will usually withstand successfully the pressures of the dentures. When the submucosal layer is thin, the soft tissues will be nonresilient, and the mucous membrane will be easily traumatized. When the submucosal layer is loosely attached to the periosteum or it is inflamed or edematous, the tissue is easily displaceable, and the stability and support of the dentures are adversely affected.

Hard Palate

The ultimate support for a maxillary denture is the bone of the two maxillae and the palatine bone. The palatine processes of the maxillae are joined together at the medial suture (Figure 13-1). The

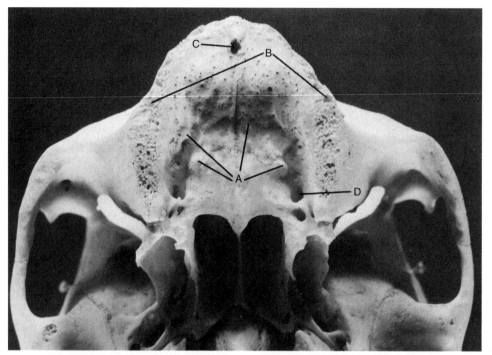

Figure 13-1 Both the maxillae and the palatine bone provide support for an upper denture. Individual differences in form determine how forces should be directed to these bones during function. *A,* Spiny projections that would irritate tissues under a denture. *B,* Rough and irregular bone of the maxillary ridges. *C,* Incisive foramen, which comes to lie closer to the crest of the ridge as resorption takes place. Thus the location of the incisive papilla, which covers the incisive foramen, in relation to the crest of the ridge is a guide to the amount of resorption that has occurred. *D,* Greater palatine foramen, which often has a spiny overhanging edge to it.

palatine processes of the maxillae and the palatine bone form the foundation for the hard palate and provide considerable support for the denture. More important, they support soft tissues that increase the surface areas of the basal seat.

A cross section of the hard palate shows that the palate is covered by soft tissue of varying thickness, even though the epithelium is keratinized throughout. In the region of the medial palatal suture, the submucosa is extremely thin, with the result that the mucosal layer is practically in contact with the underlying bone. For this reason, the soft tissue covering the medial palatal suture is nonresilient and may need to be relieved to avoid trauma from the denture base. Anterolaterally, the submucosa contains adipose tissue, and posterolaterally it contains glandular tissue. This tissue is displaceable,

and although it contributes to the support of the denture, the horizontal portion of the hard palate lateral to the midline provides the primary support area for the denture. In the area of the rugae, the palate is set at an angle to the residual ridge and is rather thinly covered by soft tissue. This area contributes to the stress-bearing role, though in a secondary capacity. The submucosa covering the incisive papilla and the nasopalatine canal contains the nasopalatine vessels and nerves.

Residual Ridge

The shape and size of the alveolar ridges change when the natural teeth are removed. The resorption following extraction of the teeth is rapid at first, but it continues at a reduced rate throughout life. If the teeth have been out for many years, the residual ridge may become small, and the crest of the ridge may lack a smooth, cortical bony surface under the mucosa. There may be large, nutrient canals and sharp bony spicules (see Figure 13-1).

The mucous membrane covering the crest of the ridge in a healthy mouth is firmly attached to the periosteum of the bone by the connective tissue of the submucosa. The stratified squamous epithelium is thickly keratinized. The submucosa is devoid of fat or glandular cells and is characterized by dense collagenous fibers that are contiguous with the lamina propria. The submucosal layer, though relatively thin in comparison with other parts of the mouth, is still sufficiently thick to provide adequate resiliency to support the denture.

The crest of the edentulous ridge is an important area of support. However, the bone is subject to resorption, which limits its potential for support, unlike the palate, which is resistant to resorption. Because of this, the ridge crest should be looked on as a secondary supporting area, rather than a primary supporting area. The inclined facial surface of the maxillary ridge provides little support,

although the peripheral tissues should be contacted to provide a border seal.

As the mucous membrane extends from the crest along the slope of the residual ridge to the reflection, it loses its firm attachment to the underlying bone (Figure 13-2). The more loosely attached mucous membrane in this region has a nonkeratinized or slightly keratinized epithelium, and the submucosa contains loose connective tissue and elastic fibers. This loosely attached tissue will not withstand the forces of mastication transmitted through the denture base as well as the mucous membrane covering the crest of the ridge and the palate.

Histological studies of the effect of wearing dentures on the keratinization of the mucosa of the crest of the residual ridges and the palate have produced conflicting results. However, most studies indicate that wearing dentures does not seem to be harmful to the epithelium, even though in denture wearers the keratinization is of reduced thickness. Cytological studies indicate that increased amounts of keratinized material are present in edentulous ridges when the clinical quality of the

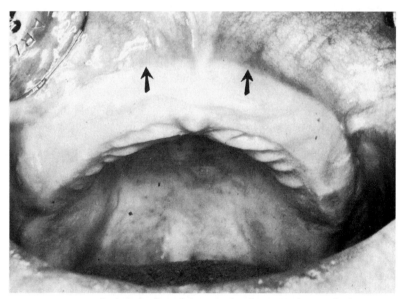

Figure 13-2 Arrows denote the line of demarcation between the attached and unattached mucous membrane. Attached mucous membrane is desirable for support. However, it is the peripheral area that contributes to the border seal. Notice the prominent incisive papilla lying anteriorly on the center of the residual ridge.

dentures is good, an indication that well-fitting dentures may be important in maintaining the normal histological condition of the mouth. Stimulation of the mucosa of the residual ridge through toothbrush physiotherapy also increases the presence of keratinized material. Histologically, removing the dentures from the mouth for 6 to 8 hours a day, preferably during periods of sleep, allows keratinization to increase and the signs of inflammation, often found in the submucosa when dentures are worn, to be dramatically reduced.

Shape of the Supporting Structure

The configuration of the bone that provides the support for the maxillary denture varies considerably with each patient. Factors that influence the form and size of the supporting bone include (1) its original size and consistency; (2) the person's general health; (3) forces developed by the surrounding musculature; (4) the severity and location of periodontal disease (a frequent cause of tooth loss); (5) forces accruing from the wearing of dental prostheses; (6) surgery at the time of removal of the teeth; and (7) the relative length of time different parts of the jaws have been edentulous. In addition, a number of anatomical features influence the shape of the hard palate and residual ridge. These are described in the following material.

Incisive Foramen   This is located beneath the incisive papilla, which is situated on a line immediately behind and between the central incisors. It lies nearer to the crest of the ridge as resorption progresses (see Figure 13-2). Thus the location of the incisive papilla gives an indication as to the amount of resorption that has taken place. The nasopalatine nerves and blood vessels pass through the foramen, and care should be taken that the denture base does not impinge on them.

Maxillary Tuberosity   The tuberosity region can hang down abnormally low because when the maxillary posterior teeth are retained after the mandibular molars have been extracted and not replaced, the maxillary teeth overerupt, bringing the process with them (Figure 13-3). These enlargements often are fibrous but can be bony. This excess tissue can prevent proper location of

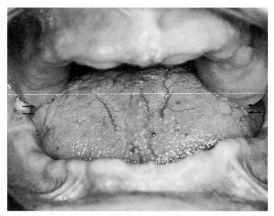

Figure 13-3   The enlarged tuberosities limit the space available and will compromise the occlusal plane and distal extension of the mandibular denture.

the occlusal plane and may interfere with the lower denture, if it is not surgically removed.

Sharp, Spiny Processes   Frequently, there are sharp, spiny processes on the maxillary and palatine bones (see Figure 13-1). These usually cause no problems because they are covered deeply by soft tissue. However, in individuals with considerable resorption of the residual ridge, these sharp spines can irritate the soft tissue left between them and the denture base. The posterior palatine foramina often have a sharp, spiny overhanging edge that may irritate the covering soft tissues as a result of pressure from the denture.

Torus Palatinus   The torus palatinus is a hard bony enlargement that occurs in the midline of the roof of the mouth and is found in about 20% of the population (Figure 13-4). It is covered by a thin layer of mucous membrane that is easily traumatized by the denture base unless a relief is provided. This relief should conform accurately to the shape of the torus because an extensive arbitrary relief robs the denture of part of its support area.

ANATOMY OF PERIPHERAL OR LIMITING STRUCTURES

The limiting structures of the upper denture can be divided into three areas: (1) the labial vestibule,

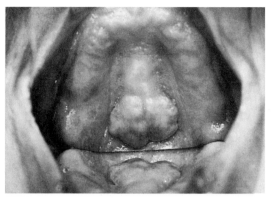

Figure 13-4　A torus palatinus is covered by a thin layer of mucous membrane, which is easily traumatized by the denture base unless a relief is provided.

which runs from one buccal frenum to the other on the labial side of the ridge; (2) the right and left buccal vestibule, which extends from the buccal frenum to the hamular notch; and (3) the vibrating line, which extends from one hamular notch to the other across the palate (Figure 13-5).

Labial Vestibule

The labial vestibule is divided into a left and right labial vestibule by the labial frenum, which is a fold of mucous membrane at the median line. It contains no muscle and has no action of its own. It starts superiorly in a fan shape and converges as it descends to its terminal attachment on the labial side of the ridge. The labial notch in the labial flange of the denture must be just wide enough and just deep enough to allow the frenum to pass through it without manipulation of the lip (Figure 13-6).

The mucous membrane lining the labial vestibule has a relatively thin mucosa. The submucosal layer is thick and contains large amounts of loose areolar tissue and elastic fibers. The mucosa of the vestibular spaces is classified as lining mucosa. It is normally devoid of a keratinized layer and is freely movable with the tissues to which it is attached because of the elastic nature of the lamina propria. Lining mucosa also forms the covering of the lips and cheeks, the alveololingual sulcus, the

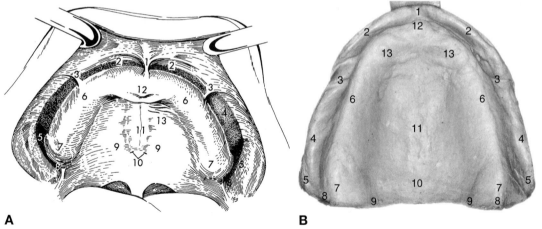

A　　　　　　　　　　　　　　　　　　　　　**B**

Figure 13-5　Correlation of anatomical landmarks. **A,** Intraoral drawing of the maxillary arch; *1,* labial frenum; *2,* labial vestibule; *3,* buccal frenum; *4,* buccal vestibule; *5,* coronoid bulge; *6,* residual alveolar ridge; *7,* maxillary tuberosity; *8,* hamular notch; *9,* posterior palatal seal region; *10,* foveae palatinae; *11,* median palatine raphe; *12,* incisive papilla; *13,* rugae. **B,** Maxillary final impression shows the corresponding denture landmarks: *1,* labial notch; *2,* labial flange; *3,* buccal notch; *4,* buccal flange; *5,* coronoid contour; *6,* alveolar groove; *7,* area of tuberosity; *8,* pterygomaxillary seal in area of hamular notch; *9,* area of posterior palatal seal; *10,* foveae palatinae; *11,* median palatine groove; *12,* incisive fossa; *13,* rugae.

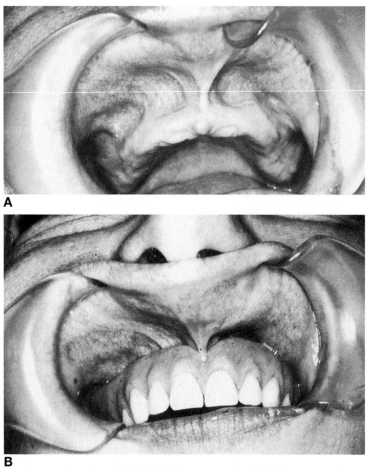

Figure 13-6   **A,** A broad maxillary labial frenum. **B,** The labial flange must fit snugly around the frenum.

soft palate, the ventral surface of the tongue, and the unattached gingiva found on the slopes of the residual ridges.

The main muscle of the lip, which forms the outer surface of the labial vestibule, is the *orbicularis oris*. Its tone depends on the support it receives from the labial flange and the position of the teeth. The fibers of the orbicularis oris pass horizontally through the lips and anastomose with the fibers of the buccinator muscle. Because the fibers run in a horizontal direction, the orbicularis oris has only an indirect effect on

the extent of an impression and hence on the denture base.

The buccal frenum forms the dividing line between the labial and buccal vestibules. It is sometimes a single fold of mucous membrane, sometimes double, and, in some mouths, broad and fan shaped. The levator anguli oris muscle attaches beneath the frenum and consequently affects the position of the frenum. The orbicularis oris pulls the frenum forward, and the buccinator pulls it backward. Thus it requires more clearance for its action than the labial frenum does (Figure 13-7).

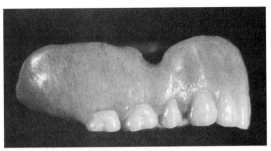

Figure 13-7 An upper denture with a properly formed notch for the buccal frenum. The buccal frenum requires more clearance than the labial frenum because it will move posteriorly as a result of the action of the buccinator muscle and anteriorly as a result of the action of the orbicularis oris.

Buccal Vestibule

The buccal vestibule lies opposite the tuberosity and extends from the buccal frenum to the hamular notch. The size of the buccal vestibule varies with the contraction of the buccinator muscle, the position of the mandible, and the amount of bone lost from the maxilla. The size and shape of the distal end of the buccal flange of the denture must be adjusted to the ramus and the coronoid process of the mandible and to the masseter muscle. When the mandible opens or moves to the opposite side, the width of the buccal vestibule is reduced. When the masseter muscle contracts under heavy closing pressures, it reduces the size of the space available for the distal end of the buccal flange. The extent of the buccal vestibule can be deceiving because the coronoid process obscures it when the mouth is opened wide. Therefore it should be examined with the mouth as nearly closed as possible. This space usually is higher than any other part of the border. The mucous membrane lining the buccal vestibule is similar to that lining the labial vestibule.

Distal to the buccal frenum lies the root of the zygoma, which is located opposite the first molar region (Figure 13-8). With increasing resorption of the ridge, it becomes more noticeable, and a denture may require relief over this area to prevent soreness of the underlying tissue.

The hamular notch, which forms the distal limit of the buccal vestibule, is situated between the tuberosity and the hamulus of the medial pterygoid plate (see Figure 13-8). The mucous membrane of the hamular notch consists of a thick submucosa made up of loose areolar tissue. This tissue, in the center of the deep part of the hamular notch, can be safely displaced by the posterior palatal border of the denture to help achieve a posterior palatal seal.

Vibrating Line

The vibrating line is an imaginary line drawn across the palate that marks the beginning of motion in the soft palate when an individual says "ah." It extends from one hamular notch to the other (Figure 13-9). At the midline, it usually passes about 2 mm in front of the fovea palatinae. These are indentations near the midline of the palate formed by a coalescence of several mucous gland ducts. They are always in soft tissue, which makes them an ideal guide for the location of the posterior border of the denture.

The vibrating line is not to be confused with the junction of the hard and soft palate because the vibrating line is always on the soft palate. It is not a well-defined line and should be described as an area rather than a line. The distal end of the denture should extend at least to the vibrating line. In most instances it should end 1 to 2 mm posterior to the vibrating line. The submucosa in the region of the vibrating line contains glandular tissue similar to that in the submucosa in the posterolateral part of the hard palate. However, because the soft palate does not rest directly on bone, the tissue for a few millimeters on either side of the vibrating line can be repositioned in the impression to improve the posterior palatal seal.

In addition, the distal end of the denture must cover the tuberosities and extend into the hamular notches. Overextension at the hamular notches will not be tolerated because of pressure on the pterygoid hamulus and interference with the pterygomandibular raphe, which extends from the hamulus to the top inside back corner of the retromolar pad in the mandible. When the mouth is opened wide, the pterygomandibular raphe is pulled forward (Figure 13-10). If the denture extends too far into the hamular notch, the mucous membrane covering the raphe will be traumatized.

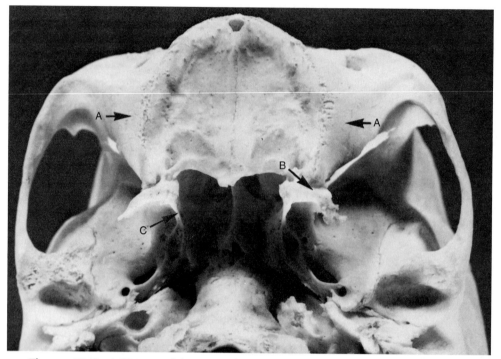

Figure 13-8 *A,* The root of the zygoma is close to the crest of the residual alveolar ridge because of the amount of resorption of the alveolar ridge. The bone is thinly covered by mucous membrane and may require relief of the denture border to prevent soreness. *B,* Hamular notch. *C,* Hamular process of the medial pterygoid plate.

PRINCIPLES AND OBJECTIVES OF IMPRESSION MAKING

The objectives of an impression are to provide support, retention, and stability for the denture. An impression also will act as a foundation for improved appearance of the lips and, at the same time, should maintain the health of the oral tissues. The impression should record all the potential denture-bearing surfaces available. To a large extent, this surface is readily identified if the biological considerations of impression making are understood correctly. However, the denture's retention is enhanced considerably if the denture extends peripherally to harness the resiliency of most of the surrounding limiting structures. An impression that records the depth of the sulcus, but not its width, will result in a denture that lacks adequate retention. Although impression techniques, methods,

and materials vary, they should be selected on the basis of biological factors. Too often techniques follow shortcuts without a consideration of the future damage that such procedures may induce.

For a successful impression to be achieved, the following concepts should be adhered to, irrespective of the selected technique:

1. The tissues of the mouth must be healthy.
2. The impression should extend to include all of the basal seat within the limits of the functions of the supporting and limiting tissues.
3. The border must be in harmony with the anatomical and physiological limitations of the oral structures.
4. A physiological type of border-molding procedure should be performed by the dentist or by the patient under the guidance of the dentist.

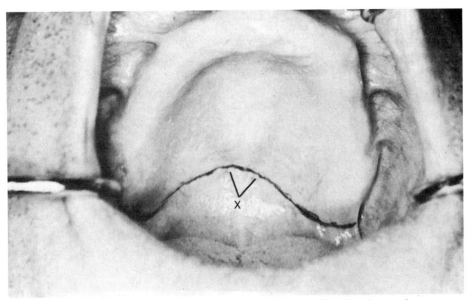

Figure 13-9   The vibrating line marked by an indelible pencil. Notice the two fovea palatinae *(X)* in the middle of the soft palate.

5. Proper space for the selected impression material should be provided within the impression tray.
6. The impression must be removed from the mouth without damage to the mucous membrane of the residual ridges.
7. A guiding mechanism should be provided for correct positioning of the impression tray in the mouth.
8. The tray and the impression material should be made of dimensionally stable materials.
9. The external shape of the impression must be similar to the external form of the complete denture.

All of these factors will contribute to a successful impression, but probably the two most important factors in making satisfactory impressions are a properly formed and accurately fitting impression tray and proper positioning of the tray within the mouth.

PREPARATION OF THE MOUTH

It is essential that the oral tissues be healthy before impressions are made. There should be no distortion or inflammation of the denture foundation tissues. These must be eliminated before the impressions are made; otherwise, the new dentures will not fit the tissues once they are no longer distorted by the swelling. The patient will then complain that the dentures, although fitting well initially, became loose after a few days. The most effective way of resolving the inflammation is to ensure that patients leave their dentures out of the mouth for at least 24 hours before the impressions are made, although a longer period often is required to resolve the problem completely. Many patients understandably object to leaving their dentures out because it is extremely disfiguring. The use of tissue conditioners is a very effective alternative, although patients should still be encouraged to leave their old dentures out as much as possible before the impressions are made. Preparation of the mouth before construction of the new dentures is discussed in detail in Chapters 7 and 8.

MAXILLARY IMPRESSION PROCEDURES

Impressions are made with a variety of materials and techniques. Some materials are more fluid than others before they harden or set. The softer materials displace soft tissue to a lesser extent and require

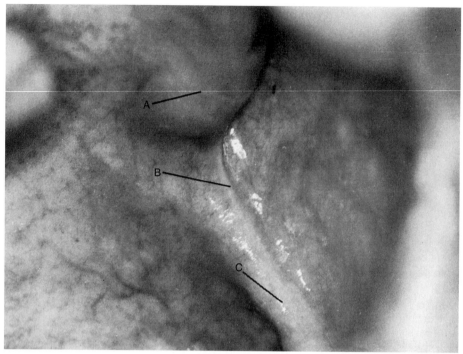

Figure 13-10 *A,* The maxillary tuberosity. *B,* The pterygomandibular raphe, which is pulled forward when the mouth is opened wide. *C,* The retromolar pad of the mandible. The cheek lies to the right in this picture and the palate to the left.

less force in their molding than do more viscous materials. These variations in the working properties of materials make it possible to devise different techniques for controlling the position and shape of the oral tissues. Some techniques are intended to record the shape of the tissues with a minimum of displacement; others are intended to displace the border tissues to a predetermined extent. Still others are devised to obtain controlled displacement of the tissues under the denture. Impressions that record the tissues with minimum displacement are described as mucostatic, whereas those that displace the tissues are classified as mucodisplacing. There is, however, no evidence to indicate that one technique produces better long-term results than another. The choice is made by the dentist on the basis of the oral conditions, concept of the function of the tissues surrounding the denture, and ability to handle the available impression materials.

Regardless of the type of impression being made, the tray is the most important part of the impression-making procedure. If the tray is too large, it will distort the tissues around the borders of the impression and will pull the soft tissues under the impression away from the bone, distorting the dimensions of the sulcus in the process. If it is too small, the border tissue will collapse inward onto the residual ridge. This too will distort the accurate recording of the border extension of the denture and prevent the proper support of the lips by the denture flange. A properly formed tray enables the dentist to carry the impression material to the mouth and control it without distorting the soft tissues that surround it.

Individual or custom trays have borders that can be adjusted so they control the movable soft tissues around the impression but do not distort them. At the same time, space is provided inside the tray so that the shape of the tissues covering the denture-bearing area may be recorded with minimal or selective displacement. Because each mouth is different, these requirements cannot be achieved successfully with stock trays. Therefore most impression procedures involve making a preliminary impression only in a stock tray. This is then poured in artificial stone and the resulting cast used to construct a custom tray. The final impression is then made with the custom tray.

PRELIMINARY IMPRESSIONS

Stock trays are constructed in either metal or plastic and may be perforated or unperforated. Although they are available in a range of shapes and sizes, they cannot fit the upper jaw of each individual without distorting the soft tissues. It is, however, important that the preliminary impression is as accurate as possible. An unsatisfactory preliminary impression will result in an unsatisfactory custom tray. This will in turn require considerable effort and time-consuming modifications before it can be used to make the final impression. Even a correctly selected stock tray will not fit the denture-bearing area perfectly. Therefore when the impression is made, it is advisable to select an impression material that has a relatively high viscosity, thereby allowing the material to compensate more easily for the deficiencies of the tray. The most suitable materials are alginate (irreversible hydrocolloid), silicone putty, or impression compound.

Silicone putty impression material has a high viscosity. It will flow beyond the tray to compensate for underextension of the stock tray, and once set, it will support itself in this position. It exhibits some degree of elasticity and so will record undercuts with reasonable accuracy. Its high viscosity means that it records surface detail poorly, and in addition, it cannot be added to if part of the impression is deficient.

The irreversible hydrocolloids record detail accurately if they are properly controlled. Because they do not absorb the mucous secretions from the palate, they can exhibit defects in the palatal part of the impression. Furthermore, the irreversible hydrocolloids lose moisture rapidly and can consequently change their size. The casts must therefore be poured soon after the impressions are removed from the mouth. The weight of the artificial stone of the cast may be sufficient to distort the borders of the impression, particularly if they are not supported by the borders of the tray.

Impression compound is a thermoplastic material with a high viscosity. Like silicone putty, the material will flow beyond the tray to compensate for underextension and will support itself in this position once it is chilled. Therefore it is not necessary to correct any underextension of the stock tray before using this material. Also, additions can be made to it if part of the impression is deficient. Its high viscosity means that it records surface detail poorly. In addition, it is nonelastic and so will not record undercuts accurately. In previous editions of this text, a technique is described whereby a preliminary compound impression is carefully and diligently "converted" into a superb custom tray. The technique has, however, been eclipsed by the one described in this chapter and in the next one on mandibular impression making. The current technique reflects a synthesis of three considerations: developments in biomaterials, a better understanding of the macroscopic and microscopic anatomy plus physiology of the edentulous milieu, and compelling clinical experiences underscoring its applied merits. The material of choice for most dentists is now a high-viscosity alginate impression material.

Tray Selection

The space available in the mouth for the upper impression is studied carefully by observation of the width and height of the vestibular spaces with the mouth partway open and the upper lip held slightly outward and downward. An edentulous stock tray that is approximately 5 mm larger than the outside surface of the residual ridge is selected. The dentist places the tray in the mouth and initially positions it by centering the labial notch of the tray over the labial frenum. The posterior extent of the tray relative to the posterior palatal seal area is maintained, and then the handle is dropped downward to permit visual inspection (Figure 13-11). Posteriorly, the tray must include both the hamular notches and vibrating line.

Alginate impression material will not support itself away from the confines of the tray, so any areas of underextension need to be corrected with soft boxing wax before the impression is made. A common site for a stock tray to be underextended is around the tuberosities and into the buccal

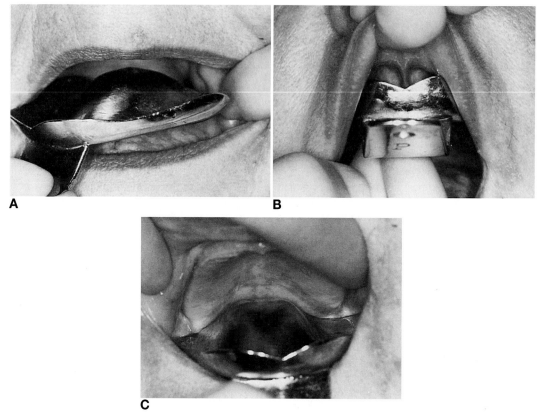

Figure 13-11   The stock tray must be of proper size and must be correctly positioned in the mouth. **A,** The patient is asked to open the mouth halfway, and the tray is rotated into the mouth in the horizontal plane using the handle. **B,** The tray is centered by positioning the labial notch over the labial frenum. **C,** The handle of the tray is dropped downward to permit visual inspection of the posterior extension across the palate and hamular notches.

vestibules. In addition, soft boxing wax can be used to line the entire border of the stock tray to create a rim that helps adapt the borders of the tray to the limiting tissues. Such a wax periphery also protects fragile border tissues from the risk of the impinging tray's hard material (e.g., metal). Across the posterior border of the tray, wax is adapted to the tissue of the posterior palatal seal area by careful elevation of the tray in this region, with the anterior part of the tray in the proper position. Again, the borders of the tray are observed visually relative to the limiting anatomical structure (Figure 13-12). The objective is to obtain a preliminary impression that is slightly overextended around the borders.

Impression Making

Before making the preliminary impression, it is advisable to practice placing the tray in position. The patient is asked to open the mouth halfway, and the tray is first centered below the upper residual ridge. The upper lip is elevated, and the tray is carried upward anteriorly into position, with the labial frenum used as a centering guide. When the tray is located properly anteriorly, the index fingers are placed in the first molar region on each side of the tray, and with alternating pressure they seat the tray upward until the wax across the posterior part of the tray comes into contact with the tissue in the posterior palatal seal area. The fingers of one hand

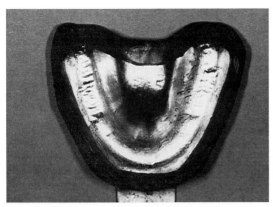

Figure 13-12 The modified stock tray is ready for making the preliminary impression.

are shifted into the middle of the tray, and border molding is carried out.

The labial and buccal vestibules can be molded by asking the patient to "suck down" onto the tray. In addition, the patient should be asked to move the mandible from side to side and then open wide. These movements will record the influence of the coronoid processes on the shape of the buccal vestibules.

The tissue surface and borders of the tray, including the rim of wax, are painted with an adhesive material to ensure that the alginate impression material adheres to the tray. The irreversible hydrocolloid is mixed according to the manufacturer's instruction and is placed in the tray and evenly distributed to fill the tray to the level of its borders. A small amount of impression material is placed in the anterior part of the palate and in the sulci opposite the tuberosities to help prevent air from being trapped in these parts of the preliminary impression (Figure 13-13, *A*). The loaded tray is then positioned in the mouth in a manner similar to that during the practice sessions (Figure 13-13, *B, C,* and *D*). Once the material has set, the cheeks and upper lip are lifted away from the borders of the impression to introduce air between the soft tissue at the reflection and the border of the impression. While the lip is elevated, the tray is removed from the mouth in one motion and inspected to ensure that all the basal seat has been recorded (Figure 13-13, *E*).

If impression compound or silicone putty is used for making the preliminary impression, the technique is the same except that the borders of the stock tray are not modified with wax. There is no need to use a tray adhesive for impression compound, although one is necessary for silicone putty. Preloading of the palate and around the tuberosities is not undertaken. The tray is loaded with the impression material and seated in the mouth in exactly the same manner as for alginate impression material.

The borders of the custom tray should now be determined. Two choices are available. Either the periphery is outlined with a disposable indelible marker on the impression at the chairside (the preferred option), or the outline is somewhat arbitrarily marked on the poured cast in the laboratory. The completed impression should be observed next to the patient's mouth and the junction of the attached and unattached mucosal tissue visually identified on the border of the impression (Figure 13-14). The impression is poured in artificial stone, and the custom tray outline should now be evident on the cast. If the outline has not been marked on the impression, it can be drawn directly on the cast. However, with the patient not present for a correlation between anatomical features and the cast, this becomes an educated guess.

Clinical experience has shown that a large number of edentulous patients seeking treatment for new complete dentures are already wearing complete dentures. If these have been worn successfully for a number of years and if the extension of the base is satisfactory, then logic suggests that these dentures can be used as a starting point for developing an accurate impression of the denture-bearing surface.

As part of the protocol for restoring the health of the supporting tissue, the denture will have been relined with a tissue conditioner. The result can be regarded as the preliminary impression and used to produce the preliminary cast by pouring artificial stone into the fitting surface of the denture. If undercuts exist on the fitting surface of the denture (e.g., around the tuberosities), then artificial stone should not be used. It would be impossible to remove the denture from the cast without damaging either the cast or, even worse, the denture. The undercuts can, of course, be removed before adding the tissue conditioner, but this means that the fitting surface of the denture has been

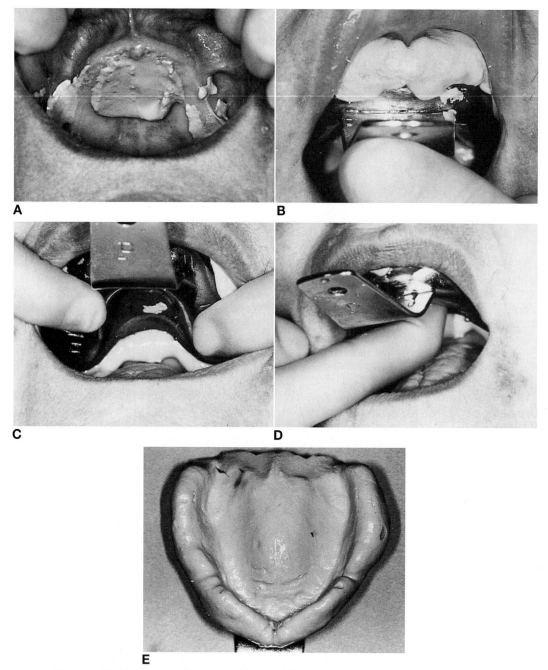

Figure 13-13 **A,** A small amount of irreversible hydrocolloid is placed into the palate and around the tuberosities. **B,** The upper lip is elevated and the tray carried upward anteriorly. The labial notch is lined up with the labial frenum. **C,** The tray is seated posteriorly by the index fingers in the region of the first molars. **D,** The tray is held in place with a finger placed into the center of the palate. **E,** The completed impression.

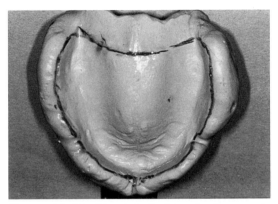

Figure 13-14 The clinically determined proposed denture base outline is drawn on with a disposable indelible marker.

irretrievably altered. This is of no consequence if the replacement denture is successful. However, if the new denture does not meet the patient's approval, then a very awkward situation can develop. If undercuts exist, the cast should be produced preferably in silicone putty, which exhibits sufficient elasticity to permit the denture to be removed but is rigid enough to allow the fabrication of a custom tray.

FINAL IMPRESSIONS

A number of materials are available for making the final impression. Plaster of Paris was once widely used as a final impression material, but it is not "user friendly" and has been superseded by other materials. These include metallic oxide impression paste, polyether and silicone impression materials, and irreversible hydrocolloids.

Metallic oxide impression pastes are rigid when set and can be used only where there are no bony undercuts. They are used in a close-fitting tray, and so the overall bulk of the impression is kept to a minimum. This is particularly useful where the denture-bearing area is considerably reduced. In these circumstances, a close-fitting tray is easier to locate correctly in the mouth compared with a spaced tray. In addition, it is easier to avoid displacing the limiting structures with a close-fitting tray. Metallic oxide impression pastes should not be used in patients with dry mouths because the paste tends to adhere to the mucous membrane.

The elastomeric impression materials and irreversible hydrocolloids are all used in spaced custom trays. To avoid displacing the border tissues, a less viscous irreversible hydrocolloid is used for making the final impression compared with that used for the preliminary impression. Irrespective of which material is selected, the optimum result will be achieved only if the custom tray has been constructed and refined correctly.

Construction of the Custom Tray

Baseplate wax, approximately 1 mm thick, is placed on the cast within the outlined border to provide space in the tray for the final impression material. The posterior palatal seal area on the cast is not covered with the wax spacer. Therefore the completed custom tray will contact the mucous membrane across the posterior palatal border, and additional stress placed here during the making of the final impression will help achieve a posterior border seal. In addition, this part of the tray will act as a guiding stop to help position the tray properly during the impression procedure (Figure 13-15, *A*). A wax spacer will not be used if a metallic oxide impression paste has been selected for making the final impression.

The custom tray should be 2 to 3 mm thick, with a stepped handle in the anterior region of the tray to facilitate removal from the mouth. The step should be of sufficient height to avoid distortion of the upper lip when the tray is in the mouth (Figure 13-15, *B*). The premise in prescribing a custom tray is that the proposed denture-bearing area of the denture will be reflected in the tray's extension.

Refining the Custom Tray

When the custom tray is removed from the preliminary cast, the wax spacer is left inside the tray (Figure 13-16). The spacer allows the tray to be properly positioned in the mouth during border molding procedures.

Border molding is the process by which the shape of the border of the tray is made to conform accurately to the contours of the buccal and labial vestibules. This essential requirement of the tray's fit ensures an optimal peripheral seal. It begins with manipulation of the border tissue against a

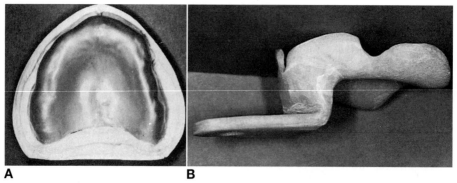

Figure 13-15 **A,** Relief wax covers the basal seat area except for the posterior palatal seal area and the labial and buccal reflections. **B,** The custom tray should be 2 to 3 mm thick and the handle shaped so that it does not interfere with the position of the upper lip.

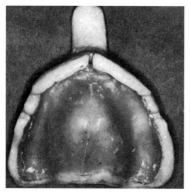

Figure 13-16 The custom tray covers the entire basal seat area. The wax spacer has been left inside the tray to allow the tray to be properly positioned in the mouth during border molding.

moldable impression material that is properly supported and controlled by the tray. The amount of support supplied by the tray and the amount of force exerted through the tissues vary according to the resistance or viscosity of the impression material.

For border molding to be carried out successfully, space must be created for the border molding material. Therefore the flanges of the custom tray should be reduced until they are 2 mm short of the reflections. Once the buccal and labial flanges of the custom tray have been adjusted, the posterior palatal border is checked. The tray must contain both hamular notches and extend approximately 2 mm posterior to the vibrating line. The vibrating

line is observed in the mouth as the patient says a series of short "ahs." The posterior border of the impression tray is marked with a disposable indelible marker, the palatal tissues are dried quickly, the tray is placed in the mouth, and the patient is asked to say "ah." The tray is removed from the mouth, and the mark that has been transferred from the tray to the mouth is compared with the vibrating line and the hamular notches. If it is underextended, the length is corrected by the addition of modeling compound.

The tray is now ready for border molding, during which the borders of the tray are molded to a form that will be in harmony with the physiological action of the limiting anatomical structures. This may be carried out in sections either recording one part of the border at a time or recording all parts of the border simultaneously.

Recording all of the border simultaneously has two general advantages: first, the number of insertions of the tray is reduced to one, and second, developing all borders simultaneously avoids propagation of errors caused by a mistake in one section affecting the border contours in another.

The requirements of a material to be used for simultaneous molding of all borders are that it should (1) have sufficient body to allow it to remain in position on the borders during loading of the tray, (2) allow some preshaping of the form of the borders without adhering to the fingers, (3) have a setting time of 3 to 5 minutes, (4) retain adequate flow while the tray is seated in the mouth,

(5) allow finger placement of the material into deficient parts after the tray is seated, (6) not cause excessive displacement of the tissues of the vestibules, and (7) be readily trimmed and shaped so excess material can be removed and the borders shaped before the final impression is made.

Stick impression compound is ideally suited for carrying out border molding in sections. However, it is unsuitable for recording all parts of the border simultaneously because it is impossible to get the material softened over the full length of the border. Polyether impression materials are well suited for border molding as they meet all of the requirements listed previously.

When border molding with polyether impression material, the following procedure should be followed:

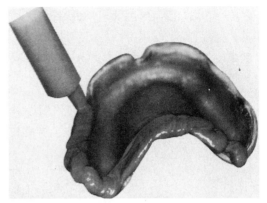

Figure 13-17   The polyether material is placed across the posterior palatal seal area and continued around the entire border of the tray.

1. An adhesive for polyether impressions is placed on the border of the tray, covering both the inside and outside of the border. The wax spacer is left inside the tray but should be cut away from the border to allow space for the impression material.
2. The polyether material is mixed and introduced into a plastic "impression" syringe. Slightly less catalyst should be used than recommended by the manufacturers to provide sufficient working time to complete the border molding.
3. The polyether material is syringed around the border and across the posterior palatal seal area (Figure 13-17). The material is quickly preshaped to proper contours with fingers moistened in cold water.
4. The tray is placed in the mouth, making certain that the lips are retracted sufficiently to avoid scraping the material from the border.
5. The border is inspected to ensure that impression material is present in the vestibule. If insufficient material is present, excess material from an adjacent site should be transferred with a finger moistened in the patient's saliva.
6. Border molding is carried out. This is accomplished in the anterior region when the lip is elevated and extended out, downward, and inward (Figure 13-18, *A*). In the region of the buccal frenum, the cheek is elevated and then pulled outward, down-

ward, and inward and moved backward and forward to simulate movement of the frenum (Figure 13-18, *B*). Posteriorly, the buccal flange is border molded by extending the cheek outward, downward, and inward. The patient is asked to open wide and move the mandible from side to side.
7. When the impression material is set, the tray is removed from the mouth.
8. The border molding is examined to determine that it is adequate (Figure 13-19). The contour of the border should be rounded. Any deficient sites can be corrected with a small mix of polyether material added to the appropriate area. Overextensions are readily detected because the tray will protrude through the polyether material and be adjusted as necessary.

The technique is basically the same if stick impression compound is used except that the border is molded in sections. The labial vestibule is molded initially, then each buccal vestibule and finally the posterior palatal area. The tray with the addition of softened compound is placed in the mouth, with the wax spacer still inside the tray, and the appropriate area is molded. The tray is carefully removed from the mouth, and the impression compound is chilled in cold water. There is no need to use an adhesive to attach the impression compound to the tray.

If the custom tray is constructed on a cast taken from the optimized previous denture, it can

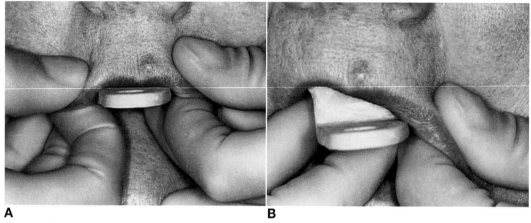

A   **B**

Figure 13-18   A, Border molding in the anterior region is achieved by moving the lip outward, downward, and inward. **B,** The left buccal flange is molded by moving the cheek outward, downward, inward, and then backward and forward to simulate movement of the frenum.

be presumed that the tray already reflects the border molding developed with the tissue conditioner that has been used to reline the denture. Thus further border molding is very likely unnecessary. This is assuming that the previous denture base is correctly extended and that care has been taken with the tissue conditioner to obtain the correct border shape. A careful scrutiny of the tray's periphery in the mouth while moving the peripheral

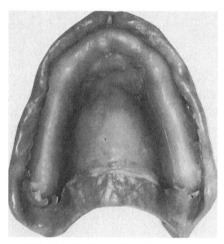

Figure 13-19   Border molding has been completed, including the posterior palatal seal area. The relief wax is still in the impression tray.

tissues will help the dentist determine whether additional segmental border molding is required. Patients are able to wear complete dentures with apparent success even though the bases are not extended correctly. Accepting an incorrectly extended base just because the denture has been worn previously is not good practice and excludes the possibility of providing something better.

Preparing the Tray to Secure the Final Impression

Space must now be created for the final impression material; otherwise, the borders will be overextended and the mucous membrane displaced unnecessarily.

The spacer wax is removed from inside the tray along with any border molding material that has flowed over it. Any excess material on the outside of the tray also is removed. The thickness of the border will vary from individual to individual, but a thick border in the anterior region results in a poor appearance. If necessary, the thickness of the labial flange should be adjusted to approximately 2.5 to 3 mm in thickness from one buccal frenum to the other. Material that extends into an undercut is reduced because this allows the tray to be seated more easily. Finally, a small amount of material is removed from those parts of the border that have not already been adjusted. Approximately 0.5 mm is removed from the inner, outer, and top surface of the border.

Stick impression compound is adjusted with a scalpel; the polyether is adjusted with either a scalpel or a bur. The material over the posterior area is not adjusted. This serves three functions. First, it slightly displaces the soft tissues at the distal end of the denture to enhance posterior border (palatal) seal. Second, it serves as a guide for positioning the tray properly for the final impression. Third, it helps prevent excess impression material from running down the patient's throat.

Finally, holes can be placed in the palate of the impression tray with a medium-sized round bur to provide escape ways for the final impression material, and the adhesive material is applied. The holes furnish relief during the making of the final impression so that the mucous membrane over the medial palatal raphe and in the anterolateral and posterolateral regions of the hard palate is not displaced excessively. Holes are also preferably placed over residual ridge sites where the soft tissues are mobile and displaceable. The objective is to avoid recording denture-bearing tissues in a displaced or distorted position.

Making the Final Impression

As with any impression, the correct positioning of the tray in the patient's mouth is essential if the final impression is to be achieved successfully. The procedure for placing the tray is the same as that used when making preliminary impressions. The tray is centered as it is carried to position on the upper ridge. This is most easily achieved by observing the position of the labial frenum relative to the labial notch in the tray. When the frenum is positioned within the notch, the index fingers of each hand are shifted to the first molar region, and with alternating pressure the tray is carried upward, without displacement of the front end of the tray downward, until the posterior palatal seal of the tray fits properly in the hamular notches and across the palate. The tray is held in position with a finger placed in the palate immediately anterior to the posterior palatal seal. This procedure should be practiced with the empty tray until the dentist feels confident of the proper position of the tray in the mouth.

The final impression material of choice is mixed according to the manufacturer's instructions and uniformly distributed within the tray. All borders must be covered. The tray is then positioned in the mouth, as described previously, and border molding is performed.

When the final impression material has set, the tray is removed from the mouth and inspected for acceptability. If it needs to be remade, the impression material is removed with particular care to preserve the border molding. Assuming the tray was formed properly, faulty positioning is the most frequent reason that a final impression must be remade. A number of reasons for remaking final impressions are described in the next chapter.

Boxing Impressions and Making the Casts

Great care is taken when making the final impression to record the functional width and depth of the sulcus. It is essential that this be preserved in the final cast. The procedure for preserving this form is called *boxing*.

A strip of boxing wax is attached all the way around the outside of the impression approximately 2 to 3 mm below the border and sealed to it with a spatula (Figure 13-20, *A*). The strip must be maintained at its full width, particularly at the distal end of the impression, to hold the vertical walls of the boxing away from the impressions and provide space for adequate thickness of the cast in this region. A thin sheet of modeling wax is then attached to the outside of the boxing strip to form the vertical wall of the boxing (Figure 13-20, *B*). The vertical wall should extend 10 to 15 mm above the impression so that the base of the cast at its narrowest point will be of this thickness. The sheet of wax should extend completely around the impression and be sealed to the boxing wax strip to prevent the escape of artificial stone when this is poured into the impression. Also, the impression should be supported in a level position by the boxing. Boxing procedures cannot be used on impressions made in hydrocolloid materials because the wax will not adhere to the impression.

Artificial stone is mixed according to the manufacturer's instructions. The stone is poured into the boxed impression level with the top of the vertical wall of the boxing and allowed to set. After

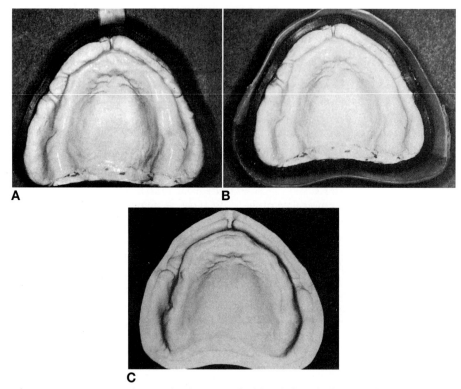

Figure 13-20   **A,** Boxing wax has been attached just below the borders of the final impression. **B,** The vertical wall of the boxing is securely attached to the boxing strip. The height of the wall will allow the base of the cast to be from 10 to 15 mm thick. **C,** The cast provides an accurate positive record of the basal seat and reflections. The thickness and form of the cast permit easy adaptation of the materials used in making the occlusion rims.

the final impression is separated from the cast, the cast must be shaped to maintain the form of the borders of the impression and yet be easily accessible for adaptation of the materials used in making the occlusion rims (Figure 13-20, *C*).

SUMMARY

1. Ensure the tissues of the mouth are healthy.
   a. Optimize the present dentures with tissue conditioners and occlusal adjustments.
   b. Encourage the patient to leave the dentures out as much as possible.
   c. Instruct the patient in oral and denture hygiene and to massage the denture-bearing tissues.
   d. Prescribe any necessary preprosthetic surgery.

2. Make preliminary impressions.
   a. Use a stock tray, modified with wax around the border, and irreversible hydrocolloid impression material.
   b. Use a stock tray with impression compound material or silicone putty impression material.
   c. On the impression's border, identify the peripheral outline of the proposed custom tray. This will conform to a line between the attached and unattached mucous membrane. Make a laboratory stone cast.
   d. If the denture has been optimized, that is, functionally border molded with a tissue conditioner, regard it as the preliminary impression. Make a laboratory cast in stone or silicone putty.

3. Fabricate a custom tray.
   a. Cover the basal seat area with wax except for the posterior palated seal area and the labial and buccal reflections
   b. Construct a custom tray that extends just past the identified junction of the attached and unattached mucosa.
4. Refine the custom tray.
   a. Try the tray in the mouth and adjust the borders as necessary. The flanges should be 2 mm short of the reflection and extend approximately 2 mm beyond the vibrating line.
   b. Develop the borders of the tray with either an incremental technique with stick tracing compound or a one-step technique with a polyether impression material.
   c. If the tray has been constructed on a cast taken from the optimized previous denture, then border molding may not be necessary.
   d. Place relief holes in the tray as required.

5. Make final impression with preferred impression material.
6. Master cast preparation.
   a. Box and pour the final impression.
   b. Trim the cast.

Bibliography

Jani RM, Bhargave K: A histologic comparison of palatal mucosa before and after wearing complete dentures, *J Prosthet Dent* 36:254–260, 1976.

Laney WR, Gonzalez JB: The maxillary denture: its palatal relief and posterior palatal seal, *J Am Dent Assoc* 75:1182–1187, 1967.

Lye TL: The significance of the fovae palatini in complete denture prosthodontics, *J Prosthet Dent* 33:504–507, 1975.

Martone AL: Clinical applications of concepts of functional anatomy and speech science to complete denture prosthodontics, *J Prosthet Dent* 13:4–33, 1963.

Watson IB, MacDonald DG: Oral mucosa and complete dentures, *J Prosthet Dent* 47:133–140, 1982.

Watson IB, MacDonald DG: Regional variations in the palatal mucosa of the edentulous mouth, *J Prosthet Dent* 50:853–859, 1983.

CHAPTER 14

Developing an Analogue/Substitute for the Mandibular Denture-Bearing Area

David M. Davis

THE MANDIBLE

The mandibular denture poses a great technical challenge for the dentist and often a significant management challenge for the patient. Nonetheless, the fundamental principles for mandibular impressions are similar to those for maxillary impressions. Both the support or stress-bearing area and the peripheral or limiting area will be in contact with the denture's fitting or impression surface. The denture base must extend as far as possible without interfering with the health or function of the tissues. The support for a mandibular denture comes from the body of the mandible. The peripheral seal is provided by the form of the denture's border as determined by the macroscopic and microscopic anatomy of the limiting structures. However, the presence of the tongue and its individual size, form, and activity complicate the impression procedure for the lower denture and also the patient's ability to manage the denture. Consequently, the retention of a mandibular denture is constantly threatened by tongue movements.

ANATOMY OF SUPPORTING STRUCTURES

Support for the lower denture is provided by the mandible and the soft tissues overlying it. The total area of support from the mandible is significantly less than from the maxillae. The average available denture-bearing area for an edentulous mandible is 14 cm^2, whereas for edentulous maxillae it is 24 cm^2. This means that the mandible is less capable of resisting occlusal forces than the maxillae are, and extra care must be taken if the available support is to be used to advantage.

Crest of the Residual Ridge

The crest of the residual alveolar ridge is covered by fibrous connective tissue, but in many mouths the underlying bone is cancellous and without a good cortical bony plate covering it (Figure 14-1).

The mucous membrane covering the crest of the residual ridge is similar to that of the upper ridge insofar as in the healthy mouth, it is covered by a keratinized layer and is attached by its submucosa to the periosteum of the mandible. The extent of this attachment varies considerably. In some people, the submucosa is loosely attached to the bone over the entire crest of the residual ridge, and the soft tissue is quite movable. In others, the submucosa is firmly attached to the bone on both the crest and the slopes of the lower residual ridge.

The mucous membrane of the crest of the lower residual ridge, when securely attached to the underlying bone, is capable of providing good soft tissue support for the denture. However, because underlying bone is often cancellous, the crest of the residual ridge may not be favorable as the primary stress-bearing area for a lower denture.

The Buccal Shelf

The area between the mandibular buccal frenum and the anterior edge of the masseter muscle is

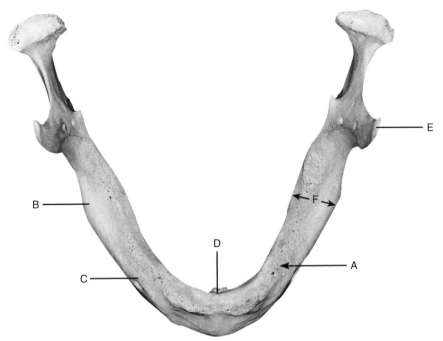

Figure 14-1 *A,* The crest of the residual ridge is often composed of cancellous bone. *B,* The buccal shelf consists of cortical bone. *C,* The mental foramen. *D,* The genial tubercles. *E,* The coronoid process. *F,* When the alveolar ridge resorbs, it results in a basal seal that becomes wider and larger. This change occurs because as resorption moves the crest of the ridge inferiorly, the width of the mandible becomes greater than that of the alveolar process at the time the teeth were removed.

known as the *buccal shelf* (Figure 14-2). It is bound medially by the crest of the residual ridge, laterally by the external oblique ridge, and distally by the retromolar pad. The total width of the bony foundation in this region becomes greater as alveolar resorption continues. The reason is that the width of the inferior border of the mandible is greater than the width at the alveolar process (see Figure 14-1).

The mucous membrane covering the buccal shelf is more loosely attached and less keratinized than the mucous membrane covering the crest of the lower residual ridge and contains a thicker submucosal layer. The inferior part of the buccinator muscle is attached to the buccal shelf, and its fibers are found in the submucosa immediately overlying the bone.

The mucous membrane overlying the buccal shelf may not be as suitable histologically to provide primary support for the denture as the mucous mem-

brane overlying the crest of the residual ridge. However, the bone of the buccal shelf is covered by a layer of cortical bone. This, plus the fact that the shelf lies at right angles to the vertical occlusal forces, makes it the most suitable primary stress-bearing area for a lower denture (Figure 14-3).

Shape of the Supporting Structure

The configuration of the bone that forms the support for a mandibular denture varies considerably among individuals. Factors that influence this form are listed in the previous chapter. Many edentulous mandibles are extremely flat, and indeed, the bearing surface can become concave, allowing the attaching structures, especially on the lingual side of the ridge, to fall over onto the ridge surface. Such conditions require displacement of these

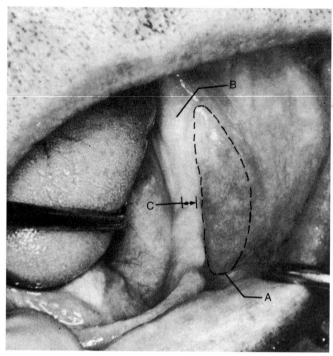

Figure 14-2 The buccal shelf is shown by the dotted line. It extends from the buccal frenum *(A)* to the retromolar pad *(B)* and from the external oblique ridge of the mandible to the crest of the residual alveolar ridge *(C)*.

tissues by the impression and make the lingual flange of the denture more difficult to adapt.

The maxillae resorb upward and inward to become progressively smaller because of the direction and inclination of the roots of the teeth and the alveolar process. The longer the maxillae have been edentulous, the smaller their bearing area is likely to be. The opposite is true of the mandible, which inclines outward and becomes progressively wider according to its edentulous age. This progressive change of the edentulous mandible and maxillae makes many patients appear prognathic (Figure 14-4).

In addition, there are a number of anatomical features that influence the shape of the supporting structure.

Mylohyoid Ridge Soft tissue usually hides the sharpness of the mylohyoid ridge. The shape and inclination of the ridge vary greatly among edentu-

lous patients. Anteriorly, the mylohyoid ridge, with its attached mylohyoid muscle, lies close to the inferior border of the mandible. Posteriorly, after resorption, it often lies flush with the superior surface of the residual ridge (Figure 14-5). The mucous membrane over a sharp or irregular mylohyoid ridge will be easily traumatized by the denture base, unless relief is provided in the denture base. The area under the mylohyoid ridge is undercut.

Mental Foramen As resorption takes place, the mental foramina will come to lie closer to the crest of the residual ridge (see Figure 14-1). In these circumstances, the mental nerves and blood vessels may be compressed by the denture base unless relief is provided. Pressure on the mental nerve can cause numbness of the lower lip.

Genial Tubercles Like the mental foramina, the genial tubercles usually lie well away from the crest

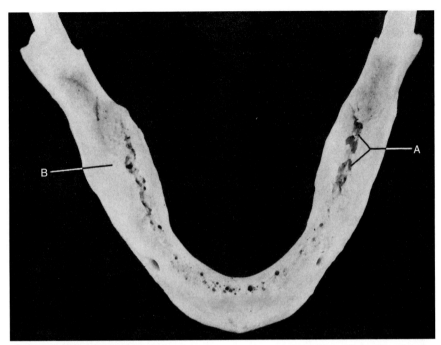

Figure 14-3 The crest of the residual alveolar ridge consists of cancellous bone *(A)*. Its porosity and roughness make it unsuitable as the primary stress-bearing area. Therefore the buccal shelf *(B)* is selected as the primary support area.

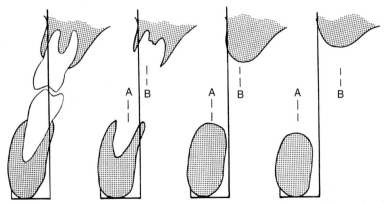

Figure 14-4 Progressive resorption of the maxillary and mandibular ridges makes the maxillae narrower and the mandible wider. The lines *A* and *B* represent the centers of the ridges. Notice how the distance between them becomes greater as the mandible and maxillae resorb.

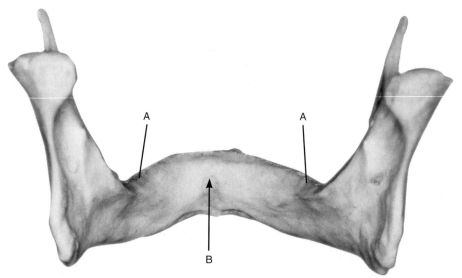

Figure 14-5 An edentulous ridge with a flat residual alveolar ridge. *A,* The mylohyoid ridges lie flush posteriorly with the crest of the alveolar ridge. The mylohyoid ridges are sharp and the area beneath them is undercut. *B,* The genial tubercles that come to lie closer to the crest of the alveolar ridge as resorption occurs.

of the ridge. However, with resorption, the genial tubercles become increasingly prominent (see Figure 14-5).

Torus Mandibularis The torus mandibularis is a bony prominence usually found bilaterally and lingually near the first and second premolars midway between the soft tissues of the floor of the mouth and the crest of the alveolar process. In edentulous mouths, where considerable resorption has taken place, the superior border of the torus may be flush with the crest of the residual ridge (Figure 14-6). The torus mandibularis is covered by an extremely thin layer of mucous membrane. It often needs to be removed surgically because it can be difficult to provide relief within the denture for the torus without breaking the border seal.

ANATOMY OF PERIPHERAL OR LIMITING STRUCTURES

The influence of the limiting structures in the mandible is more difficult to record than in the maxillae. The reason is that the structures on the lingual side must be considered, as well as those around the labial and buccal surfaces of the denture. The structures on the lingual side of the mandible are more complicated to control than those on the buccal and labial sides. The problem is the greater range of their movement and the speed of their actions.

Labial Vestibule

The labial vestibule runs from the labial frenum to the buccal frenum (Figures 14-7 and 14-8). The length and thickness of the labial flange vary with the amount of tissue that has been lost. The extent of the denture flange in this area often is limited because of the muscles that are inserted close to the crest of the ridge. The mentalis muscle is a particularly active muscle in this region. The depth of the flange will be determined by the turn of the mucolabial fold, which is the line of flexure of the mucous membrane as it passes from the mandible to the lip.

The mandibular labial frenum contains a band of fibrous connective tissue that helps attach the orbicularis oris muscle. Therefore the frenum is

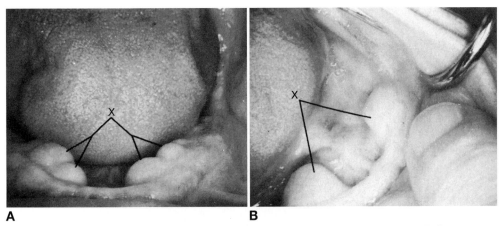

Figure 14-6   Tori mandibulari (X). Surgical reduction of these will be necessary before a satisfactory seal can be developed.

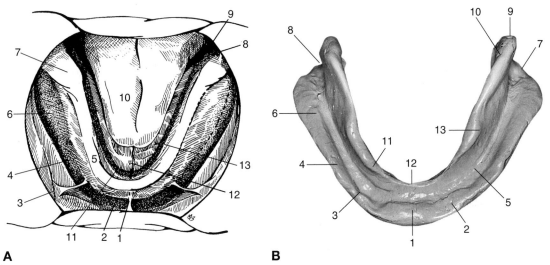

Figure 14-7   Correlation of anatomical landmarks. **A,** Intraoral drawing of the mandibular arch: *1,* labial frenum; *2,* labial vestibule; *3,* buccal frenum; *4,* buccal vestibule; *5,* residual alveolar ridge; *6,* buccal shelf; *7,* retromolar pad; *8,* pterygomandibular raphe; *9,* retromylohyoid fossa; *10,* tongue; *11,* alveololingual sulcus; *12,* lingual frenum; *13,* region and premylohyoid eminence. **B,** Mandibular final impression showing the corresponding denture landmarks: *1,* labial notch; *2,* labial flange; *3,* buccal notch; *4,* buccal flange; *5,* alveolar groove; *6,* buccal flange, which covers the buccal shelf; *7,* retromolar pad; *8,* pterygomandibular notch; *9,* lingual flange with extension into retromylohyoid fossa; *10,* inclined plane for the tongue; *11,* lingual flange; *12,* lingual notch; *13,* premylohyoid eminence. (Adapted from Martone AL: *J Prosthet Dent* 13: 4-33, 1963.)

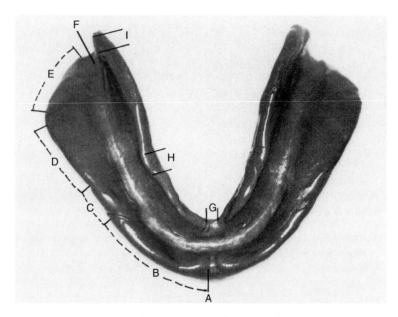

Figure 14-8   A completed final impression with border outline landmarks. *A,* Mandibular labial notch. *B,* Mandibular labial flange. *C,* Mandibular buccal notch. *D,* Buccal flange. *E,* Area influenced by the masseter. *F,* Retromolar pad area. *G,* Lingual notch. *H,* Premylohyoid eminence. *I,* Retromylohyoid fossa. Notice the S curve of the lingual flanges and also that in the molar region, the flanges slope toward the tongue and extend below the attachment of the mylohyoid muscles on the mylohyoid ridges. The slope of the lingual flanges allows the mylohyoid muscles to contract and raise the floor of the mouth without displacing the lower denture. The length of the lingual flange in the molar region allows it to reach the mucolingual fold of tissue in the floor of the mouth to maintain the seal of the lower denture. The posterior end of the lingual flange bends laterally toward the mandible to fit into the retromylohyoid fossa. This part of the denture guides the tongue onto the top of the lingual flange.

quite sensitive and active, and the denture must be fitted carefully around it to maintain a seal without causing soreness.

The muscles of the lower lip pull actively across the denture border, polished surfaces, and teeth. When the patient's mouth opens wide, the orbicularis oris muscle becomes stretched, narrowing the sulcus. This would displace the mandibular denture if the flange was unnecessarily thick. Mandibular dentures and, hence, impressions will always be narrowest in the anterior labial region (see Figures 14-7 and 14-8).

The mucous membrane lining the labial vestibule and all limiting structures in the mandible is similar to that lining the vestibule in the upper jaw. The epithelium is thin and nonkeratinized, and the submucosa is formed of loosely arranged connective tissue fibers mixed with elastic fibers and muscle fibers, depending on the site of histological examination.

Buccal Vestibule

The buccal vestibule extends posteriorly from the buccal frenum to the outside back corner of the retromolar pad. The buccal flange, which starts immediately posterior to the buccal frenum, swings wide into the cheek and is nearly at right angles to the biting force. The impression is always widest in this region (see Figures 14-7 and 14-8).

The extent of the buccal vestibule is influenced by the buccinator muscle, which extends from the modiolus anteriorly to the pterygomandibular raphe posteriorly and has its lower fibers attached to the buccal shelf and the external oblique ridge. The external oblique ridge does not govern the extension of the buccal flange because the resistance, or lack of resistance, encountered in this region varies widely. The buccal flange may extend to the external oblique ridge, up onto it, or even over it, depending on the location of the mucobuccal fold. However, palpation of the external oblique ridge is a valuable landmark in helping to ascertain the relative amount of resistance, or lack of resistance, of the border tissues in this region.

The denture should cover completely the buccal shelf, despite the fact that it will rest directly on fibers of the buccinator muscle. The bearing of the denture on muscle fibers would not be possible except for the fact that the fibers of the buccinator muscle run parallel to the base and, hence, its pull, when in function, is parallel to the border and not at right angles to it. Thus its displacing action is slight. More resistance is encountered in this region when the denture is first inserted than is manifested a few weeks after the denture has been worn. Thus it is possible to stretch and displace these tissues and so increase the area available for support and stability.

The distobuccal border, at the end of the buccal vestibule, must converge rapidly to avoid displacement by the contracting masseter muscle, whose anterior fibers run outside and behind the buccinator muscle in this region (see Figure 14-8). When the masseter muscle contracts, it pushes inward against the buccinator muscle and produces a bulge into the mouth. The extent to which the masseter muscle influences the distobuccal edge of the mandibular impression and, hence the denture, varies from individual to individual. If the ramus of the mandible has a perpendicular surface and the origin of the muscle on the zygomatic arch is situated medially, the muscle pulls more directly across the distobuccal denture border. This forces the buccinator muscle inward, reducing the space in this area. If the opposite is true, greater extension is allowed on the distobuccal portion of the mandibular impression. The extent of its effect will be recorded only when the masseter muscle contracts.

Distal Extension

The distal extension of the mandibular denture is limited by the ramus of the mandible, by the buccinator muscle fibers that cross from the buccal to the lingual side as they attach to the pterygomandibular raphe and the superior constrictor muscle, and by the sharpness of the lateral bony boundaries of the retromolar fossa, which is formed by a continuation of the internal and external oblique ridges ascending the ramus. If the impression extends onto the ramus, the buccinator muscle and adjacent tissues will be compressed between the hard denture border and the sharp oblique ridges. This will not only cause soreness but also limit the function of the buccinator muscle. The desirable distal extension is slightly to the lingual of these bony prominences and includes the pear-shaped retromolar pad, which provides a soft tissue border seal (Figure 14-9).

The retromolar pad is a triangular soft pad of tissue at the distal end of the lower ridge. Its mucosa is composed of a thin, nonkeratinized epithelium, and in addition to loose alveolar tissue, its submucosa contains glandular tissue, fibers of the buccinator and superior constrictor muscles, the pterygomandibular raphe, and the terminal part of the tendon of the temporalis muscle. The action of these muscles limits the extent of the denture and prevents placement of extra pressure on the distal part of the retromolar pad during impression procedures. Because of this, the denture base should extend approximately one half to two thirds over the retromolar pad.

Lingual Border

The lingual tissues under the tongue exhibit less direct resistance than the labial and buccal borders do and are distorted easily when the impression is being made. Such extension will cause tissue soreness and dislodgement of the denture by tongue movements. For success to be achieved with a lower impression, it is important to understand the action of the mylohyoid muscle.

Mylohyoid Muscle The floor of the mouth is formed by the mylohyoid muscle, which arises from the whole length of the mylohyoid ridge. This ridge is sharp and distinct in the molar region and becomes almost indiscernible anteriorly. Medially,

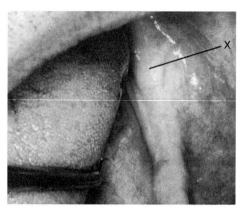

Figure 14-9 The retromolar pad *(X)* is the posterior landmark for a mandibular denture.

the fibers join those from the mylohyoid muscle of the opposite side, and posteriorly they continue to the hyoid base (Figure 14-10). The muscle lies deep to the sublingual gland and other structures in the anterior region and so does not affect the border of the denture in this region except indirectly.

However, the posterior part of the mylohyoid muscle in the molar region affects the lingual impres-

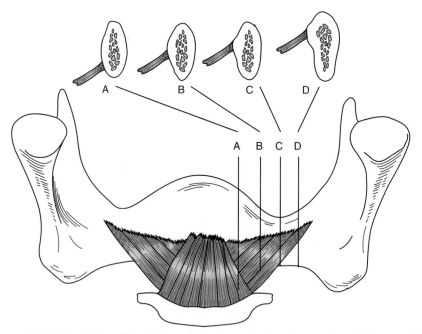

Figure 14-10 Relationships of the mylohyoid muscle in various regions. The letters with prime signs denote cross sections of the designated areas. *A,* Canine region. *B,* Premolar region. *C,* First molar. *D,* Third molar. At point *D,* notice that the mylohyoid ridge approaches the level of the alveolar crest. The angle of the posterior lingual flange in the molar region is affected by this muscle; anteriorly, only the length of the flange is affected.

sion border in swallowing and in moving the tongue. During swallowing, the mylohyoid muscles contract, raising the floor of the mouth. During impression taking, it is very easy to carry the impression material into the undercut below the mylohyoid ridge because the mylohyoid muscle is a thin sheet of fibers that, in a relaxed state, will not resist the impression material. Extension of the lingual flange under the mylohyoid ridge cannot be tolerated in function because it will interfere with the action of the mylohyoid muscle when it contracts, and this will displace the denture, causing soreness. For the denture to be successful, the flange must be made parallel to the mylohyoid muscle when it is contracted.

Fortunately, in this posterior region, the lingual flange can go beyond the mylohyoid muscle's attachment to the mandible because the mucolingual fold is not in this area. Thus the impression may depart from the stress-bearing area of the lingual surface of the ridge, moving away from the body of the mandible to be suspended under the tongue in soft tissue on both sides of the mouth, thereby reaching the mucolingual fold of soft tissue for a border seal (see Figures 14-7 and 14-8). The distance that these lingual borders can be away from the bony areas will depend on the functional movements of the floor of the mouth and by the amount that the residual ridge has resorbed.

An extension of the lingual flange well beyond the palpable position of the mylohyoid ridge, but not into the undercut, has other advantages. The lack of direct pressure on the sharp edge of the ridge will eliminate a possible source of discomfort. If the impression is made with pressure on or slightly over this ridge, displacement of the denture and soreness are sure to result from lateral and vertical stresses. On the other hand, if the border stops above the mylohyoid ridge, vertical forces will cause soreness, and the border seal will be easily broken. If the flange is properly shaped and extended, it will provide border seal and guide the tongue to rest on top of the flange.

Retromylohyoid Fossa

The retromylohyoid fossa, as its name implies, is the area posterior to the mylohyoid muscle. As the lingual flange moves into this fossa, it ceases to be influenced by the action of the mylohyoid muscle

and so can move back toward the body of the mandible producing the typical S curve of the lingual flange (see Figures 14-7 and 14-8).

The retromylohyoid fossa is bounded by the retromylohyoid curtain. The posterolateral portion of the retromylohyoid curtain overlies the superior constrictor muscle, and the posteromedial portion covers the palatoglossal muscle plus the lateral surface of the tongue. The inferior wall overlies the submandibular gland, which fills the gap between the superior constrictor muscle and the most distal attachment of the mylohyoid muscle. The denture border should extend posteriorly to contact the retromylohyoid curtain when the tip of the tongue is placed against the front part of the upper residual ridge. Protrusion of the tongue causes the retromylohyoid curtain to move forward.

The medial pterygoid muscle lies behind the superior constrictor muscle (Figure 14-11). Contraction of the medial pterygoid muscle can cause a bulge in the wall of the retromylohyoid curtain in the same way that contraction of the masseter muscle can cause a bulge in the buccinator muscle.

Sublingual Gland Region

In the premolar region, the sublingual gland rests above the mylohyoid muscle. When the floor of the mouth is raised, this gland comes quite close to the crest of the ridge and reduces the vertical space available for the extension of the flange in the anterior part of the mouth (Figure 14-12). The sublingual gland may be pushed down and laterally out of position by resistant impression material. This can be avoided by shaping this part of the flange of the tray to slope inward toward the tongue and making the final impression with a low-viscosity impression material.

The lingual frenum area is also rather shallow. It should be registered in function because at rest the height of its attachment is deceptive. In function, it often comes quite close to the crest of the ridge, even though when at rest it is much lower.

Alveololingual Sulcus

The alveololingual sulcus, which is the space between the residual ridge and the tongue, extends from the lingual frenum to the retromylohyoid curtain. Part of it is available for the lingual flange

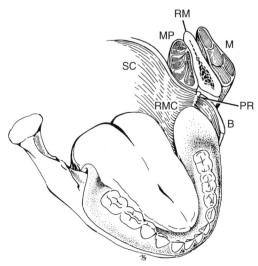

Figure 14-11 Diagram shows the relationship of the medial pterygoid muscle to the superior constrictor muscle. *B*, Buccinator muscle; *M*, masseter muscle; *MP*, medial pterygoid muscle; *PR*, pterygomandibular raphe; *RM*, ramus of the mandible; *RMC*, posterolateral portion of the retromylohyoid curtain formed by the mucous membrane covering the superior constrictor muscle *(SC)*.

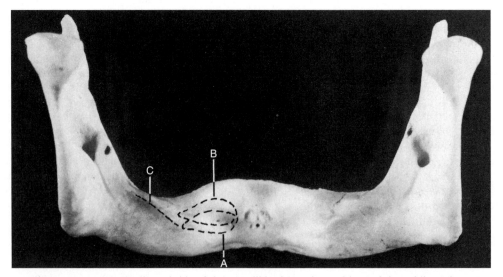

Figure 14-12 The lingual side of the mandible shows the positions of the sublingual gland relative to the mylohyoid muscle, at rest *(A)* and when contracted *(B)*. The mylohoid ridge is denoted by *C*.

of the denture. From the preceding discussion on the functional anatomy of the floor of the mouth, the shape of the lingual border of the denture should now be clear.

The border can be considered in the following three regions:

1. *The anterior region.* This extends from the lingual frenum back to where the mylohyoid ridge curves above the level of the sulcus. Here a depression, the premylohyoid fossa, can be palpated and a corresponding prominence, the premylohyoid eminence, seen on impressions (see Figures 14-7 and 14-8). The lingual border of the impression in this anterior region should extend down to make contact with the mucous membrane floor of the mouth when the tip of the tongue touches the upper incisors. The lingual flange will be shorter anteriorly than posteriorly. At the premylohyoid fossa, the flange becomes larger as it extends below the level of the mylohyoid ridge.

2. *The middle region.* This part extends from the premylohyoid fossa to the distal end of the mylohyoid ridge, curving medially from the body of the mandible. This curvature is caused by the prominence of the mylohyoid ridge and the action of the mylohyoid muscle (see Figures 14-7 and 14-8).

   When the middle of the lingual flange is made to slope toward the tongue, it can extend below the level of the mylohyoid ridge. In this way, the tongue rests on top of the flange and aids in stabilizing the lower denture on the residual ridge. In addition, this slope of the lingual flange provides space for the floor of the mouth to be raised during function without displacing the lower denture. The seal of the lower denture is maintained during these movements because the lingual flange remains in contact with the mucolingual fold in the alveololingual sulcus. Therefore in this area, the flange rests not on mucous membrane in contact with bone but on soft tissue. When the mylohyoid muscle is relaxed, there is a space between the flange and the floor of the mouth, but contact is reestablished when the floor of the mouth is raised.

3. *The posterior region.* Here the flange passes into the retromylohyoid fossa. As it does, it is no longer influenced by the action of the mylohyoid muscle, and so the flange can turn laterally toward the ramus to fill the fossa and complete the typical S form of the correctly shaped lingual flange (see Figures 14-7 and 14-8).

MANDIBULAR IMPRESSION PROCEDURES

The same principles of impression making are used for lower impressions as for upper impressions (see Chapter 13). As for the upper jaw, it is essential that the oral tissues are healthy before impressions are made.

Making the Preliminary Impression

The space available in the mouth for the lower impression is studied to determine the general form and size of the basal seat. An edentulous stock tray is selected that will provide for approximately 5 mm of bulk of impression material over the entire basal seat area. Posteriorly, the retromolar pads should be covered by the tray. The tray is raised anteriorly for observation of the relation between the lingual flanges and the lingual slope of the lower residual ridge (Figure 14-13). If the stock tray is made from metal, the lingual flanges can be reshaped, if necessary, by bending to allow for the action of the mylohyoid muscle (Figure 14-14). Any areas of underextension need to be corrected with soft boxing wax before the impression is made. A common site for stock trays to be under-extended is over the retromolar pads and down into the retromylohyoid fossae. In addition, soft boxing wax can be used to line the entire border of the stock tray to create a rim, which helps adapt the borders of the tray to the limiting tissues (see Figure 14-14).

Before the preliminary impression is made, it is advisable to practice placing the tray in position and to rehearse with the patient. The patient is asked to open the mouth halfway, and the tray is rotated into the mouth in the horizontal plane with the handle (see Figure 14-13) until it is centered over the residual ridge, with the tongue raised slightly so

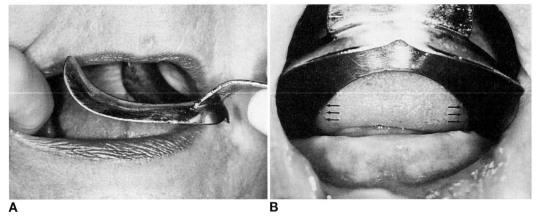

A   **B**

Figure 14-13 Preliminary impression making. **A,** A lower stock tray is placed in the mouth by extension of one corner of the mouth with the index finger. The side of the tray is placed in the opposite corner and the tray is rotated into position. **B,** The tray is raised anteriorly for observation of whether there is adequate space between the lingual flanges *(arrows)* and the lingual slope of the residual ridge to accommodate sufficient bulk of impression material.

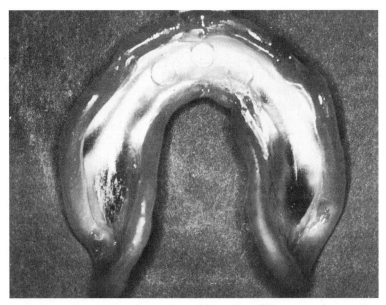

Figure 14-14 A rim of wax helps conform the borders of the tray to the mouth and confines the impression material in the tray. Note the lingual shape of the tray to accommodate the action of the mylohyoid muscles and to fit into the retromylohyoid fossae.

that it is positioned in the tongue space of the tray. As the tray is seated gently by alternating pressure from an index finger on either side of the tray in the first molar region, the patient is asked to let the tongue relax. Once the tray is seated, the borders of the impression are molded. A description of the movements necessary for molding the borders of the impression is given in the section on refining the custom tray.

The tissue surface and borders of the tray, including the rim of wax, are painted with an adhesive material to ensure that the irreversible hydrocolloid adheres to the tray. The irreversible hydrocolloid is mixed according to the manufacturer's instructions and evenly distributed to fill the tray to the level of the border. The loaded tray is then positioned in the mouth in a manner similar to that during the practice session and held in position while the impression material sets (Figure 14-15, *A*). Once the material has set, the cheeks and lower lip are lifted away from the borders of the impression, and the tray is removed from the mouth in one motion.

If impression compound is used for making the preliminary impression, the technique is the same except that the borders of the stock tray are not modified with wax, and there is no need to use a tray adhesive. Impression compound has a high viscosity, and unless care is taken, it is very easy to displace the mylohyoid muscle while making the impression. Silicone putty can be used as an alternative to impression compound.

Once the preliminary impression has been removed from the mouth, the borders of the custom tray should be identified. As with the upper preliminary impression, this is best done at the chairside with a disposable indelible marker to outline the periphery on the impression before it is poured in artificial stone (Figure 14-15, *B*).

A preliminary cast also can be obtained from the fitting surface of the patient's existing lower denture, provided the extension is satisfactory.

Constructing the Custom Tray

A wax spacer, approximately 1 mm thick, is placed over the crest and slopes of the residual ridge, leaving the borders uncovered. The buccal shelf on each side also may be left uncovered so that the completed custom tray contacts the mucous membrane in the region of the buccal shelves. This helps to position the tray correctly in the mouth and to place additional pressure on this primary stress-bearing area when the final impression is made. Extra wax can be placed over the lingual slopes of the cast below the level of the mylohyoid ridge to provide additional space for the action of the mylohyoid muscle.

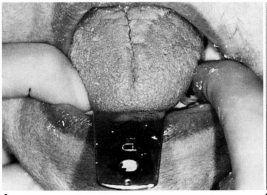 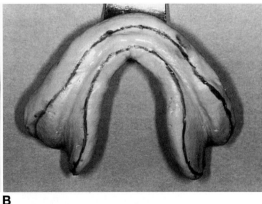

A   **B**

Figure 14-15 **A,** The stock tray is held in the mouth by an index finger from either hand placed on top of the tray in the region of the first molar. The tongue should be raised and protruded by the patient. **B,** The outline for the custom tray should be marked on the impression at the chairside with a disposable indelible marker.

The custom tray should be 2 to 3 mm thick, with an anterior handle centered over the labial flange in the approximate position of the anterior teeth, and shaped so as not to interfere with the position of the lip. This may be achieved with either a stepped handle of sufficient height to avoid distortion of the lower lip or a straight handle, approximately 20 mm in height, which runs vertically and parallel to the lip. Two additional handles, one on each side, are placed in the first molar region. These are centered over the crest of the residual ridge and are approximately 20 mm in height (Figure 14-16).

The anterior handle is used to carry the tray into the mouth and position it over the residual ridge. The posterior handles are used as finger rests to complete the placement of the tray and to stabilize the tray in the correct position, with minimal distortion of the soft tissues by the fingers as they hold the tray in position. The flanges of the tray should be contoured like the flanges of the complete denture. Thus while the impression is made, the limiting border tissues will be in a position similar to the one they will be in when the denture is in the mouth.

Refining the Custom Tray

When the custom tray is removed from the preliminary cast, the wax spacer is left inside the tray. This allows the tray to be positioned correctly on the residual ridge for border molding procedures.

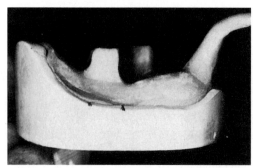

Figure 14-16   The completed tray shows the anterior handle shaped to avoid interfering with the lower lip and the two finger rests in the molar region.

For border molding to be carried out successfully, space must be created for the border molding material. The flanges of the custom tray should be reduced until they are approximately 2 mm short of the limiting structures. This is easier to achieve and check for the labial and buccal flanges than the lingual flange, where direct observation of the relationship is difficult to observe.

Border molding can be achieved with either an incremental technique with stick tracing compound or a one-step technique with a rubber material such as polyether impression material. When an incremental technique is used, stick tracing compound is added and molded initially along the border of the labial flange, followed in turn by each buccal flange. Lingually, the same sequence is followed. The anterior lingual border is molded first, followed by the left and right posterior lingual extension, including the retromolar pads.

The one-step technique for border molding the lower custom tray is similar to that used for the upper tray. See Chapter 13 for a description (Figure 14-17).

Irrespective of which method is used, the same border molding movements are carried out by the dentist and the patient. These are the following:

1. The labial flange is molded by lifting the lower lip outward, upward, and inward.
2. In the region of the buccal frenum, the cheek is lifted outward, upward, inward, backward, and forward to simulate movement of the frenum.
3. Posteriorly, the cheek is pulled buccally to ensure that it is not trapped under the tray, and then the cheek is moved upward and inward. The effect of the masseter muscle on the border of the impression is recorded by asking the patient to exert a closing force while the dentist exerts a downward pressure on the tray.
4. The anterior lingual flange is molded by asking the patient to protrude the tongue and then to push the tongue against the front part of the palate. Protruding the tongue determines the length of the lingual flange of the tray in this region, whereas pushing the tongue against the anterior part of the palate causes the base of the tongue to spread out

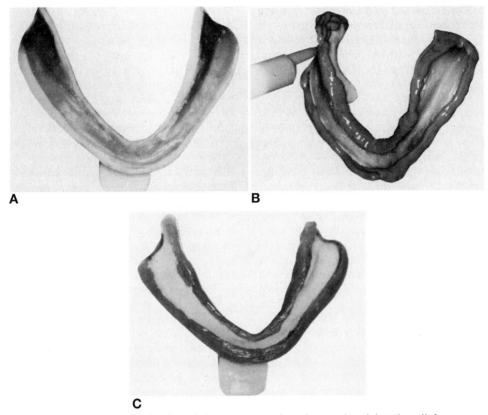

Figure 14-17 A, The borders of the custom tray have been reduced, but the relief wax remains in place. **B,** The polyether impression material is syringed around the borders of the tray until they are all covered. **C,** The completed border molding with the relief wax removed.

and develop the thickness of the anterior part of the flange.

5. Protruding the tongue activates the mylohyoid muscle, which raises the floor of the mouth. This helps the dentist determine the length and slope of the lingual flange in the molar region. The lingual flange must slope toward the tongue more or less parallel to the direction of the fibers of the mylohyoid muscles. It is important to ensure that the tongue moves bodily forward when it is protruded. Apparent protrusion of the tongue can be achieved by contraction of the intrinsic muscles of the tongue, but this does not raise the floor of the mouth. Because of

this, some clinicians get the patient to make a "k" sound because this activates the mylohyoid muscle.

If border molding material builds up on the inside of the lingual flange in this region, it must be removed; otherwise, it will interfere with the action of the mylohyoid muscle. It is better to have the tray contoured with too much slope toward the tongue in the molar region than with too little because the final impression material will fill the excess space.

6. The distal end of the lingual flange is molded by again asking the patient to protrude the tongue. This action activates the

superior constrictor muscle, which supports the retromylohyoid curtain. The patient is then asked to close the mouth as the dentist applies downward force on the impression tray. This records any effect that the contraction of the medial pterygoid muscle has on the retromolar curtain.

7. Finally, the patient is asked to open wide. If the tray is too long, a notch will be formed at the posteromedial border of the retromolar pad, indicating encroachment of the tray on the pterygomandibular raphe, and the tray must be adjusted accordingly.

The final border molded tray should be so formed that it supports the cheeks and lip in the same manner as the finished denture will do. The lingual surface of the tray should be shaped so that it guides the tongue into the same position it will occupy in relation to the finished denture. It should be possible for the patient to wipe the top of the tongue across the vermilion border of the upper lip, with the tray in place in the mouth, without noticeable displacement of the tray.

If the custom tray is constructed on a cast taken from the optimized previous denture, it can be presumed that the tray already reflects the border molding developed with the tissue conditioner and, thus, further border molding is unnecessary.

Preparing the Tray to Secure the Final Impression

Space must now be provided for the final impression material; otherwise, the borders will be overextended and the mucous membrane displaced unnecessarily. The wax spacer is removed from inside the tray along with any border molding material that has flowed over it. Any excess material on the outside of the tray is removed, and approximately 0.5 mm of border molding material is removed from around the border.

Finally, small holes can be drilled through the tray, approximately 10 mm apart, in the center of the alveolar groove and over the retromolar pads. These will provide escapeways for the final impression material and relieve pressure over the crest of the residual ridge and the retromolar pads when the final impression is made.

Making the Final Impression

A good final impression cannot be made unless a properly fitting tray is in the correct position on the residual ridge. Therefore this procedure should be practiced before making the final impression. The procedure is the same as that used when making preliminary impressions. The tray is rotated into the mouth in the horizontal plane with the anterior handle until it is over the residual ridge. At this time, the patient is asked to raise the tongue slightly, and the tray is moved downward toward its final position. The dentist's index fingers of each hand are placed on top of the posterior handles, and, with alternating gentle pressure, the tray is seated until the buccal flanges come into contact with the mucosa covering the buccal shelf. With the tray held steadily and not moving on the residual ridge, the borders of the impression are formed in the manner already described.

Once the patient and dentist are familiar with the procedure, the final impression material of choice is mixed according to the manufacturer's instructions and evenly distributed within the tray. All borders must be covered. Before the custom tray is placed into the mouth, any gauze that has been placed under the tongue to help dry the mouth must be removed. The tongue must be kept forward, touching the upper lip, while the impression material sets.

When the final impression material has set, the tray is removed from the mouth and inspected for acceptability (Figure 14-18). If it needs to be remade, the impression material is removed with particular care to preserve the border molding.

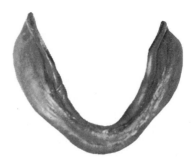

Figure 14-18   The completed final impression.

Boxing Impressions and Making the Casts

A wax form is developed around the border of the final impression to preserve the shape of the periphery and to simplify making casts. This procedure is called *boxing* and has already been described for the upper impression. The technique is the same for the lower impression, with the addition that the tongue space is filled with a sheet of wax that is attached to the superior surface of the boxing wax (Figure 14-19).

REMAKING THE FINAL IMPRESSION

Impression making is not easy. It requires great attention to details and a thorough understanding of the anatomy and physiology of oral tissues. The extra time that may be spent in making impressions not only means the difference between success and failure, but also means less time spent in making adjustments to the finished dentures.

Patients should be told that often it is necessary to make more than one impression before a final impression is acceptable. If the tray is correctly positioned in the mouth, errors in the impression indicate that the tray needs to be modified before another impression is made. The tray should not be modified unless it was positioned correctly when the impression was made.

The most common reason for having to repeat an impression is due to incorrect positioning of the tray. The following are some possible errors:

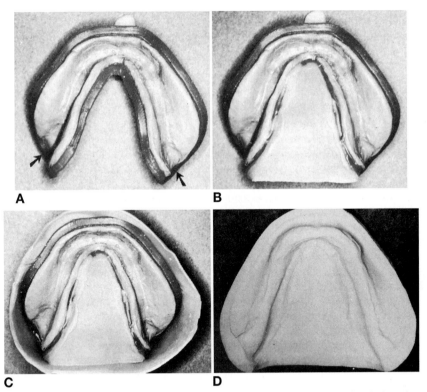

Figure 14-19   Boxing the impression. **A,** Boxing wax has been attached just below the borders of the impression. It extends for the full width at the posterior ends of the impression *(arrows)* to hold the vertical walls of the boxing in the proper position. **B,** The tongue space is filled with wax. **C,** The wall of the boxing is securely attached to the strip of boxing wax and to the posterior extent of the tongue space filler. **D,** The final cast is formed so that posterior ends of the residual ridges are well supported, with artificial stone providing the needed strength in these regions.

1. A thick buccal border on one side with a thin buccal border on the opposite side. This indicates that the tray was out of position in the direction of the thick border.
2. A thin labial border with the tray showing on the inside surface of the labial flange. This indicates that the tray was placed too far posteriorly and not centered correctly over the anterior ridge.
3. A thick lingual border on one side with a thin lingual border on the opposite side. This indicates that the lower tray was out of position in the direction of the thin border.
4. A thin anterior lingual border with the tray showing on the inside surface of the lingual flange. This suggests that the lower tray was too far forward in relation to the residual ridge. It will be accompanied by a thick labial border. In a similar manner thick labial border in the upper arch with the tray showing through over the anterior slope of the palate indicates that the tray was too far forward in relation to the residual ridge.
5. Excess thickness of impression material over the fitting surface of the tray and material unsupported by the borders of the tray. This indicates that the tray was not seated down sufficiently on the residual ridge. The correct thickness of material over the fitting surface of the tray, but with material extending beyond the border of the tray so that it is unsupported by the tray, suggests that the tray is underextended in that area.
6. The tray showing through the impression material over the fitting surface of the tray and the borders showing through the final impression material. This indicates that the tray has been seated on the residual ridge with too much pressure. The correct thickness of material over the fitting surface of the tray, but with the border showing through the final impression material, suggests that the tray is overextended in that area.

Other reasons for having to repeat an impression include the following:

1. Voids or discrepancies that are too large to be corrected accurately

2. Incorrect consistency of the final impression material when the tray was positioned in the mouth
3. Movement of the tray while the final impression material was setting
4. Incorrect border molding procedures (e.g., an excess bulk of impression material in the anterior lingual region and impression material unsupported by the tray at the distal end of the lingual flange indicates that the tongue was allowed to drop back from its anterior position and so did not correctly mold the lingual border)
5. The use of either too much or too little impression material

SUMMARY

1. Ensure that the tissues of the mouth are healthy.
   a. Optimize the present denture with tissue conditioners and occlusal adjustments.
   b. Encourage the patient to leave the denture out as much as possible and to massage the proposed supporting tissues.
   c. Ensure that oral and denture hygiene protocols are observed.
   d. Prescribe any necessary preprosthetic surgery.
2. Make the preliminary impression.
   a. Use a stock tray, modified with wax around the border, and irreversible hydrocolloid impression material, or
   b. Use a stock tray and either impression compound or silicone putty.
   c. Identify the peripheral outline of the custom tray. Mark the junction of the attached and unattached mucous membrane on the preliminary impression. Make a laboratory stone cast.
   d. If the denture has been optimized, that is, functionally border molded with a tissue conditioner, regard it as the preliminary impression. Make a laboratory cast in stone or silicone putty.
3. Make a custom tray.
   a. Outline the stress-bearing surface for the denture and lay down a wax spacer as appropriate.
   b. Construct a custom tray that extends just past the identified junction of the attached and unattached mucous membrane.

4. Refine the custom tray.
   a. Try the tray in the mouth and adjust the borders as necessary. The flanges should be 2 mm short of the reflection and should allow for the action of the mylohyoid muscles when the floor of the mouth is raised.
   b. Develop the borders of the tray with either an incremental technique with stick tracing compound or a one-step technique with a rubber material.
   c. If the tray has been constructed on a cast taken from the optimized previous denture, then border molding may not be necessary or else required at an individual site or sites.
5. Make the final impression with the preferred impression material.

6. Master cast preparation.
   a. Box and pour the final impression.
   b. Trim the cast.

Bibliography

Barrett SG, Wheeler HR: Structure of the mouth in the mandibular molar region and its relation to the denture, *J Prosthet Dent* 12:835-847, 1962.

Martone AL: Clinical applications of concepts of functional anatomy and speech science to complete denture prosthodontics, *J Prosthet Dent* 13:4-33, 1963.

Pietrokovski J, Massler M: Alveolar ridge resorption following tooth extraction, *J Prosthet Dent* 17:21-27, 1967.

Schwarz WD: The lingual crescent region of the complete lower denture, *Br Dent J* 144:312-314, 1978.

Shannon JL: The mentalis muscle in relation to edentulous mandibles, *J Prosthet Dent* 27:477-484, 1972.

Chapter 15

Identification of Shape and Location of Arch Form: The Occlusion Rim and Recording of Trial Denture Base

George A. Zarb, Yoav Finer

Many years ago, the distinguished British scholar Sir Wilfred Fish described a denture as having three surfaces: an impression, an occlusal, and a polished surface. Each surface (Figure 15-1) is developed separately in complete denture prosthodontics, but the dentist integrates all three to create a stable, functional, and esthetic result. The impression surface rests on the residual ridges and transmits forces directly to the denture-bearing tissues. The occlusal surface consists of the articulating surfaces of the prosthetic teeth that make contact during most functional and parafunctional activity. The polished surface comprises the nonarticulating parts of the teeth (buccal and lingual surfaces) along with the labial, buccal, lingual, and palatal parts of the denture base material. Both design and orientation of the polished surface are determined by its relationship to the functional role of the tongue, lips, and cheeks (Figure 15-2, *A* to *C*). The polished surface occupies a position of equilibrium among these groups of muscles and is frequently referred to as the *neutral zone* (Figure 15-2, *D*). The dentist determines the neutral zone's location by reconciling intraoral anatomical landmarks with a clinical assessment of lingual and circumoral activity. This three-dimensional planned location of a planned denture's polished surface is first established in the occlusion rims.

Occlusion rims are used as provisional substitutes for the planned complete dentures or implant-supported prostheses and are used to record first the neutral zone and then the maxillomandibular relations. They are made on the stone cast that represents the denture-supporting tissues and consist of a trial denture base (TDB), which is a provisional substitute for the eventual denture base, and a wax rim.

The TDB must be rigid, accurate, and stable. It is made of hard baseplate wax or, preferably, autopolymerizing (cold-curing) or light-cured acrylic resin. Such a TDB will be used at both the maxillomandibular registration and the try-in appointments. Infrequently, the TDB is made of processed acrylic resin, after final impressions are made, and eventually the selected teeth are also processed onto it. The rim itself is made preferably of baseplate wax because it is a convenient and easy material to manage.

TDBs made in wax (Figures 15-3 and 15-4) are usually reinforced with wire. These bases are occasionally bulky and brittle, but dentists and technicians frequently find them easier to work with when setting up teeth, especially when a restricted interarch distance exists. Autopolymerizing or light-cured resin TDBs also are extensively used. Undercuts are first blocked out on the cast to avoid possible cast surface damage, and the resin in its doughlike state is molded onto the cast. Alternatively, a wax template is lined with autopolymerizing resin (Figure 15-5), though this is slightly more time-consuming. An autopolymerizing resin base also can be made by the "sprinkle-on" method (Figure 15-6). In both cases, the monomer and polymer are applied alternately until a relatively even thickness of resin base is achieved, and in both cases the casts are placed in hot water in a pressure cooker for 10 minutes under 30 lb of pressure. This produces rapid polymerization, and excess monomer

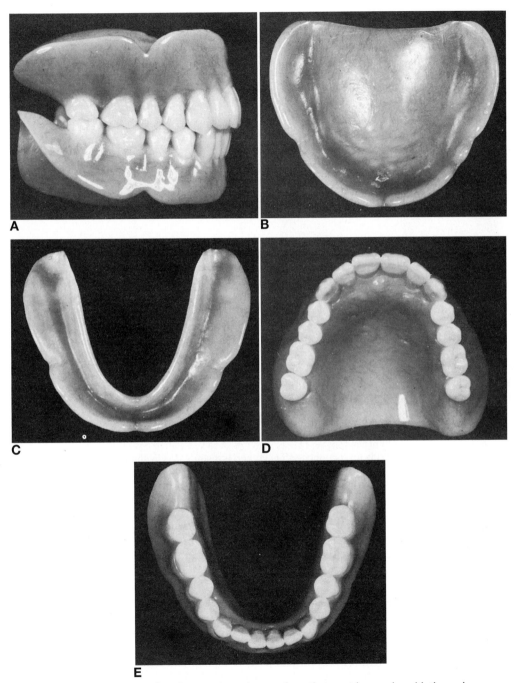

Figure 15-1   Complete dentures have three surfaces that must harmonize with the oral biological environment. **A,** The dentures' polished surfaces are so contoured as to support and contact the cheeks, lips, and tongue. **B** and **C,** The impression or basal surfaces are fitted to the basal seats. **D** and **E,** The occlusal surfaces of one denture must fit those of the opposing denture.

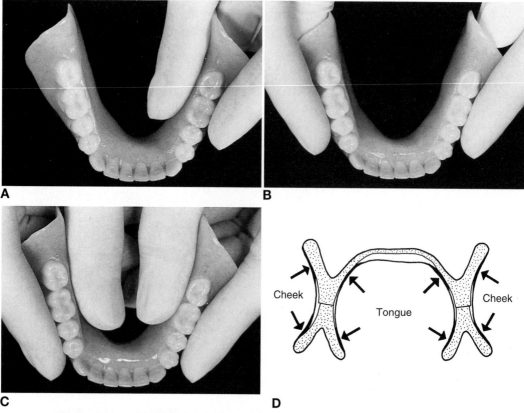

Figure15-2 The design and orientation of the denture's polished surface are influenced by functional activities of the tongue, cheeks, and lips. **A** to **C,** Relative positions of the groups of muscles making up the tongue, cheeks, and lips simulated by the fingers. **D,** Arrows indicate the direction of muscular activity in a coronal plane through the molar region of the two occlusion rims. Shaded areas denote the neutral zone.

is eliminated. Both methods produce a base that is rigid, stable, and easily contoured and polished. Acrylic resin bases are excellent for making maxillomandibular relation records. They fit accurately and are not easily distorted. Their only disadvantage is that they may take up space needed for setting the teeth, necessitating some grinding of the acrylic resin base in required areas. They may also be loose because of the necessary blockout of undercuts in the cast. A TDB and occlusion rim made of extra-hard baseplate wax are easiest for subsequent teeth arrangement (see Figures 15-3 and 15-4). The wax can be softened all the way through to the cast, so the teeth can be set directly against the cast if necessary. For many patients,

"hard" baseplate materials must be cut away to allow the teeth to be set in their proper places when restricted interarch space is present.

OCCLUSION RIMS

The occlusion rims are used to establish (1) the level of the occlusal plane, (2) the neutral zone or arch form (which is related to the activity of the lips, cheeks, and tongue and includes preliminary circumoral and facial support), and (3) the preliminary maxillomandibular relation records, which include the vertical and horizontal jaw relationships and an estimate of the interocclusal distance. Unfortunately, none of these determinations can

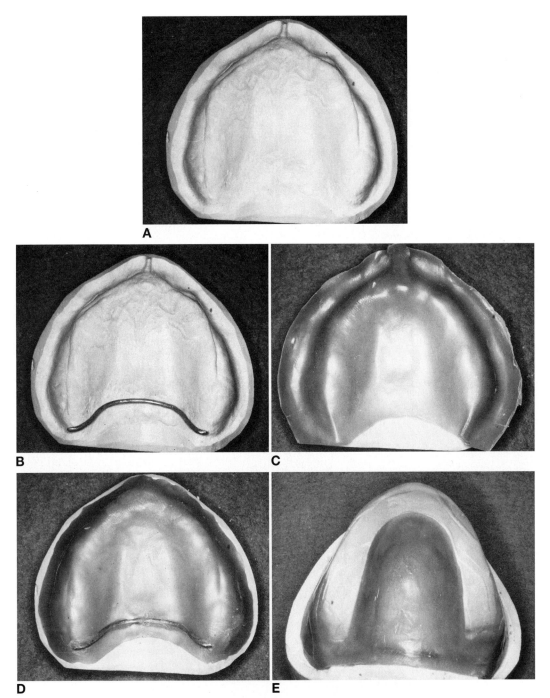

Figure 15-3 Construction of an extra-hard wax occlusion rim. **A,** The maxillary cast is dusted with talcum powder as a separating medium. **B,** Ten-gauge reinforcement wire is adapted to the posterior palatal area to extend through the hamular notches, 2 mm in front of the vibrating line. **C** and **D,** A sheet of softened baseplate wax is pressed firmly against the cast to form the recording base. **E,** The roll of softened wax is sealed to this base and contoured to the desired arch form. The rim is built to a height slightly greater than the total length of the teeth and the amount of residual alveolar ridge shrinkage.

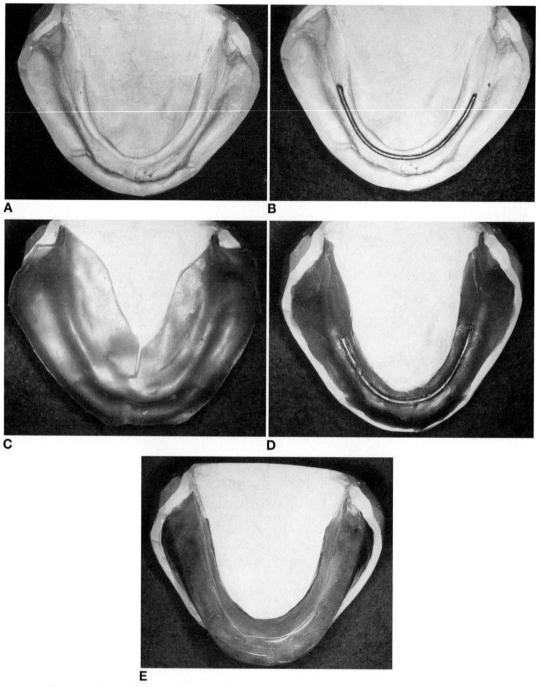

Figure 15-4 This mandibular cast (**A**) has a reinforcing wire adapted on the lingual of the residual ridge (**B** to **D**). A sheet of softened baseplate wax is closely adapted to the potential denture-bearing area of the cast to form the recording base. **E,** The roll of softened wax is sealed to the base and contoured to the desired form.

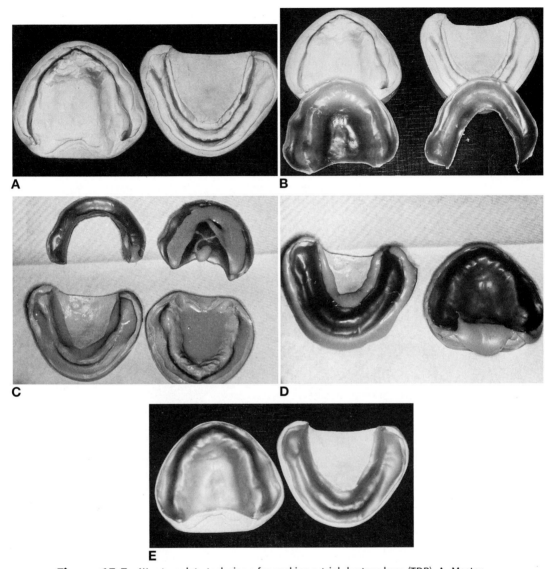

Figure 15-5 Wax template technique for making a trial denture base (TDB). **A,** Master casts prepared by waxing out the undercuts and applying a separating medium. **B,** Wax templates are formed and lined with autopolymerizing acrylic resin (**C** and **D**). **E,** The completed (well-fitting and stable) trial base is ready for the addition of occlusion rims.

be made in a precise scientific way, and most of the knowledge concerning them is theoretical. However, clinical experience has provided successful directions or protocols, which are used to help achieve the clinical objectives. The preferred

clinical sequence to follow is (1) design the arch form on each wax occlusion rim, (2) establish the level/height of the occlusal plane on the mandibular occlusion rim, (3) modify the maxillary rim to meet the mandibular rim evenly at the desired vertical

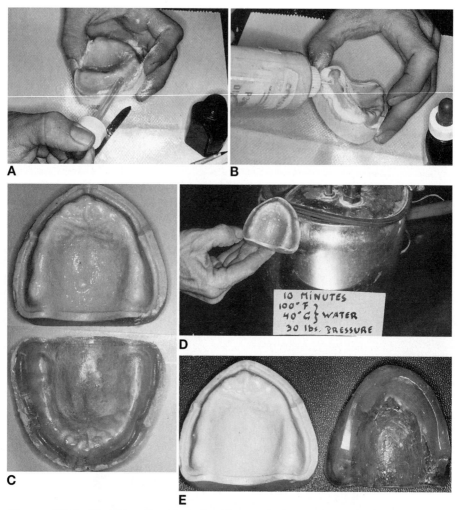

Figure 15-6 "Sprinkle-on" method of making a resin denture base. **A** and **B,** Monomer and polymer are applied alternately until an evenly thick base is developed. The base (**C**) and cast (**D**) are placed in a pressure cooker to complete polymerization. **E,** The denture base is trimmed and polished, and a wax rim is sealed onto it.

dimension of occlusion (VDO), and (4) make a preliminary centric relation (CR) record.

Arch Form

Both the width of the occluding surfaces and the contour of the arch form of the occlusion rims should be individually established for each patient to simulate the desired arch form of the artificial teeth. This is an integral part of the neutral zone determination objective. Such an analogue of the missing teeth and their supporting tissues will enable the dentist or technician to accurately follow instructions for arranging the artificial teeth. This can serve to reduce the amount of time spent with the patient by the dentist at the try-in appointment and allow more time for perfecting the arrangement of the teeth.

Fish drew the profession's attention to the concept of a neutral zone in complete denture construction. He argued that the natural teeth occupy a zone of equilibrium, with each tooth assuming a position that is the resultant of all the various forces acting on it. This is usually a stable position unless actual changes in the dentition have occurred. When natural teeth are replaced by artificial teeth, it is logical to set the artificial teeth in a position as close as possible to the one the natural teeth occupied. The same forces that stabilized the natural teeth can then be used to stabilize the dentures. In the treatment of partially edentulous patients, it is common to find that sufficient natural teeth remain to provide a guide for the positions of the artificial teeth. When the patient is edentulous, it is not always easy to determine where the natural teeth were in relation to the partially or totally resorbed alveolar ridges. Clinical judgment must be brought to bear in such situations, and this may be quite challenging.

Certain types of dentitions are accompanied by specific patterns of soft tissue behavior. Clinical observation of patients with dentures suggests that these characteristic types of soft tissue movements persist into old age and offer a clue to the location of the preexisting natural teeth. The best guide for determining and designing the arch form is to consider the pattern of bone resorption where the teeth are lost and the use of anatomical landmarks that are relatively stable in position. Furthermore, documented clinical experience confirms that the denture space or neutral zone can be reproduced with minor variations that lie within the range of clinical acceptability.

Mandibular Arch   The occlusion rim is designed to conform to the arch form that, in the dentist's judgment, the patient had before the natural teeth and alveolar bone were lost. In the lower jaw, a larger proportion of bone loss occurs on the labial side of the anterior residual ridge. The loss occurs equally on the buccal and lingual sides of the residual ridge in the premolar region, but in the molar region the loss appears to be primarily from the lingual side of the ridge because of the cross-sectional shape of the mandible (which is wider at its inferior border than at the ridge crest). Thus the residual ridge almost invariably becomes more lingually placed in the anterior region and more buccally placed in the posterior region. Most often, the occlusion rim is contoured as a guide for placing artificial teeth labial to the ridge in the anterior region, over the ridge in the premolar region, and slightly lingual to the ridge in the molar region. The curvatures of the occlusion rims, which simulate the arch form of the posterior teeth, follow the curvature of the mandible itself when seen from above. Lines are drawn on the cast to provide a tangible guide for shaping/designing the arch form. One line is drawn from the lingual side of the retromolar pad and extended anteriorly to a point just lingual to the crest of the ridge in the premolar region. This line aids in positioning the lingual surfaces of the posterior teeth, and it establishes the lingual extent of the occlusion rim (Figure 15-7). This lingual line can be curved similar to the curvature of the body of the mandible.

The anterior part of the occlusion rim is contoured to compensate for the estimated bone loss in this region, and the corners of the mouth are used as guides for determining an approximate location for the canines and first premolars. The experienced dentist learns to visualize the artificial teeth (represented at this state by the contoured rim) as growing out of the alveolar bone and following the curvature of the bone. The end result is an arch form that is frequently not on the residual ridge but anterior or labial to it. Several techniques employ soft waxes, impression materials, and tissue conditioners as adjunctive efforts to functionally establish a correct neutral zone for the arch form. When advanced anterior ridge reduction has been accompanied by an upward migration of the mentalis muscle attachment to the crest of the ridge, a certain amount of compromise is essential, and the rim is trimmed very thin and placed on, or lingual to, the ridge crest (note the risk of the denture's encroachment on the tongue space). If this sort of compromise creates an intolerable situation for the patient, surgical labial sulcus deepening in this area or the provision of implants may be considered to provide adequate support for the anterior segment of the denture. Some dentists and technicians have subscribed to a tooth-on-the-ridge philosophy, which has seriously undermined efforts for denture

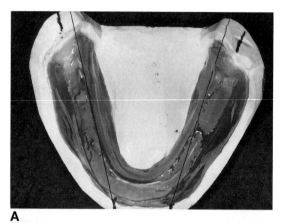

A

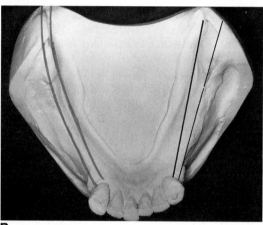

B

Figure 15-7 **A,** A straight line drawn from lingual of the retromolar pad to a point just lingual to the crest of the ridge in the premolar region can act as a guide for positioning artificial posterior teeth. **B,** A partially edentulous cast with a straight line on the right and a curved line on the left, showing the curvature of the body of the mandible.

stability and esthetics. The concept of a neutral zone in the context of a keen understanding of patterns of alveolar ridge resorption enables the dentist to determine the arch form for the patient receiving treatment.

Maxillary Arch The tongue's size and positions during function do not appear to have as profound an impact on the stability of the maxillary denture as on the mandibular one. However, optimal neutral

zone determination is still mandatory for speech and esthetic purposes, with a little more leeway available for the latter consideration. Bone reduction usually occurs on the labial and buccal areas of the maxillary residual ridge. Consequently, the residual edentulous ridge is usually palatal to the original location of the natural teeth. The maxillary teeth should be labial and buccal to the residual edentulous ridge if they are to be placed in the neutral zone and occupy the position of their predecessors. If this pattern of bony reduction is ignored, the dentist ends up with a contracted maxillary arch form within the confines of the mandibular arch form. This oversight guarantees inadequate labial support.

The incisive papilla appears to occupy a stable locale on the palate, unless it is modified surgically. Clinical experience and anthropometric measurements indicate that the incisal edges of the maxillary central incisors are usually 8 to 10 mm anterior to the center of the incisive papilla. The tips of the canines are also related to the center of the papilla, and a high percentage of canines are 61 mm in front of the papilla (Figure 15-8, *A*). The papilla is circled and used as a rough guide in locating the anteroposterior position of the maxillary anterior teeth (Figure 15-8, *B*). Also, after the natural teeth are lost the canines should be located in a coronal plane passing through the posterior border of the papilla. A patient's old dentures, preextraction photographs, or diagnostic casts and photographs made before the dentition deteriorated should be used to assist both selection of artificial teeth and establishment of the optimal labial support for the patient. The simulated position of the posterior teeth is really a clinical judgment call. An assessment of the amount of resorption that has occurred, coupled with realization that the posterior teeth's inclinations are buccal to the ridge shape, is the guide to be followed. Furthermore, the position of the posterior maxillary teeth will, to a varying extent, also be influenced by the size of a patient's smile, as well as the position of the mandibular teeth. The latter's positions tend to be more rigidly determined.

If the patient has been wearing inadequate dentures, tooth loss will have a pronounced effect on the appearance of the lips and adjacent tissues. As a result of the loss of substance and the reduction

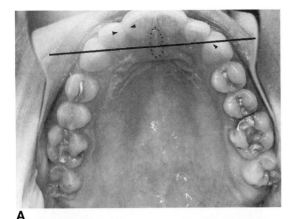

A

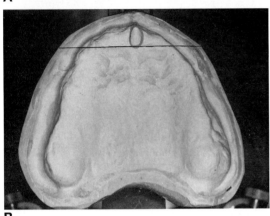

B

Figure 15-8 **A,** In the natural dentition, the tips of the maxillary canines are frequently 61 mm anterior to the center of the incisive papilla *(dotted circle).* **B,** On an edentulous cast, the papilla is circled because it provides a rough guide to positioning the maxillary canines.

in elastic properties, the connective tissue will not provide sufficient resistance to the activities of the orbicularis oris and associated muscles. Consequently, the effect of the degenerative changes in the skin becomes exaggerated, and the lips appear to have aged to a much greater extent than the surrounding parts. The skin becomes roughened, and deep vertical lines appear in the body and margins of the lips. There is a noticeable shortening/thinning of the lips because of a tendency for the lip margins to roll inward. The nasolabial fold changes direction to become almost continuous with the

groove at the corner of the mouth, and the lips and cheeks are no longer distinctly separated (Figure 15-9). Such a loss of well-defined demarcation tends to produce a generally disordered appearance of the lower half of the face. At this stage, it may be difficult to visualize proper lip support in an attempt to counter the changes just described. However, the dentist can and should use the occlusion rim to achieve the best balance between neutral zone determination and harmonious labial support.

Altering labial support probably does not affect cheek support as much as it affects lip support because the buccinator muscle is stretched between the pterygomandibular raphe and the modiolus muscles. It must be remembered that the longer the period of edentulism, the greater will be the loss of the muscle tone. Consequently, the relearning of the original muscle patterns and recovery of tone is likely to be insufficient even if the best dentures are provided. The more accurate the position of teeth replacement and the sooner it occurs, the easier will be the task of relearning and reacquiring optimal cheek and lip support.

Another useful average value is an approximate measurement between the peripheries of the denture flanges in the regions of the maxillary and mandibular canines. A 40-mm figure is a good place to start, with an average measurement of 20 mm for each occlusion rim. These values are not fixed, and they are modified depending on clinical assessment of the particular patient being treated (Figure 15–10).

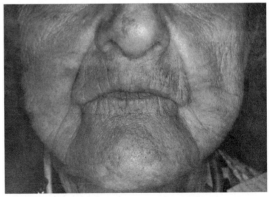

Figure 15-9 Degenerative skin changes create virtual continuity between the nasolabial fold and the corner of the mouth.

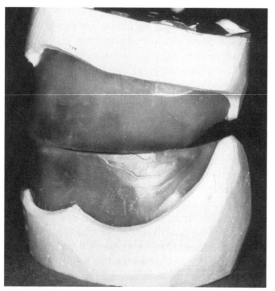

Figure 15-10   Two occlusion rims have been contoured and adjusted and are now ready to be used for making the preliminary centric relation record. The trimmed and contoured wax rims serve as an analogue for the mouth's neutral zone. They can be used to indicate position of the prosthetic teeth.

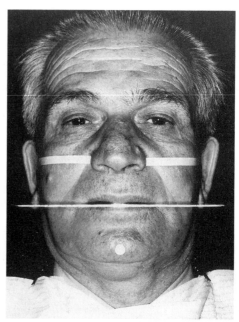

Figure 15-11   For demonstration purposes, the ala-tragus line on this patient has been bilaterally taped on. The occlusal plane is established when the wax occlusion rim is made parallel to this line. A Fox plane-guide or similar device may be used for the paralleling.

Level of the Occlusal Plane

Many dentists use a technique whereby the starting point for establishing the occlusal plane is the maxillary occlusion rim. The procedure entails shaping the occlusion rim so the incisal plane is parallel to the interpupillary line and is at a height that allows for the length of the natural tooth plus the amount of tissue resorption that has occurred. The upper lip can also be a guide if it is of average length. The occlusal plane, posteriorly, is made to parallel the ala-tragus line on the basis of the position of most natural occlusal planes (Figure 15-11). Then the lower occlusion rim is adjusted to meet evenly with the upper rim and reduced until sufficient interocclusal distance has been obtained. This procedure is adequate for many patients and usually results in satisfactory dentures. It certainly cannot be regarded as applicable to all patients, however.

There are other approaches to occlusal plane determination. The preferred method is to first seek to reconcile tongue function and its relation to the occlusal plane and mandibular denture stability. When this approach is related to Fish's description of the neutral zone and the activity of the modiolus muscles as described below, a rational and clear guide for occlusal plane determination evolves. The food bolus is triturated while resting on the mandibular occlusal surfaces (occlusal table). This table is an area bounded by the cheek tissues buccally, the tongue lingually, the pterygomandibular raphe and its overlying tissues distally, and the contraction of the corner of the mouth mesially. The mesial boundary is a point where eight muscles meet at the corner of the mouth. The meeting place, called the *modiolus* ("hub of a wheel" in Latin), forms a distinct conical prominence at the corner of the mouth (Figure 15-12). If the thumb is placed inside the corner of the mouth and the finger outside on the prominence, and then the lip and cheek are contracted, the modiolus feels like a knot. The modiolus becomes fixed every time the buccinator muscle contracts, which is a natural accompaniment of all chewing efforts. The contraction of the modiolus presses the corner of the mouth against the premolars so the occlusal table is closed in front. Food is crushed by the premolars and molars and does not escape at the corner of the mouth unless seventh nerve damage has occurred (as in Bell's palsy). A good reminder of the significance of this observation is the drooling that frequently occurs when a patient with an inferior alveolar local anesthesia block attempts to drink.

The practical application of this approach lies in establishing the height of the occlusal plane and developing the polished surface of the denture in the occlusion rims. The corners of the mouth are marked on the occlusion rims to provide the dentist and technician with anterior landmarks for the height of the first premolars (Figure 15-13, *A* to *C*). The retromolar pads are relatively stable posterior landmarks, even in patients with advanced ridge reduction. The mandibular first molar is usually at a level corresponding to two thirds of the way up the retromolar pad (Fig. 15-13, *D*). The retromolar pads are circled on the final casts, and the land of

the cast (edge) is marked at points one half to two thirds of the height of the pad. These points will aid in determining the height of the distal end of the occlusal plane. The anterior and posterior landmarks are joined when the wax is melted to this level with a hot spatula. The resultant occlusal plane is almost invariably parallel to the residual alveolar ridges and to the interpupillary line. Its height will conform to activities of the tongue, cheek, and corner of the mouth (Figure 15-13, *E*), which tend to enhance mandibular denture stability.

Tests to Determine Vertical Dimension of Occlusion

The maxillary occlusion rim is next adjusted to meet evenly with the mandibular rim, and they are augmented or reduced until an adequate functionally determined interocclusal distance is obtained.

The anterior position of the maxillary occlusion rim is so modified that the lower lip gently caresses the rim during pronunciation of the letter *F*. The rim is usually parallel to the interpupillary line and is at a height that accommodates the length of the natural tooth plus the amount of assessed bone reduction that has occurred. It is possible to simulate (though rather difficult to visualize) proper length and lip support by contouring the labial aspect of the maxillary occlusion rim. It would be preferable, and in fact easier, for the dentist to select the anterior teeth for the patient's denture at the examination appointment and set them for proper length and lip support in the occlusion rims. Further characterization of the anterior arrangement could then be done at the patient's next appointment.

The tests that aid the dentist in establishing the correct VDO by means of occlusion rims are reviewed in Chapter 16, and the following are the tests most frequently used:

1. Judgment of the overall facial support
2. Visual observation of the space between the rims when the jaws are at rest
3. Measurements between dots on the face when the jaws are at rest and when the occlusion rims are in contact
4. Observations when the "s" sound is enunciated accurately and repeatedly—the average speaking space

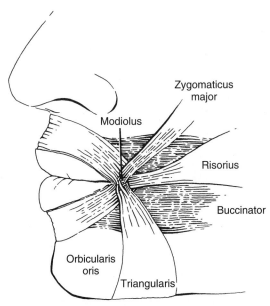

Figure 15-12 The modiolus.

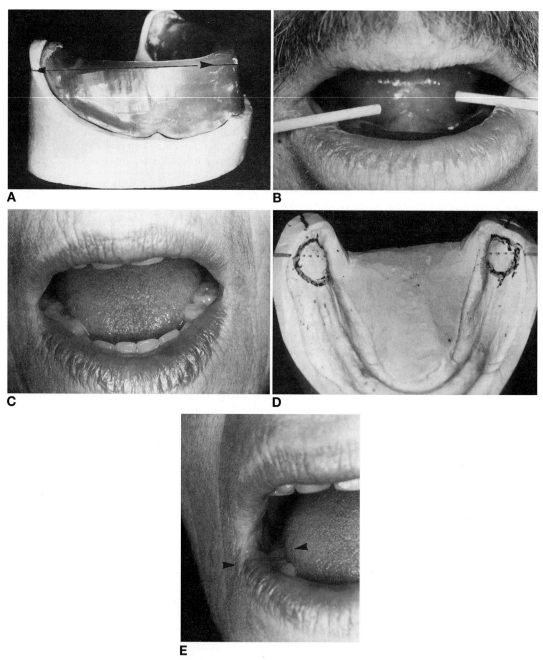

Figure 15-13 A mandibular occlusion rim (**A**) is trimmed to conform to two pairs of landmarks: the right and left corners of the mouth (**B** and **C**) and a point two thirds of the way up the retromolar pads (**D**). The wax rim is melted with a hot spatula to the level indicated by the *arrows* in **A**. Mandibular teeth set to this level (**E**) will conform to the tongue and cheeks and to activities of the corners of the mouth *(arrowheads)*.

The last test ensures that the occlusion rims come close together but do not contact. It must be emphasized that the interocclusal (interim) or speaking space that exists between the posterior teeth when the patient is enunciating "s" sounds is unrelated to the interocclusal space of rest position. Clinical experience suggests that this space is about 1.5 to 3 mm for most patients. However, patients with a Class II occlusion tend to have a larger speaking space, and patients with a Class III occlusion have a smaller space.

Both tests 1 and 2 are particularly effective if the patient's old dentures are used for comparison. Old dentures can be valuable for prognostic purposes, especially if they are used with treatment liners to recover an optimal VDO. Old dentures can also have their facial surfaces selectively augmented with a soft wax to assist the dentist in assessing the required cosmetic support from the dentures' polished surfaces. This is a useful step when the shape of the dental arch form is determined, as it should be, by the dentist.

The next clinical step is creating a preliminary CR record, which is made after the height of the mandibular occlusal plane has been determined and the occlusion rims have been contoured to simulate the position that will be occupied by the artificial teeth and tissues of the complete dentures (see Figure 15-10) and the preferred interocclusal space established. The occlusion rims are used to establish a preliminary CR record and to transfer it by means of a face bow, or an arbitrary mounting, to a semiadjustable articulator.

The vertical and horizontal relations of the jaws are integral components of the CR position in edentulous patients. The provisional VDO is first established (as already described). The horizontal jaw relation record is then made at this level, and the occlusion rims are transferred to an articulator.

An articulator is used in complete denture construction to simulate very simple jaw movements, for convenience and to provide a solid base in the patient's mouth. The use of a semiadjustable articulator permits three jaw relations be transferred from the patient to the instrument: (1) the relation of the jaws to the opening axis (face bow transfer); (2) the vertical separation of the jaws (VDO determination) and the horizontal relation of the lower to the upper jaw in CR; and (3) the relation of the

lower jaw to the upper jaw when the mandible is protruded so the incisor teeth will be edge to edge. Obviously, the dentist makes all these records. However, many dentists prefer to use an articulator with average setting of the condylar guidance (see Chapter 16) and use a CR record exclusively.

Interocclusal Centric Relation Records

Most clinical educators agree that the actual method of transferring a centric jaw relation record to the dentist's articulator of choice is arguably irrelevant. Several excellent methods or techniques are available, but what counts is that the record is correctly mounted on the articulator before proceeding with the setting up of the prosthetic tooth. Therefore this next clinical step, making an interocclusal CR record, is a crucial one. It must be carried out impeccably if time-consuming clinical repeat activities are to be avoided. Interocclusal records are described as static, graphic, or functional. Static records are made with a soft material interposed between the two rims. The material used (e.g., wax) hardens to provide a "checkbite" record, which is stable and very easy to use. Graphic recordings are done with intraoral or extraoral tracing devices, with a central bearing point secured to the trial denture or record bases. Functional records are made with pantographic tracing devices. All these methods are very useful. However, the graphic and functional records are infrequently used. The preferred method is the static technique because of its ease of reproducibility and repeatability. The technique is carried out as follows:

1. Prepare small (3 to 4 mm deep) V-shaped grooves in the maxillary occlusion rim. There are usually two grooves that are placed bilaterally in the first molar–second premolar region, in areas touched by the opposing wax rim. These areas are lubricated with a petroleum jelly, and the maxillary occlusion rim is placed in the mouth. If the anterior rims are also in contact, it is possible to prepare a similar groove in the region of the maxillary central incisor.
2. Prepare box-shaped areas (2 to 3 mm deep) in the corresponding opposing areas of the mandibular occlusion rim. Fill these areas with the chosen registration material (e.g.,

softened beeswax), and place the mandibular occlusion rim in the mouth.

3. The comfortably seated and upright patient has his or her head supported by a suitable headrest. The dentist guides the patient's mandible into a CR position. Stabilize the mandibular trial base with the forefinger and thumb of one hand and use the thumb and fingers of the other hand to guide the mandible. The fingers stabilizing the base also can be moved upward to stabilize the maxillary base, if required. In this manner, the bases' stability is ensured, and the mandible can be guided while visibility is retained. Alternative hand positions are advocated by different clinicians.

4. The patient and bases must be kept immobile while the material is setting. This may simply not be possible for some patients, especially where mandibular residual ridge resorption is extensive or neuromuscular control is compromised. Clearly, implant-stabilized occlusion rims solve this problem quite easily. The advantage of a wax recording medium lies in its allowing the operator to guide mandibular opening and closure into the soft wax to verify the record's accuracy.

It is prudent to rehearse the previously described maneuvers before the recording medium is actually introduced. The trial bases should be taken out of the mouth, excess recording material removed, and the distal areas of the bases checked to ensure that they do not contact distally. This is a frequent site for recording errors. The accuracy of this record should be checked and rechecked before proceeding to an articulator mounting. The use of frequent trial closures, plus a practical and meticulously applied technique, will yield accurate results. Any additional checks or tests that ensure an accurate CR record are strongly endorsed. An ingenious technique for this purpose is the use of centric checkpoints.

Infrequently, the preliminary CR record is an incorrect one and undiagnosed at this appointment. It will, however, become apparent at the try-in appointment when a new record and remount will have to be made. This is a time-consuming step and should hopefully not be required. However, it must be recalled that clinical determination of occlusal discrepancies is more discernible with prosthetic teeth in place than with wax occlusion rims. The problem can be rectified, although additional chairside and laboratory time is required.

SUMMARY

1. Ensure well-fitting, retained, and stable TDBs. The retention may have to be aided with a denture adhesive. The stability will be enhanced after design of the arch form, or neutral zone.
2. Establish the neutral zone by considering the following:
   a. Arch forms' location in previous dentures (if present)
   b. An assessment of the amount and pattern of bone loss
   c. Use of anatomical landmarks
   d. Preliminary esthetic evaluation
3. Determine the height of the occlusal plane in the mandibular occlusion rim
   a. Use corners of the mouth as the anterior landmarks
   b. Use the retromolar pads (two thirds up) as the posterior landmarks
   c. Join all four points with a hot, broad wax spatula
4. Establish the VDO by modifying the height of the occlusion rim while ensuring the following:
   a. An even meeting of both rims in CR position
   b. An interocclusal distance that the dentist judges as being functionally adequate for the patient in question
5. Prepare rims for a CR registration with grooves in the maxillary wax and opposing box-shaped areas in the mandibular wax
6. Return the occlusion rims to the mouth for repeated trial closures. The CR record is made with the dentist's selected medium. The CR record is confirmed and remade, if requested, until a repeatable CR record is established.

Bibliography

Barrenäs L, Ödman P: Myodynamic and conventional construction of complete dentures: a comparative study of comfort and function, *J Oral Rehabil* 16:457-465, 1989.

Beresin VE, Schiesser FJ: *The neutral zone in complete and partial dentures*, ed 2, St Louis, 1978, Mosby.

Berry DC, Wilkie JK: *An approach to dental prosthetics, vol 2, Pergamon series on dentistry*, London, 1964, Pergamon Press.

Fish EW: An analysis of the stabilizing factors in full denture construction, *Br Dent J* 52:559-570, 1931.

Fish EW: *Principles of full denture prosthesis*, ed 4, London, 1948, Staples Press Ltd.

Karlsson S, Hedegård B: Study of the reproducibility of the functional denture space with a dynamic impression technique, *J Prosthet Dent* 41:21-25, 1979.

Lee JH: *Dental esthetics*, Bristol, 1962, John Wright & Sons Ltd.

Lott F, Levin B: Flange technique: an anatomic and physiologic approach to increased retention, function, comfort, and appearance of denture, *J Prosthet Dent* 16:394-413, 1966.

Nairn RI: The circumoral musculature: structure and function, *Br Dent J* 138:49-56, 1975.

Neill DJ, Glaysher JKL: Identifying the denture space, *J Oral Rehabil* 9:259-277, 1982.

Pound E: Controlling anomalies of vertical dimension and speech, *J Prosthet Dent* 36:124-135, 1976.

Tallgren R: The continuing reduction of the residual alveolar ridges in complete denture wearers: a mixed longitudinal study, *J Prosthet Dent* 27:120-132, 1972.

Watt DM, Likeman PR: Morphological changes in the denture bearing area following the extraction of maxillary teeth, *Br Dent J* 136:225-235, 1974.

Wright CR: Evaluation of the factors necessary to develop stability in mandibular dentures, *J Prosthet Dent* 16:414-430, 1966.

Wright SM: The polished surface contour: a new approach, *Int J Prosthodont* 4:159-163, 1991.

CHAPTER 16

Biological and Clinical Considerations in Making Jaw Relation Records and Transferring Records from the Patient to the Articulator

James D. Anderson

The different components of the masticatory system are closely related and can be regarded as a functional unit. They are composed of the jaws and teeth; the temporomandibular joints (TMJs) and associated ligaments; the muscles of mastication; the tongue, cheeks, and lips; and the sensory and motor innervation (and vasculature) to these structures. In the edentulous patient, the teeth and their associated periodontal ligament nerves are lost. It is the aim of prosthodontic treatment to provide (complete denture) replacement function for the lost teeth. For these rather unnatural acrylic (denture) replacements to function successfully in the physiological environment to which they are so intimately related, knowledge is needed of the functional anatomy; the control and limits of jaw and joint motion; and the relationships and control of the lips, tongue and other structures. This includes some understanding of the neurophysiological, behavioral, and psychological mechanisms involved.

In the identification of the elements of jaw relations for the treatment of edentulous patients, the aim is to facilitate adaptation of the complete dentures to the rest of the masticatory system. For this goal to be achieved, it is necessary to find a vertical dimension of occlusion that is appropriate, stable occlusal contacts that are harmonious with the existing TMJs and masticatory muscles, and contours that are consistent with the surrounding facial soft tissues and musculature. All of these features can, in theory, be simulated in properly trimmed occlusion rims.

If it were practical, virtually all the steps to create these features could be done by the dentist at the chairside with the patient. Not only could the denture teeth be arranged to be esthetically pleasing and biologically compatible, but they could also be arranged so that the occlusal surfaces contact and glide over one another smoothly, without dislodging the denture bases. However, it is extremely inconvenient to perform intraorally the procedures involved in the construction of complete dentures. The difficulties posed by the presence of saliva, movement of the denture bases, the surrounding soft tissues, and the patient's ability to cooperate all make it impractical to do many of the steps intraorally. Instead, the occlusion rims are used to transfer the jaw relation information to an articulator so that trial tooth arrangements can be set up in the laboratory where working conditions are much more easily controlled.

This chapter discusses the biological considerations in identifying the important aspects of jaw relations and details methods of transferring that information to the articulator.

REGULATION OF MANDIBULAR MOVEMENT

Before the identification of vertical and horizontal jaw relations, a short description of mandibular movements of relevance for jaw recordings is presented. Mandibular movements are complex in nature and vary greatly among persons and within each person. Many different mandibular movements occur during mastication, speech, swallowing, respiration, and facial expression. When parafunctional movements (bruxism and clenching) are also added, the complexity of mandibular movements is obvious. It is essential that the dentist be knowledgeable of mandibular movements to understand various aspects of occlusion, to arrange artificial teeth, and to select and adjust recording devices and articulators. Ideally, the articulator should exactly reproduce jaw movements within the range of contacts between opposing teeth so that the planned occlusion on the instrument will function properly in the patient's mouth. However, no such perfect articulator is available. Therefore regardless of the methods and instruments chosen, the dentist needs to know about their inherent inaccuracies to inform the clinical adjustments needed after their use.

Factors That Regulate Jaw Motion

When opposing teeth are in contact and mandibular movements are made, the direction of the movement is controlled by the neuromuscular system and limited by the movement of the two condyles and the guiding influences of the contacting teeth. When the opposing teeth are not in contact and mandibular movements occur, the direction of movement is controlled by the mandibular musculature and limited by condylar movements alone. The condyles and teeth modify mandibular movements initiated by the neuromuscular system.

Influence of Opposing Tooth Contacts

An important aspect of many jaw movements includes the contacts of opposing teeth. The manner in which the teeth occlude is related not only to the occlusal surfaces of the teeth themselves but also to the muscles, TMJs, and neurophysiological components including the patient's mental well-being. When patients wearing complete dentures bring their teeth together in centric or eccentric positions within the functional range of mandibular movements, the occlusal surfaces of the teeth should meet evenly on both sides. In this manner, the mandible is not deflected from its normal path of closure, nor are the dentures displaced from the residual ridges. In addition, when mandibular movements are made with the opposing teeth of complete dentures in contact, the inclined planes of the teeth should pass over one another smoothly and not disrupt the influences of the condylar guidance posteriorly and the incisal guidance anteriorly.

Research has shown that condylar movement is limited not solely by the anatomy of the TMJs but also by the contacts of opposing teeth. Variations in condylar movement have been observed concomitantly as deflective occlusal contacts or steep incisal guidance from opposing canines change the pathway of mandibular movement. Thus the inclined planes of artificial teeth must be so positioned that they will be in harmony with the other factors that regulate jaw motion. A failure to develop this kind of occlusion can disturb the stability of complete dentures and cause denture bases to move on the soft tissues of the residual ridges.

Several dentists have observed that patients adapt to complete dentures by avoiding eccentric tooth contacts during mastication and by chewing on both sides at the same time. Such a chewing pattern will presumably reduce the risk of denture dislodgment. It may also explain why patients appear to function well with dentures even in the absence of a balanced occlusion. Such an occlusal change, loss of balancing contacts in lateral excursion, has been reported to occur in patients already within a year or two after denture insertion.

Influence of Temporomandibular Joints

All mandibular motion is either rotation or translation (or more commonly a combination of these, Figure 16-1). A rotational movement is one in which all points within a body describe concentric circles around a common axis. A translatory movement is one in which all points within a body are moving at the same velocity and in the same direction. Rotational movements of the mandible take place in the lower compartment of the TMJ between the superior surface of the condyle and the inferior surface of the articular disk. Translatory, or gliding, movements of the mandible take place in the upper compartment of the TMJ between the superior surface of the articular disk as it moves with the condyle and the inferior surface of the glenoid fossa. Mandibular movements, except opening and closing

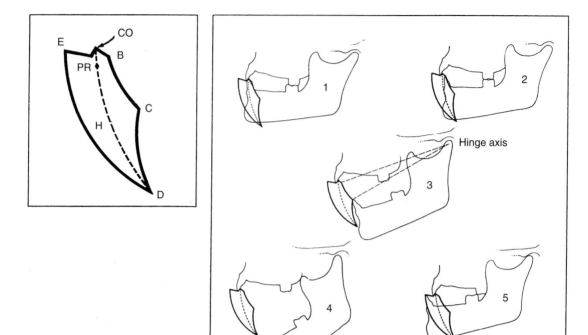

Figure 16-1 Mandibular border movements in the sagittal plane. The mandibular position in centric occlusion *(CO)* is depicted in *1,* and centric relation or the most retruded position *(B)* in *2.* Rotation, the terminal hinge movement *(3)* takes place between *B* and *C,* from which the translation phase of the posterior opening occurs to *D,* the maximum opening position *(4).* The most protrusive closure from *D* ends in *E,* maximum protrusion with tooth contacts, *5.* The postural rest position *(PR)* and the habitual closure *(H)* are located well inside the borders. (Redrawn from Mohl ND, Zarb GA, Carlsson GE et al. editors: *A textbook of occlusion,* Carol Stream, IL, 1988, Quintessence Publishing.)

when the mandible held by the patient or dentist in its most posterior position (posterior terminal hinge movement), are combinations of rotation and translation. This terminal hinge movement is of specific interest in complete denture construction because it is the basis for recording centric relation.

Muscular Involvement in Jaw Motion

The muscles responsible for mandibular movement generally show increased activity during any jaw movement. This increase in activity may be associated with movement of the mandible, fixation on a given position, or stabilization so movement will be smooth and coordinated from one position to another. The activity and interaction of the muscles for a series of jaw movements have been studied extensively by researchers with electromyography (EMG). In clinical practice, however, muscle palpation and observation of the movement pattern usually are enough for evaluation of the muscular involvement in jaw motion.

Neuromuscular Regulation of Mandibular Motion

Mastication is a programmed event residing in a "chewing center" located within the brain stem (probably in the reticular formation of the pons) (Figure 16-2). The cyclic nature of mastication (jaw opening and closure) is the result of the action of this central pattern generator. Conscious effort may either induce or terminate chewing, but it is not required for the continuation of chewing. In a similar manner, sensory impulses from the orofacial region may modify the basic cyclic pattern of the chewing center to achieve optimal function (see Figure 16-2). The alteration of chewing characteristics (rate, force, duration) as related to the consistency of a bolus of food is an example of this type of influence. Finally, central influences from areas of the brain associated with other patterned or "learned" behavior, emotion, and stress may inhibit or excite the chewing center.

The muscles that move, hold, or stabilize the mandible do so because they receive impulses from the central nervous system. The impulses that regulate mandibular motion may arise at the conscious level and result in voluntary mandibular activity. They also may arise from subconscious levels as a result of the stimulation of oral or muscle receptors or of activity in other parts of the central nervous

system. The impulses initiated at the subconscious level can produce involuntary movements or modify voluntary movements. At any one time the cell body of the motor nerve may be influenced by these various sources to inhibition or excitation (Figure 16-3). Impulses from the subconscious level, including the reticular activation system, also regulate muscle tone, which plays a primary role in the physiological rest position of the mandible.

The Envelope of Motion

In an explanation of the clinical implications of mandibular movements, it is helpful to define the limits of possible motion and certain mandibular reference positions. Figure 16-3 shows one method that may be used to record and study mandibular movements. Tests indicate that edentulous patients can make reproducible lateral border movements

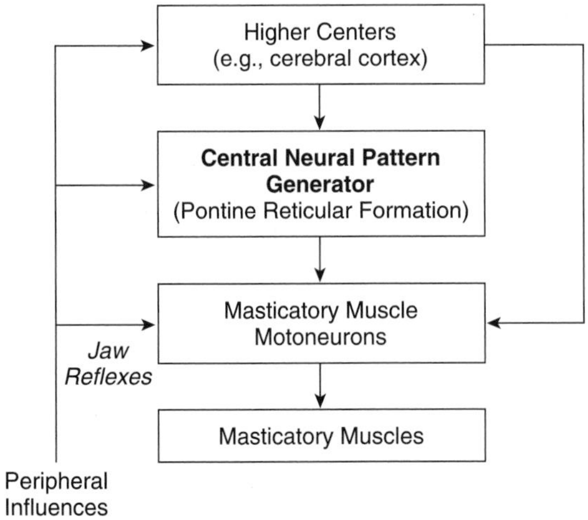

Figure 16-2 The masticatory muscle motoneurons are primarily influenced by the central neural pattern generator but may be initiated or modified by the higher centers in the cerebral cortex. All three structures are influenced by impulses received from the peripheral nerves. (From Orchardson R, Cadden SW: Mastication. In Linden RWA, editor: *The scientific basis of eating: Taste and smell, salivation, mastication, and swallowing and their dysfunctions* [Frontiers of oral biology, vol. 9] Basel, Switzerland, 1998, S. Karger AG.)

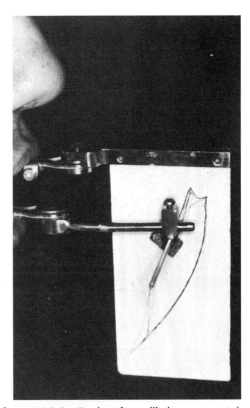

Figure 16-3 Tracing of mandibular movements in the saggital plane. For further explanation see Figure 16-1.

when stabilized baseplates are used to support the pantographic recording device. Envelopes of motion (maximum border movements) in the sagittal and frontal planes as scribed by a dentate subject are shown in Figures 16-4 and 16-5. The dotted line represents the masticatory cycle. This functional movement takes up only a small part of the maximum movement area. Mastication is very

seldom a pure hinge movement but involves simultaneous translatory and rotary movements.

Rest Position

The rest position (or physiological rest, or the vertical dimension, or postural position of the mandible) is established by muscles and gravity. There have

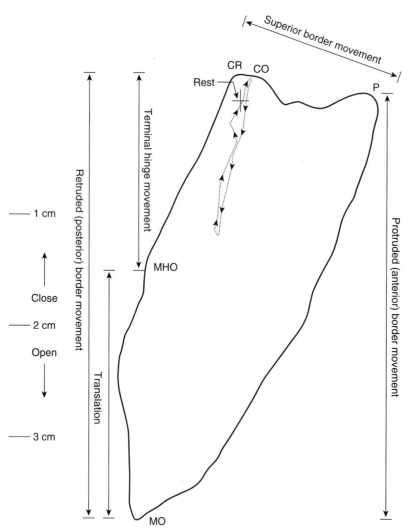

Figure 16-4   Envelope of motion (mandibular border movement area) in the sagittal plane. *CO,* Centric occlusion; *CR,* centric relation; *MHO,* maximum hinge-opening position; *MO,* point of maximum opening of the jaws; *P,* most protruded position of the mandible with the teeth in contact; *Rest,* postural rest position.

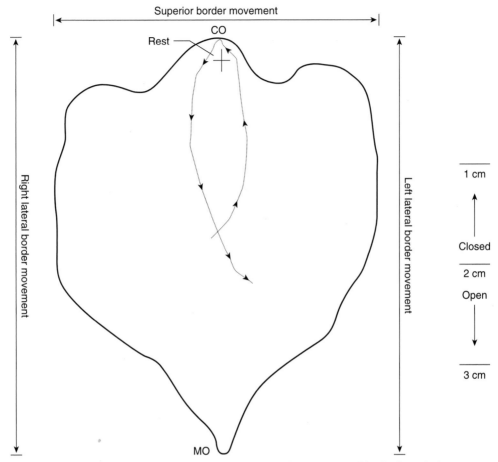

Figure 16-5 Envelope of motion (mandibular border movements) in the frontal plane. *CO,* Centric occlusion; *MO,* point of maximum opening of the jaws; *Rest,* postural rest position.

been two main hypotheses about the postural rest position of the mandible. One involves an active mechanism and the other a passive mechanism. According to the first hypothesis, this position is assumed only when the muscles that close the jaws and those that open the jaws are in a state of minimal contraction to maintain the posture of the mandible. The second hypothesis holds that the elastic elements of the jaw musculature, and not any muscle activity, balance the influence of gravity. However, numerous studies have shown evidence of EMG activity in patients at postural rest position. It also is well known that the jaw drops when one falls asleep, and muscle tension is reduced further. The current consensus is that the physiological rest position is actively determined. The clinically recorded rest position, usually 2 to 4 mm below the maximum intercuspation position, does not correspond to recorded minimal EMG activity. The mandible in the EMG rest position is usually several millimeters lower than in the clinical rest position. A range of reduced muscle tension, up to an interocclusal distance of about 10 mm, has been reported (Figure 16-6). It is therefore more accurate to refer to a "range of posture" rather than to a single rest position.

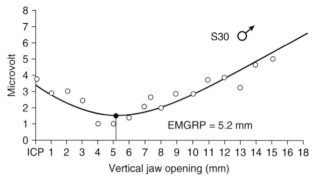

Figure 16-6 Nonspecific electromyographic (EMG) activity in the masseter and anterior temporalis areas at different vertical dimensions with an interpolated best fit parabola. The lowest point on the parabola indicates an "EMG rest position" of 5.2 mm of jaw opening. (From Michelotti A, Faralle M, Vollaro S et al.: Mandibular rest position and electrical activity of the masticatory muscles, *J Prosthet Dent* 78:48-53, 1997.)

Study results of growth and development have shown that the rest position of the mandible tends to remain relatively stable for reasonable lengths of time. However, short- and long-term intraoral and general factors can influence the postural rest position, such as wear and loss of teeth, aging, and general health factors. The physiological rest position also is influenced by the position of the head. This position can be verified by reclining and inclining the head. When the patient's head is reclined, the distance between the teeth is less than when the head is held in a normal alert position. When the head is inclined, the distance is greater. Therefore the patient's head should be upright and unsupported when observations of physiological rest position are being made.

IDENTIFYING THE MAXILLOMANDIBULAR RELATIONS FOR COMPLETE DENTURES

Determining the Vertical Dimension

The vertical jaw relations are expressed in the amount of separation of the maxillae and mandible under specified conditions. They are classified as the vertical dimensions of *occlusion* and *rest*. The vertical dimension of occlusion is established by the natural teeth when they are present and in occlusion. In patients who have lost their natural teeth and must wear dentures, the vertical dimension of occlusion is established by the vertical height of the

two dentures when the teeth are in contact. Thus the vertical dimension of occlusion must be established for edentulous patients so their denture teeth will come into contact at the appropriate height.

The natural teeth establish the occlusal vertical dimension during jaw development and in place. In the course of a person's lifetime, many things happen to the natural teeth. Some are lost, some are so worn that they lose their clinical crown length, some are attacked by dental caries, and in some a restoration fails to maintain their full clinical crown length. Consequently, even patients who have retained their natural teeth may have a reduced occlusal vertical dimension. The preextraction vertical measurement may not reliably indicate the dimension to be incorporated in complete dentures. Information about occlusal vertical dimension with natural teeth, or with previous dentures, should not be ignored, however, because it is probably better than not having any values or record at all as in a totally edentulous subject. Modifications from preextraction values or previous dentures should be made as indicated when the information is available.

The methods for determining vertical maxillomandibular relations can be grouped roughly into two categories. The *mechanical* methods include use of preextraction records and measurements, ridge parallelism, and others. The *physiological* methods include the use of physiological rest position, the swallowing phenomenon, and phonetics as a means for determining the facial dimension at which occlusion should be established. The use of esthetics and patient-reported comfort adds to the mechanical and physiological approaches to the problem.

All estimates of the vertical dimension must be considered tentative until the teeth are arranged on their trial bases, and observations of phonetics and esthetics can be used as a check against the vertical relations established by mechanical or physiological means.

Mechanical Methods

Preextraction Records

Profile Radiographs Profile radiographs of the face have been much used in research of verti-cal dimension of occlusion (Figure 16-7), but because of radiation risks they cannot be considered adequate today for routine clinical use in prostho-dontic treatment for edentulous patients.

Casts of Teeth in Occlusion A simple method of recording the vertical overlap relation and the size and shape of the teeth is to use diagnostic casts mounted on an articulator (Figure 16-8). The casts give an indication of the amount of space required between the ridges for teeth of this size.

Facial Measurements Various devices for making facial measurement have been used in many different forms. Devices have been made to record the relation of the head to the central incisors

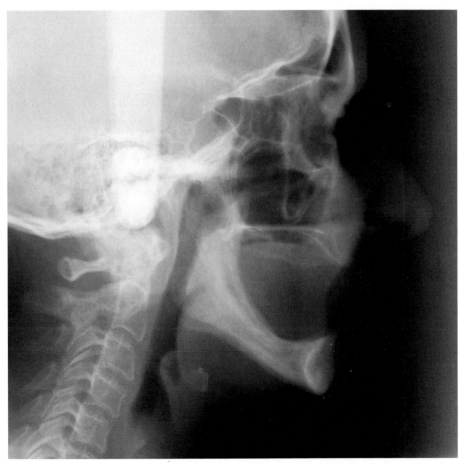

Figure 16-7 Cephalometric radiograph that could be used to help determine vertical dimension of occlusion.

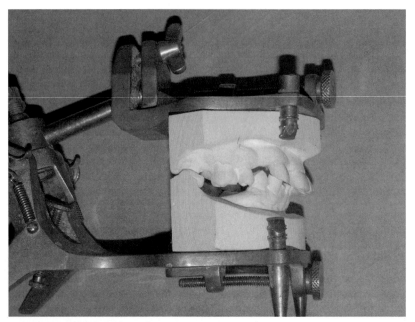

Figure 16-8   Preextraction study models mounted to measure estimates of size, shape, arrangement, and overlap of teeth.

vertically and anteroposteriorly by placement of a face bow with auditory meatus plugs and with spectacle suspension. Another method is to record the distance from the chin to the base of the nose by means of a pair of calipers or dividers before the teeth are extracted (Figure 16-9).

Ridge Relations

Incisive Papilla to Mandibular Incisors   The incisive papilla is a stable landmark that changes comparatively little with resorption of the alveolar ridge. The distance of the papilla from the incisal edges of the mandibular anterior teeth on diagnostic casts averages approximately 4 mm in the natural dentition. The incisal edges of the maxillary central incisors are an average of 6 mm below the incisive papilla. Therefore the mean vertical overlap of the opposing central incisors is about 2 mm (Figure 16-10). It is important to remember that these are average measurements around which there is considerable individual variation. They should be used with caution, and they do not appear to be relevant in patients with severe resorption.

Parallelism of the Ridges   Parallelism of the maxillary and mandibular ridges, plus a 5-degree opening in the posterior region, often gives a clue as to the appropriate amount of jaw separation.

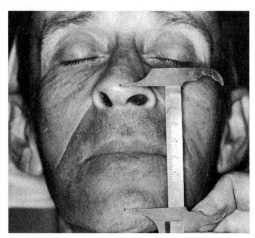

Figure 16-9   A measurement is made between two points on the face when the mandible is in physiological rest position.

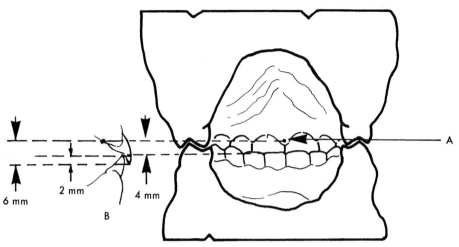

Figure 16-10 Sectioned casts, posterior view. *A,* When the teeth are in centric occlusion, the incisal edges of the mandibular central incisors are on average 4 mm from the incisive papilla. *B,* Sagittal view of the central incisors; the vertical overlap is about 2 mm.

Because the clinical crowns of the anterior and posterior teeth have nearly the same length, their removal tends to leave the residual alveolar ridges nearly parallel to each other. This parallelism is natural, provided there has been no abnormal change in the alveolar process such as previous advanced periodontal disease or gross overeruptions (Figure 16-11).

This parallelism of the ridges is favorable from a mechanical point of view because occlusal loading on the dentures is less likely to cause them to slide anteriorly or posteriorly. However, in most people, the teeth are lost at different times, and when a person finally becomes edentulous, it often is observed that the residual ridges are no longer parallel. In addition, the edentulous ridges of the mandible and maxillae will become progressively more discrepant from the standpoint of width (Figure 16-12).

Measurement of the Former Dentures Dentures that the patient has been wearing can be measured, and the measurements can be correlated with observations of the patient's face to determine the amount of change required. These measurements are made between the ridge crests in the maxillary and mandibular dentures with a Boley gauge (Figure 16-13). Then, if the observations of the patient's face indicate that this distance is too

short or too long, a corresponding change can be made in the new dentures.

Physiological Methods

Physiological Rest Position Registration of the jaw in physiological rest position gives an indication of the appropriate vertical dimension of occlusion. This is possible because the difference between the occlusal vertical dimension and the rest vertical dimension is the interocclusal distance (formerly referred to as the "freeway space"). The interocclusal distance is the distance or gap existing between the upper and lower teeth when the mandible is in the physiological rest position. It usually is 2 to 4 mm when observed at the position of the first premolars. This may not be an exact guide; however, when used with other methods, it will aid in determining the vertical relation of the mandible to the maxillae. One method is to have the patient relaxed, with the trunk upright and the head unsupported. After insertion of the wax occlusion rims, the patient swallows and lets the jaw relax. When relaxation is obvious, the lips are parted to reveal how much space is present between the occlusion rims. The patient must allow the dentist to separate the lips without moving the jaws or lips or trying to help the dentist. The interocclusal distance

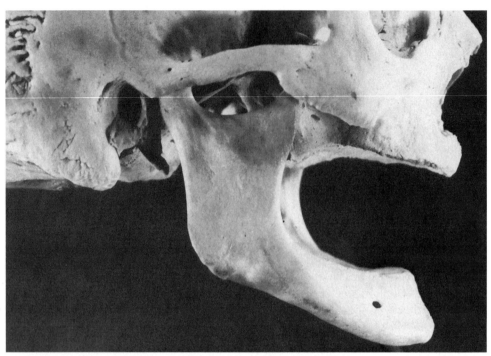

Figure 16-11 The crest of the lower residual ridge will be approximately parallel to the crest of the upper ridge when the jaws are positioned at the vertical dimension of occlusion. This relationship is regarded as ideal for the stability of dentures.

at the rest position should be between 2 and 4 mm when viewed at the premolar region. The interarch space and rest position can be measured by means of indelible dots or adhesive tape on the face. If the difference is greater than 4 mm, the occlusal vertical dimension may be considered too small; if less than 2 mm, the dimension is probably too great. The occlusion rims are adjusted until the dentist is satisfied with the amount of interarch space and until other requirements of an acceptable vertical dimension have been obtained, such as patient comfort and phonetic and esthetic considerations (Figure 16-14). It is worth noting that the presence or absence of dentures or occlusion rims and the vertical dimension of these can affect the physiological rest position. The method used for determining the position (e.g., relaxation, swallowing, or phonetics) also may modify its vertical level (see Figure 16-14). Dentists must keep this in mind when using the rest position as a guide for establishing vertical maxillomandibular relations.

It is essential that an adequate interocclusal distance exist when the mandible is in its physiological rest position. However, results of experimental research have shown that a rapid adaptation takes place after changes of the vertical dimension, leading to another rest position and creation of a new interocclusal distance. This has been found to occur even after an increase that was greater than the original interocclusal distance. Such findings indicate that the rest position alone is not a reliable basis for the determination of maxillomandibular relations and that small variations of the vertical dimension are not so critical because the adaptive capacity of the masticatory system usually is great. It should be combined with other evaluations, such as patient comfort, phonetics, and esthetics.

Phonetics Phonetic tests of the vertical dimension include listening to speech sound production and observing the relationships of teeth during speech. The production of *ch*, *s*, and *j* sounds brings

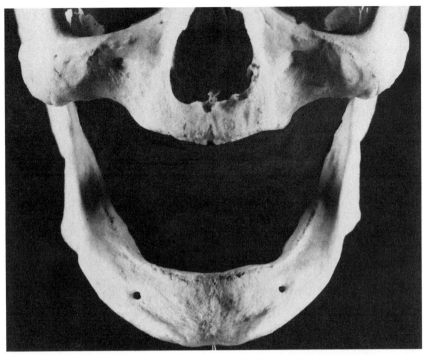

Figure 16-12   It is a common finding in edentulous patients that the mandibular ridge becomes progressively wider, and the maxillary ridge narrower, as bone resorption continues. This is exemplified in this edentulous skull.

the anterior teeth close together. When correctly placed, the lower incisors should move forward to a position nearly directly under and almost touching the upper incisors. If the distance is too large, it means that too small a vertical dimension of occlusion may have been established. If the anterior teeth touch when these sounds are made, the vertical dimension is probably too great. Likewise, if the teeth click together during speech, the vertical dimension is probably too great.

Esthetics   The vertical relation of the mandible to the maxillae also affects esthetics. A study of the skin of the lips compared with the skin over other parts of the face can be used as a guide. Normally the tone of the facial skin should be the same throughout. However, it must be realized that the relative anteroposterior positions of the teeth are at least equally as involved in the vertical relations of the jaws as in the restoration of skin tone. The

contour of the lips depends on their intrinsic structure and the support behind them. Therefore the dentist must initially contour the labial surfaces of the occlusion rims so they closely simulate the anteroposterior tooth positions and the contour of the base of the denture. This contoured surface must replace or restore the tissue support provided by the natural structures (Figure 16-15). If the lips are not properly supported anteriorly, they will be more nearly vertical than when supported by the natural tissues. In such a situation, the tendency is to increase the vertical dimension of occlusion to provide support for the lips, and this can lead to excessive lower face height. The esthetic guide to an appropriate vertical maxillomandibular relation is, first, to select teeth that are the same size as the natural teeth and, second, to estimate the amount of tissue lost from the alveolar ridges. However, recent evidence suggests that this method of estimating the appropriate vertical dimension is a

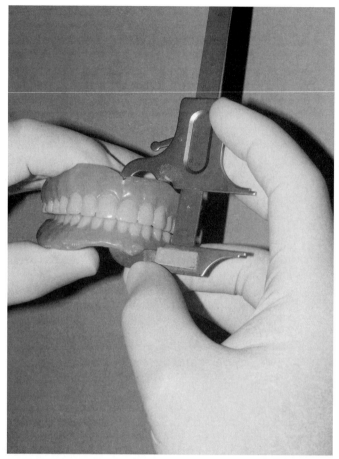

Figure 16-13 Boley gauge measuring the distance between the ridge crests as indicated by the previous dentures.

relatively unreliable one. In a study of young dentate individuals (where the issue of lip support is eliminated), dentists gave relatively poor estimates of the effects of changes in vertical dimension from facial photos when the vertical dimension was artificially opened between 2 and 6 mm. This method should therefore be used with caution or in combination with other methods.

Swallowing Threshold The position of the mandible at the beginning of the swallowing act has been used as a guide to the vertical dimension of occlusion. The theory is that the teeth come together with a very light contact at the beginning

of the swallowing cycle. If denture occlusion is continually missing during swallowing, the dimension of occlusion may be insufficient (too far closed). On this basis, a record of the relation of the two jaws at this point in the swallowing cycle is used as an indicator of the vertical dimension of occlusion. The technique involves building cones of wax on the lower denture base in such a way that they contact the upper occlusion rim when the jaws are open too wide (Figure 16-16). Then the flow of saliva is stimulated by food, such as a piece of candy. The repeated action of swallowing the saliva will gradually reduce the height of the wax cones to allow the mandible to reach the level of

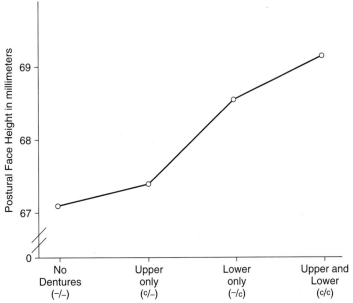

Figure 16-14   Change in postural face height with insertion (or removal) of dentures.

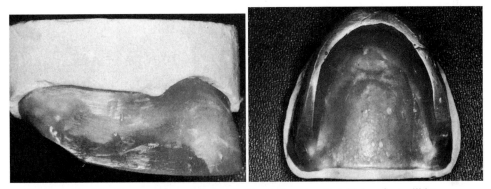

Figure 16-15   The maxillary occlusion rim is contoured so its labial surface will be similar to that of the finished denture base and the artificial teeth. Lateral *(A)* and occlusal *(B)* views show the contour and dimensions of the neutral zone, which have been approximated in this occlusion rim. Identical principles are used in contouring mandibular occlusion rims. (From Heath MR, Boutros MM: The influence of prosthesis on mandibular posture in edentulous patients, *J Prosthet Dent* 51: 602-604, 1984.)

the vertical dimension of occlusion. The length of the time to complete this action and the relative softness of the wax cones will affect the results. No consistency in the final vertical positioning of the mandible has been found with this method.

Tactile Sense and Patient-Perceived Comfort
The patient's tactile sense can be used as a guide for the determination of the occlusal vertical dimension. With this method, an adjustable central bearing screw is attached to one of the occlusion rims, and a central bearing plate is attached to the

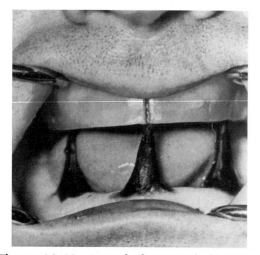

Figure 16-16 Cones of soft wax attached to the mandibular base form an interocclusal record as they are forced against the maxillary occlusion rim when the patient swallows. Swallowing should establish the proper horizontal and vertical relations of the mandible to the maxillae.

other one (Figure 16-17). The central bearing screw is adjusted first, so it is obviously too long. Then, in progressive steps, the screw is adjusted downward until the patient indicates that the jaws are closing too far. The procedure is repeated in the opposite direction until the patient indicates that the teeth feel too long. The screw then is adjusted downward again until the patient indicates that the length is about right. The adjustments are reversed alternately until the height of the contact feels comfortable to the patient. The problem with this method relates to the presence of foreign objects in the palate and the tongue space. There are also some conflicting results on the precision of this method. Patient participation in the decision to establish a vertical dimension record should be considered, however, because there are both physiological and psychological advantages to this approach.

Testing the Vertical Jaw Relations with the Occlusion Rims None of the methods just listed, used alone, will yield an appropriate vertical

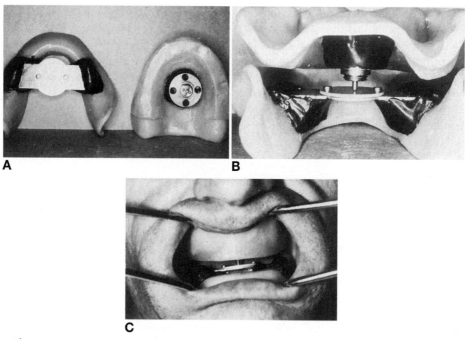

Figure 16-17 A to C, An intraoral tracing instrument (the Coble device) that can be used both for recording of the vertical dimension by means of the adjustable central bearing point and for horizontal jaw relation by tracing mandibular movements from side to side. The apex of the tracing should indicate the position of centric relation.

dimension of occlusion reliably in all patients. It is appropriate therefore to use one or more of the methods to approximate the relationship and then to use other methods to independently test the appropriateness of the relationship initially estimated, before the record is sent for the set-up of teeth.

When multiple independent methods used for determining the vertical dimension appear to yield similar results, this (still preliminary) estimate can be taken as the vertical height at which teeth should be set. When the horizontal jaw relations have been established, the centric relation record will be taken at this vertical dimension for transfer to the articulator.

Of course a further review of this tentative determination will occur later at the try-in appointment, when teeth are set in the wax trial dentures and the vertical dimension is verified in the mouth. At that time these methods will be used again collectively to confirm the vertical dimension before completion of the dentures.

DETERMINING HORIZONTAL JAW RELATIONS

The principles of good occlusion apply to both dentate and edentulous patients. The problem is, however, that there is no consensus on the definition of good occlusion. It also is most probable that the requirements of the occlusion for complete dentures differ from those of a natural dentition. For stability of complete dentures to be maintained, the opposing teeth must meet evenly on both sides of the dental arch when the teeth contact anywhere within the normal functional range of mandibular movement. Dentists usually agree that such a *balanced occlusion* is preferable for complete dentures. (In the natural dentition, a *mutually protected occlusion* is frequently observed, with the modifications *canine protected occlusion* and *group function occlusion* as equally acceptable variations.)

The basic horizontal relationship is centric relation. It is a reference relationship that must be recognized in any prosthodontic treatment. Other horizontal jaw relations are at points of movement away from centric relation in the horizontal plane. Collectively they are referred to as eccentric relations and include protrusive positions, right and left lateral excursions, and all intermediate positions.

Confusion in Terms and Concepts

The term *centric relation* is given a number of different meanings in its application to the development of dental restorations. In the dental literature, centric relation has been associated with, among other things, the neuromuscular reflex learned when the primary teeth are in occlusion, the posterior terminal hinge position, the physiological rest position, and the position of the mandible during swallowing.

The "Glossary of Prosthodontic Terms" (1999) lists no less than seven different definitions of centric relation. Although these definitions are somewhat different, all of them indicate that centric relation is determined by the TMJ structures and not by the dentition. Most of them relate to the terminal hinge axis, some of them mention the retruded or posterior position, and others emphasize the uppermost position of the condyles. The condylar position (an anatomical relationship) cannot be determined with certainty at clinical examination, but the terminal hinge axis (a relationship defined by jaw *movement*) can be demonstrated. The physiological transverse hinge axis is located by a series of controlled opening and closing movements of the jaws when the mandible is held in its most retruded position relative to the maxillae. These mandibular movements are called *terminal hinge movements* and are part of the posterior border movement that occurs without translation (see Figure 16-1).

Several studies have shown that the terminal hinge axis and a mandibular position on that axis can be recorded with good precision. The small differences found with various techniques for recording centric relation do not seem to be of clinical significance, especially not for complete dentures with their tendency to move on the soft tissues of the residual ridges.

The confusion in terminology has been aggravated by controversy over the connection between centric relation and centric occlusion. The current definition of *centric occlusion* is the occlusion of opposing teeth when the mandible is in centric relation. This may or may not coincide with the maximum intercuspation position. The most common concept in construction of complete dentures is to have the maximum intercuspation position coinciding with centric relation. Another concept maintains that in many patients a broader area of stable contacts near centric relation is necessary, the so-called freedom in centric or long centric.

Some authors have argued in favor of the "muscular position" on the grounds that it is the most frequently used in function. It has been defined as the position reached after a relaxed mandibular closure from the rest position, and it usually coincides with the maximum intercuspation or intercuspal position in a healthy natural dentition. Research has shown that the muscular position is more variable than a retruded position and cannot be recorded with the same predictability as centric relation is. It is true, however, that most patients' teeth occlude in a position that is slightly anterior, 0.5 to 1.0 mm, to the centric relation. This fact would speak in favor of a limited range of continuous tooth contact in occlusion anterior and lateral to centric relation, even when that position is used for the recording of the horizontal jaw relation. Another argument for this concept concerns the repeated findings in clinical studies that the distance between the maximum intercuspation position and centric relation is increased in long-term complete denture wearers, even if the relationships coincided when constructed. This increase is most probably caused by movements of the dentures over time as a consequence of changes in the denture-supporting tissues.

Significance of Centric Relation

There is extensive dental literature in which concepts, definitions, and methods for recording the horizontal jaw records are discussed. Even if there are many varying opinions on details, there seems to be a consensus that a correct registration of centric relation is essential in the construction of complete dentures. Many dentures fail because the occlusion is not planned or developed to include this position. Centric relation is the horizontal reference position of the mandible that can be routinely assumed by edentulous patients under the direction of the dentist. It is possible for dentists to verify the relationship of casts on the articulator when they are mounted in centric relation. If the hinge axis record has been properly transferred, an accurate centric relation record will orient the lower cast to the opening axis of the articulator in the same relationship as the patient's mandible relates to his/her

opening axis. Clinical experience, however, suggests that good function is possible when an arbitrary face bow or even no face bow is used during denture construction. It appears that the most critical factor is an appropriate centric relation record, whereas the face bow is of minor importance. Therefore it is recommended that when an arbitrary face bow, or no face bow is used, the centric relation record should be made at or very close to the selected vertical dimension of occlusion. In this way, the potential errors of not having recorded the true hinge axis will be greatly reduced.

Eccentric Relation Records

As the mandible moves forward in protrusive excursion, the condyles move downward and forward. Similarly, as the mandible moves laterally to one side, the condyle on the opposite side moves downward, forward, and inward. These downward movements of the posterior part of the mandible have the effect of moving the mandibular posterior teeth downward, creating space between them and the maxillary posterior teeth or occlusion rims. This effect is known as the *Christensen phenomenon*. Because dentists seek to provide the patient with smooth, continuous contact of the denture teeth throughout the functional range of jaw motion, the Christensen phenomenon should be included in the development of the occlusion, particularly in the posterior segments of the dentition. A registration of the condyle paths can be performed by means of a variety of intraoral and extraoral methods and the articulator adjusted accordingly. However, such recordings are associated with extremely great variations, and the clinical value of them is not supported by convincing documentation. Therefore they are not regarded as necessary for achieving clinically acceptable results.

TRANSFERRING RECORDS FROM THE PATIENT TO THE ARTICULATOR

For the articulator to provide accurate interocclusal relationships, the casts on the articulator must relate to the hinge axis of the instrument in as nearly as possible the same way as the jaws relate to the patient's arc of closure. The dentist must record the relationship between the upper jaw and arbitrary points near the condyles and then transfer that relationship to the instrument. As noted earlier, these locations near the condyles are serving as an approximation of the hinge axis of mandibular motion. Relating the maxillary and mandibular casts just as the jaws relate puts the mandibular cast in the correct position on the articulator so that it will move appropriately. The mandibular cast is thus related indirectly to the hinge axis only through the maxillary cast, which in turn relates directly to the guidances. The articulator can then be programmed with the eccentric records if needed to yield a reasonable estimate of jaw motion and resulting occlusal relationships.

TYPES OF PATIENT RECORDS

Both the vertical and horizontal relationships of the mandible to the maxillae can be transferred from the patient to the articulator with three general classes of records: hinge axis records; interocclusal records, such as the centric relation and eccentric records; and graphic records. The simplest articulators are designed to accept only interocclusal records, whereas the more sophisticated instruments are capable of providing adjustments in response to all three types of records.

Hinge Axis Records

As the patient's jaw opens and closes, the posterior border of its movement, at least in the earliest phases, is the arc of a circle in the sagittal plane around an imaginary transverse axis passing through or near the condyles. The same is true of the articulator. Similarly, other movements of the jaws occur in arcs. For an accurate reproduction of those movements, the axes of those arcs should be coincident between patient and instrument, particularly where the patient's vertical dimension is to be changed. The axis of the arcs can be located when the mandible is in its most posterior position by means of a kinematic face bow or hinge bow, or it can be approximated by use of an arbitrary type of face bow. There is evidence that the kinematic record cannot be transferred to the articulator reliably, even in dentate patients. It is even more difficult in the edentulous patient. Consequently, the kinematic record of the hinge axis is usually ignored in complete denture construction,

in favor of an arbitrary location with facial landmarks. This method provides a substantially less accurate estimate of the location of the true hinge axis, but evidence suggests that there is no clinical impact from this loss accuracy.

The Face Bow

The face bow is a calliper-like device that is used to record the relationship of the jaws to the opening axis of the jaws and to orient the casts in this same relationship to the opening axis of the articulator. It is important to note that this is a relationship between the jaws and the axis of movement, not an anatomical relationship between the jaws and the TMJs, except to the extent that the axis of movement might happen to be near the TMJs. (Some dentists and dental technicians also consider the face bow a convenient instrument for supporting the casts while they are being attached to the articulator.) The instrument consists of a U-shaped frame or assembly that is large enough to extend from the region of one TMJ around the front of the face (5 to 7.5 cm in front of it) to the other TMJ and wide enough to avoid contact with the sides of the face. The parts that contact the skin near the TMJs are the condyle rods, and the part that attaches to the occlusion rim is the fork. The fork attaches to the face bow by means of a locking device (which also serves to support the face bow, the maxillary occlusion rim, and the maxillary cast while the casts are being attached to the articulator) (Figure 16-18). The fork of the arbitrary face bow is attached to the maxillary occlusion rim, so the record is a simple relationship between the upper jaw and the approximate axis of the jaw opening.

Some face bows are designed to fit directly into the external auditory meatus. This type of design is easier to manipulate clinically than holding the condylar rods over the hinge axis markings while the bite fork is tightened in position (Figure 16-19). An average distance from the external auditory meatus to an arbitrary hinge axis is built into the face bow design. This distance is compensated for in the articulator by offsetting the mounting points an equivalent amount (Figure 16-20).

There is much in the prosthodontic literature that maintains that a face bow transfer is essential for avoiding errors in the occlusion of finished dentures.

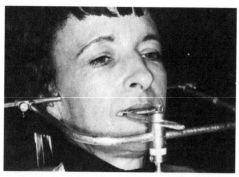

Figure 16-18 Patient with upper occlusion rim and bite fork held in place with the lower occlusion rim. The ear rods are over the markings on the side of the face.

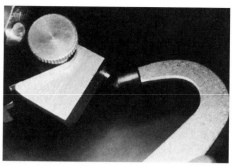

Figure 16-20 The ear rod of an articulator fitting to a point on the condylar housing that compensates for the use of the external auditory meatus.

Indeed it is easy to acknowledge the theoretical advantages of using a face bow to orient the casts to the hinge axis of the articulator (Figure 16-21). It should be remembered, however, that these theoretical advantages to the use of a face bow might not necessarily produce a better clinical end result. Results of one of the few systematic studies made to compare patient response to variations in dentures technique failed to show any significant differences between a "complex" technique involving hinge-axis location for a face bow transfer to the articulator and a "standard" technique without face bow and with an arbitrary mounting. Similar clinical results with dentures constructed by the two techniques were found at both short- and long-term recall assessments. The investigation included dentists' evaluation of occlusion, denture stability, retention, and condition of the denture-bearing tissues, with patients' satisfaction and adaptation. The results indicated that the success of denture treatment involves many factors, and the use of a face bow is not an essential one. These results have been supported by similar findings in the context of constructing stabilization appliances. Such documentation and extensive clinical experience

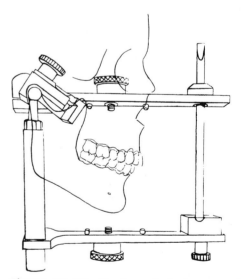

Figure 16-21 The theoretical advantages of using a face bow include the anatomical similarity of the resulting relationship between the teeth and the condyles. However, this relationship does not ensure that the movements of the articulator will result in a better clinical result for the patient with dentures.

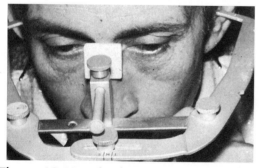

Figure 16-19 A face bow related to a patient's external auditory meatus and nasion.

have caused many practicing dentists to stop using a face bow. It is also clear that imperfections may exist with both complex and standard techniques. Any type of face bow and all articulators suffer from errors and can only approximate conditions in the patient's masticatory system. This is, of course, no excuse for abandoning impeccable technique and sound principles of denture construction. Consequently, scrupulous clinical control and the acceptance of a need for adjustments are necessary with any method.

The argument that a face bow is helpful in supporting the maxillary cast while it is being mounted on the articulator may be true. However, an arbitrary mounting of the maxillary cast can be accomplished on any articulator with any convenient support material by aligning the occlusal plane of the wax occlusion rim horizontally and parallel to the arms of the articulator.

Interocclusal Records

Virtually all articulators will accept at least some interocclusal records. An interocclusal record simply provides a measure of one single positional relationship of the lower jaw to the upper jaw. That position might be centric relation, maximum intercuspation position, or any eccentric point in lateral or protrusive excursions. Although the centric relation position establishes a "static" relationship of the jaws, the protrusive and lateral records permit adjustment of the articulator components to perform variations in the *movement* pattern of the casts over one another. The instrument then interpolates between records (with varying degrees of accuracy) to provide a representation of the full range of jaw movement. As noted earlier, these eccentric records are highly variable, to the extent that their clinical value has not been demonstrated, and they are therefore regarded as unnecessary for clinically acceptable results.

Graphic Records

A shortcoming of the interocclusal records is that they provide accurate relations between the casts only at the jaw positions where they were taken. The articulator must interpolate the movements between the record points. Because the border

movements of the jaw are typically curved, an articulator programmed with only interocclusal records is likely to be inaccurate. Graphic records capture these curved limits, and an articulator capable of curved movements can be programmed to accept these records, thus yielding a more accurate reproduction of the jaw movements.

However, obtaining accurate records from the patient requires that the graphic writing apparatus be firmly fixed to the jaws. This is not difficult where teeth are present but is very problematic when the patient is edentulous and the attachment can only be made through occlusion rims. The graphic records are inaccurate as a result and therefore offer no advantage over the more arbitrary interocclusal records. The extra capability of an articulator that will reproduce curved movements is therefore of no use.

Clinical Steps

Maxilla The face bow is the instrument that carries the relationship between the maxillae and the condyles from the patient to the articulator. The arbitrary face bow is placed on the face, with the condyle rods located approximately in the region of the hinge axis, which will be near the condyles.

The first step in this process is to mark the approximate location of the hinge axis on the skin on each side of the patient's face. One frequently recommended method is to position the condyle rods on a line extending from the outer canthus of the eye to the top of the tragus of the ear and approximately 13 mm in front of the external auditory meatus. This placement generally locates the rods within 5 mm of the true center of the opening axis of the jaws. The imaginary line joining the two points is an approximate hinge axis.

The occlusion rim is trimmed to the position that will be occupied by the teeth as described in the previous chapter. The second step is to ensure that the occlusion rim (with bite fork attached) is stable and tightly adapted to the maxillary ridge. The patient can help hold the occlusion rim firmly seated by biting against it using the mandibular occlusion rim. This biting or closed position is only used for the practical purpose of holding the maxillary rim firmly seated. This is not a record of interocclusal relationships.

In the final clinical step, the condylar rods of the face bow are positioned over the condylar markings, thus recording the approximate hinge axis (see Figure 16-18). The patient can help by holding the condylar rods in place while the clinician locks the bite fork to the face bow. This locks the relationship between the maxillae and the approximate hinge axis through the occlusion rim, the bite fork, and the face bow. This relationship can now be carried to the articulator (Figure 16-22).

Mandible   The relationship of the mandible to the articulator hinge axis is achieved indirectly by relating the mandible to the maxilla. In the edentulous patient, this relationship is recorded by means of a centric relation record taken between the occlusion rims.

Recording Centric Relation

The registration of centric relation is considered difficult, and it is true that it requires training and experience to achieve reliable results. There are biological difficulties that arise from a lack of coordination of mandibular musculature, psychological difficulties that are due to a patient or dentist who is uncertain or tense because of the importance of the recording, and mechanical difficulties that are due to unstable and sometimes poorly fitting baseplates and varying tissue resiliency. As a result, even consistently repeatable centric relation records can, in fact, be in error.

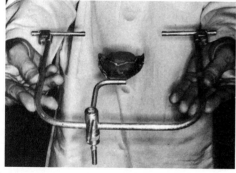

Figure 16-22   The completed face bow record ready to be matched to the articulator.

The following instructions can assist the patient in retruding the mandible:

1. Instruct the patient by saying, "Let your jaw relax, pull it back, and close slowly and easily on your back teeth."
2. Instruct the patient by saying, "Get the feeling of pushing your upper jaw out and closing your back teeth together."
3. Instruct the patient to protrude and retrude the mandible repeatedly while holding his or her fingers lightly against the chin.
4. Instruct the patient to turn the tongue backward toward the posterior border of the upper denture.
5. Instruct the patient to tap the occlusion rims or back teeth together repeatedly.
6. Tilt the patient's head back while the various exercises just listed are carried out.
7. Palpate the temporal and masseter muscles to relax them.

The instructions should be given in a calm and confident manner. When the patient is responding properly, the dentist should say so. When the patient is not responding properly, there should be no criticism. In this manner, the patient's awareness of the desired position is reinforced while avoiding tension.

Such recommendations have a long tradition in clinical practice. However, their effectiveness is not supported by documented evidence. Patient-governed activity to close in centric relation has proven to yield extremely variable results. On the other hand, research has shown that the most reproducible recording of a retruded mandibular position in dentate subjects is achieved by gently guiding the mandible backward with the subject relaxing the jaws. This also can be effective in helping record centric relation in edentulous patients. Many clinicians have obtained good results by training the patients to perform a hinge-axis rotation before the actual registration, by having the patient as relaxed and passive as possible, and by actively guiding the mandible in small movements up and down. By maintaining finger contact with the mandible, the dentist can usually feel when the hinge movement is performed.

There is probably no best method for recording centric relation. A method favored by one dentist will fail for another. Both accurate and erroneous records of centric relation have been made by these methods. Therefore it cannot be overemphasized that, irrespective of the method used, subsequent clinical checking and rechecking must be done throughout the denture construction phases.

The consistency of the recording material is of significance: it must not offer resistance during mandibular closure, or it will inadvertently guide the path of the mandible as it approaches the point of the static record. On the other hand, once set, the recording material must have sufficient strength and rigidity to retain the relationship between the occlusion rims and support the models during the mounting process. Silicone bite registration materials are acceptable.

Recording Eccentric Records

The methods for recording eccentric records are analogous to the methods for recording centric relation. Similarly, the instructions to the patient are analogous. However, given the enormous variation in the accuracy of these records and the absence of evidence for their usefulness in the clinical result, little can be gained by taking such records.

Laboratory Steps

Maxilla   The first step in relating the maxilla to the articulator is to ensure that the articulator is locked in the centric relation position. The condylar balls are thus immobilized in their housings during the steps that follow.

The next step is to attach the face bow ear rods to the instrument with special connections that match one to the other (see Figure 16-20). This usually is done either by altering the distance between the ear rods until they fit the width of the articulator hinge pin, or the reverse, by altering the width between the articulator condylar housings until they fit the distance between the ear rods (Figure 16-23). The latter arrangement is theoretically advantageous because altering the width between the condylar balls will change the arc of rotation of the nonworking side condyle. This may be significant in fixed prosthodontics, but probably irrelevant for complete denture construction.

The ear rods on the hinge axis represent two points of attachment between the face bow and the articulator. To hold the maxillary occlusion rim and cast firmly in three dimensions, a third point of reference must be set. Some face bows use an infraorbital pointer, set to approximate the infraorbital foramen on the patient, with a matching indicator on the articulator. Others use a nasion relater for

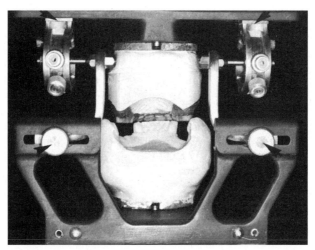

Figure 16-23   The width between the articulator condylar elements can be adjusted to fit the intercondylar width recorded on the face bow.

the same purpose. The intent of these "third point" recording devices is to position the occlusal plane on the articulator so that the arms of the instrument are approximately parallel to the patient's Frankfort plane (see Figure 16-21). However, because the articulator is designed to reproduce the *movement* of the mandible and not the *anatomy* of the maxillomandibular relations, the need for the third point becomes moot. The articulator will be programmed to move relative to the occlusal plane at any angulation within the mechanical limits of the instrument. As a practical matter, it is easiest to work with the instrument if the occlusal plane is positioned about halfway between the upper and lower members, with the midline of the models in line with the incisal pin. The face bow can be supported on the lab bench at this level while the plaster is

poured on the maxillary cast to join it to the upper member of the articulator (Figure 16-24).

Given that the use of a face bow has been found not to be essential for successful denture construction and that the articulator reproduces the movement of the mandible, not the anatomical facial relationships, the cast of the maxilla can be mounted by any convenient arbitrary method that is within the working limits of the articulator. The maxillary occlusion rim supporting the maxillary cast could be held in place by an easily moulded ball of clay, while the plaster is added to the upper member to lock the cast in place. As just noted, it is usually easiest to work with the articulator if the occlusal plane is roughly parallel to the upper and lower members and about halfway between them, and the midline is approximately coincident with the incisal pin.

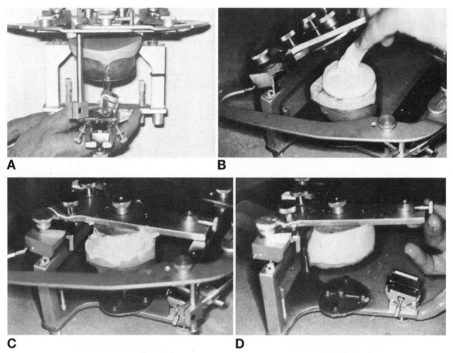

Figure 16-24 **A,** Face bow, occlusion rim, and cast, and upper member of the Whip Mix articulator, supported by the lower member to facilitate mounting of the upper cast. The lower member is used in this procedure for convenience only. **B,** With the upper member raised, plaster is distributed over the top of the upper cast. **C,** The upper member of the articulator has been closed back into position, bringing the mounting plate into the plaster. **D,** Mounting of the upper cast on the articulator completed. Notice the neat appearance of the plaster that attaches the upper cast to the mounting ring.

Mandible   As noted earlier, the relationship of the mandibular cast to the lower member of the articulator is established indirectly by the relationship between the mandible and the maxilla—the centric relation record. This relationship is achieved very simply by inverting the articulator and relating the mandibular occlusion rim to the maxillary with the CR record (Figure 16-25). This provides support for the mandibular cast while plaster is placed to join it to the lower member.

ARTICULATORS

Articulators are instruments that attempt to reproduce the range of movement of the jaws. Maxillary and mandibular casts are attached to the articulator so that the functional and parafunctional contact relations between the teeth can be studied. Diagnosis, the arrangement of artificial teeth, and the development of the occlusal surfaces of cast fixed restorations are common uses.

Some articulators are very simple, consisting of nothing more than a simple hinge (Figure 16-26). These articulators do little more than simulate the hinge motion of the mandible and hold the casts in centric relation. At the other extreme, complicated articulators, which require very complex recording apparatus, aim to simulate all the nuances of jaw movement. No articulator exactly reproduces the full range of jaw movement, nor is the reproduction

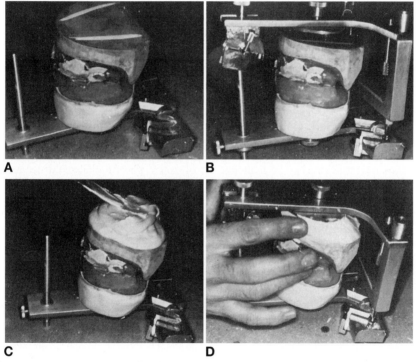

Figure 16-25   **A,** The occlusion rims and lower cast are placed in position on the upper cast, which is attached to the upper member of the articulator. **B,** The lower member of the articulator is positioned on the inverted upper member, leaving adequate space between the mounting ring on the lower member and the lower cast. **C,** With the lower member of the articulator removed, plaster is distributed over the surface of the lower cast. **D,** The lower member is placed on the upper member. The condylar spheres must be firmly seated in the condylar housings, and the incisal guide pin must be firmly seated in the incisal table. The lower cast is attached to the mounting ring on the lower member of the articulator by the plaster.

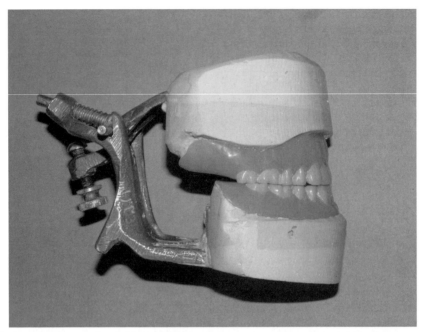

Figure 16-26 A simple hinge articulator.

of such a range required for fabricating any kind of prosthesis. In between is a series of several instruments that provide a more or less accurate reproduction of movement (Figure 16-27). The challenge for the dentist is to choose an articulator that is suitable for the purpose at hand, neither more nor less complicated than necessary. This requires an understanding of what the instrument will and will not do, as well as a grasp of the treatment objectives for the given patient.

Early articulators were based on individual theories of occlusion. However, the normal variation in mandibular movement between patients, and even the variable movement of the joints within one patient, soon made it necessary to design adjustable articulators. An emerging understanding of the neurophysiology of mandibular movement and the influence of several morphological and behavioral considerations led to the notion that each patient is his or her own best articulator. Therefore the diverse, and frequently subtle, variations required for each individual occlusion could be more easily achieved with an adjustable articulator that accepted a variety of records. The final "individualization" of an occlusion can then be done intraorally as required.

Most articulators in common use today are adjustable and attempt to reproduce jaw *movement* of each patient's jaw by trying to reproduce the *anatomy* of the jaw joints and related structures. Although this approach has the benefit of being intuitive, it ignores certain realities of the biological system. For example, the great variation in movements at the TMJs within the envelope of motion is virtually impossible to reproduce mechanically. Furthermore, the movement of the occlusion rims on the underlying ridges is not reflected on the instrument. It is important then to recognize that the adjustments made on an articulator are not attempts to make the instrument more *anatomically* correct, but rather they are attempts to more closely simulate the *motion* of the mandible regardless of the settings that result.

Selecting the Articulator for Fabricating Complete Dentures

The large number and great range in complexity of modern articulators can mislead the dentist into thinking that the choice of a suitable instrument is a potentially difficult one. However, the choice is greatly simplified if one considers what records

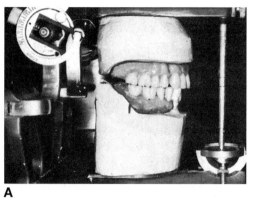

A

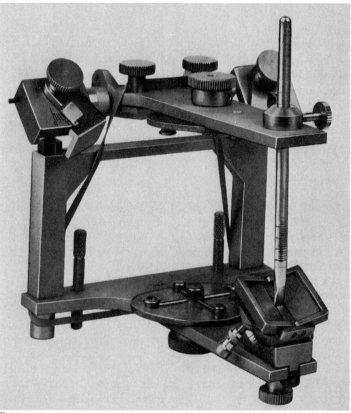

B

Figure 16-27   Examples of two semiadjustable arcon articulators. **A,** Hanau Model 130-28. **B,** Whip Mix.

can be obtained accurately, what the instrument will be required to do, and the fact that articulator technology is not a substitute for a biological understanding of the masticatory system.

As noted earlier, it would be extremely difficult to obtain accurate graphic records, so sophisticated, fully adjustable articulators that reproduce the curves of the border movements are unnecessarily complex. Similarly, instruments that require a kinematic face bow transfer to locate the hinge axis offer no advantage.

At the other extreme, the simple hinge articulator can be relied on to preserve the centric relation position precisely, provided the original interocclusal record is accurate and the instrument itself is rigid. Occlusal contacts in centric relation can thus be perfected with confidence. However, this instrument cannot be used to relate the occlusal surfaces in excursive movements because it cannot accept even simple eccentric interocclusal records. Refining nonworking side contacts for balanced occlusion is thus not possible on this type of instrument.

Between the extremes is the semiadjustable articulator, which will accept an arbitrary face bow record, and interocclusal records. This instrument has individually adjustable condylar guidances both horizontally and vertically. The majority of such instruments in use today are *arcon** instruments, meaning that the condylar guidance is located in the upper (cranial) member on the articulator and the ball (condylar analogue) is located in the lower (mandibular) member (see Figure 16-21).

Programming the Articulator

The centric relation record is the first essential record that is used to mount the casts on the articulator. The instrument is thus programmed already in two significant respects: the casts are related together in centric relation and at the selected vertical dimension of occlusion (provided by the trimmed occlusion rims). It remains then, to program the posterior (condylar) and anterior (incisal) elements of the articulator.

Whether or how the articulator is programmed beyond these basic parameters will depend on the clinical records that are taken, their demonstrated value, and the ability of the articulator to accept these records. It will also depend on the plans of the clinician, particularly the choice of posterior tooth mould and the overbite-overjet relations. Because both graphic records and eccentric records are of limited value, as noted earlier, there is little reason to program an articulator beyond the centric

relation record and the vertical dimension. On the assumption that there is an intention to program the articulator to more than the first two basic parameters, two elements need to be considered.

Condylar Elements   As the mandible moves forward in protrusive excursions, the condyles typically move downward, separating the posterior teeth. Therefore the amount by which the posterior teeth are separated is a measure of the amount the condyles move downward as they move forward (ignoring for the moment the effect of the incisal guidance). As noted earlier, interocclusal records that attempt to capture that downward and forward movement are highly variable and therefore of limited value. An arbitrary setting of the condylar elements will therefore provide an entirely satisfactory representation of the condylar movement. Average settings of the condylar inclination on the articulator can be used. (The average values given in early studies were 33 degrees for sagittal and 15 degrees for lateral condyle path inclination.)

With the adjustment of these two settings, the condylar elements of semiadjustable articulators will be programmed. The instrument interpolates the movements among the centric, protrusive, and lateral positions with limited precision to provide a representation of the range of mandibular movement. As noted earlier, although the accuracy may be limited, clinical experience suggests that such accuracy is not needed for the patient needing complete dentures.

Incisal Elements   The overbite-overjet relations of the anterior teeth are determined primarily by esthetics and phonetics. However, the resulting incisal guidance also influences the separation of the posterior teeth during excursions. Therefore the functional consequences of the incisal guidance relationship must be considered. These factors determine how the incisal elements of the articulator will be programmed.

Where no overbite is planned between the anterior teeth, the incisal guide table will be left perfectly flat (Figure 16-28). When the table is set this way, the anterior teeth will have to be arranged so that they contact only on the incisal edges (or not at all). Any posterior disclusion will be the result of the descending condyles.

---

*Arcon is a contraction of the words ARticulator and CONdyle.

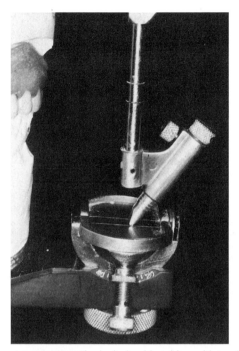

Figure 16-28 The incisal guide table and lateral plates set perfectly flat.

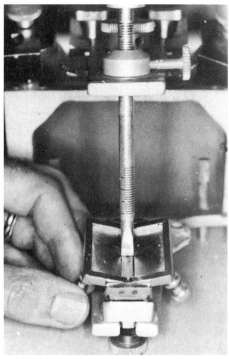

Figure 16-29 The incisal guide table and lateral plates raised.

Whereas esthetics or phonetics require overlapping incisors, an incisal guidance will likely be created (which will have an impact on the posterior disclusion). The dentist has control over the steepness of that guidance by setting the incisal table: where an incisal guidance is needed in protrusion, the table is rotated to an elevated position. As the incisal pin travels along the table, the models are separated anteriorly. Tooth contact then can only be maintained in protrusion by arranging the teeth in an overlapped position. Where a lateral guidance is sought (more common in fixed than complete denture prosthodontics), the lateral plates of the tables can be elevated in a similar way. The result is an overlapping of lateral cusps and tooth guidance that was intended by the clinician when the tables were set (Figure 16-29). An alternative approach is to set the preferred esthetically influenced anterior teeth set-up to create a customized incisal guidance in acrylic resin on the incisal guide table. This technique is very usefully employed in fixed prosthodontics, but rarely so when rehabilitating edentulous patients.

Arbitrary Settings　All articulators suffer from errors and can only approximate conditions in the patient's masticatory system. Consequently, careful adjustments must be performed at insertion of most prostheses, especially dentures, regardless of the occlusal system or articulator used. Many dentists have recognized this fact and have abandoned the use of a face bow, adopting instead a technique of mounting casts arbitrarily. (Some dentists may even have developed a troubled conscience as a result.)

Recognizing that the denture bases move on the tissues under load, the dentist can make an arbitrary setting of the condylar elements at zero degrees. This will yield an artificially diminished separation of the posterior teeth. However, when combined with a neutral (zero) incisal guidance and cuspless teeth, with or without a compensating curve or a second molar ramp, the tooth arrangement becomes perfectly flat with bilateral nonworking contact (Figure 16-30). When the

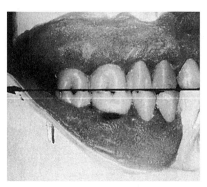

Figure 16-30   The condylar guide inclination and incisal guide table set at zero degrees, with the cuspless teeth set on a flat plane.

dentures are inserted in the mouth, the natural separation of the posterior teeth is largely compensated for by the compression of the tissues under the denture bases, the compensating curve, or the molar ramp, if necessary. The articulator is thus reduced to a simple hinge, and the arranging of the teeth is greatly simplified. The appropriateness of this tooth arrangement (and thus the choice of the articulator used) is a clinical judgment that should be made in advance. A more complex instrument is thus not necessarily a better choice.

Bibliography

Anonymous: The glossary of prosthodontic terms, *J Prosthet Dent* 81:39-110, 1999.

Bakke M: Mandibular elevator muscles: physiology, action, and effect of dental occlusion, *Scand J Dent Res* 101:314-331, 1993.

Becker CM, Kaiser DA: Evolution of occlusion and occlusal instruments, *J Prosthodont* 2:33-43, 1993.

Bowley JF, Bowman HC: Evaluation of variables associated with the transverse horizontal axis, *J Prosthet Dent* 68:537-541, 1992.

Bowley JF, Michaels GC, Lai TW et al: Reliability of a facebow transfer procedure, *J Prosthet Dent* 67:491-498, 1992.

Bowley JF, Pierce CJ: Reliability and validity of a transverse horizontal axis location instrument, *J Prosthet Dent* 64:646-650, 1990.

Brill N, Fujii H, Stoltze K et al: Dynamic and static recordings of the comfortable zone, *J Oral Rehabil* 5:145-150, 1978.

Broekhuijsen ML, van Willigen JD, Wright SM: Relationship of the preferred vertical dimension of occlusion to the height of the complete dentures in use, *J Oral Rehabil* 11:129-138, 1984.

Carlsson GE, Ericson S: Postural face height in full denture wearers: a longitudinal x-ray cephalometric study, *Acta Odontol Scand* 25:145-162, 1967.

Ellinger CW, Somes GW, Nicol BR et al: Patient response to variations in denture technique, part III: five-year subjective evaluation, *J Prosthet Dent* 42:127-130, 1979.

Goldberg LJ, Chandler SH: Central mechanisms of rhythmical trigeminal activity. In Taylor A, editor: *Neurophysiology of the jaws and teeth,* Basingstoke, 1990, MacMillan Press.

Gross M, Nissan J, Ormianer Z et al: The effect of increasing occlusal vertical dimension on face height, *Int J Prosthodont* 15:353-357, 2002.

Hiiemae KM, Heath MR, Heath G et al: Natural bites, food consistency and feeding behaviour in man, *Arch Oral Biol* 41:175-189, 1996.

Keshvad A, Winstanley RB: An appraisal of the literature on centric relation, part III, *J Oral Rehabil* 28:55-63, 2001.

Lavigne G, Kim JS, Valiquette C et al: Evidence that periodontal pressoreceptors provide positive feedback to jaw closing muscles during mastication, *J Neurophysiol* 58:342-358, 1987.

Manns A, Miralles R, Guerrero F: The changes in electrical activity of the postural muscles of the mandible upon varying the vertical dimension, *J Prosthet Dent* 45:438-445, 1981.

Mohl ND, Zarb GA, Carlsson GE et al, editors: *A textbook of occlusion,* Chicago, 1988, Quintessence Publishing.

Morneburg TR, Pröschel PA: Predicted incidence of occlusal errors in centric closing around arbitrary axes, *Int J Prosthodont* 15:358-364, 2002.

Muller F, Heath MR, Kazazoglu E et al: Contribution of periodontal receptors and food qualities to masseter muscle inhibition in man, *J Oral Rehabil* 20:281-290, 1993.

Olsson KA, Westberg KG: Interneurons in the trigeminal motor system. In van Steenberghe D, De Laat A, editors: *Electromyography of jaw reflexes in man,* Leuven, 1989, Leuven University Press.

Palla S: Occlusal considerations in complete dentures. In: McNeill C, editor: *Science and practice of occlusion,* Chicago, 1997, Quintessence Publishing Co. Inc.

Rugh JD, Drago CJ: Vertical dimension: a study of clinical rest position and jaw muscle activity, *J Prosthet Dent* 45:670-675, 1981.

Schwartz G, Enomoto S, Valiquette C et al: Mastication in the rabbit: a description of movement and muscle activity, *J Neurophysiol* 62:273-287, 1989.

Sessle BJ: Mastication, swallowing and related activities. In Roth GI, Calmes R, editors: *Oral biology,* St Louis, 1981, Mosby.

Shodadai SP, Turp JC, Gerds T et al: Is there a benefit of using an arbitrary facebow for the fabrication of a stabilization appliance? *Int J Prosthodont* 14:517-522, 2001.

Simpson JW, Hesby RA, Pfeifer DL et al: Arbitrary mandibular hinge axis locations, *J Prosthet Dent* 51:819-822, 1984.

Thexton AJ, Hiiemae KM: The effect of food consistency upon jaw movement in the macaque: a cineradiographic study, *J Dent Res* 76:552-560, 1997.

Toolson LB, Smith DE: Clinical measurement and evaluation of vertical dimension, *J Prosthet Dent* 47:236-241, 1982.

Walker PM: Discrepancies between arbitrary and true hinge axes, *J Prosthet Dent* 43:279-285, 1980.

Wiskott HW, Belser UC: A rationale for a simplified occlusal design in restorative dentistry: historical review and clinical guidelines, *J Prosthet Dent* 73:169-183, 1995.

Wood DP, Korne PH: Estimated and true hinge axis: a comparison of condylar displacements, *Angle Orthod* 62:167-175; discussion 176, 1992.

Zarb GA: Oral motor patterns and their relation to oral prostheses, *J Prosthet Dent* 47:472-478, 1982.

Zarb GA, Carlsson GE, Sessle BJ et al, editors: *Temporomandibular joint and masticatory muscle disorders,* Copenhagen, 1994, Munksgaard.

CHAPTER 17

Selecting and Arranging Prosthetic Teeth and Occlusion for the Edentulous Patient

Aaron H. Fenton

A knowledge and understanding of a number of physical and biological factors directly related to the patient are required to appropriately select artificial teeth to rehabilitate the occlusion. The goals for this phase of therapy are to construct complete dentures that (1) function well, (2) allow the patient to speak normally, (3) are esthetically pleasing, and (4) will not abuse the tissues over residual ridges. The dentist is the best person to accumulate, correlate, and evaluate the biomechanical information so that the artificial teeth selected will meet the individual needs of the patient. The selection of artificial teeth is a relatively simple non–time-consuming procedure, but it requires the development of experience and confidence. The setting of the selected teeth in wax according to a concept of occlusion is a laboratory procedure that requires the use of accurate record bases and articulator mountings of models. These record bases permit the dentist to transfer the tooth arrangement or occlusal scheme back from the articulator to the patient's mouth for a final examination of the maxillomandibular jaw relationships, an evaluation of the occlusal concept, and the philosophy of occlusion to be fulfilled. These activities are performed during what is termed the *try-in appointment*.

ANTERIOR TOOTH SELECTION

A smile is the most visible record of a dentist's care of an edentulous patient. It is present for all to see. Anterior tooth selection (ATS) has been based on theories that tooth shape relates to head shape, and tooth appearance is influenced by a patient's age, sex,

and personality. If no other information about ATS is available, these systems can be used to select teeth.

The dentist's professional obligation is to give the patient adequate information, guidance, and opportunity to choose their teeth. ATS is the area of prosthodontic care in which the patient should be given a primary responsibility to determine the esthetic outcome.

ATS for dental prostheses has both psychological and dental considerations that are influenced by the societal values for youth and health. Patients may wish to have teeth that look whiter and less restored than what would normally be expected in persons their age. The dentist's task is to assist a patient in making the best decision.

Tooth manufacturers provide a variety of shade guides, mold guides, and measurement charts to assist dentists in the selection of anterior teeth (Figure 17-1). Because each system can produce satisfactory results, select a manufacturer based on local availability and reliable delivery. Future tooth repairs are easier if the prosthetic teeth are readily matched.

Although the dental profession seeks to realistically replace the missing dentition, prosthetic teeth are often smaller in size and lighter in color than the range of the natural dentition. This does not seem to be a problem because patients most often object to teeth being too large or too dark. They often prefer teeth that are lighter. Ask your local laboratory which tooth sizes and colors are selected most often. Find out if the laboratory has problems with a manufacturer's tooth color and size matching or if frequent repairs are needed.

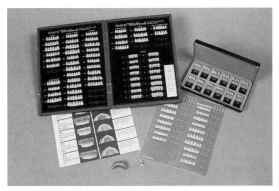

Figure 17-1   Shade and mold guides assist in tooth selection.

Psychology of Acceptance: Give Patients What They Want

The United States is a consumer-oriented society, yet patients leave many dental decisions to the dentist, such as the posterior palatal seal or the retromylohyoid extension. Dentists have knowledge of oral anatomy and esthetics and the physiology of speech and mastication. Teeth can be selected without the patient's input. This is dentally feasible, but therapeutically dangerous.

Everyone sees the anterior teeth, and everyone has an opinion. Patients should be given enough information and assistance and should be guided toward a limited selection of anatomically possible tooth selections so that they can choose the teeth that make them happy. Let the patient decide; then both the patient and dentist will get what each wants.

Patients, and perhaps their close personal friends, know what they think teeth should look like, so get them involved in the decision making. Psychologically, this is effective therapy. Patients more readily accept prosthetic care if they have had some input. Satisfied patients tell their friends who treated them; dissatisfied patients tell everyone.

The first step in ATS is to listen to the patient. What the patient wants is the reason that she or he came to your office. Do not miss it. Too often, dentists are so keen to make impressions and all those dental things that they alone know about that they underestimate the value of hearing what the patient wants.

At the first appointment, ask your patient for his or her opinion about the existing teeth. Write it down in the patient's own words (e.g., "My teeth don't show anymore.") Then restate it in your words to clarify what the patient expects (e.g., "If we make teeth of the same size, but lighter in color, and a little longer at the front, would that make them show the way you want?") Listen much and talk little. We cannot hear when we are talking.

Let the decision maker choose the teeth. A patient may have another person such as a spouse, relative, or friend whose opinion is valued. Ask them. That person may be more the reason why the patient is seeking treatment than the patient. It takes only a few seconds to find out if there is someone else with whom the patient would like to check regarding tooth color and size. You may devote hours of laboratory and chairtime only to find out that the setup that you and the patient agree on in the office is not liked by their spouse, and they demand that you change the teeth or set-up. This will have to happen only once for you to remember it.

People vary in how much they value the appearance of their teeth. The importance of ATS to patients can range from the indifferent "it doesn't matter" to unrealistic expectations that cannot be satisfied. Fortunately, almost all patients are well between these two extremes. Your most important task is to quickly find out where your patients are on this spectrum of interest in the appearance of their smiles. Their responses will indicate how interested they are in change and how much time you will devote to tooth appearance. This affects your cost of providing the service of complete denture treatment.

Second, get records of existing and previous teeth and find out the patient's opinion of them. Ask patients what their teeth looked like before the existing dentures. Explain that to get the best result for them, you need to know what their teeth were like before. Their mouth has probably changed, and present appearances can be misleading. Ask the patient to bring any models, old dentures, and photographs that show them happy and smiling, to the next appointment. The patient will give you credit for trying to provide the best personal service, and you will get some indication of what the teeth were like. Make alginate impressions and plaster models of the dentures that best satisfy the patient, and with the patient's permission, make a photocopy of any relevant pictures (Figure 17-2). You may make good dentures, but patients will never forget if a favorite wedding picture gets too close to a Bunsen burner.

If your patients are happy with the appearance of their teeth, use these records to provide a denture service that has similar teeth, but a better vertical dimension of occlusion and adaptation to the tissues. This has been identified as a "conformative approach" to prosthodontic care. The message that you are interested in making their teeth as natural as possible can be personalized further by asking if their teeth were like their direct descendents: their children. Photographs or dental models of adult children are sometimes the best way to create a smile that your patient appreciates. At least ask. The patient can always decline (Figure 17-3).

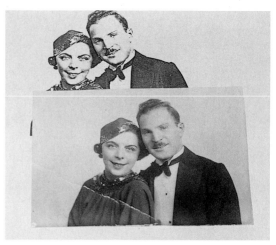

Figure 17-2 Photocopy a patient's photograph to help in selecting tooth size and positioning.

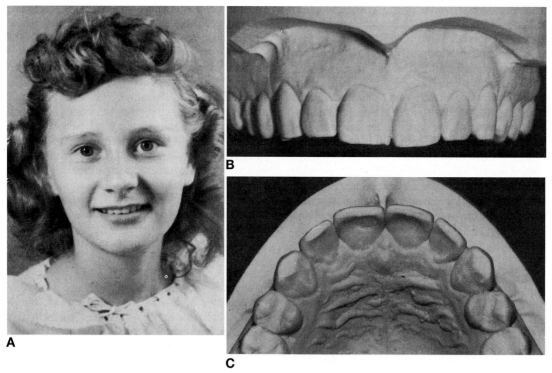

Figure 17-3 **A,** This patient's childhood photograph provided assistance in selecting denture teeth for her at age 54. **B** and **C,** Diagnostic casts made of her 30-year-old daughter furnished additional assistance. The daughter's tooth shade (Vita A1 for the centrals and laterals, A2 for the canines) also substantiated her mother's request for a light tooth shade.

On the other hand, your patients may not like their present teeth. Often the most important thing to find out is how *not* to make teeth because of the patients' dislike of their own teeth or previous dentures. If the teeth are the wrong color, size, shape, or position, plan on improvements. Also, the teeth may be excessively worn, or tissue changes may be so advanced that making teeth similar to what the patient has would be of little benefit. In these situations, consider a *reorganized approach* where you plan to change the prostheses to improve them. Even though you are planning improvements, improvements are a change. Assess the tolerance and motivation of your patients for change and work within the range that they can accept. The pleasure of prosthodontics is blending the interpersonal aspects of patient care with the biology of the mouth and the science of dental materials.

Third, arrange your practice for ATS. Make it easy for you and your patients to view their faces in good light. Your patient should be able to stand before a north-facing window, and you should have adequate color-corrected lighting. Tall or short patients should stand so that you can see their face and smile as others see them. Position yourself so that the window light comes over your shoulder and onto your patient's face. Make sure your patients put their glasses on if they need them. Give your patients a hand mirror of about 6 inches (or 15 cm) in diameter so that they can see how their face looks. A smaller mirror does not give an adequate image to the patient; a larger mirror makes it difficult for you to see around it.

Fourth, allow your patients to select the color of teeth they prefer. Dentists are familiar with an array of tooth shades and mold guides and charts, but these can be too confusing for patients to decide. They beg off making a decision and tell the dentist to decide what is best for them. Then you are responsible. If your patients like your decision, that is fine. If they, or anyone else, are at all skeptical, suddenly it is your teeth that are the problem, not theirs. Avoid this roadblock by tactfully insisting that your patients decide which teeth are best for them. This is easily done in a nonthreatening manner by giving the patients a simple choice with two options (i.e., a Method of Pair Comparison).

Tell your patients that you need their help to get the best results. Explain that you have many colors

and sizes of teeth to best treat your patients, but only a few are appropriate for them. A display of all of your shade and mold guides at this point is impressive but confusing to a patient untrained in dental anatomy. Reassure your patients that any required decisions will be simple. They will only have to tell which one of two things they prefer; in other words, make a simple choice.

Color is the easiest thing for a patient to decide about teeth. Show the patient a complete shade guide and select the two tabs that are lightest and darkest (Figure 17-4). Point out how different these two are and satisfy yourself that the patient can see the difference and agree. Hold them against the patients' lips and ask them to note how different they are. Then ask them to point to the one that they prefer. Delete the rejected color. On the basis of the decision, select another shade in the preferred half of the shade guide and repeat the pair comparison. After two selections by the patient, you will probably have a pair of shades that are very close to what the patient wants. To confirm the patient's decision, reverse the sides of the pair so that the preferred shade is presented on the opposite side. Try another shade that is close to the preferred shade. By now the psychology of decision making is as important as the physiology of color perception. Usually patients can still select the same shade even when you move it from side to side in the pair, but sometimes they are unwilling to state a preference.

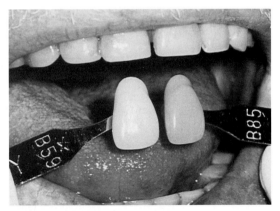

Figure 17-4 A pair of tooth shades to compare. Ask your patient to point to the one that he or she prefers.

If patients are unable or unwilling to decide on a shade, their powers of perception can still help to select a tooth color. Ask them to point out which one of the pair of tabs they notice. By default, the tab that they do not notice is less conspicuous and therefore a better color.

In the rare situations in which patients still cannot decide, advise them that they are correct. Both shades are appropriate, and a pleasing appearance could be made with either one of them. However, you would still like them to be happy, so they should choose between the two shades when you have the actual teeth. Order two sets of teeth so that the patient can compare them side by side and select the best before they are needed for setup.

Fifth, choose a size of tooth that is appropriate. Existing dentures, models of previous teeth, and photographs all give valuable input for selection of the size and shape of teeth. Teeth can be measured in millimeters and teeth of similar size selected (Figure 17-5). Even so, patients may have a clear perception of how large a tooth they prefer. Coupled with actual measurement, again use the Method of Pair Comparison to assist patients to decide what size of tooth they prefer. Set two different sizes of teeth on a piece of wax rope or on the tooth selector rim that some companies provide. Place this under the upper lip and find out which one the patient prefers. The decision is often not one of preference, but rejection. People note and reject the teeth that are, for example, too large,

small, long, or short. By default they prefer the other set of teeth.

Sixth, select the mold of the teeth. Teeth of a similar size can have a different appearance because of differences in the crown taper and labial curvature. This is the least obvious of the three judgments to be made, yet it can provide the "finishing touch" to replicate a realistic appearance for your patient. Mold determination requires previous models or photographs for guidance. If the patient is to receive immediate insertion complete dentures, the actual teeth are the best indicator of mold. If teeth are unavailable, allow the patient to select between molds of the same size but different shapes. Set two different molds on the right and left sides of a piece of wax rope and ask patients which they prefer (Figure 17-6).

Anterior tooth selection should be completed early in treatment, preferably before final impressions are made. This gives ATS appropriate significance and allows time for judgment of the result before the teeth are needed. Order all of the teeth (1×28) because the premolars are part of the smile. Their color, size, and shape should complement the anterior teeth. Show patients the actual teeth at the impression appointment and secure their agreement (Figure 17-7). If the teeth are not what patients think they will be, based on the shade and mold guide estimations, they can be reordered and exchanged before they are needed for setup in

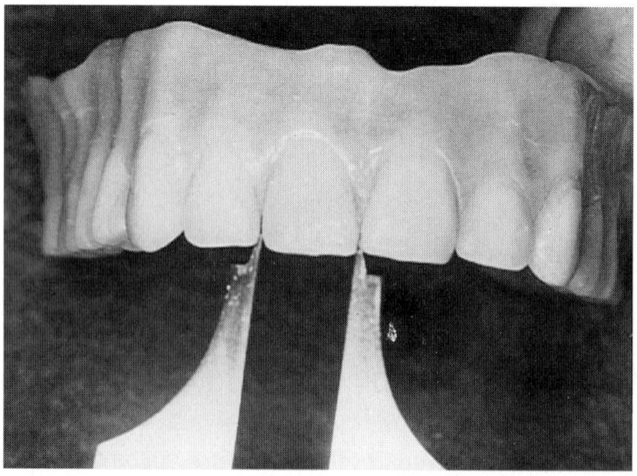

Figure 17-5 Use a Boley gauge to determine the size of teeth in millimeters. A similar-sized tooth can be selected based on this evidence.

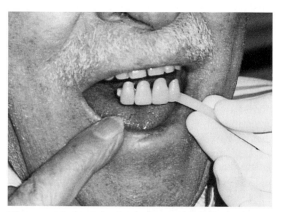

Figure 17-6 Pair comparison to identify the best mold of teeth. The two teeth on the left and the two teeth on the right are from different molds. The patient can see them in the mirror, and he is pointing to the ones that he prefers.

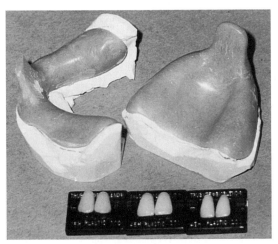

Figure 17-7 Order the selected teeth early so that the patient can see them at the impression appointment. Confirm their acceptability before they are needed for setup.

wax. Otherwise, it is expensive for your laboratory fees and office chairtime to exchange and reset a second set of teeth.

Additional Clinical and Technical Considerations in Anterior Tooth Selection

Patient preferences, local anatomy, and the opposing dentition can affect the ATS of materials or mold.

Patient Preference   Patients may want teeth to be porcelain or acrylic, depending on various reasons that they have heard: "Acrylic teeth stain," "Porcelain teeth are real," "Porcelain teeth are noisy for chewing," or "Porcelain teeth are heavy." There are a variety of opinions. Listen and respond with your knowledge of dental materials, but do not be disheartened if the patient is skeptical. Facts are not always as accepted as opinions. If the denture is not compromised by patients' requests, you can perhaps accede to their wishes. Make patients aware that you are modifying your therapy personally for them and make a note in the chart. Again, this is an opportunity for patients to accept responsibility for their decisions.

Highly Visible Gingiva   Select squarer teeth with a long contact point rather than highly tapered teeth. This will minimize the interproximal display

of pink gingival acrylic. It is harder to make realistic-appearing gingival acrylic compared with teeth. Therefore make a smile with slightly more dental and less gingival display.

Limited Interocclusal Space   Use acrylic teeth. They can be ground thin, yet they will still chemically bond to the underlying denture base acrylic. Porcelain teeth lose their mechanical retention if the palatal pins are ground off.

Opposing Natural Teeth   Porcelain can be very abrasive. Use acrylic teeth for dentures that oppose natural teeth to minimize their wear. The acrylic teeth will wear, but they can be replaced. This is preferable to the porcelain destruction of enamel. Also, acrylic teeth are less brittle than porcelain when additional adjustment is required to match natural occlusion.

Overdentures   The tooth positioned just over a retained tooth root or implant abutment has to be "hollow-ground," and a little extra tooth volume is needed for strength. Use a square flat mold in a standard nonlaminated acrylic. Tapered or curved teeth get too thin and weak in the gingival areas. Highly characterized or laminated teeth may become translucent or separate their veneers when ground thin over tooth roots or implants.

The Personal Touch: Characterization of Selected Teeth

Explain to patients that smiles are more realistic with subtle chips, wear, or restorations. These hint at the presence of a dentition for many years, as opposed to looking "brand new." Although this service is offered to all patients, lately, more patients seem to prefer an undamaged appearance of light-colored teeth. Fewer patients opt for too-visible characterization. Nevertheless, anterior tooth characterization can produce strikingly realistic effects that make the patient's smile look as if it is enamel, dentin, and gingiva. Teeth can be modified to create a personal smile in a number of ways and combinations, such as changes in color and position (Figure 17-8), individual grinding and placement (Figure 17-9), placement of restorations and worn appearance (Figure 17-10), and natural proportion and subtle variations in position (Figure 17-11).

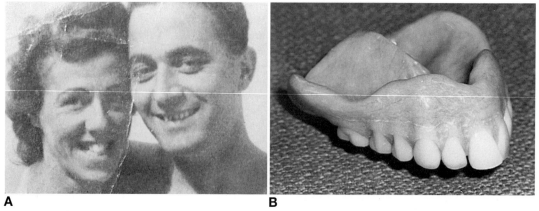

Figure 17-8 Characterization with colors: use different tooth colors to create the best effect. **A,** The prominent position and color of this patient's maxillary right central were identified from a photograph. **B,** The maxillary central incisors were Dentsply shade 102; the rest of the smile was Dentsply shade 114. This emphasized the tapered arch form and created the illusion of more prominence for the upper right central incisor than was prosthetically possible. The smile appears real to this patient.

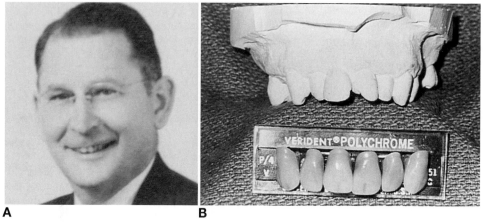

Figure 17-9 Characterization by grinding: immediate dentures allow for realistic tooth selection and shaping. **A,** A previous photograph hints at the prominence of the maxillary central incisors, their overlap of the lateral incisors, and the Angle Class II relationship. **B,** A study model allows selection of the best available mold.

Continued

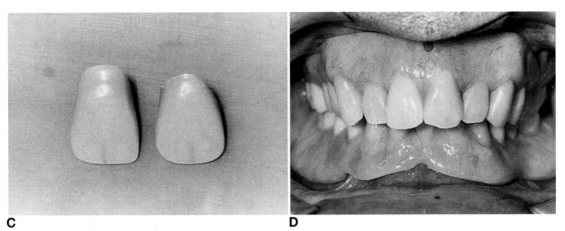

C   D

Figure 17-9 *cont'd* **C,** The acrylic teeth are trimmed to recreate the actual tooth shape. It could not be found in any mold guide. **D,** The completed prosthesis faithfully replicates the irregularity of tooth color, size, mold, and Angle Class II position. This patient's smile looks real.

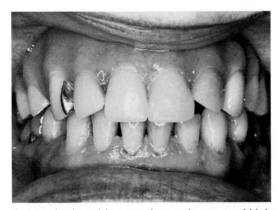

Figure 17-10 Characterization with restorations and wear. A gold inlay is in the mesial of the upper right canine, the upper left lateral incisor is rotated prominently, and the incisal is chipped, with an Angle Class II Division 2 tooth arrangement. The teeth are a single uncharacterized shade, but all the other natural effects make them appear real.

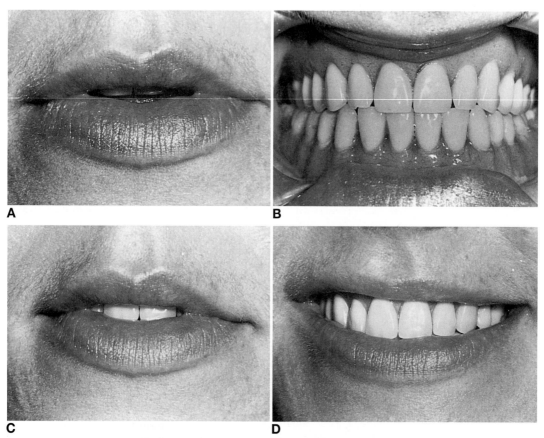

Figure 17-11   Characterization by natural arrangement: a standard anterior tooth shade and mold is made to look real by the subtle natural irregularity of tooth positioning. **A,** The patient's presenting smile with teeth that are too small and hardly visible. **B,** The maxillary teeth are a single uncharacterized color, too small, out of proportion to the lower teeth, and too uniform in position. **C,** The new smile has better lip support and visibility at rest. The midline of the teeth is different from the lip at rest because it is set for the more visible asymmetrical smile. **D,** The patient's smile is in proportion to the surrounding tissues. Each tooth has an individual identity because of subtle variations in angle and rotation. The central incisors are at the midline of the smile, but they are not a mirror image of each other. The patient's left lateral incisor is rotated out at the mesial. The canines and visible premolars vary in gingival prominence and angulation. The gingiva is inconspicuous. This smile is perceived to be real and gives the patient self-confidence.

POSTERIOR TOOTH SELECTION

Until the middle 1920s, most posterior denture teeth were anatomical in design and represented the forms of natural teeth. In the mid 1920s, dentists began to experiment with tooth forms that, were designed for a specific functional purpose rather than merely reproducing natural forms. Thus emerged a number of nonanatomical denture teeth. The occlusal surfaces of these teeth are not copies from the natural form but are given forms that, in the opinion of the tooth carver, were designed to meet specific patient needs, such as denture base stability and improvements in mastication. Some nonanatomical posterior denture teeth were designed completely without cusps, whereas others were mechanical in design, possessing metal cutters to increase masticatory efficiency. The maintenance of hard and soft tissues of the dental arches has been difficult to relate to tooth forms and occlusal schemes. Other factors, such as (1) properly fitted bases; (2) correct jaw relation records that are transferred to an instrument capable of accepting what is recorded; and (3) the arrangement of teeth for the best stability and other functional and non-functional activities, are considered to have an influence on the maintenance of these tissues.

Posterior teeth are selected for color, buccolingual width, total mesiodistal width, cusp tip to cervical collar height, material, and the cuspal inclination needed for the concept of occlusion to be used in restoring the patient.

Buccolingual Width of Posterior Teeth

The buccolingual widths of artificial teeth should be less than the widths of the natural teeth they replace. Artificial posterior teeth that are narrow enhance the development of the correct form of the polished surfaces of the denture by allowing the buccal and lingual denture flanges to slope away from their occlusal surfaces. These narrower forms, especially in the lower denture, assist the cheeks and tongue in maintaining the dentures on the residual ridge.

Mesiodistal Length of Posterior Teeth

The length of the mandibular residual ridge from the distal of the canine to the retromolar pad will dictate the dimensions of the posterior teeth selected. Artificial posterior teeth are manufactured with varying widths and lengths that easily accommodate the needs of the patient.

After the six anterior mandibular teeth have been placed in their final position, a point is marked on the cast landing area at the distal of the canine. A second mark is placed on the landing area of the cast at the point where the mean residual ridge begins to ascend to the retromolar pad. Posterior teeth are not positioned on this inclined plane. The available space will dictate whether three or four posterior teeth are used. The arrangement of only three posterior teeth is more often the norm and will reduce the

potential for placement of the second molar too far posterior. Maxillary posterior teeth that extend too close to the posterior border of the maxillary denture may cause the patient to bite the cheek.

Vertical Height of the Facial Surfaces of Posterior Teeth

It is best to select posterior teeth corresponding to the interarch space and to the height of the anterior teeth. Artificial posterior teeth are manufactured in varying occlusal-cervical heights. The height of the maxillary first premolar should be comparable with that of the maxillary canines to have the proper esthetic effect. Without this relationship, the denture base material will appear unnatural distal to the canines. Ridge lapping the posterior teeth can be done without sacrificing leverage or esthetics. The form of the dental arch should copy, as nearly as possible, the arch form of the natural teeth they replace.

Types of Posterior Teeth According to Materials

For many years, porcelain was the favorite tooth material because of the rapid wear of acrylic resin. However, with the tendency for porcelain to chip and fracture, acrylic resin teeth have gained in popularity. Improved acrylic resin teeth and newer composite resin teeth are more wear resistant, and they have supplanted porcelain during the past two decades.

Acrylic resin or composite resin posterior teeth are specifically called for when they oppose natural teeth or teeth whose occlusal surfaces have been restored with gold. These resin teeth reduce the possibility that the artificial teeth will cause unnecessary abrasion and destruction of the natural or metallic occlusal surfaces of the opposing teeth. Acrylic resin teeth also are desirable when the tooth must be excessively reduced in height because of a small interarch distance. The chemical bonding of the resin teeth with the denture base prevents these teeth from breaking away from the denture base.

Types of Posterior Teeth According to Cusp Inclines

The cuspal inclines for posterior teeth were described earlier in great detail. Posterior artificial teeth are manufactured with cusp inclines that vary from steep to flat. Selecting the tooth to be used is based on the concept of occlusion to be developed, the philosophy of occlusion to be fulfilled, and the accomplishment of both of these goals with the least complicated approach (Table 17-1).

ARRANGING TEETH FOR COMPLETE DENTURE OCCLUSION

Once the master casts have been mounted on the articulator, the teeth are set in the occlusion rims so a more accurate observation of the jaw relationship can be recorded, and eventually the

---

Table 17-1
Comparison of Denture Tooth Molds and Occlusal Concepts

Tooth Mold	Occlusal Concept	Advantage	Disadvantage
20- or 30-degree cusped teeth	• Centric jaw record, face bow, protrusive records to semiadjustable articulator • Set upper anterior and posterior teeth, then lowers to cross-arch contact or "balanced occlusion"	• Reported slightly more efficient in chewing tests • Posteriors appear more natural	• Most time and complexity of records • Limitations of anterior tooth positions • Restriction of posterior tooth positions to that allowed by cuspal anatomy
Monoplane 0-degree teeth	• Centric relation jaw record only • Simple articulator • Set 12 anterior teeth with overjet but no overbite • Set lower teeth in flat plane to middle of retromolar pad • Set upper to match; no attempt on contact on excursions	• Simplest of all recordings • Simplest articulator • Quick arrangement of teeth • Wide range of posterior tooth positions possible • No lateral stresses on mucosa with parafunction • Easier for patients with uncoordinated closures (e.g., patients with dyskinesias, Parkinson's disease, or stroke)	• Flat premolars may appear less esthetic • Reported as less efficient in chewing tests • Anterior esthetics need more overjet and no overbite
Flat teeth with compensating curve or second molar ramp	• Centric relation jaw record • Semiadjustable articulator • Anterior teeth with overjet and slight overbite • Posteriors set to contact on at least 1 point on nonworking or balancing contact	• Simple to set up; allows for more esthetic overlap of anterior teeth • The posterior point contact maintains denture base stability on excursions or parafunction	• Slightly more laboratory setup time than flat teeth • Premolars appear flat if visible
Combinations or "lingualized" occlusion	• Centric jaw record • Monoplane lower posterior teeth set to retromolar pad • Anatomical upper posterior teeth set with only lingual, not buccal cusps touching	• Upper premolars appear natural • Some range of posterior tooth position allowed • Reported slightly better chewing than monoplane teeth	• Some grinding needed to create upper cusp tip/lower fossa contacts (some manufacturers are now producing molds for this occlusal concept)

occlusion established. Most dentists carve the wax occlusion rims as accurately as they can for determining the desired amount of lip support and have their technician make the preliminary arrangement of teeth. The carved occlusion rims provide the technician with reliable guides for placement of the anterior teeth in the wax occlusion rims. Subsequently, these dentists make corrections in the tooth positions when the wax trial dentures are observed in the mouth at the try-in appointment.

The incisive papilla is a valuable guide to anterior tooth placement because it has a constant relationship to the natural central incisors (see Figure 17-3, Figure 17-12). The incisive papilla is found in the lingual embrasure between these incisors. Naturally, it should serve to position the midline of the upper denture or, more specifically, the central incisors in the dental arch. However, the mesial surfaces of the central incisors of some people are not exactly in the center of their face or mouth. Therefore information on the center of the upper

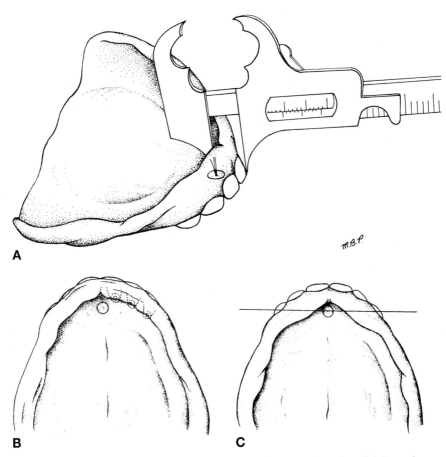

A

B   **C**

Figure 17-12   Indications of correct anteroposterior positioning of artificial anterior teeth. **A,** By measurement from the middle of the incisive fossa on the trial denture base to the labial surfaces of the central incisors. **B,** By visualization of the imaginary roots of artificial anterior teeth. The imaginary roots will be further in front of the residual ridge when a great amount of resorption has occurred. **C,** By determining the relationship of a transverse line extending between the middle of the upper canines and the incisive fossa.

lip or face should be recorded on the carved wax occlusal rim.

A line marking the center of the incisive papilla on the wax rim can be extended forward onto the landing area of the cast (Figure 17-13). The central incisors set on either side of this line will have positions similar to those of the natural teeth insofar as right and left orientations are concerned. The incisive papilla is also a good guide for the anteroposterior positioning of the teeth (see Figure 17-13). The labial surfaces of the central incisors are usually 8 to 10 mm in front of the papillae. This distance, for obvious reasons, will vary with the size of the teeth and the labiolingual thickness of

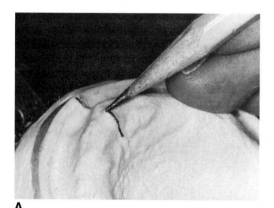

A

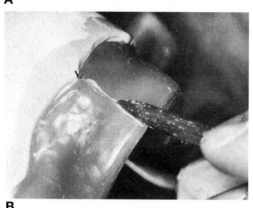

B

Figure 17-13   The incisive papilla is used to help locate the midline of the dental arch. **A,** A mark is made on the cast through the center of the papilla. **B,** The mark is transferred to the occlusion rim as a guide to placement of the maxillary incisors.

the alveolar process carrying the natural teeth, so it is not an absolute relationship. Furthermore, as severe resorption of the residual ridge in a vertical direction occurs, the incisive papilla may be located more posteriorly to the position of the replacement teeth. Thus the distance from the papilla to the labial surface of the teeth may become greater for those patients with excessive bone loss in the maxillary anterior region.

Another guide to positioning the central incisors is their relationship to the reflection of soft tissues under the lip or as recorded in the maxillary impression. The labial surfaces and incisal edges of the teeth are anterior to the tissues at the reflection, where the denture borders would be placed. This fact must be kept in mind when placing an artificial incisor in the wax occlusion rim. The root of the natural tooth extends into the alveolar process, with a relatively thin layer of bone over it labially. This means that in some situations the residual ridge can be used as a guide to determine the proper inclination of anterior teeth. However, the accuracy of this guide decreases as resorption of the residual ridge progresses. Clinical judgment is essential in the evaluation and application of these guides.

The anteroposterior position of the dental arch should be governed chiefly by consideration of the orbicularis oris muscle and its attaching muscles and by the tone of the skin of the lips. Superficially, this means the position and expression of the lips. The orbicularis oris muscle affects, and is affected by, the following seven muscles: the quadratus labii superioris, caninus, zygomaticus, quadratus labii inferioris, risorius, triangularis, and buccinator. These muscles control expression and reflect the personality and appearance of every person wearing complete dentures. The tone and action of these muscles depend on the anteroposterior support provided by the teeth and the denture base material.

Setting teeth over the maxillary anterior ridge may undermine the esthetic result. The greatest harm is done when the maxillary anterior teeth are set too far back on the ridge or under the ridge. In other words, the tooth's direction is upward and backward. In the resorbed situation, the crest of the ridge is considerably more posterior than it is in a patient with recent extractions. If the rule of setting teeth over the ridge is followed after the residual ridge has resorbed, a prematurely aged appearance will result.

If the wax occlusion rims have been accurately carved to support the lips and the maxillomandibular jaw relationship, they will provide an excellent guide to correct anteroposterior tooth positioning in the dental arch. If they have not been accurately carved, the dentist must decide what alterations will be necessary when the teeth are arranged. For example, if the lip needs more support when the occlusion rims are in the mouth, the incisors should be set in front of the labial surface of the wax rim. If the lips are too full at that time, more of the labial surface of the occlusion rims should be cut away before the teeth are set.

Arranging the Maxillary Anterior Teeth

After selecting the anterior molds for the maxillary and mandibular teeth, the arrangement is left to the discretion of the individual dentist to achieve the esthetic needs of the patient. Remove the maxillary wax occlusion rim on one side from the midline around the arch for a distance of approximately 1 inch (about 25 mm). For the maxillary anterior teeth to be set with the appropriate labial orientation, it may be necessary to grind the acrylic resin to reduce the thickness of the record base. This is a common occurrence in clinical practice and should always be performed before grinding on the neck of the tooth. A longer tooth clinically will provide a better esthetic result. Short, stubby teeth are not natural in appearance. Do not be concerned should you create a hole in the record base because it will be covered with wax in setting the anterior teeth. Often it is helpful to set both central incisors and thus establish the midline before setting the lateral and canine.

Maxillary Central Incisor Place a small portion of soft, pink wax on the neck of the maxillary central incisor and attach the tooth to the record base over the anterior region of the residual ridge. Make certain that the long axis of the tooth is perpendicular to the horizontal, with the incisal edge 0.5 mm below the wax occlusal rim. Seal the tooth into position with pink wax, using the no. 7 spatula. Try to use only the amount of wax needed for securely attaching the teeth to the record base. Excess wax should be removed from the teeth. The

maxillary central incisor is the most difficult tooth to set because it establishes the midline and the esthetic support of the patient's lip. The proper arrangement of the maxillary and mandibular anterior and posterior teeth relies on the setting of the maxillary central incisors.

Maxillary Lateral Incisor Place the maxillary lateral incisor next to the central incisor, with the neck slightly depressed. Arrange the incisal edge in symmetry with the central incisor and with the remaining anterior occlusal rim. This incisal edge is even with the remaining maxillary wax occlusal rim and is therefore slightly elevated from the central incisor. The incisal edge is parallel with the mandibular wax occlusal rim. After this tooth is arranged in the normal position for a lateral incisor, it may be repositioned with spacing, lapping, or rotation to meet the individual esthetic requirements for the patient.

Maxillary Canine Place the maxillary canine so that the anterior one half of the incisal edge is in symmetry with the lateral and central incisors as it curves around the labial contour of the wax occlusal rim. The neck of the tooth must be prominent and the tooth tilted slightly to the distal. Like the central incisor, the incisal tip of the canine must be 0.5 mm below the maxillary wax occlusal rim. Again, after initially setting the tooth to these guidelines, any individual changes necessary for the creation of naturalness for the patient should be performed.

Remaining Maxillary Anterior Teeth Arrange the remaining maxillary anterior teeth on the other sides of the arch to complete the anterior setup. The wax supporting the teeth must be heated and sealed both to the teeth and to the record base to maintain the set teeth in position.

Arranging the Mandibular Anterior Teeth

The wax occlusal rim is removed from the area of the lower midline around the arch for approximately 1 inch (around 25 mm). This is similar to the procedure you performed on the maxillary wax occlusal rim when the maxillary anterior teeth were set.

Mandibular Central Incisor   Position the central incisor next to the midline and tip it slightly to the labial. Direct the long axis of the tooth toward the residual ridge. Be certain that the necks of the teeth are depressed so that they are in from the edge of the record base. The incisal edges of these teeth must be at the height of the mandibular wax occlusal rim. This will result in a 0.5-mm vertical overlap with the maxillary central and canine teeth. A 1- to 2-mm horizontal overlap must exist between the lingual surface of the maxillary anterior teeth and the labial surface of the mandibular anterior teeth. Such an arrangement will create a

low incisal guidance, which is exactly what one should achieve for the patient (Figure 17-14).

Mandibular Lateral Incisor   Position the lateral incisor next to the central incisor, with the long axis of the tooth directed toward the residual ridge. The incisal edge should be at the height of the wax occlusal rim. The 1 to 2 mm of horizontal overlap between the maxillary and mandibular anterior teeth should be continued.

Mandibular Canine   Place the mandibular canine with the anterior one half of the incisal edge in

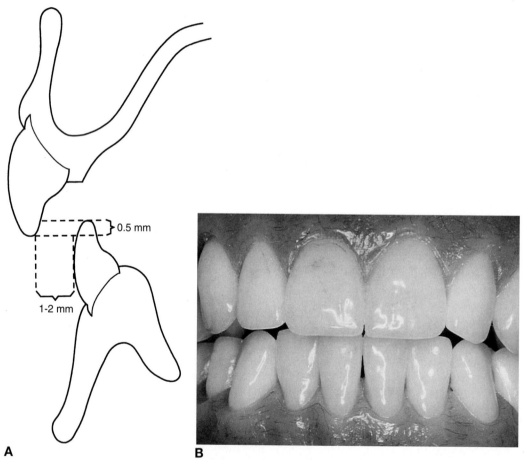

A   **B**

Figure 17-14   **A,** 0.5 mm of vertical overlap and 1 to 2 mm of horizontal overlap must exist between the maxillary anterior teeth and their mandibular antagonists to achieve a low incisal guidance, which is needed for the anterior teeth to function in harmony with most posterior tooth forms. **B,** The low incisal guide angle is both esthetic and functional.

symmetry with the lateral and central incisors. Place the incisal tip at the same level as the lateral and central incisors. The neck of the tooth is slightly prominent and tilted to the distal. After these teeth are adjusted to this ideal arrangement, they may be altered by rotation, spacing, and tilting the teeth to achieve the naturalness requirement of the patient.

Remaining Mandibular Anterior Teeth Arrange the remaining anterior teeth on the other side of the arch to complete the anterior setup. Again, be sure to seal all the teeth to the record base with pink baseplate wax and the no. 7 spatula. It is at this point in the clinical management of a patient that you may wish to evaluate the esthetics of all anterior teeth by a try-in with the patient.

Anterior artificial teeth should be placed in essentially the same positions previously occupied by the natural teeth, and the labial surface of the denture base material should duplicate, as nearly as possible, the contour and position of the mucous membrane covering the alveolar ridge. Reducing the horizontal and vertical overlaps of the anterior teeth is necessary to reduce the incisal guide angle. It should be recognized that this reduction may have an impact on esthetics. The dangers from a high incisal guidance far exceed the possible impact on esthetics that might be produced when the teeth are set with less horizontal and vertical overlaps. It is not necessary for the anterior teeth to contact in maximum intercuspation. In fact, it is better that they be set just out of contact.

If the mandibular ridge is forward of the maxillary ridge (as in a prognathic jaw relationship), the upper anterior teeth should be set end to end, with the incisal edges in light contact with the mandibular anterior teeth. When the prognathism is extreme, it may not be possible to have tooth contact in the incisor region because the maxillary incisors will be placed too far anteriorly and will put the upper lip under too much tension. In such situations, an anterior crossbite is the only alternative.

Extremely high ridges may seem to create a problem unless it is realized that natural teeth once projected from these ridges. Insufficient space between the residual ridges is an indication that either the artificial teeth selected are longer than the

natural teeth or the vertical dimension of the face may be closed. However, if only parts of the ridges are too close together, the cause may be an incomplete alveolectomy during tooth extraction. Surgical removal of small bony projections may be indicated.

Arranging the Posterior Teeth

The preliminary arrangement of posterior teeth involves the application of principles similar to those applied in the arrangement of anterior teeth. The artificial posterior teeth should be placed near to where the natural teeth were positioned. This is easier said than done, however, because there are only a few guides for posterior tooth position. The final position of the occlusal plane, the occlusal contacts, and even the number of posterior teeth cannot be determined until the jaw relations are evaluated and found correct.

The orientation of the anterior occlusal plane is determined initially by the wax occlusal rim. The anatomical guides most often used in developing the anterior plane of occlusion are the corners of the mouth. In general, the plane should be located either at or slightly below the corners of the mouth. During the arrangement of the mandibular anterior teeth, the position of the incisal edges of the mandibular anterior teeth eventually establishes the level of the anterior plane of occlusion. The posterior plane of occlusion is an extension of this anterior plane level with the junction between the middle and upper third of the retromolar pads bilaterally. These posterior references (retromolar pads) will place the overall plane at a level that is familiar to the tongue. If the plane is located higher or lower, for whatever reason, the dentures will interfere with normal tongue action. This will adversely influence denture base stability (Figure 17-15).

The inclination of the occlusal plane is important to the stability or instability of dentures. If the plane is too low in the anterior region or too high in the posterior region, the maxillary denture will tend to slide forward. Ideally, the plane of occlusion should parallel the mean mandibular residual ridge.

The height of the occlusal plane is not simply a matter of dividing the maxillomandibular denture space equally. This space is governed by the relative amount of bone lost from the two ridges. More bone may have been lost from the maxillae than from the mandible, and the occlusal plane should not be placed an equal distance between the two ridges. It also should not be at a level that would favor the weaker of the two ridges (basal seats). The most reliable guides are esthetics or anterior tooth placement and the retromolar pads.

The buccolingual position of the posterior teeth and the posterior arch form are determined anteriorly by the position of the canine and posteriorly by the shape of the basal seat and the location of the retromolar pads. The curvature of the arch of anterior teeth should flow pleasingly toward the posterior teeth. The posterior teeth are positioned in such a way that they are properly related to the bone that supports them and to the soft tissues that contact their facial and lingual surfaces. In the final tooth arrangement, the posterior form of the arch will be determined largely by the "neutral zone" between the cheeks and tongue. This is the space resulting from the removal of the posterior teeth and the loss of bone from the residual ridges. The pressure of the cheeks and tongue against the facial and lingual surfaces of the erupting natural teeth was strong enough to influence their alignment in the dental arch. These forces also are applied against dentures. Therefore the final arrangement of the arch must be developed with respect for the tongue and cheek (see Figure 17-15).

The solution to the problem is to position the teeth along a line extending from the tip of the canine to the middle of the retromolar pad. This arbitrary line should pass through the central fossa of the mandibular premolars and molars (Figure 17-16).

The basic principle for the buccolingual positioning of posterior teeth is that they should be positioned over the residual ridge. The canine and retromolar pad should provide guides for this arrangement.

OCCLUSAL SCHEMES FOR COMPLETE DENTURE OCCLUSION

The occlusal scheme or the tooth molds selected for occlusal rehabilitation will depend on the concept of occlusion that has been selected to satisfy the needs of the patient. The posterior teeth, arranged according to the occlusal concept selected, should fulfill the dentist's philosophy of occlusion as well appear esthetically pleasing. Posterior tooth forms have aroused a great deal of controversy among clinicians and researchers. Chewing efficiency tests have shown a slight advantage to cusped teeth. Cuspal anatomy has not been shown to have any significant effect on the supporting tissues. Patient preference surveys have been inconclusive. Prosthetic tooth anatomy seems to be more important to dentists than to the patients who use the teeth. In the absence of clear evidence of the benefits of one tooth anatomy compared with others, dentists should use the least complicated procedures and tooth forms that will satisfy their con-

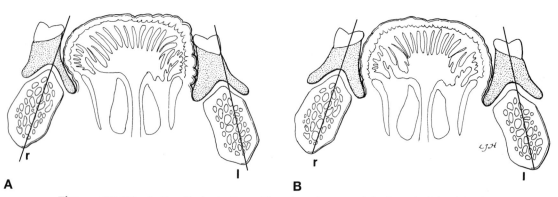

Figure 17-15 **A,** Mandibular teeth positioned too far toward the buccal of the ridge *(r)* and too far toward the lingual *(l).* **B,** Positions of the mandibular teeth corrected from those shown in **A.**

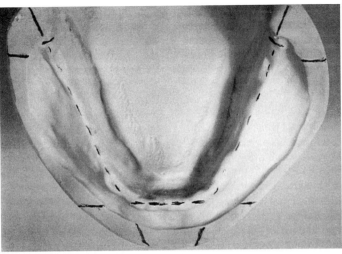

A

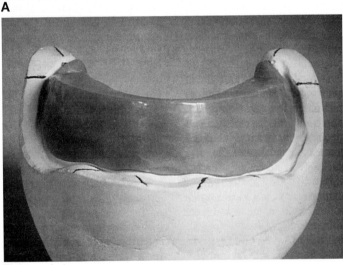

B

Figure 17-16 **A,** The mean residual ridge, as well as selected anatomical landmarks, provides the guidances used in the buccolingual and anteroposterior positioning of the mandibular posterior teeth. **B,** Centering the wax occlusal rim on the mandibular record base with the anatomical guides is essential to the appropriate placement of the artificial teeth. The basal seat, or mean residual ridge, and the retromolar pads bilaterally are used to develop the positioning and height of the wax occlusal rim.

cepts of occlusion and articulation of a mucosal supported dentition.

There are several schools of thought on the choice of occlusal forms of posterior teeth for the three concepts of occlusion most often selected, namely, (1) bilateral balance, (2) monoplane or nonanatomical, and (3) lingualized articulations. Anatomical molds usually are selected for bilateral balanced articulation; however, nonanatomical teeth can be used in a balanced concept with the use of compensating curves. Nonanatomical or cuspless teeth are generally the choice for monoplane articulation, although teeth with cusps also can be used. For the lingualized occlusal concept, a combination of upper anatomical and lower non-anatomical molds has been introduced by several tooth manufacturers.

Arranging Anatomical Teeth to a Balanced Articulation

The anterior teeth are set with a minimal vertical overlap of 0.5 to 1 mm and 1 to 2 mm of horizontal overlap to establish a low incisal guidance (see Figure 17-14). After these requirements are satisfied, the teeth may be rotated, tipped, overlapped, or spaced to achieve naturalness. In the arrangement of the posterior teeth, most clinicians set the mandibular teeth before the maxillary because this provides better control of the orientation of the plane of occlusion both mediolaterally and superoinferiorly.

Number of Posterior Teeth Set   The decision on the number of teeth to use will depend on the available space for posterior teeth from the distal of the canine to the retromolar pad. Placing teeth on the residual ridge incline as it ascends to the pad should be avoided. If only three teeth are to be arranged, it is more convenient to drop the first premolar and place the second premolar and the first and second molars into the available space. Eliminating the first premolar is a logical choice because this tooth has less occlusal surface for the mastication of food.

Setting the Mandibular Teeth First   The primary consideration in positioning the premolars is that they follow the form of the residual ridge. The facial surface of the premolars should be perpendicular to the occlusal rim, and yet slightly facial to the canine, but never farther facially than the buccal flange.

In the ideal situation, the mandibular first and second premolars, with their central grooves, are positioned on a line from the canine tip to 1 to 2 mm below the top of the retromolar pad (Figure 17-17). Before the first premolar is positioned, a small section of the mandibular wax occlusal rim is removed to accommodate the first and second premolars. A small cone of soft pink baseplate wax is attached to the neck of the first premolar tooth, and

it is positioned in the arch in contact with the canine and with its central grooves on the reference line from the tip of the canine to the retromolar pad. The long axis of the tooth is positioned so that the cusp tips are level with the remaining mandibular wax occlusal rim. The second premolar is set in a similar manner. When these lower teeth have been arranged, a segment of the maxillary occlusal rim is removed to accommodate the first maxillary premolar, which is set into maximum intercuspation with the two lower premolars. If a space develops between the maxillary canine and first premolar, the maxillary first premolar is aligned with the canine, and the maxillary second premolar is positioned in the upper arch. Then the two mandibular premolars are repositioned to achieve maximum intercuspation with the maxillary premolars. The mandibular first premolar may need to be adjusted mesiodistally to fit into the available space. Reshaping of the tooth by grinding usually will satisfy the space requirements. Maintenance of the occlusal plane by positioning the mandibular teeth at the appropriate height is of paramount importance as is the placement of their central grooves on the reference line from the tip of the canine to the retromolar pad. The first three premolars set (two mandibular and one maxillary) are the key to the relative anteroposterior intercuspation of all the remaining posterior teeth. Once the premolars are set and properly related to each other, positioning of the remaining mandibular posterior teeth is easily accomplished.

In the positioning of the mandibular first molar, the central groove is placed on the canine to retromolar pad reference line. The vertical height of the tooth is adjusted by positioning the cusp tips on the occlusal plane. After these adjustments are completed, the maxillary first molar is articulated with the mandibular first molar. A small segment of the wax occlusal rim is removed, and the tooth is attached to the record base with a small cone of soft baseplate wax. After the tooth is positioned, it is sealed to the record base with molten wax and the hot no. 7 spatula. After the maxillary first molar is positioned, the articulator is closed so that the mandibular tooth will assist in seating the maxillary tooth into maximum intercuspation. The index finger is used to hold the cervical neck of the maxillary tooth in place while the articulator is closed.

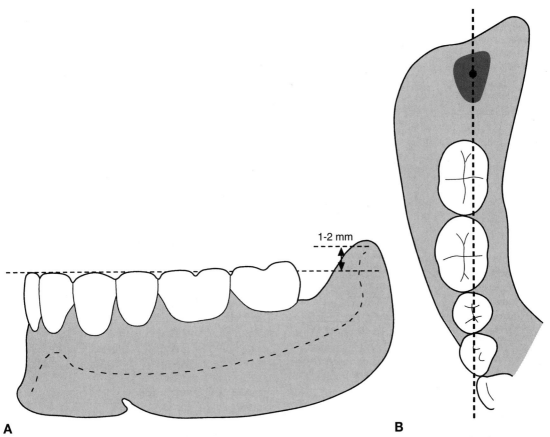

Figure 17-17   **A,** A point 1 to 2 mm below the top of the retromolar pad and the tip of the positioned mandibular cuspid are guides used in the placement of the mandibular posterior teeth. **B,** The central grooves of the posterior teeth are positioned on a line between the cuspid tip and the middle of the retromolar pad. When only three posterior teeth are arranged, it is essential that the central grooves of the molars be positioned slightly to the buccal to avoid crowding the tongue.

This will develop the desired lingual cusp contact of the maxillary molar in the central fossa of the mandibular antagonist. The same procedure is used for setting the remaining maxillary teeth. The teeth on the opposite side of the dental arches are arranged in a similar manner.

Setting the Maxillary Teeth First   In arranging the maxillary posterior teeth first, start with the maxillary first premolar and continue the arrangement of the teeth through to the second molar. During the positioning of these teeth, the maxillary lingual cusps are aligned with the reference line that

has been scribed on the mandibular wax occlusal rim from the mandibular canine tip to the middle of the retromolar pad. Positioning the maxillary teeth with a slight opening of the contact points between these teeth allows the mandibular teeth to better assume their correct mesiodistal position as they are interdigitated with the maxillary posterior teeth. Because this intercuspation is very exacting, it is best done by placing the mandibular first molar in position first. For the first molar to be placed and still preserve the reference line on the wax occlusal rim, a block of wax approximately the size of the mandibular molar tooth is all that is removed from the mandibular wax occlusal rim. When the mandibular first molar is placed in position without adjoining teeth, it is possible to determine its correct anteroposterior position more easily. If the mandibular first premolar is positioned first, the inconstant vertical overlap might crowd the tooth into difficult intercuspation with the maxillary teeth, and this would be continued throughout all the mandibular posterior teeth. Therefore placement of the mandibular first premolar is left until last to take up all the variation in vertical and horizontal overlap of the anterior teeth. The first premolar is then ground to fit the remaining space.

The second mandibular molar is placed after the positioning of the first molar, thereby assuring its anteroposterior correctness. The mandibular second premolar is next placed, after another block of wax has been cut away from the occlusal rim. The mandibular first premolar is the last tooth to be placed. It frequently needs to be ground because of the minimal space remaining between the second premolar and the canine after these teeth have been arranged in maximum intercuspation. For this reason, the tooth must be ground and shaped to fit the space available. The teeth on both sides of the dental arches are arranged in a similar manner.

Evaluating Bilateral Balanced Articulation   The presence of a balanced articulation can be inspected after all the maxillary and mandibular teeth have been arranged. However, it must be remembered that unless the teeth are positioned in exactly the same location in the articulator as they were when their primordial forms were carved in the cutting instrument, they will not balance. Furthermore, if the end-controlling factors recorded from the patient and transferred to the instrument are also not the same as those used in developing the tooth molds, one should not expect a perfect bilateral balance to be present. With luck, what one will see during this exercise is that some minor deflections are observed and that some tooth material is available for selective reshaping after processing to achieve the required balanced articulation during the various movements. The amount of movement of the articulator in a lateral direction during this evaluation process should be minimal, usually bringing the maxillary and mandibular canines into an end-to-end relation to each other will suffice.

Arranging Nonanatomical Mandibular Posterior Teeth to Balanced Articulation

The arrangement of nonanatomical posterior teeth with both anteroposterior and mediolateral compensating curves permits the establishment of a balanced articulation. In such arrangements, the mandibular teeth usually are arranged first followed by the maxillary teeth. The contours established in the wax occlusal rim and the use of the several reference lines and guides developed for the anatomical arrangement also are used with the nonanatomical teeth. The major difference is in the positioning of the mandibular posterior teeth to develop the compensating curves.

Number of Posterior Teeth Set   Most often, the number of posterior teeth used in balanced articulation with nonanatomical teeth will be limited to three. It is more convenient to drop the first premolar and place the second premolar and the first and second molars into the available space. Eliminating the first premolar is a logical choice because this tooth has less occlusal surface for the mastication of food. With the elimination of the first premolar and with the use of only three posterior teeth, it often is necessary to position the two molars slightly to the facial.

Anteroposterior Compensating Curve   The anteroposterior compensating curve begins at the distal marginal ridge of the first posterior replacement tooth (which is usually the second premolar) and continues through the second molar (Figure 17-18). The amount of curvature developed is dependent on the steepness of the condylar guidance, but it rarely requires more than a combined 20-degree elevation of the occlusal surfaces of the posterior teeth from the horizontal plane of orientation established by the anterior and posterior reference points. The anteroposterior curve is developed to provide the needed tooth structure for balancing contacts in the protrusive movement.

Mediolateral Compensating Curve   A mediolateral compensating curve also is needed to provide the needed tooth structure to achieve balanced articulation during lateral movements. This curve also is initiated with the first replacement tooth and continues through the second molar. The degree to which the facial cusps are elevated in relation to the lingual cusps to establish this curve will vary with the condylar and incisal guidances. The curve usually does not exceed 5 to 10 degrees from the horizontal plane of orientation when viewed in the frontal plane (Figure 17-19).

First Premolar The position of the first mandibular replacement tooth (second premolar) will be dictated by the position of the lower anterior teeth. The second premolar should be positioned immediately next to the canine, with no space allowed to detract from pleasing esthetics. The central fossa of the mandibular premolar tooth is aligned with the

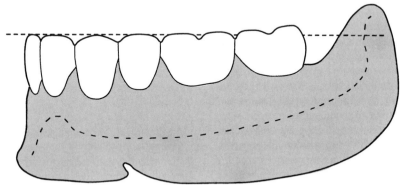

Figure 17-18 The anteroposterior compensating curve involves the cuspid tips and the retromolar pads as the anatomical guides. The curve begins with the mesial of the molar positioned level with the plane of occlusion and the distal surface slightly elevated. The curve continues with the placement of the second molar with the distal surface located at or above the top of the retromolar pad. The extent of the curve rarely exceeds 20 degrees.

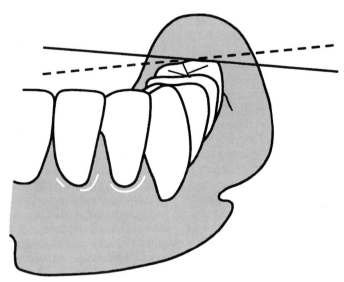

Figure 17-19 The mediolateral curve is formed by slightly elevating the buccal cusps of the posterior teeth above the lingual cusps. The curve usually does not exceed 10 degrees from the horizontal plane.

reference line from the tip of the canine to the middle of the retromolar pad. The long axis of the tooth is perpendicular to the occlusal plane, and the facial cusp is slightly elevated above the lingual cusp.

First Molar Position the mandibular first molar next to the premolar with the mesial marginal ridge at the same level as the distal marginal ridge of the premolar and its distal marginal ridge slightly elevated. This will position the tooth with its long axis directed anteriorly. The anteroposterior compensating curve begins with this tooth. The distal of the first molar should be elevated approximately 1 mm above the occlusal plane that was established by the anterior and posterior reference points. The amount of elevation may need to be increased or decreased, depending on the mechanical equivalent recorded for the horizontal condylar guidance. A high, condylar guidance will require a greater compensating curve. The central fossa of the first molar should be slightly to the facial in relation to the reference line from the canine to the retromolar pad. This will avoid possible crowding of the tongue. When viewed in the frontal plane, the mediolateral compensating curve, initiated with the setting of the premolar, should be maintained by a slight elevation of the facial cusp above the lingual cusp. The tooth is sealed with the hot no. 7 spatula and pink wax when its arrangement has been achieved.

Second Molar The mandibular second molar is positioned with the mesial marginal ridge at the same level as the distal marginal ridge of the first molar. The anteroposterior compensating curve is continued posteriorly by elevating the distal of this second molar tooth approximately 2 mm above the occlusal plane established by the reference points. The long axis of this tooth also will be anteriorly directed. The central fossa of the second molar also will be positioned slightly to the facial of the reference line. The facial cusps of both the first and second molars should be in a straight line when viewed from the occlusal surface. The teeth should not be positioned "around" the remaining residual ridge. The mediolateral compensating curve should be continued as viewed in the frontal plane. When the arrangement is completed, the tooth is sealed to the record base with the hot no. 7 spatula.

Remaining Mandibular Posterior Teeth The mandibular posterior teeth are arranged for the other side of the arch with the same criteria and procedures as just outlined. As the remaining teeth are positioned, they should be evaluated in relation to the teeth on the opposite side of the arch. This is extremely important, especially in trying to maintain (1) the appropriate level of the occlusal plane and (2) the same degree of anteroposterior and mediolateral compensating curves for both sides of the mandibular arch. When all teeth have been properly positioned, they are sealed to the record base with pink baseplate wax.

Arranging Nonanatomical Maxillary Posterior Teeth to Balanced Articulation

First Premolar For most patients, only three maxillary posterior teeth will be used. In such instances, only one premolar and two molars are the customary teeth selected. The premolar selected is usually the maxillary first premolar because of its longer occlusal cervical height, which provides a more esthetic arrangement. After some of the wax occlusal rim distal to the canine is removed, the first premolar is set. Place a small portion of soft, pink wax on the neck of the maxillary premolar and attach the tooth to the record base. Carefully close the articulator and establish contact between the occlusal surface of the maxillary tooth and the central fossa or marginal ridges of the mandibular antagonist. There should be approximately 1 to 2 mm of horizontal overlap of the maxillary facial cusp in relation to the mandibular facial cusp. This relationship will help prevent cheek biting and also will contribute to the attainment of a balanced articulation.

First Molar Position the maxillary first molar tooth alongside the premolar, aligning their marginal ridges and facial surfaces. Carefully close the articulator and establish contact between the maxillary occlusal surface and the central fossa or marginal ridges of the mandibular antagonist. Maintain maximum contact between the maxillary occlusal surface with the central fossa of the lower tooth and the 1 to 2 mm of horizontal overlap of the maxillary facial cusp in relation to the mandibular facial cusps. View the tooth-to-tooth relationships from the lingual by turning the instrument around and looking through the tongue space. Seal the tooth with pink wax.

Second Molar Position the maxillary second molar tooth with a small cone of pink wax. Again, carefully close the articulator and establish the tooth contacts as you did with the first molar. Seal the tooth to the record base.

Remaining Maxillary Posterior Teeth The maxillary posterior teeth are arranged for the other side of the arch with the same criteria and procedures as previously outlined for maxillary posterior teeth. As the remaining teeth are positioned, they should be evaluated for the required contacts between the maxillary occlusal surfaces and the central fossae and marginal ridges of the mandibular antagonists. When all teeth have been properly positioned, they are sealed to the record base with pink wax and evaluated. Bilateral balanced articulation between the maxillary and mandibular teeth will be developed and refined after the dentures are processed with the selective occlusal reshaping procedures.

Arranging Nonanatomical Teeth to Monoplane Articulation

The technique for arranging cuspless teeth in a flat plane or monoplane occlusal concept is a distinct departure from what has been previously described. With this concept of occlusion, there is no attempt to eliminate deflective occlusal contacts in lateral or protrusive excursions. The dentist's desire to achieve an optimal esthetic result will require some vertical overlap of the anterior teeth. However, this can generally be accommodated for with sufficient horizontal overlap to permit a range of anterior and lateral movements without anterior tooth contacts. Basically, the patient can clench and grind in and around maximum intercuspation during both functional and nonfunctional activities. However, some deflective occlusal contacts of the posterior teeth will be experienced.

When the nonanatomical teeth are arranged to satisfy the monoplane occlusal concept, the condylar inclinations on the articulator are set at 0 degrees. The articulator is reduced to a simple hinge articulator. With the mandibular wax occlu-

sion rim positioned on its cast on the articulator, a small segment of the rim is removed from the posterior tooth area. The maxillary posterior teeth are positioned one at a time with the mandibular wax occlusal rim and its references and guides for tooth placement. The maxillary teeth are positioned to occlude with the flat surface of the mandibular wax occlusion rim and to approximate the position of the maxillary occlusion rim contour that was previously determined. There should be approximately 1 to 2 mm of horizontal overlap of the maxillary facial cusp in relation to the mandibular wax occlusal rim. When completed, the occlusal surfaces of the maxillary posterior teeth should be flat against the mandibular wax occlusal rim.

The mandibular teeth are arranged so they will maximally contact the upper teeth. A segment of the mandibular wax occlusal rim is removed to accommodate each tooth. Each tooth, in turn, is placed with a small cone of wax, and the articulator is closed while the wax is still warm. The tooth is arranged in maximum contact with the flat lingual cusp of the maxillary tooth contacting the central groove area of the flat mandibular posterior tooth. The anteroposterior relation of the upper and lower teeth is not critical because of the absence of cusps. Any combination of premolars or molars can be used to fill the available space. The posterior limit of the extent of these teeth is the point at which the mandibular ridge begins to curve upward toward the retromolar pad.

Arranging Mandibular Posterior Teeth to Lingualized Articulation

Lingualized articulation has been advocated by many practitioners over the past 70 years, and in most instances these clinicians have done so with a variety of tooth molds. However, what has been lacking for the practitioner are tooth molds designed specifically for this concept. Myerson Lingualized Integration (MLI) molds represent an occlusal scheme designed for this concept. It has been suggested that these molds will provide maximum intercuspation, an absence of deflective occlusal contacts, adequate cusp height for selective occlusal reshaping, and a natural and pleasing appearance.

The MLI teeth are available in two posterior tooth molds: (1) controlled contact (CC) and

(2) maximum contact (MC) molds. The primary difference in the two molds is the maxillary posterior teeth. The mandibular teeth are the same for both molds. The mandibular teeth were designed with lower cusp heights and multiple occlusal spillways to assist in mastication. The selection of one or the other mold (CC or MC) is dependent on the patient's ability to consistently reproduce their centric jaw relation position. Judgments regarding this capability are generally made during several appointments before and after the maxillomandibular record appointment. For those patients in whom uncertainty exists in the registration and reproducibility of the centric jaw relation position, the CC mold is suggested because it provides for greater freedom of movement around maximum intercuspation. For those patients in whom muscle control is not a problem and jaw relation records are easily repeated, the MC mold may be the tooth selection of choice.

In the MC mold, the maxillary teeth are more anatomical in appearance with greater cusp heights. This form demands some minor reshaping and refinement of the occlusal fossae and marginal ridges of the mandibular teeth during the arrangement of the teeth to accept the lingual cusps of the maxillary teeth. With the MC mold, a more exacting occlusion can be attained in maximum intercuspation, and bilateral balanced articulation can be developed over a greater range of movement both anteroposteriorly and mediolaterally. Lingualized integration is based on the maxillary lingual cusp functioning as the main supporting cusp in harmony with the occlusal surfaces of the lower teeth. From the position of maximum intercuspation, the maxillary lingual cusps glide over the opposing teeth with an absence of deflection during nonrestrictive lateral and protrusive movements.

The maxillary cusp heights in the CC mold are lower and permit greater flexibility around maximum intercuspation. The tooth contacts in eccentric positions remain as bilateral balanced articulation, even though the range of contact is less because of the reduced height to the maxillary lingual cusps. However, a greater range of contact is probably not necessary for most edentulous patients, and the bilateral balanced articulation achieved with the CC mold is very acceptable.

A natural appearance to the "buccal corridor" is provided by both MLI molds. The facial surfaces and cusps for the maxillary tooth forms provide the illusion of naturalness because of their anatomical form.

In the arrangement of the teeth for lingualized articulation, the mandibular teeth are set first to establish the occlusal plane. The MLI tooth scheme calls for anteroposterior and mediolateral compensating curves arranged in the mandibular arch, thereby permitting balanced articulation between the maxillary lingual cusps and the mandibular teeth during various jaw movements. The superoinferior position of the mandibular teeth in relation to the tongue and the medial roll of the buccinator muscle is again an important consideration during the arrangement of the teeth. The mediolateral positioning of the mandibular teeth in relation to the tongue and cheek interactions also is considered.

Number of Posterior Teeth Set   The decision on the number of teeth to use with lingualized articulation will depend on the available space for posterior teeth. Most often, the number of posterior teeth will be limited to three. The second premolar, with its wider occlusal surface, and the first and second molars are the teeth most often selected for the arrangement.

Anterior and Posterior Reference Points   The anterior references that assist in tooth positioning are the same as those described earlier. A line drawn between the anterior and posterior reference points will establish the plane of occlusion and serve as the starting point for the setting of the teeth.

Buccolingual Positioning of the Teeth   A line that extends from the tip of the canine to the middle of the retromolar pad will help in determining the buccolingual positioning of the teeth. Eliminating a premolar in the tooth arrangement places the first molar in a more anterior position. The wider first molar in the anterior position will crowd the tongue if it is not positioned properly. Both the first and second molars should be positioned slightly to the facial of the reference line to increase the space available to the tongue.

Anteroposterior Compensating Curve The anteroposterior compensating curve begins with the distal marginal ridge of the first premolar tooth and continues through the last replacement tooth or the second molar. The amount of curvature is dependent on the condylar guidance mechanical equivalent established by the protrusive interocclusal record. Only rarely will the condylar guidance be more than 30 degrees if the maxillary cast has been mounted with a face bow. Obviously, the third point of reference used with the face bow will influence the mounting. It is recommended that the bite fork, positioned parallel to the mean residual ridge of the maxillary arch, be used as the third point of reference. The anteroposterior curve is established to permit a balanced articulation along the protrusive pathway.

Mediolateral Compensating Curve A mediolateral compensating curve is established to provide balanced articulation during lateral movements. The curve is initiated with the first replacement tooth (second premolar) in the mandibular arch and continues through the second molar. This curve is created by positioning the facial cusp slightly above the lingual cusp. A mediolateral compensating curve usually will not exceed 5 to 10 degrees from the horizontal plane of occlusion as viewed in the frontal plane.

Premolar The first premolar tooth is positioned in contact with the canine and with its long axis perpendicular to the occlusal plane. The occlusal surface is positioned on the occlusal plane; however, the facial cusp is elevated slightly above the lingual cusp to establish the mediolateral compensating curve. The second premolar is eliminated from the arrangement.

First Molar The mesial marginal ridge of the first molar is placed in contact with the distal margin of the premolar. The distal marginal ridge of this tooth is elevated slightly above the mesial marginal ridge to create the anteroposterior compensating curve. The mediolateral compensating curve is maintained by elevating the facial cusp of the molar slightly above the lingual cusp. The central fossa of the first molar is positioned slightly to the facial of

the reference line connecting the canine with the middle of the retromolar pad.

Second Molar The mesial marginal ridge of the second molar is placed level with the distal of the first molar, and the anteroposterior compensating curve is continued by elevating the distal marginal ridge of this tooth. In general, the distal of the second molar will be at the height of the top of the retromolar pad. The central fossa of the second molar is positioned to the facial of the buccolingual reference line and in a straight line with the first molar. The mediolateral compensating curve is continued by elevating the facial cusps above the lingual cusps.

Remaining Mandibular Posterior Teeth The mandibular posterior teeth are arranged for the other side of the arch with the same criteria and procedures, as previously outlined. As the remaining teeth are positioned, it is extremely important to maintain (1) the appropriate level of the occlusal plane and (2) the same degree of anteroposterior and mediolateral compensating curves for both sides of the mandibular arch.

Arranging Maxillary Posterior Teeth to Lingualized Articulation

Premolar The first tooth arranged in the maxillary arch is the first premolar. This tooth is selected because of its cusp tip to cervical margin height. A longer tooth will provide a more esthetic expression of naturalness along the buccal corridor. The tooth is positioned in contact with the canine and with its long axis perpendicular to the occlusal plane. The lingual cusp is positioned to contact the marginal ridge or occlusal fossa of its mandibular antagonist. No attempt is made at this time to balance the facial or lingual cusps in lateral or protrusive movements. Maximum interdigitation of the lingual cusp against the occlusal surface of the mandibular tooth is the primary consideration.

First Molar The mesial marginal ridge of the first molar is placed in contact with the distal margin of the premolar. The lingual cusp is positioned in the central fossa of the mandibular tooth, and maximum interdigitation is assured. Often, a Class I molar relationship will not be present. Such a relationship is not necessary, and positioning of the teeth to establish such a relationship is discouraged. Integration of the lingual cusps with the marginal ridge or fossa of the mandibular antagonist is the primary consideration. Position of the tooth emphasizing maximum intercuspation will continue the mediolateral compensating curve established in the arrangement of the mandibular teeth.

Second Molar   The mesial marginal ridge of the second molar is placed level with the distal of the first molar. The anteroposterior compensating curve is continued when the tooth is closed into contact with the mandibular tooth. Again, maximum intercuspation is essential, as is the maintenance of the mediolateral compensating curve.

Arranging the Maximum Contact Mold   In the arrangement of the MC mold, the maxillary teeth are positioned with the incisal pin slightly open when the lingual cusps are in contact with their mandibular antagonists. The prominence of the maxillary lingual cusps will require some occlusal reshaping of the central fossae and marginal ridges of the lower teeth to establish maximum intercuspation. After each maxillary tooth is positioned, a thin sheet of articulating paper is interposed between the tooth and its mandibular antagonist. The articulator is closed, marking the first contact point. The contact point on the occlusal surface of the mandibular tooth is enlarged by grinding with a round bur to permit the lingual cusp to obtain positive seating with the lower tooth. This process is continued until maximum interdigitation is achieved and the incisal pin is in contact with the incisal table.

Remaining Maxillary Posterior Teeth   The remaining maxillary posterior teeth are arranged for the other side of the arch with the same criteria and procedures, as previously outlined.

OCCLUSAL MODIFICATIONS AND THE SELECTIVE RESHAPING PROCESS

Processing changes, coupled with the lack of occlusal balance before processing, requires a remount procedure to correct occlusal discrepancies and to obtain a balanced articulation. The occlusal reshaping procedures usually are performed at the denture delivery appointment.

Establishing Maximum Intercuspation

It is much easier to develop maximum intercuspation at the centric jaw relation position when the prostheses are on the articulator. Once maximum intercuspation is achieved, balanced articulation in the several eccentric movements may be attained in the mouth.

After the clinical remount of the maxillary and mandibular complete dentures, small strips of articulating paper are placed on the occlusal surfaces of the mandibular teeth. With the articulator locked in the hinged position, all occlusal prematurities are marked. Using a Brasseler carbide trimming and finishing bur no. 7010, remove tooth structure in all areas of contact except the maxillary lingual cusps. Premature contacts most often are at the central fossae or marginal ridges of the lower teeth and on the lingual inclines of the maxillary facial cusps. Continue marking the contacts and reshaping the teeth until all lingual cusps in the maxillary posterior teeth demonstrate maximum intercuspation with their mandibular antagonists (Figure 17-20). Remember this procedure is one that establishes the maxillary lingual cusp as the main supporting cusp in the occlusal contact pattern. The dentures are returned to the oral environment after the occlusal reshaping procedures to verify that maximum intercuspation has been achieved at centric jaw relation position (Figure 17-21).

Adjusting the Working and Balancing Contacts

Working side interferences will result from contact between the lingual inclines of the maxillary facial cusps and the facial inclines of the facial cusp of the mandibular tooth in lateral excursions. Balancing side interferences will occur between the lingual cusps of the maxillary teeth as they move across the lingual inclines of the facial cusps of the mandibular teeth in lateral excursions. Balancing contacts are the direct result of the compensating curves

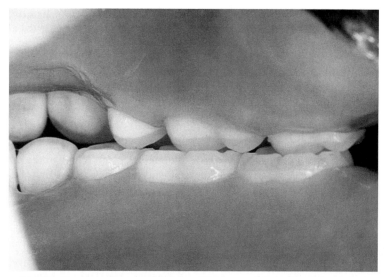

Figure 17-20   The lingual cusps of the maxillary posterior teeth are the main supporting cusps that interdigitate with the central fossae and marginal ridges of the mandibular posterior teeth.

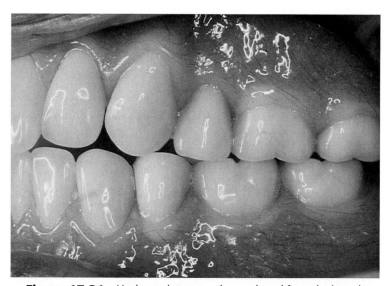

Figure 17-21   Maximum intercuspation as viewed from the buccal.

being out of harmony with the lingual cusps, and the refinement of the occlusal contacts between the maxillary lingual cusp and the occlusal surface of the mandibular teeth is required.

The development of a harmonious working and balancing occlusion will require the judicious reduction of heavy working side contacts. These heavy working contacts are created during the adjustment of maximum intercuspation when the premature contacts were eliminated. After the working and balancing contacts are marked, careful selective grinding procedures are performed. Adjusting the working and balancing contacts is a clinical procedure to be completed after the complete dentures are positioned over their residual ridges. With articulating paper positioned between the posterior teeth bilaterally, carefully guide the patient into a lateral movement. The extent of the movement will be approximately 2 to 3 mm in the molar region. Working interferences will appear as markings on the lingual inclines of the facial cusps of the maxillary teeth as they pass over the facial inclines of the mandibular facial cusps. Occlusal reshaping procedures with the use of the Brasseler carbide trimming and finishing bur no. 7010 are completed by gently grinding the lingual inclines of the maxillary facial cusp that demonstrate interferences.

Balancing interferences and maximum intercuspation contacts may occur very near to each other on the occlusal surfaces of the mandibular teeth. The maximum intercuspation stop is generally in the central portion of the tooth, whereas balancing contacts begin in the same area and move in a distal facial direction onto the lingual inclines of the mandibular facial cusps. The width of the balancing contact markings may be very small, and care must be used in reducing balancing interferences. If the balancing contact must be reduced, it will be only the facial portion of the mandibular

marking that is altered. Selective grinding of the entire contact area will result in the loss of maximum intercuspation. The selective occlusal reshaping procedures should be continued until a smooth, free-gliding movement is observed (Figures 17-22 and 17-23).

Adjusting the Protrusive Contacts

Protrusive contacts result from the maxillary lingual cusps gliding over the distal lingual "cusp" of the mandibular tooth in a straight protrusive movement (Figure 17-24). Should deflective protrusive contacts be observed, as evidenced by heavy occlusal markings, their refinement will be necessary. Position articulating paper between the posterior teeth bilaterally and guide the mandible into a protrusive movement from maximum intercuspation. Premature protrusive contacts also may appear between the lingual inclines of the maxillary facial cusps and the facial inclines of the mandibular facial cusps during this movement. Such contacts may be eliminated by grinding on the mandibular facial cusp with the Brasseler bur. When heavy maxillary facial cusp contacts occur, their removal or the modification of the opposing deflective contacts on the mandibular teeth must be

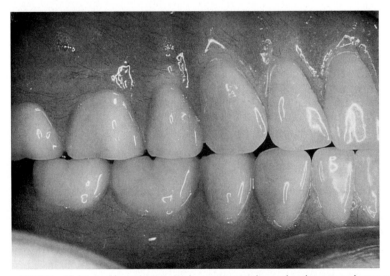

Figure 17-22 Right working movement demonstrates the occlusal contacts between the maxillary buccal cusps and the mandibular posterior teeth during this lateral movement.

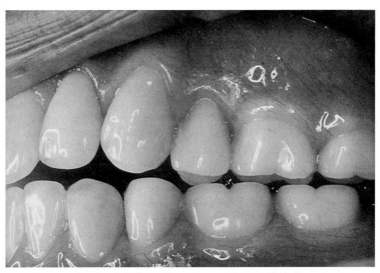

Figure 17-23 During the right lateral movement, the maxillary lingual cusps contact the lingual inclines of the mandibular buccal cusps to create a balanced articulation.

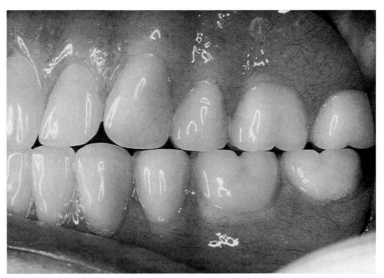

Figure 17-24 During the protrusive movement, a balanced articulation is achieved by contact between the maxillary buccal cusps of the posterior teeth and the buccal cusps of their mandibular antagonists.

accomplished without disturbing any of the contacts required in the other movements.

When the anterior teeth are brought into contact in a protrusive movement, it is desirable to have the posterior teeth contact bilaterally to prevent tilting and dislodgment of the dentures. If the anterior teeth contact prematurely in the protrusive movement, the anterior mandibular teeth are the teeth usually modified, keeping the esthetics of the dentures in mind.

With the occlusal reshaping procedures accomplished for maximum intercuspation and working, balancing, and protrusive movements, the occlusion is examined for holding contacts in centric jaw relation position. The occlusion also is examined for an absence of deflective occlusal contacts during all of these mandibular movements.

SUMMARY OF TOOTH SELECTION AND ARRANGEMENT

Treatment of edentulous patients is enjoyable when one has empathy, listening skills, and an appreciation of dental esthetics. Impressions and recordings of healthy tissues need to be made and accurately transferred to an articulator. Teeth should be positioned in harmony with intraoral and circumoral muscle activity and adjusted so that they occlude and articulate evenly. Several different prosthetic tooth molds have been produced, and each has some purported advantages. In the absence of a clear advantage, dentists should use tooth molds that are esthetically pleasing and have a simple procedure for setup.

Bibliography

Academy of Prosthodontics: Glossary of prosthodontic terms, ed 6, *J Prosthet Dent* 71:41-112, 1994.

Beck HO: Occlusion as related to complete removable prosthodontics, *J Prosthet Dent* 27:246-256, 1972.

Clough HE, Knodle JM, Leeper SH et al: A comparison of lingualized occlusion and monoplane occlusion in complete dentures, *J Prosthet Dent* 50:176-179, 1983.

Davies SJ, Gray RMJ, McCord JF: Good occlusal practice in removable prosthodontics, *Br Dent J* 191:491-502, 2001.

Frush JP: Linear occlusion, *Ill Dent J* 35:788-794, 1966.

Frush JP, Fisher RD: Dentogenics: its practical application, *J Prosthet Dent* 9:914-921, 1959.

Hirsch B, Levin B, Tiber N: The effect of patient involvement and esthetic preference on denture acceptance, *J Prosthet Dent* 28:127-132, 1972.

Hirsch B, Levin B, Tiber N: Effects of dentist authoritarianism on patient evaluation of dentures, *J Prosthet Dent* 30:745-748, 1973.

Jones PM: The monoplane occlusion for complete dentures, *J Prosthet Dent* 85:94-100, 1972.

Khamis MM, Zaki HS, Rudy TE: A comparison of the effect of different occlusal forms in mandibular implant overdentures, *J Prosthet Dent* 79:422-429, 1998.

Lang BR: Complete denture occlusion, *Dent Clin N A* 40:85-101, 1996.

Lang BR, Razzoog ME: A practical approach to restoring occlusion for edentulous patients, Part I: guiding principles of tooth selection, *J Prosthet Dent* 50:455-458, 1983.

LaVere AM, Marcroft KR, Smith RC et al: Denture tooth selection: size matching of natural anterior tooth width with artificial denture teeth, *J Prosthet Dent* 72:381-384, 1994.

Levin B: Monoplane teeth, *J Am Dent Assoc* 85:781, 1972.

Levin B: A review of artificial posterior tooth forms including a preliminary report on a new posterior tooth, *J Prosthet Dent* 38:3-15, 1977.

Lombardi RE: The principles of visual perception and their clinical application to denture esthetics, *J Prosthet Dent* 29:358-382, 1973.

Lombardi RE: A method for the classification of errors in dental esthetics, *J Prosthet Dent* 32:501-513, 1974.

Pleasure MA: Anatomic versus non-anatomic teeth, *J Prosthet Dent* 3:747-754, 1953.

Pound E: Utilizing speech to simplify a personalized denture service, *J Prosthet Dent* 24:586-600, 1971.

Sproull RC: Color matching in dentistry. I. The three dimensional nature of color, *J Prosthet Dent* 29:416-424, 1973.

Sproull RC: Color matching in dentistry. II. Practical applications of the organization of color, *J Prosthet Dent* 29:556-567, 1973.

18

The Try-in Appointment

Charles L. Bolender

The vertical dimension and centric relation (CR) of edentulous jaws are tentatively established with the occlusion rims, as described in Chapter 16. After the preliminary arrangement of the artificial teeth on the occlusion rims, it is essential that the accuracy of the jaw relation records made with the occlusion rims be tested, perfected if incorrect, and then verified to be correct. The dentist must assume that the preliminary jaw relation records were incorrect until they can be proven correct. This mental attitude of the dentist—attempting to prove that the jaw relation records are wrong—is essential in perfecting and verifying jaw relation records.

Patients should be advised to leave existing dentures out of the mouth for a minimum of 24 hours before the jaw relation records are perfected and verified at the time of the try-in appointment. Unfortunately, most patients will find this to be an unreasonable request. An acceptable alternative is to have the existing dentures relined with a soft temporary material. Whichever approach is taken, the soft tissues of the basal seat will be rested and in the same form as they were when the final impressions were made. If this procedure is not followed, the distorted condition of the soft tissue can prevent the registration of accurate interocclusal records.

It is almost impossible to overemphasize the importance of perfection and verification of jaw relation records. The appearance and comfort of the patient, occlusion of the teeth, and health of the supporting tissues are all directly related to the accuracy of jaw relation records.

VERIFYING THE VERTICAL DIMENSION

The maxillary and mandibular trial dentures are placed in the patient's mouth. The patient is instructed to close lightly so the maxillary labial frenum can be checked to see that it is absolutely free. This is necessary before the relation of the lip to the teeth can be observed. If the denture border causes binding of the frenum, the labial notch should be deepened.

Next, a tentative observation of the centric occlusion (CO) is made. The mandible is guided into CR by a thumb placed directly on the anteroinferior portion of the chin with patient instructions to "open and close until you feel the first feather touch of your back teeth." At first contact, the patient opens and repeats this closure, only this time stopping the instant a tooth touch is felt and then closing tight. The procedure will reveal errors in CR by the touch and slide of teeth on each other. Errors in CR can interfere with tests for vertical relations.

The vertical dimensions of occlusion and of rest must now be given careful consideration because the final positions of the anterior and posterior teeth will depend to a great extent on the amount of space that is available vertically. Unfortunately, there is no precise scientific method of determining the correct occlusal vertical dimension. The acceptability of the dentures' vertical relations depends on the experience and judgment of the dentist. Nevertheless, the factors that govern final determination of this relation can be said to hang on careful consideration of the following:

1. Preextraction records
2. The amount of interocclusal distance to which the patient was accustomed, either before the loss of natural teeth or with old dentures

3. Phonetics and esthetics
4. The amount of interocclusal distance between the teeth when the mandible is in its rest position
5. A study of facial dimensions and facial expression
6. Lip length in relation to the teeth
7. The interarch distance and parallelism of the ridges as observed from the mounted casts
8. The condition and amount of shrinkage of the ridges

A combination of these factors and considerations may be used to aid in determining an acceptable vertical dimension.

VERIFYING CENTRIC RELATION

After the vertical dimension has been determined, CR is verified. This can be done by intraoral observation of intercuspation or by an extraoral method on the articulator.

Intraoral Observation of Intercuspation

The test for accuracy of the preliminary CR record involves the observation of intercuspation when the mandible is pulled back by the patient as far as it will go and closure is stopped at the first tooth contact. The patient is guided into CR by a thumb placed on the anteroinferior portion of the chin and the index fingers bilaterally on the buccal flanges of the lower trial denture (Figure 18-1). With the index fingers, the dentist checks that the lower trial denture is seated in an inferoanterior direction. The patient pulls his lower jaw back as far as it will go and closes just until the back teeth make a "feather touch." As tooth contact approaches, the dentist's index fingers should rise off the buccal flanges. Pressure on the buccal flanges, or stretching the lip with the index fingers, will create the risk of posteriorly displacing the lower trial denture. Then the patient closes tightly. Any error in CR will be apparent when the teeth slide over each other, especially if anatomical teeth are used (Figure 18-2). A second closure made with the same instructions

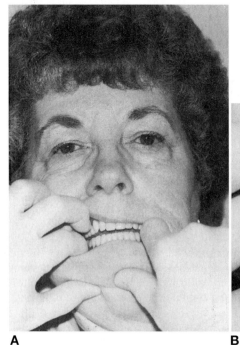
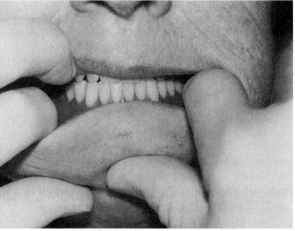

A   **B**

Figure 18-1 **A,** Hand and finger positions for checking the accuracy of centric relation records. **B,** As tooth contact approaches, the index fingers are raised off the buccal flanges to avoid displacement of the lower denture.

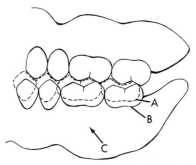

Figure 18-2 An error in centric occlusion (CO) that is due to an error in centric relation mounting will produce contact of the inclined planes of the cusps (**B**). Further closure will allow the teeth to slide into CO (**A**). The path of closure is an arc (**C**) about the posterior terminal hinge axis.

and a stop at first tooth contact will permit visual observation of any error.

Errors in the mounting may prevent intercuspation of some teeth when the first contact is made. If the patient stops the closure at the instant the first teeth touch, an error will be indicated by the space between the lower tooth or teeth and the teeth they were supposed to touch. The amount of error observed in this manner will be magnified by the effect of the inclined plane contacts. All the teeth that occluded uniformly on the articulator must have equally uniform contacts in the mouth; if they do not, the touch and slide observation will prove the mounting incorrect.

Once it is determined that the mounting is incorrect, a preliminary observation of esthetics is made. If the anterior teeth are not placed to support the lip properly, their positions are corrected. Then vertical overlap of the anterior teeth is carefully noted. This is important because the amount of vertical overlap will be a guide to the amount of closure permitted when the next interocclusal record is made.

Because complete dentures rest on movable soft tissues, it is difficult to detect anything other than gross occlusal errors by visual observation of the occlusion. As a result, one should not rely on visualization for the final determination of cast mounting accuracy.

The posterior teeth are removed from the lower occlusion rim, and both occlusion rims are placed in the mouth. Impression plaster (or an interocclusal registration paste), is mixed, and with the hands in the same position as for testing the previ-

ous record, the selected recording medium is placed on both sides of the lower occlusion rim in the molar and premolar regions. This may be done with a narrow plaster or cement spatula. Then the patient is instructed to pull the lower jaw back and close slowly until requested to stop and hold that position. The closure is stopped when the anterior teeth have the same vertical overlap as they had before the posterior teeth were removed. Thus the vertical relation of the two jaws will not have changed. When the plaster or registration paste is set, the new record is removed with the two occlusion rims, and the lower cast is remounted on the articulator.

In an alternate technique an abbreviated beeswax occlusion rim is used to replace the removed posterior teeth. (The rim may replace all the posterior teeth, or else a "tripod" of beeswax stops can be used [Figure 18-3].) The patient is

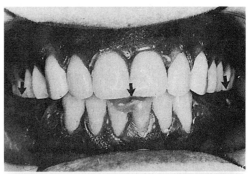

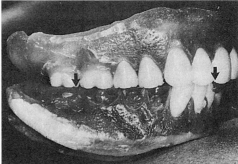

Figure 18-3 A modified beeswax interocclusal record of centric relation (CR) is made to correct an error in the preliminary mounting of casts. The lower posterior teeth are removed so there will be no contact between upper and lower trial dentures. The vertical overlap of anterior teeth is a guide to the vertical dimension at which CR will be recorded. Arrows indicate the beeswax tripod of stops.

guided into the most retruded mandibular position at the selected vertical dimension when the upper posterior teeth will indent the softened opposing wax rims. The lower cast is remounted on the articulator, and the lower posterior teeth are reset in CO.

The occlusion rims, with the teeth in good tight CO, are returned to the mouth, and the same tests are made as before. If the teeth occlude perfectly and uniformly when the lower jaw is drawn back as far as it will go, the CR mounting may be assumed to be correct. There should be uniform simultaneous contact on both sides of the mouth, in the front and back and without any detectable touch and slide.

It is essential with this procedure that the dentist tries to find an error in the previous record. The record must be assumed to be incorrect unless no touch and slide can be detected. The entire procedure is repeated until all doubt as to the correctness of the relationship of the casts is gone.

Extraoral Articulator Method

CR can be checked or verified by an extraoral method in which observations are made on the articulator rather than in the mouth. The technique is easy and thus attractive, but its use depends on taking one or two liberties. A CR registration in soft wax is placed between the opposing teeth. The teeth do not contact through the wax; thus the record is made at a slightly increased vertical dimension. Although clinical experience endorses this technique, a purist might argue that such verification is likely to work correctly only if a kinematic hinge axis, rather than an arbitrary face bow recording, is used originally. Because conclusive research to support such an argument is absent and because extensive clinical application of the technique has led to predictable and reproducible results, it deserves description.

Remember: The purpose of the extraoral method is to determine whether the position of the teeth on the articulator (Figure 18-4) is the same as that in the patient's mouth (Figure 18-5). As mentioned previously, it is difficult to detect occlusal errors by clinical observation, so wax, plaster, or a bite registration paste must

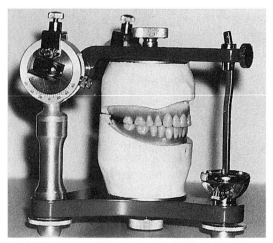

Figure 18-4 Artificial teeth positioned on a Dentatus ARH articulator.

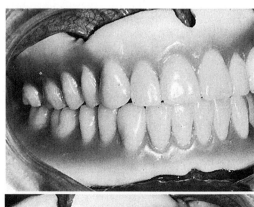

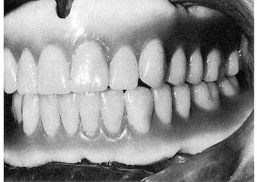

Figure 18-5 The same trial dentures as shown in Figure 18-4 being evaluated for proper occlusion. Clinical observation of tooth contacts is not as accurate as the extraoral method.

be used as the recording medium in this technique.

Impression material (e.g., two pieces of Aluwax) is placed over the posterior mandibular teeth (Figure 18-6). A thickness is chosen that will eliminate the danger of making contact with the opposing teeth when biting pressure is exerted. No wax is placed on the anterior teeth because anterior tooth contact tends to cause the patient to protrude his lower jaw. The teeth must be completely dry and the wax pressed firmly on the teeth to elimi-

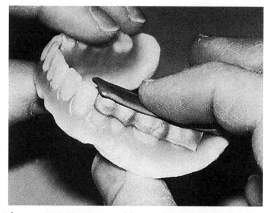

Figure 18-6 A second layer of warmed Aluwax is applied to the first layer, which has been carefully adapted to the posterior teeth.

nate voids between it and the teeth. The two thicknesses of wax are sealed with a warm spatula (Figure 18-7). The chilled upper trial denture is placed in the patient's mouth. Next, just the wax portion is immersed in a water bath of 130° F (54° C) for 30 seconds (Figure 18-8). Both the temperature and the time are critical in achieving a uniformly softened wax. (Aluwax retains heat longer than baseplate wax, which provides more working time for the next step.)

The mandibular trial denture is seated with the index fingers bilaterally positioned on the buccal flanges. The mandible is guided into CR by a thumb on the anteroinferior portion of the chin to direct some guidance toward the condyles. The thumb must be on the point of the chin, not under it; the patient is guided in a hinge movement, closing lightly into the wax (Figure 18-9). As contact with the wax approaches, the index fingers are raised from the buccal flanges. The patient then closes into the wax until a good index is made (Figure 18-10). Care must be taken that the patient does not penetrate the wax and make tooth contact. If one method of suggested retrusion does not work, another may. In any case, a minimum amount of occlusal pressure should be exerted on the wax.

The lower trial denture is then carefully removed from the mouth and placed in ice water to chill the wax thoroughly (Figure 18-11). Next, the trial dentures are removed from the ice water and

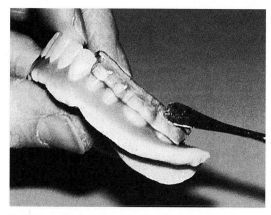

Figure 18-7 The two layers of Aluwax are sealed with a warm spatula.

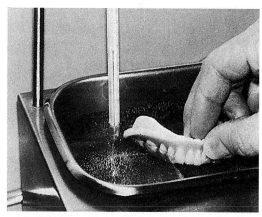

Figure 18-8 Only the Aluwax is immersed in 130° F (54° C) water for 30 seconds.

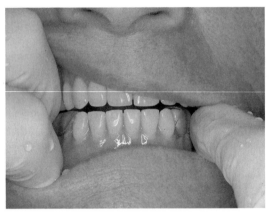

Figure 18-9 The mandible is guided into centric relation with the thumb on the anteroinferior portion of the chin and the index fingers seating the lower trial denture in a downward and forward direction.

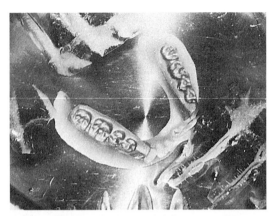

Figure 18-11 The lower trial denture and attached Aluwax are chilled in ice water for several minutes.

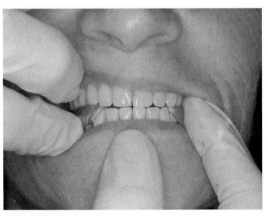

Figure 18-10 The patient is instructed to close lightly into the softened wax. The index fingers should be slightly raised from the buccal flanges at this point.

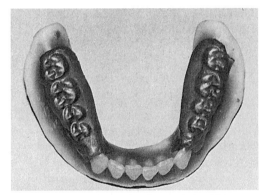

Figure 18-12 The occlusal record should be approximately 1-mm deep and free of any penetration by the underlying teeth.

dried. It is important that the imprint of the opposing teeth be crisp and about 1 mm deep, with no penetration of the wax by a maxillary tooth (Figure 18-12). If penetration occurs, it will likely deflect the occlusal contact as well as shift the bases or change the maxillomandibular relation horizontally and vertically. The chilled dentures are returned to the patient's mouth, and the patient is guided into CR. The record is acceptable if there is no tilting or torquing of the trial dentures from initial contact to complete closure (Figure 18-13). Underlying soft tissue displacement may cause a slight movement of the bases and must be taken into account when evaluating the contact. If the record is unacceptable, the procedure must be repeated.

After the wax has been chilled, the trial dentures are placed on their casts, and the locked articulator is closed in CR; the opposing teeth should fit into the indentations in every way (anteriorly, posteriorly, laterally, and vertically) (Figure 18-14). When the original CR interocclusal record and the check are both correct, these teeth will fit into the indentations surprisingly well.

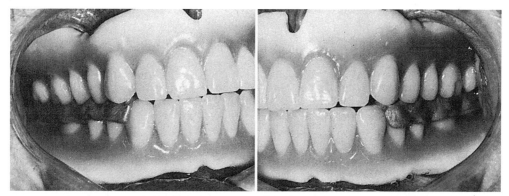

Figure 18-13 Checking the accuracy of the interocclusal wax record clinically.

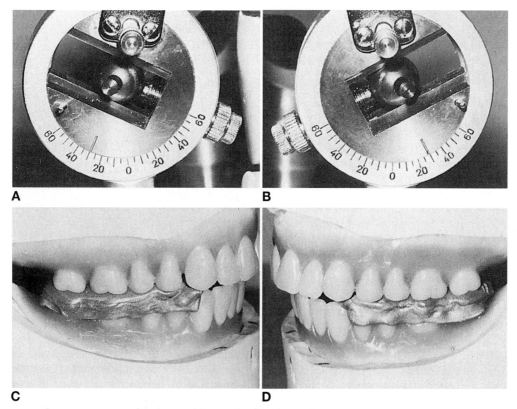

Figure 18-14 With the condylar mechanisms locked in a centric position (*A* and *B*), the upper teeth should fit accurately into the wax index (*C* and *D*). When this occurs, it means that the original recording was correct.

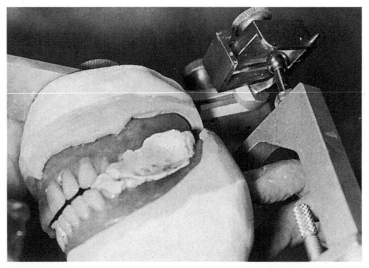

Figure 18-15 A plaster interocclusal centric relation (CR) record is used to test the accuracy of preliminary mounting on the articulator. The location of the condylar sphere in contact with the posterior, lateral, and superior elements of the condylar housing indicates that the preliminary record and test record are clinically identical. Thus the casts on the articulator are assumed to be in CR.

If the opposing teeth do not fit exactly into the indentations in the new record, it means that the original mounting was incorrect or that the patient did not bite cleanly into the interocclusal wax. To evaluate this, the dentist must return the chilled trial dentures and wax record to the mouth and reevaluate their accuracy, as previously described. If the record still appears to be correct in the patient's mouth, then the original CR registration, mounting, or both were incorrect. In these cases, the mandibular cast must be separated from the mounting ring and the cast remounted by means of the last interocclusal wax record. The new mounting is again checked to prove or disprove its correctness.

If the initial registration (preliminary CR record) was made in plaster or a bite registration paste, the same recording medium should be used to verify the accuracy of the mounting on the articulator. Likewise, if wax was used, wax should be the verifying medium. However, it is easier to distort wax when the record is removed from the mouth and tested on the articulator (Figure 18-15).

SECTION II: ECCENTRIC JAW RELATION RECORDS, ARTICULATOR AND CAST ADJUSTMENT, ESTABLISHMENT OF THE POSTERIOR PALATAL SEAL

When the final occlusion is developed and corrected on the articulator, it is essential that the movements of the articulator simulate mandibular positions or movements of the patient within the range of normal functional contacts of teeth. Thus the condylar elements of the articulator must be adjusted so that they approximate the condylar-guiding factors within the temporomandibular joints (TMJs). These adjustments of the condylar elements of the articulator are made by means of interocclusal eccentric records.

PROTRUSIVE AND LATERAL RELATIONS

There seems to be confusion in the minds of many dentists as to what a protrusive registration is intended to attain. The idea that the angle and lines of the bony fossa completely govern the path of the condyle is erroneous. A study of the anatomy and function of the joint reveals that the condylar path is governed partly in its shape and function by the meniscus. The meniscus is attached in part to the lateral pterygoid and moves forward during opening and lateral mandibular movements. The path is controlled further by the shape of the fossa, the attachments of the ligaments, the biting load during movement (muscular influence), and the amount of protrusion. Variation in registrations can be caused by several factors. The registration may vary according to the biting pressure exerted after the mandible has been protruded. The condyle, not being locked on a path, is subject to change in its path with a variation of pressure. Undoubtedly, there is some leeway for adaptability to conform to the changing conditions of the teeth. Many parts of the body are phenomenal in their ability to adapt to unusual conditions, and the TMJ is one of them. Not many complete dentures could be worn if this were not true. However, registration of a normal comfortable movement of the condyle in its path, with subsequent harmonious eccentric occlusion and CO to conform to this, greatly augments lasting function of dentures. Therefore there does not seem to be much excuse for failure to register this path because it is not difficult or time-consuming in proportion to the results obtained.

CONTROLLING FACTORS OF MOVEMENT

Edentulous patients bring only one controlling factor to the movement of the mandible, a fact that seems to be misunderstood generally. The misconception exists because many dentists think the condyle paths control the movement of the mandible entirely. In the laws of articulation, the incisal guidance provided by the anterior teeth is an important part of the control. This guidance is always decided by the dentist, consciously or not. With semiadjustable articulators like the Dentatus, Hanau, and Whip Mix, incisal guidance is controlled by the inclination of the incisal guidance mechanism, which is determined by the horizontal and vertical overlap of the anterior teeth. The incisal guidance is more influential in controlling movements of the mandible than the condylar paths are because the

condylar paths are farther away from the cusp inclines, which both the incisal angle and the condyle angle influence.

ECCENTRIC RELATION RECORDS

A previous chapter underscored the fact that eccentric relation records are rarely used in the fabrication of complete dentures. They are referred to in this chapter mainly for historical purposes. Their consideration also provides interesting insights into the complexity of mechanical simulation of jaw movement. Skipping over this section is certainly an option for the reader.

The path of the condyle in protrusive and lateral movements is not on a straight line. The shape of the mandibular fossa is an ogee curve as viewed in the sagittal plane. This double curve will cause the apparent path of the condyle to be different with varying amounts of mandibular protrusion. The ideal amount of protrusion for making the record is the exact equivalent of the amount of protrusion necessary to bring the anterior teeth end to end. However, the mechanical limitations of most articulators require a protrusive movement of at least 6 mm so the condylar guidance mechanisms can be adjusted.

Methods of registering the condyle path may be classified as intraoral and extraoral. Extraoral methods are generally exemplified by the Gysi and McCollum techniques. The intraoral methods may be listed as (1) plaster and carborundum grind-in, (2) chew-in by teeth opposing wax, (3) chew-in modified by a central bearing point, (4) Needles's styluses cutting a compound rim, (5) Needles's technique modified by a Messerman tracer, (6) protrusive registration in softened compound, (7) protrusive registration in plaster, and (8) protrusive registration in softened wax.

Lateral and protrusive condylar inclinations may be registered when straight protrusive movements are made. Many dentists consider these short-range lateral movements sufficiently indicative for practical purposes. However, for a complete registration, lateral records are necessary to indicate the limit of the range of movement, as shown by the Gothic arch (needle point) tracings.

Wax interocclusal records may be made on the occlusion rims before the teeth are set up or on the posterior teeth at the try-in appointment. Records made on occlusion rims must be considered tentative because the vertical and horizontal overlaps of the anterior teeth have not as yet been determined and the exact amount of protrusion and the level at which the anterior teeth are to contact are still unknown. These preliminary records permit tentative adjustment of the condylar guidances on the articulator.

Plaster interocclusal records are made after the anterior teeth have been arranged for esthetics and after both CR and the vertical dimension have been verified. If the horizontal overlap is sufficient to obtain enough protrusive movement of the lower jaw that the articulator can be adjusted, this record will be adequate. It also will be an accurate record of the relation of the jaws during incision. If the horizontal overlap of the incisors is too small to permit sufficient mandibular movement for adjustment of the condylar guidance, the patient must be instructed to protrude the jaw farther when the record is made. The minimum amount of protrusion for condylar guidance adjustment is 6 mm. This limitation is necessary because of mechanical deficiencies of most articulating instruments.

Lateral interocclusal records can be made to set the condylar inclination and the mandibular lateral translation on the articulator. However, with complete dentures, it is more difficult to secure accurate and reproducible lateral records than protrusive records, in part because of the displaceability of the ridge mucosa. In addition, most semiadjustable articulators are not able to accept many lateral eccentric records. It is therefore generally accepted that making lateral interocclusal records for patients with complete dentures is not practical and probably not warranted.

Eccentric interocclusal records may be made with the guidance of extraoral tracings. While the tracing device is still attached to the occlusion rims, the amount of protrusive movement is determined by observation of the distance between the apex of the tracing and the needle point. The amount and direction of the lateral movement can be determined by observing the distance of the needle point from the apex of the tracing while the needle is on one of the arcs of the tracing. When the needle point is 6 mm from the apex, the mandible in the first molar region will be approximately 3 mm lateral to its position in CR. The molar tooth will have moved laterally 3 mm because it is approximately midway between the tracing and the working-side condyle.

Protrusive Interocclusal Records for the Whip Mix Articulator (Arcon Type)

After try-in, the trial dentures are placed on the articulator. The lateral condylar guidances are set at 0 degrees so the articulator will be moved in a straight protrusive direction. The horizontal condylar guidances are set at 25 degrees to give an indication of the space that will exist between the posterior teeth when the mandible is protruded.

The lower member of the articulator is moved forward approximately 6 mm, with the teeth out of contact and then closed, until the incisal edges of the lower anterior teeth reach the vertical level of the incisal edges of the upper anterior teeth. The 6 mm of forward movement that is necessary to permit proper adjustment of the horizontal condylar path of the articulator may bring the lower anterior teeth several millimeters in front of the upper anterior teeth.

The horizontal relation of the lower to the upper anterior teeth and the relationship of the midlines of the upper and lower anterior teeth are observed carefully because they will be the guides to the dentist that the patient has closed in approximately the proper position when the protrusive record is made in the mouth (Figure 18-16, *A*). Interfering opposing posterior teeth that contact before the lower anterior teeth reach the desired vertical relation should be removed from the wax occlusion rim.

When the dentist has become familiar with the relation of the lower to the upper anterior teeth in the protrusive position, the trial dentures are removed from the articulator and placed in the patient's mouth. The trial dentures are held in position by the dentist in the same way as for making the interocclusal CR record.

The patient is instructed to move his jaw straightforward and then to bite lightly on his front teeth. The dentist determines the amount and nature of the forward protrusion by the previous observation of the relationship of the anterior teeth on the articulator. The patient practices closing in

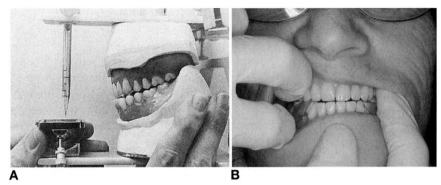

A   **B**

Figure 18-16   **A,** The articulator (Whip Mix) in a protrusive position to show the amount of forward movement necessary to adjust the condylar elements. This relationship will guide the dentist when a protrusive record is made in the patient's mouth. **B,** The patient rehearses closing in protrusive position, and the dentist observes the anteroposterior relation of the opposing anterior teeth and their alignment (between the upper and lower central incisors); this will be used as a guide for the amount and direction of protrusive movement. The movement should be similar to that observed on the articulator.

the protrusive position under the guidance of the dentist until both become familiar with the procedure (Figure 18-16, *B*).

A small amount of recording material that does not distort easily when set (impression plaster) is placed on the occlusal surfaces of the lower posterior teeth. Then, as in the practice sessions, the patient protrudes his mandible and closes into the recording material. The patient is instructed to stop the closure before the opposing teeth make contact and to hold the jaw lightly and steadily in the desired position until the recording material sets. The relationship of the lower to the upper anterior teeth in the patient's mouth should closely approximate the relationship observed on the articulator and during the rehearsal sessions.

The trial dentures and interocclusal record are removed from the mouth. The lateral condylar guidances on the upper member of the articulator are set at 20 degrees so they will not interfere if the mandible has not moved forward in straight protrusion and the horizontal condylar guidances are set at 0 degrees. Then the trial dentures and interocclusal protrusive record are returned to the articulator (Figure 18-17, *A*). The horizontal condylar housings are rotated individually until the guidance plates contact the condylar spheres (Figure 18-17,

B and *C*) and the angulation of the protrusive movement for both sides is recorded.

The advantages of the protrusive registration made in plaster, or a recording material of similar consistency, are that the resistance to the biting force is minimal and uniform and there is nothing that guides the patient's mandible except the memory patterns of mandibular protrusion and the instructions by the dentist. Also, the recording material will not be distorted during adjustment of the articulator. The disadvantage of plaster is related to the difficulty many patients experience in holding their mandibles in a steady protrusive position long enough for the material to set.

Protrusive Interocclusal Record for the Dentatus Articulator (Non-Arcon Type)

Three thicknesses of Aluwax are placed over the occlusal surfaces of the mandibular posterior teeth, rather than the two described for CR verification. The edges of the wax are sealed on both the buccal and the lingual sides with a warm spatula (Figure 18-18). The chilled upper trial denture should be placed in position on the upper cast mounted in the articulator.

Next, only the Aluwax portion of the lower trial denture is immersed in a water bath of 130° F (54° C)

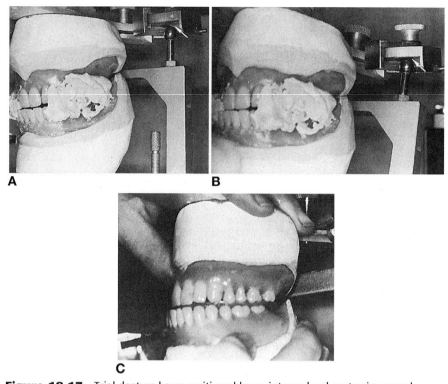

A   B

C

Figure 18-17 Trial denture bases positioned by an interocclusal protrusive record (impression plaster) are returned to the Whip Mix articulator. **A,** The horizontal condylar guidance mechanism is not in contact with the condylar sphere *(arrow).* **B,** The condylar mechanism is rotated into contact with the condylar sphere *(arrow),* thus establishing horizontal condylar guidance on the articulator. **C,** An interocclusal protrusive record has been made in wax, with the articulator adjusted as in **B.**

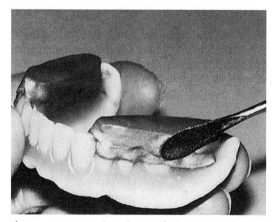

Figure 18-18 Three layers of Aluwax sealed with a warm spatula.

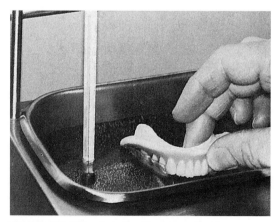

Figure 18-19 Only the Aluwax portion is immersed in 130° F (54° C) water for 30 seconds.

for 30 seconds (Figure 18-19). The lower trial denture is placed on the lower cast, and the articulator is set a quarter of an inch (6 mm) in protrusion with the condyle paths, registering 25 degrees. At this position, the upper member of the articulator is pressed into the warm wax to approximately a third of its depth. The mandibular trial denture is removed from the cast, and the wax record is chilled thoroughly.

Both trial dentures are now placed in the patient's mouth, and the patient is taught how to protrude into these indentations. The patient rehearses this protrusive action to prepare for making such a protrusive movement later when the wax is softened.

The mandibular trial denture is now removed from the mouth and the wax record is resoftened in hot water. Care is taken not to destroy the indentations.

The trial denture is reinserted into the mouth, and the patient is told to feel carefully and move into these markings in the manner rehearsed previously (Figure 18-20). (Instructions have already been given not to exert occlusal pressure into these indentations until told to do so.)

The position of the teeth relative to the indentations is carefully observed, and when the teeth coincide with these markings, the patient is instructed to bite, but not to bite through the wax.

As an alternative the patient can be instructed to relax his jaw muscles while the dentist elevates the mandible with the index finger placed beneath the inferior portion of the chin. With either approach, the anterior teeth should remain slightly out of contact to avoid any tooth interference.

The wax record is chilled in the mouth, removed, and examined for any contact between the teeth. The trial dentures are replaced on the articulator, and the articulator is protruded so the maxillary teeth will fit partially into the indentations. The locknuts for the condylar guidance slot adjustments are loosened. While pressure is exerted on the upper articulator member with one hand and the condylar guidance slot is worked back and forth with the other hand, a condylar path inclination is found that permits the teeth to stay in contact with the wax throughout (Figure 18-21). This adjustment is repeated for the opposite side. It will readily be seen that too steep a path prevents contact in the posterior part of the arch, and too horizontal a path prevents contact in the anterior part of the arch. As stated earlier, the correct degree of condylar path incline can be attained by tooth contact of the wax throughout the arch; the condylar guidance slot is locked in the position thus obtained.

A protrusive record is first made on the articulator so the correct amount of protrusive distance (which is also centered) will guide the patient's

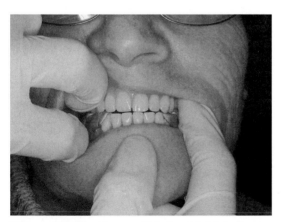

Figure 18-20   The mandible is guided into the index previously made on the articulator.

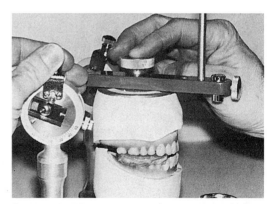

Figure 18-21   Pressure on the Dentatus articulator with one hand and back and forth movement of the condylar guidance slot with the other permit a condylar path inclination to be found that gives uniform contact of the wax index and opposing teeth.

mandible to the desired protrusive position. Unless the patient has a guide and has rehearsed, it will be extremely difficult to keep the mandible from closing too far or not far enough in protrusive occlusion, to the right or left in lateral occlusion, or in a combination of protrusion and lateral occlusion. Such a record will give an unsatisfactory setting to the articulator. The record is made with a protrusive distance a quarter of an inch (6 mm) because it is thought that with a shorter distance the condyle will not move down its path sufficiently to be recorded on the instrument. A protrusive movement of more than a quarter of an inch is usually beyond the range of the patient, and registration of a greater distance is not necessary.

An alternative procedure involves the use of impression plaster for making the protrusive interocclusal record, as described for the Whip Mix articulator.

ESTABLISHMENT OF THE POSTERIOR PALATAL SEAL

The posterior palatal seal is completed before the final arrangement of the posterior teeth because this final arrangement is a laboratory procedure and is done in the absence of the patient.

The posterior border of the denture is determined in the mouth, and its location is transferred onto the cast. A T burnisher, or mouth mirror, is pressed along the posterior, angle of the tuberosity until it drops into the pterygomaxillary (hamular) notch (Figure 18-22). The locations of the right and left pterygomaxillary notches are marked with an indelible pencil. On the median line of the anterior part of the soft palate are two indentations formed by the coalescence of ducts known as the foveae palatinae. The shape of these depressions varies from round or oval to oblong. The dentist can make them more readily discernible by having the patient hold his nose and attempt to blow through it (Valsalva maneuver). This will accentuate the foveae palatinae and vibrating line.

The vibrating line of the soft palate, normally used as a guide to the ideal posterior border of the denture, usually is located slightly anterior to the foveae palatinae. However, it may be on or slightly posterior to the foveae palatinae. The slight devia-

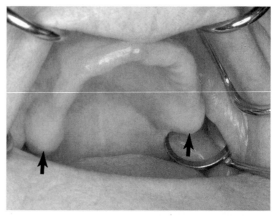

Figure 18-22   The pterygomaxillary (hamular) notch *(arrow)* in the mouth often is deceiving. To be certain of its location, the dentist can palpate it with a mouth mirror placed posterior to the tuberosity *(arrow)*.

tion from these markings is estimated by having the patient say "ah" and thus vibrate the soft palate. The dentist observes closely and marks the vibrating line with an indelible pencil (Figures 18-23 and 18-24). The two pterygomaxillary notch markings are joined to the median line mark. The trial denture base is now inserted so the indelible pencil line will

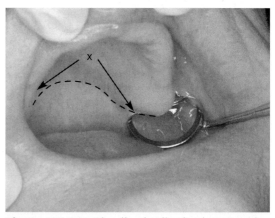

Figure 18-23   The vibrating line has been traced on the palatal tissues with indelible pencil. The *X* with arrows marks where it passes through the hamular notch on both sides slightly anterior to the foveae palatinae.

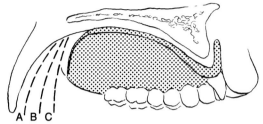

Figure 18-24 The vibrating line and width of the posterior palatal seal depend on the soft palate form (**A, B,** or **C**). Form **C** allows only a narrow posterior palatal seal; **A** allows the widest seal.

be transferred from the soft palate to the trial denture base, and the excess baseplate is reduced to this line (Figure 18-25). The trial denture base is placed on the cast, and a knife or pencil is used to mark a line following the posterior limits of the baseplate (Figure 18-26). This line should extend laterally 3 mm beyond the crest of the hamular notch.

The anterior line that indicates the location of the posterior palatal seal is drawn on the cast in front of the line indicating the end of the denture (Figure 18-27). The width of the posterior palatal seal itself is limited to a bead on the denture that is 1- to 1.5-mm high and 1.5-mm broad at its base (Figure 18-28). A greater width creates an area of tissue placement that will have a tendency to push the denture downward gradually and to defeat the purpose of the posterior palatal seal. In other words, the posterior palatal seal should not be made

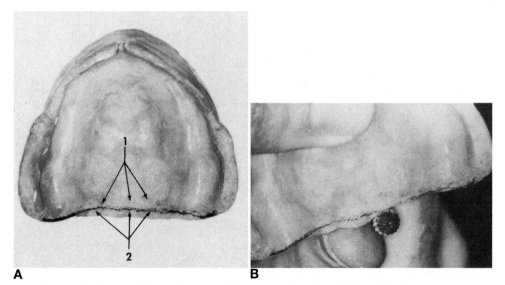

A
B

Figure 18-25 **A,** The indelible pencil line across the palate in Figure 18-23 has been transferred to the denture base and can be seen rather indistinctly *(1)*, anterior to the solid line marking the end of the denture *(2)*. **B,** The trial denture base is shortened posteriorly with an acrylic bur as far as this line.

Continued

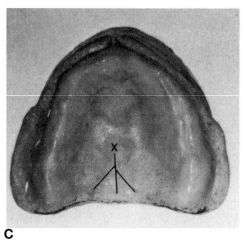

Figure 18-25 *cont'd* **C,** The trial denture base shows the anticipated length of the completed denture. *X* denotes the location of the vibrating line that was transferred from the patient's mouth.

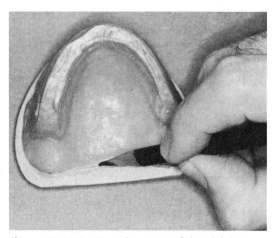

Figure 18-26 Posterior extent of the trial denture base traced on the cast.

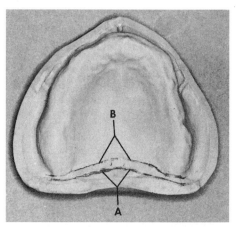

Figure 18-27 The posterior line *(A)* indicates the end of the denture posteriorly across the palate. The anterior line *(B)* marks the location of the posterior palatal seal that will be carved into the cast and transferred as a bead onto the denture.

too wide. Placement of tissue should be such that when the dentures move in function, as they always do, the placed tissue will move with the dentures and not break the seal.

A V-shaped groove 1- to 1.5-mm deep is carved into the cast at the location of the bead. A large, sharp scraper is used to carve it, passing through the hamular notches and across the palate of the

cast (Figures 18-29 and 18-30). The groove will form a bead on the denture that provides the posterior palatal seal (Figure 18-31). The bead will be 1- to 1.5-mm high, 1.5-mm wide at its base, and sharp at its apex. The depth of the groove in the cast will be determined by the thickness of the soft tissue

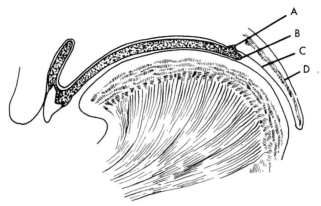

Figure 18-28   Sagittal diagrammatic view of denture in place in the mouth. A bead on the posterior extent *(A)* is 1 to 1.5-mm high and 1.5-mm broad at the base, and 2-mm anterior to the end of the denture *(B)*. *C*, Movable soft palate. *D*, Muscles of the soft palate.

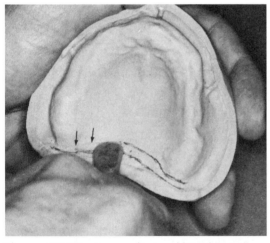

Figure 18-29   A groove is carved into the cast *(arrows)* with a large, sharp scraper to form the posterior palatal seal.

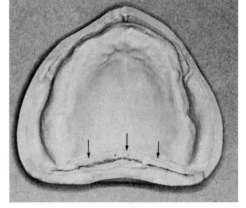

Figure 18-30   The groove in the cast *(arrows)* forms a bead on the finished denture (Figure 18-28).

against which it is placed and will establish the height of the bead.

The narrow and sharp bead will sink easily into the soft tissue to provide a seal against air being forced under the denture. If the bead has been made too high, the sharpness will make this apparent within 24 hours of the insertion of the dentures, and it can be easily relieved. The narrowness of the bead makes the seal with minimal downward pressure on the denture.

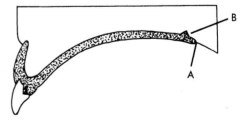

Figure 18-31   The denture ends on the cast at *A*. The bead *(B)*, located 2 mm in front of the vibrating line, is extended laterally through the center of the hamular notches.

SECTION III: CREATING FACIAL AND FUNCTIONAL HARMONY WITH ANTERIOR TEETH

The anatomical structures that collectively form the face normally develop concurrently and are interdependent during function throughout life. Disruptive events in this homeostatic complex can range from relatively minor changes, such as a deflective occlusal contact to major alterations in bodily form, such as removal of the natural teeth, which drastically affects the form and function of the remaining living parts.

In this context of homeostasis, creating facial and functional harmony with anterior teeth becomes a biological challenge of utmost significance. Not only must the teeth be of proper form, size, and color to harmonize with the face, but they also must become a functioning component in a living environment that depends on their proper position for its normal physiological activity. This proper position allows patients to preserve their facial identities as they existed when natural teeth were present. The ability of patients to maintain their normal facial expressions will likely be the most important psychological factor in acceptance of the dentures.

ANATOMY OF NATURAL APPEARANCE AND FACIAL EXPRESSION

The dentist who is treating a patient with complete dentures has as much to do with the beauty of the face as has any other medical specialist. The

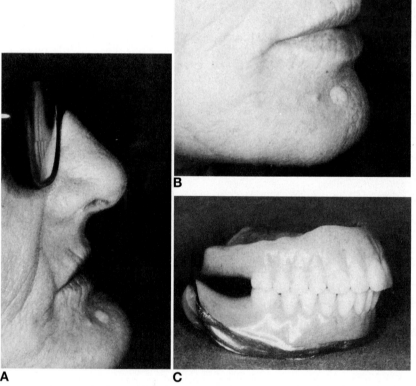

A   **C**

Figure 18-32 **A,** The lower part of this face lacks proper contour because of inadequate support for the orbicularis oris muscle and muscles related to it. **B,** Facial contours have been properly restored. The improvement in appearance is directly related to the position of the artificial teeth and the form of the suporting base material of the complete dentures **(C).**

appearance of the entire lower half of the face depends on the dentures. It is usually not difficult on casual meeting to detect the person who is wearing poorly constructed dentures (Figure 18-32). The characteristic thin, drooping upper lip that appears lengthened and has a reduced vermilion border is typical of malpositioned anterior teeth and probably a reduced vertical dimension of occlusion. Tense, wrinkled lips often reveal the patient's efforts to hold the denture in place. The drooping corners of the mouth tell the story of the misshapen and misplaced dental arch form of the anterior teeth, the thin denture borders, and often the reduced occlusal vertical dimension. The appearance of premature aging may be caused not by age itself but by the lack of support for the lips and cheeks due to the loss or improper replacement of teeth. The apparent extra fullness of the lower lip may be the result of too broad a mandibular dental arch or the elimination or reduction of the mentolabial sulcus. This may indicate that the lower anterior teeth have been placed too far lingually or that the labial flange of the lower denture base is overextended or too thick.

Normal Facial Landmarks

One must study normal facial landmarks before attempting to achieve the goal of a natural and pleasing facial expression with complete dentures. The facial landmarks of the lower third of the face have a direct relationship to the presence of the natural teeth (Figure 18-33). The contours of the lips depend on their intrinsic structure and the support for them provided by the teeth and the soft tissues or denture bases behind them. When the natural teeth are lost, these landmarks and surrounding facial tissues become distorted. To reestablish normal appearance and function, the dentist must replace the artificial teeth in the same position as the natural teeth that were lost.

The lips vary in length, thickness, shape, and mobility in different patients. Such variance accounts for the degree of visibility of the upper and lower anterior teeth during speech and other facial expressions. When the mandible is in the resting position, the lips usually contact each other and turn slightly outward, exposing the vermilion border. The vertical groove in the middle of the

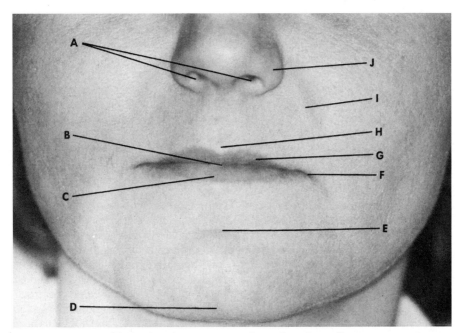

Figure 18-33   Facial landmarks. *A*, Nares; *B*, rima oris; *C*, lower lip; *D*, mentum; *E*, mentolabial sulcus; *F*, angulus oris; *G*, upper lip; *H*, philtrum; *I*, nasolabial sulcus; *J*, ala nasi.

upper lip is called the *philtrum,* and the horizontal depression midway between the lower vermilion border and the bottom of the chin is called the *mentolabial sulcus,* or groove (see Figure 18-33). Incorrect positioning of the anterior teeth or supporting base material of complete dentures will alter the normal appearance of the vermilion border, the philtrum, and the mentolabial sulcus in edentulous patients.

The *nasolabial sulcus,* or groove, is a depression in the skin on each side of the face, which runs angularly outward from the ala of the nose to approximately just outside the corners of the mouth (anguli oris) (see Figure 18-33). The zygomaticus muscle originates on the zygomatic bone and angles downward and forward to insert at the corner of the mouth into the orbicularis oris muscle. The action of the two zygomatici muscles in elevating the corners of the mouth for smiling produces the nasolabial sulcus (Figure 18-34). Many older patients want to have the nasolabial sulcus obliterated because it becomes a wrinkle as the skin loses resilience. Removal of the nasolabial fold has been attempted by thickening the denture base under the fold, but the extra bulk in this location causes a very unnatural appearance. The sulcus is normal and should not be eliminated. The proper treatment is to bring the entire upper dental arch forward to its original position when the natural teeth were present and to maintain the original arch form of the natural teeth and their supporting structures. Thus the prominence of the nasolabial sulcus will be restored to its original contour. In many patients, the corners of the lip line (rima oris) will be as high as the center portion, but the lip line will not necessarily be straight all the way across.

The upper lip rests on the labial surfaces of the upper anterior teeth, and the lower lip on the labial surfaces of the lower anterior teeth and incisal edges of the upper teeth. For this reason, the edge of the lower lip should extend outward and upward from the mentolabial sulcus. A reproduction of the horizontal overlap of the natural anterior teeth in the denture is essential to maintaining proper contour of the lips (Figure 18-35).

A study of the inclination of the osseous structure supporting the lower anterior teeth indicates that in most patients the clinical crowns of the lower teeth are labial to the bone that supports them. Likewise, a study of the inclination of osseous structure and the inclination of maxillary anterior teeth reveals that the upper lip functions on an incline (Figure 18-36). Neglect of these factors in the replacement of natural teeth often will cause the lip to be ill formed and, in time, lead to the formation of vertical lines in the lip.

Maintaining Facial Support and Neuromuscular Balance

The orbicularis oris muscle and its attaching muscles are important in denture construction inasmuch as the various contributing muscles have bony origins and their insertions are into the modioli and orbicularis oris muscle at the corners of the mouth (Figure 18-37). Thus the functioning length of all these muscles depends on the function of the orbicularis oris. The muscles that merge into the orbicularis oris are the zygomaticus, the quadratus labii superioris, the caninus (levator anguli oris), the mentalis, the quadratus labii inferioris, the triangularis (depressor anguli oris), the buccinator, and the risorius.

The orbicularis oris is the muscle of the lips. It is sphincterlike, attaching to the maxillae along a median line under the nose by means of a band of fibrous connective tissue known as the maxillary labial frenum and to the mandible on a median line by means of the mandibular labial frenum. The buccinator is a broad band of muscle forming the entire wall of the cheek from the corner of the mouth and passing along the outer surface of the maxilla and mandible until it reaches the ramus, where it passes to the lingual surface to join the superior constrictor of the pharynx at the pterygomandibular raphe (see Figure 18-37, *B*). The two buccinators and the orbicularis form a functional unit that depends on the position of the dental arches and the labial contours of the mucosa or the denture base for effective action. With the loss of teeth, the function of the orbicularis, buccinator, and attaching muscles is impaired. Because these muscles of expression are no longer supported at their physiological length, contraction of the unsupported fibers does not produce normal facial expression because the lips and face no longer move naturally or maybe even at all. Contraction simply takes up the droop in the fibers. However,

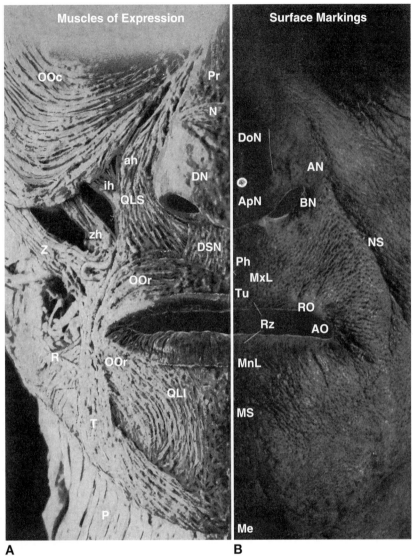

Figure 18-34   The polyfunctional pyramid. **A,** Underlying superficial musculature. *Ah,* Angular head; *DN,* dilator naris; *DSN,* depressor septi nasi; *ih,* infraorbital head; *N,* nasalis; *OOC,* orbicularis oculi; *OOR,* orbicularis oris; *P,* platysma; *Pr,* procerus; *QLI,* quadratus labii inferioris; *QLS,* quadratus labii superioris; *R,* risorius; *T,* triangularis; *Z,* zygomaticus; *ZH,* zygomatic head. **B,** Surface anatomy. *AN,* Ala nasi; *AO,* angulus oris; *ApN,* apex nasi; *BN,* basis nasi; *DoN,* Dorsum nasi; *Me,* mentum; *MnL,* mandibular lip; *MS,* mentolabial sulcus; *MxL,* maxillary lip; *NS,* nasolabial sulcus; *Ph,* philtrum; *RO,* rima oris; *RZ,* red zone or vermilion border; *Tu,* tubercle. (From Martone AL, Edwards : *J Prosthet Dent* 11:1009-1018, 1961.)

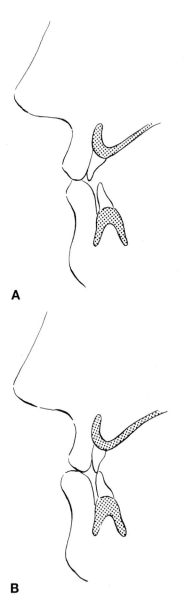

A

B

Figure 18-35 **A,** Reproduction of a patient's former horizontal overlap with the correct facial contour. **B,** Horizontal overlap changed so the maxillary anterior teeth contact the mandibular teeth, with resultant damage to the upper lip.

when these muscles are correctly supported by complete dentures, impulses coming to them from the central nervous system cause a shortening of the fibers that allows the face to move in a normal

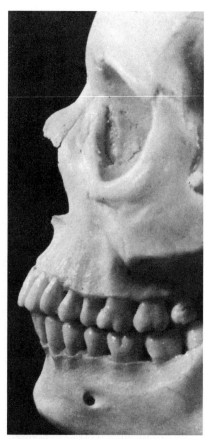

Figure 18-36 The incisal edges and labial surfaces of the lower anterior teeth are labial to the bone supporting them. The inclination of the labial plate of bone and the labial surfaces of the upper anterior teeth causes the upper lip to function on an incline. It is easy to observe the lack of support of the lip that will result when artificial anterior teeth are positioned over the crest of the residual ridge. Resorption of the alveolar process in the mandibular anterior region after removal of the anterior teeth will move the residual bony ridge lingually at first and then labially as resorption continues.

manner. Thus the memory patterns of facial expression developed within the neuromuscular system when the patient had natural teeth are continued or reinforced so the patient's original appearance is maintained (Figure 18-38).

Three factors affect the face in repositioning the orbicularis oris with complete dentures: (1) the thickness of the labial flanges of both dentures, (2) the anteroposterior position of the anterior teeth, and (3) the amount of separation between the mandible and the maxillae (Figure 18-39). If the jaws are closed too far, and the dental arch is located too far posteriorly, the upward and backward positioning of the orbicularis oris complex will move the insertions of these muscles closer to their origins. This will cause the muscles to sag when at rest and to be less effective when contracting. Such positions automatically drop the corners of the mouth, with a resultant senile edentulous expression, and may lead to atrophy of the muscle fibers.

The correct width of the maxillary denture borders plays a great part in supporting these muscles and lengthening the distance that they must extend to reach their insertion. If the mouth has

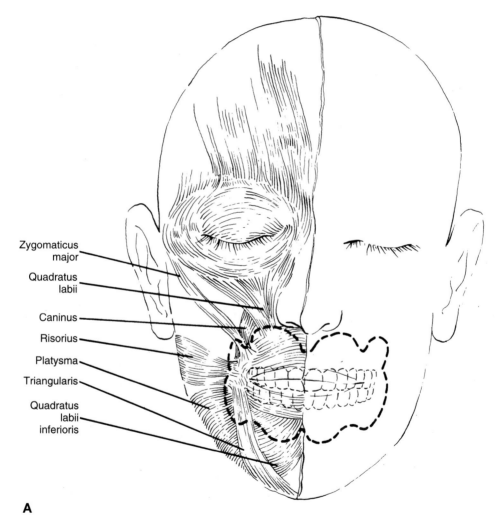

Zygomaticus major

Quadratus labii

Caninus

Risorius

Platysma

Triangularis

Quadratus labii inferioris

A

Figure 18-37 **A,** Muscles that maintain facial support. When artificial teeth and the denture base material restore the lips to their correct contour, the facial muscles will be at their physiological length, and contraction will create the normal facial expression of the patient.

Continued

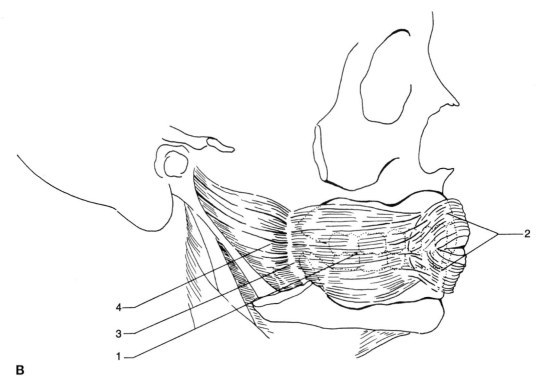

B

Figure 18-37 *cont'd* **B,** Functional unit of the buccinator. This muscle *(1)* and the orbicularis oris muscle *(2)* depend on the position of the upper denture for their proper action. *(3)* is the pterygomandibular raphe, and *(4)* is the superior constrictor of the pharynx.

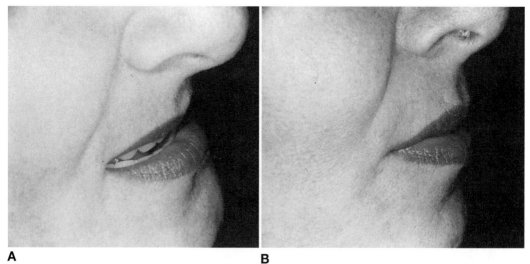

A   **B**

Figure 18-38 **A,** These lips are incorrectly contoured and are not moving naturally during speech. The lack of facial expression results from inadequate support of the lips by the anterior teeth, improper thickness of the labial flanges, and an inadequate vertical dimension of occlusion. **B,** The lips have been restored to correct contour with new dentures.

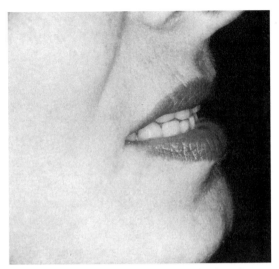

Figure 18-39 Notice the activity of the lips during speech when they are properly supported by new dentures. Compare this with the lack of activity in the same patient (Figure 18-38, A).

been edentulous a long time, with considerable resorption of the residual ridges, the borders need to be thick to restore the position of the muscles (Figure 18-40).

Repositioning anterior teeth that are protruding or slightly protruding to reduce their horizontal overlap and improve the appearance of the patient is a serious mistake. The muscles, teeth, and all associated structures grew simultaneously; therefore the physiological length of the muscles was determined early. In fact, the muscles of the face, cheeks, tongue, and lips helped align the natural teeth in the dental arches. To move teeth back in dentures is to invite a loss of

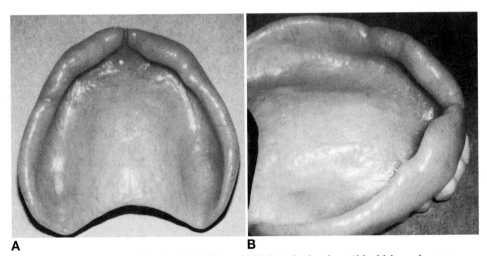

A   **B**

Figure 18-40 **A** and **B,** The labial flange is thick at the borders. This thickness harmonizes with the available space in the patient's mouth because of resorption of the upper residual ridge.

Continued

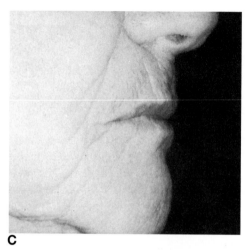

C

Figure 18-40 *cont'd* **C,** The bulk is needed for correct support of the upper lip.

facial expression that may be more damaging to the appearance of the patient than the slightly protruding teeth. Individual pronounced irregularities may be improved, as long as the position of the dental arch in its support of the orbicularis oris muscle and attaching muscles is not perceptibly altered.

Thus normal facial expression and proper tone of the skin of the face depend on the position and function of the facial muscles. These muscles can function physiologically only when the dentist has positioned and shaped the dental arches correctly and has given the mandible a favorable vertical position. In addition, the dentures themselves must have a pleasing and natural appearance in the patient's mouth, a condition that is dependent on arranging the artificial teeth in a plan that simulates nature. This, then, is the challenge of creating facial and functional harmony with anterior teeth.

BASIC GUIDES TO DEVELOPING FACIAL AND FUNCTIONAL HARMONY

After an acceptable vertical dimension of occlusion has been determined and the horizontal relation of the casts on the articulator has been verified for CR, the appearance of the patient is studied and modifications are made in the arrangement of the teeth to obtain a harmonious effect with the patient's face.

The guides that are considered in developing facial and functional harmony include the following:

1. The preliminary selection of artificial teeth
2. The horizontal orientation of anterior teeth
3. The vertical orientation of anterior teeth.
4. The inclination of anterior teeth
5. Harmony in the general composition of anterior teeth
6. Refinement of individual tooth positions
7. The concept of harmony with sex, personality, and age of the patient
8. The correlation of esthetics and incisal guidance

Although these factors are discussed individually, for simplicity they are interrelated in the actual clinical situation.

Preliminary Selection of the Artificial Teeth

The preliminary selection of teeth must be critically evaluated for size, form, and color as they have been arranged in the trial denture. The six upper anterior teeth, when properly supporting the upper lip, should be of sufficient overall width to extend in the dental arch to approximately the position of the corners of the mouth and still allow for individual irregularities of rotation, overlapping, and spacing. The canines should extend distally so they can be the turning point in the dental arch. The form of the teeth should be harmonious with the face but not necessarily identical with the outline form of the face. The color of the teeth should blend with the face so the teeth do not become the main focal point of the face. The anterior teeth are the principal ones to be considered in esthetics, although the posterior teeth, involving height of plane and width of arch, play their part also. Any records used in the initial selection of teeth should be consulted at this time to ensure that the desired result has been achieved (Plate 18-1). The dentist must make changes in the selection of teeth if such changes will improve the appearance of the dentures.

Horizontal Orientation of the Anterior Teeth

The position and expression of the lips and the lower part of the face are the best guides for determining the proper anteroposterior orientation of anterior teeth. The other guides or measurements are secondary and must be ultimately related to the appearance of the patient.

The greatest harm done in esthetics is setting the maxillary anterior teeth back to or under the ridge, regardless of the amount of resorption that has taken place. A study of the anterior alveolar process will disclose that its direction is upward and backward from the labial surface of the maxillary incisors (see Figure 18-36). Therefore the crest of the upper ridge is considerably more posterior in a resorbed

ridge than it was when the teeth were recently removed (Figure 18-41).

Insufficient support of the lips resulting from anterior teeth that are located too far posteriorly is characterized by a drooping or turning down of the corners of the mouth, a reduction in the visible part of the vermilion border, a drooping and deepening of the nasolabial grooves, small vertical lines or wrinkles above the vermilion border, a deepening of the sulci, and a reduction in the prominence of the philtrum (Figure 18-42, *A*).

A striking difference occurs when the anterior teeth are in proper position (Figure 18-42, *B*). The

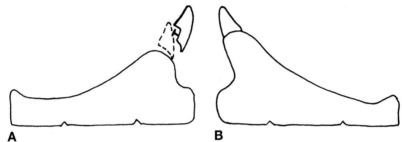

Figure 18-41 **A,** Correct positioning of an artificial central incisor to restore the physiological length of muscles for proper functioning. Dotted outline shows the tooth incorrectly positioned to follow the residual ridge. **B,** Position of the original natural central incisor.

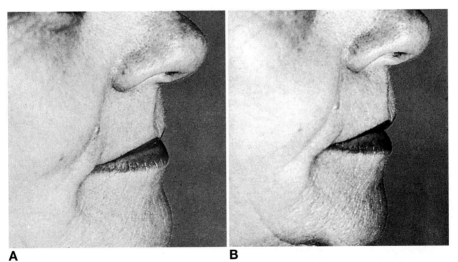

Figure 18-42 **A,** Artificial anterior teeth positioned too far posteriorly. Notice the lack of tone in the skin of the upper lip. **B,** Artificial anterior teeth positioned correctly in an anteroposterior direction. Notice the improved skin tone.

vermilion borders become visible, the corners of the mouth assume a normal contour, many of the small vertical lines above the vermilion of the upper lip are reduced or eliminated, and the tone of the skin surrounding the dentures takes on a character similar to that of the skin in other parts of the face not affected by the position of the teeth. Although the nasolabial groove will still be present, the drooping appearance often can be considerably reduced. Nasolabial grooves should not be eliminated, and the dentist must be careful about the information the patient receives in this regard. However, patients should be informed as to the other improvements that can be made by the dentures that will produce a more youthful appearance.

Excessive lip support resulting from anterior teeth located too far anteriorly is characterized by a stretched tight appearance of the lips, a tendency for the lips to dislodge the dentures during function, elimination of the normal contours of the lips, and distortion of the philtrum and sulci (Figure 18-43). A photograph of the patient with natural teeth can be most helpful in the placing of artificial teeth. The teeth can be so arranged that the appearance and contours of the lips and lower part of the face resemble those seen in the picture (see Plate 18-1, *C*).

The relation of the maxillary and mandibular anterior ridges to each other has an influence on the anteroposterior position of both the maxillary and the mandibular anterior teeth. A common error is to attempt to establish a standard vertical and horizontal overlap without regard to the ridge relation. This should not be done because the anteroposterior position of the teeth must correspond to the positions of the ridges. If the mandibular ridge is forward of the maxillary ridge, as in prognathism, the upper anterior teeth should be placed lingual to the mandibular teeth. The anterior teeth can then be set end to end, with the incisal edges at an angle that produces a seating action on the maxillary denture (Figure 18-44).

A study of the position of natural teeth on diagnostic casts will provide information that can be transferred to the arrangement of artificial anterior teeth. As mentioned previously, the upper lip functions on an incline produced by the labial plate of the alveolar process and the crowns of the upper anterior teeth. The position of the natural anterior teeth makes their labial surfaces at least as far forward as the labial most part of the reflection (Figure 18-45, *A*). This information can be transferred to the position of the artificial anterior teeth on the trial denture base. Such a guide also will be helpful in con-

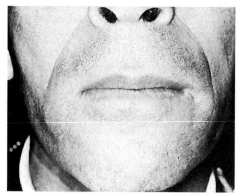

Figure 18-43   A stretched appearance of the lips and philtrum indicates that artificial anterior teeth are positioned too far anteriorly.

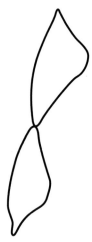

Figure 18-44   Correct inclination of the teeth and incisal edges in a moderate prognathic relation.

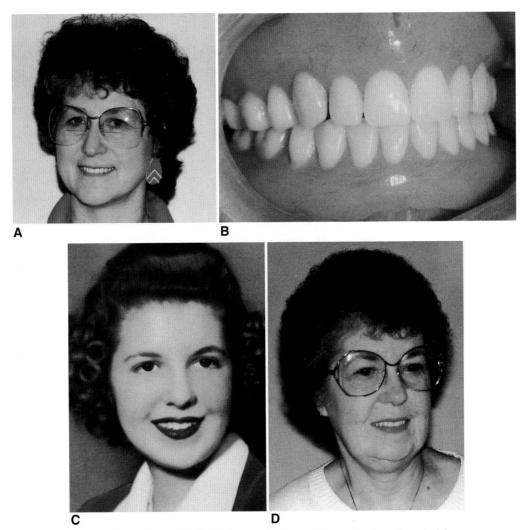

Plate 18-1 The teeth used for both these patients are Vitapan hard acrylic resin (Vita Zahnfabrik, Bad Säckingen, FRG). **A** and **B,** With preextraction records as a guide, this patient's upper canines are shade A3.5, but her other anterior and posterior teeth are A2. Frequently, the upper natural canines will be darker than the other teeth. **C** and **D,** Her high school graduation picture, showing her natural teeth, was used as a guide in selecting arranging the anterior teeth for replacement dentures at age 64.

Continued

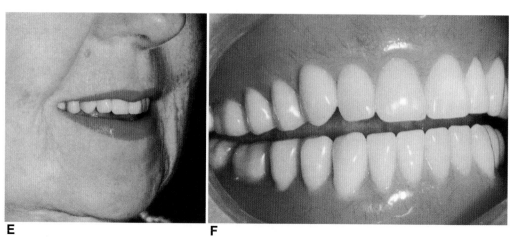

Plate 18-1 *cont'd* **E** and **F,** She requested a light shade, which was used, with a pleasing result.

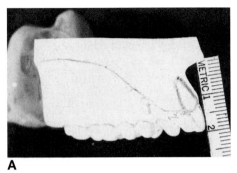

A

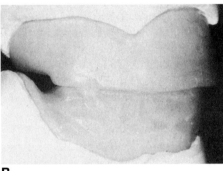

B

Figure 18-45   A, Relation of the labial surface of the natural central incisor to the reflection in a sectioned cast. **B,** The inclination of the labial surfaces of wax occlusion rims should simulate the inclination observed in the natural situation. When the occlusion rims slope lingually toward the occlusal surface in the anterior region, they will rarely if ever provide proper support for the lips.

touring the occlusion rims (Figure 18-45, *B*) and in developing the preliminary arrangement of anterior teeth.

Observing the position of the anterior teeth when the trial denture base is out of the mouth can be helpful. The labial surfaces of many natural upper central incisors are approximately 8 to 10 mm in front of the middle of the incisive papilla. Measurements with a Boley gauge from the middle of the incisive fossa on the trial denture base to the labial surfaces of the artificial central incisors will show the relationship of these teeth to the incisive papilla (Figure 18-46, *A*).

When the trial denture bases are viewed from the tissue-contacting surface, the labial portions of the

anterior teeth should be apparent, and a visualization of their imaginary roots can be helpful. If the imaginary roots appear to be on the labial side of the residual ridge (with allowance made for bone loss from that part of the ridge), the anterior teeth will be very near to their correct labiolingual positions. If the imaginary roots appear to extend into the crest of the residual ridge, the artificial teeth are positioned too far posteriorly on the trial denture base (Figure 18-46, *B*). The location of the incisive fossa in relation to the crest of the ridge gives an indication of the amount of resorption of the upper residual ridge: the greater the resorption, the farther in front of the crest the imaginary roots should appear.

An imaginary transverse line between the upper canines, as viewed from the tissue-contacting surface of the upper trial denture base, should cross near the middle of the incisive fossa when anterior teeth of the proper size are located correctly in the anteroposterior position (Figure 18-46, *C*). If the line falls anterior to the incisive fossa, the overall width of the anterior teeth may be too small or the teeth may be positioned too far forward. If the line falls posterior to the papilla, the overall width of the anterior teeth may be too large or the teeth positioned too far back.

Vertical Orientation of the Anterior Teeth

The amount of the upper anterior teeth seen during speech and facial expression depends on the length and movement of the upper lip in relation to the vertical length of the dental arch. If the upper lip is relatively long, the natural teeth may not be visible when the lip is relaxed or even during speech (Figure 18-47, *A*); however, in this situation some teeth may be exposed when the person smiles. In other patients, with a relatively short upper lip, the full crowns may be visible below the upper lip (Figure 18-47, *B*). In some of these patients, a large amount of the mucous membrane (or denture base), in addition to the teeth, may be exposed when they smile.

Furthermore, the movement of the lips during function varies considerably among patients. Therefore when artificial teeth are placed in the same position as the natural teeth, the amount of

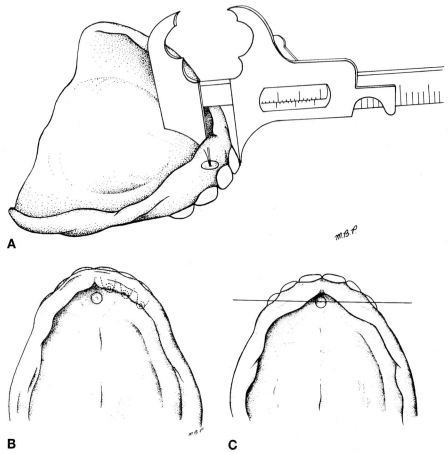

Figure 18-46 Indications of correct anteroposterior positioning of artificial anterior teeth. **A,** By measurement from the middle of the incisive fossa on the trial denture base to the labial surfaces of the central incisors. **B,** By visualization of the imaginary roots of artificial anterior teeth—the imaginary roots will be farther in front of the residual ridge when a great amount of resorption has occurred. **C,** By determining the relationship of a transverse line extending between the middle of the upper canines and the incisive fossa.

upper teeth visible will vary for each patient. During a normal smile, the incisal and middle thirds of the maxillary anterior teeth are visible in almost all patients and the cervical third in approximately half the patients. The incisal third of the mandibular anterior teeth will be visible in most patients. Mandibular anterior teeth are seen to a greater extent than maxillary anterior teeth in about half the patients during speaking. In addition, mandibular anterior teeth become more visible in persons

40 years of age and older and are seen to a greater extent in men than in women.

A simple test can be used to estimate the length of the upper lip in relation to the residual ridges. The index finger is placed on the incisive papilla with the relaxed upper lip extending down over the finger (Figure 18-47, *C*). The amount of the finger covered by the upper lip gives an indication of the length of the lip relative to the residual ridge and the extent to which it will cover the upper anterior teeth (Figure 18-47, *D*). An estimation of the amount of residual ridge resorption must be included in the calculation. Knowing the length of time the natural teeth have been out will help make this estimate.

However, the lower lip is a better guide for the vertical orientation of anterior teeth than the upper lip is. In most patients, the incisal edges of the natural lower canines and the cusp tips of the lower first premolars are even with the lower lip at the corners of the mouth when the mouth is slightly open (Figure 18-48, *A*). If artificial lower anterior teeth are located above or below this level, their vertical positioning will probably be incorrect

(Figure 18-48, *B*). In addition to any changes in position of the lower teeth, the position of the upper teeth and the vertical dimension of occlusion must be considered because these are all closely interrelated. When the lower teeth are above the lip at the corners of the mouth, any one or a combination of the following may exist: (1) the plane of occlusion may be too high; (2) the vertical overlap of the anterior teeth may be too much; and (3) the vertical space between the jaws may be excessive. When the lower teeth are below the lip at the corners of the mouth, the opposite situations may exist. The use of other observations and guides will help in deciding what corrections should be made.

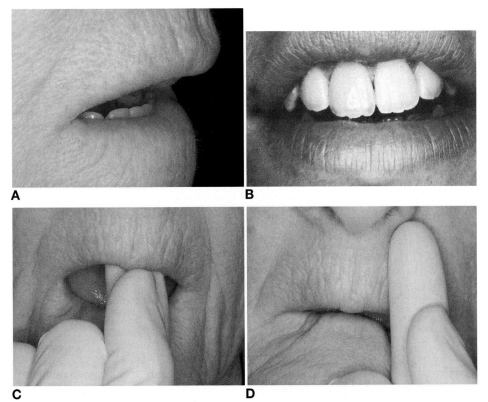

A   **B**   **C**   **D**

Figure 18-47   A, This long upper lip obscures the natural upper anterior teeth even during speech. **B,** A relatively short upper lip exposes almost all the crowns of the upper central and lateral incisors. **C,** The upper lip is allowed to drape over the index finger, which has been placed on the incisive papilla. The thumb is in contact with the vermilion border. **D,** The amount of index finger that has been covered by the upper lip is an indication of the length of the upper lip relative to the upper residual ridge.

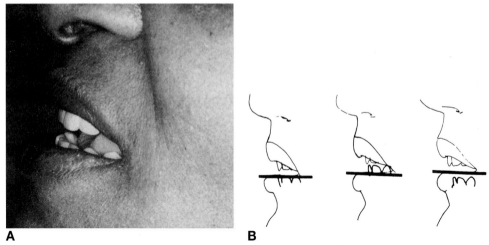

Figure 18-48 **A,** Incisal edge of the natural lower canine at the level of the lower lip. **B,** Relationship of artificial lower teeth to the lower lip. *Left,* correct height; *middle,* too high; *right,* too low.

Observing the size of the trial denture bases can give clues to the vertical orientation of the anterior teeth. In most patients, the lower and upper natural teeth occupy approximately the same amount of interarch space. If the dimensions of the lower trial denture, from the border of the base to the incisal edges of the teeth, appear to be significantly different from the same measurements on the upper trial denture, then the plane of occlusion may need to be raised or lowered to make the trial dentures more similar in height (Figure 18-49). These measurements are made from the incisal edges to the denture borders. The vertical space between the jaws (vertical dimension of occlusion) must also be considered because of its close interrelationship with the plane of occlusion. If there has been more shrinkage from one jaw than from the other, the amounts of base material between the incisal ends of the teeth and the basal surface of the denture may be different, even though the overall dimensions are similar.

A study of the location of artificial anterior teeth and their imaginary roots, in relation to the residual ridges on the trial denture bases, can help determine the position of the teeth. The artificial anterior teeth should be located vertically in the same positions as were previously occupied by the natural teeth. When it appears as though there is insufficient interarch space to accommodate the upper and lower anterior teeth without significantly reducing their size by grinding, it is good to remember that at one time there was space for the natural teeth, with an adequate interocclusal distance in the patient's mouth. Insufficient space between the residual ridges is an indication that either the artificial teeth are longer than the natural teeth or the vertical dimension of the face is too short.

Inclination of the Anterior Teeth

In some patients, the upper anterior teeth are inclined labially relative to the frontal plane when the head is erect (Frankfort plane parallel to the floor). In others, they are inclined more lingually (Figure 18-50, *A*). Diagnostic casts, photographs, and the patient's memories about the "slant of the upper front teeth" can help solve the problem concerning the inclination of the natural teeth.

A study of teeth in human skulls indicates that the roots of the anterior teeth are parallel to and very close to the labial surface of the bone. Usually, there is an obtuse angle between the bone and the labial surfaces of the teeth. In some skulls, the labial

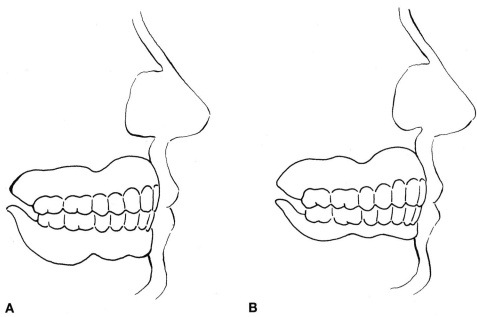

Figure 18-49 **A,** Upper and lower dentures of approximately the same height. **B,** Upper denture considerably larger than the lower. Often this discrepancy in size indicates an incorrect vertical positioning of the artificial teeth.

surfaces of the teeth are parallel to the bone but also slope labially. When the labial surfaces are curved from cervical to incisal, the cervical third may appear to be continuous with the inclination of the labial plate of bone (Figure 18-50, *B*). Diagnostic casts support this premise. When the natural teeth are removed with no unnecessary surgery, the original inclination of the labial plate of bone is preserved and will remain until considerable resorption has occurred, thus providing a guide to the inclination of the anterior teeth (Figure 18-50, *C*). The inclination of the labial surface of the residual ridges as seen on edentulous casts can supply this information.

The profile form of the patient's face often is representative of the natural anterior tooth inclination within the oral cavity. The lips supply the pressures from the outside that help determine the anteroposterior position and inclination of the anterior teeth. Therefore it is logical to assume that the inclination of the anterior teeth parallels the profile line of the face (Figure 18-51). Suggestions for individual tooth position to provide harmony between the inclination of the teeth and the profile line of the face are described later.

Harmony in the General Composition of Anterior Teeth

A number of factors are interrelated in the general composition of the anterior teeth for a normal and pleasing appearance. Although these factors vary among patients, there is sufficient constancy to warrant individual attention. The topics to be discussed in providing harmony within the general composition of the anterior teeth include (1) harmony of the dental arch form and the form of the residual ridge, (2) harmony of the long axes of the central incisors and the face, (3) harmony of the teeth with the smiling line of the lower lip, (4) harmony of the opposing lines of the labial and buccal surfaces, (5) harmony of the teeth and profile line, and (6) harmony of incisal wear and age.

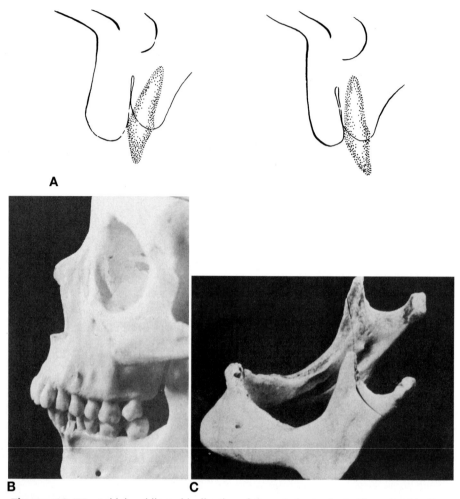

Figure 18-50 Labial and lingual inclination of the anterior teeth. **A,** The natural teeth have varying degrees of inclination. **B,** Notice the inclination and position of the anterior teeth in relation to the inclination of the labial plate of bone. **C,** The inclination of this lower residual ridge provides the information that the lower anterior teeth, which it once supported, had a labial inclination.

Harmony of the Dental Arch Form and Form of the Residual Ridge The anterior arches may be classified in a general way as square, tapering, and ovoid, to follow the form of the dental arch when the teeth are present (Figure 18-52). However, they cannot be closely classified as such because of the frequent intermingling of the characteristics of one form with those of another.

The central incisors in the square arch assume a position more nearly on a line with the canines than in any other setup. The four incisors have little rotation because the square arch is wider than the tapering arch. This gives a broader effect to the teeth and should harmonize with a broad, square face (Figure 18-53, *A*).

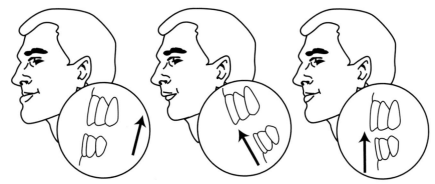

Figure 18-51   The inclination of anterior teeth often parallels the profile line of the lower third of the face.

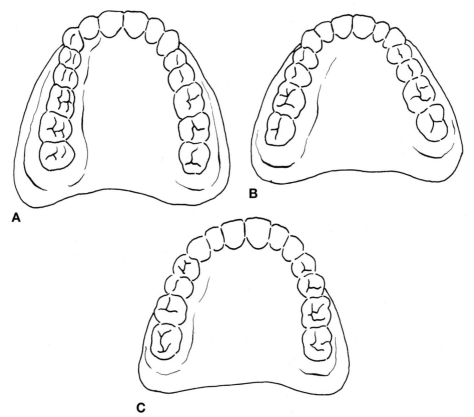

Figure 18-52   Varying shapes of the natural dental arch. **A,** Square. **B,** Tapering. **C,** Ovoid.

The central incisors in the tapering arch are a greater distance forward from the canines than in any other arch. There usually is considerable rotating and lapping of the teeth in the tapering arch because of less space. Therefore crowding results. The rotated positions reduce the amount of tooth surface showing, and the teeth do not appear as wide as in other setups. This narrowed effect is usually in harmony with a narrower tapering face (Figure 18-53, B). In fact, the very narrowness of the tapered arch contributes to the narrowness and taper of the face. Natural teeth move in function, and this frictional movement wears the contact areas. Artificial teeth need to be ground on these corresponding contact areas to allow the necessary rotational positions and give the desired effect of a tapering setup.

The central incisors in the ovoid arch are forward of the canines in a position between that of the square and that of the tapering arch. The teeth in this form of arch are seldom rotated, and they therefore show a greater amount of labial surface than in the tapering setup and, as a result, have a broader effect that should harmonize with an ovoid face (Figure 18-53, C).

The form of the palatal vault gives an indication as to the original form of the dental arch before removal of the natural teeth and resorption of the residual ridge. A broad and shallow edentulous palatal vault indicates that the dental arch form originally may have been square; a high, V-shaped edentulous vault probably indicates a tapering dental arch, and a rounded vault of average height may indicate an ovoid dental arch. Most patients exhibit some combination of these classifications.

The arch form of the artificial anterior teeth should be similar in shape to the arch form of the residual ridge, if one assumes there was no unnecessary surgery when the anterior teeth were removed (Figure 18-54). This simple anatomical fact often is neglected, but it should be observed carefully. When the anterior teeth are arranged in an arch form that corresponds to the form of the residual ridge, natural-appearing irregularities that may have been present in the patient's mouth will often be reproduced.

Changing the shape and position of the artificial dental arch away from the form of the natural arch causes a highly unsatisfactory loss of face form and expression. A square arch form where the natural arch was more tapering will cause a stretching of

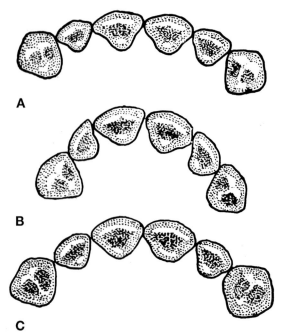

Figure 18-53   Anterior arch forms. **A,** Square. **B,** Tapering. **C,** Ovoid.

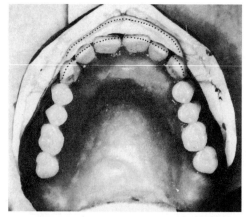

Figure 18-54   Dotted lines indicate that the arch form of artificial anterior teeth on the trial denture base is basically similar to that of the anterior part of the residual ridge.

the lips, with elimination of the natural philtrum. A tapering arch form where the natural dental arch was square will not adequately support the corners of the mouth for proper facial expressions.

The shape and position of the dental arch determine the size of the buccal corridor. The buccal corridor is the space between the buccal surfaces of the upper teeth and the corners of the mouth visible when the patient smiles. It varies considerably among patients, and its size is not critical. However, the presence of the buccal corridor helps eliminate an appearance of too many teeth in the front of the mouth. When the arch form of the posterior teeth is too wide or the lips do not move to their full extent during smiling because of improper support, the size of the buccal corridor will be reduced or perhaps eliminated (Figure 18-55).

Patients may request a change in the position or form of their dental arch, but the dentist should not compromise on this point because the unfavorable consequences can be laid to no one else.

Harmony of the Long Axes of the Central Incisors and Face

One of the early observations that

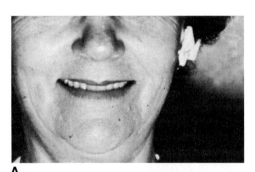

A

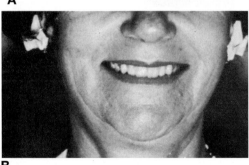

B

Figure 18-55 **A,** Buccal corridor inadequate because of improper placement of the upper teeth. **B,** Anterior teeth in proper position to support the upper lip. Notice the adequate buccal corridor.

should be made in developing the arrangement of anterior teeth for the patient is the relationship of the long axes of the central incisors to the long axis of the face. When the long axes of these teeth are not in harmony with the long axis of the face, the arrangement will not blend with the face because the incisal plane of the anterior teeth will not be parallel to the interpupillary line (Figure 18-56, *A*). This will cause an unpleasant disharmony of lines. It is a simple task to reset the central incisors to make their long axes harmonize with the long axis of the face (Figure 18-56, *B*). If the central incisors must be divergent at their incisal edges, the midline of the dental arch should be at the center of the face. Then the lateral incisors and canines will almost automatically fall into their proper alignment, and the incisal plane will be in balance with the interpupillary line.

The long axes of the central incisors should be parallel to the long axis of the face, and the midline of the dental arch (the contact area between the central incisors) should be located near the middle of the face. This is determined by dropping an imaginary perpendicular line from the midpoint on the interpupillary line. The midline position of the natural central incisors can be estimated also by observing the position of the incisive papilla on the cast and the corresponding fossa in the upper trial denture base because the incisive papilla was located lingually and between the natural upper central incisors before their extraction.

The midline of the mandibular dental arch is between the central incisors and usually is aligned with the midline of the maxillary central incisors. When the lower anterior teeth are correctly located anatomically in the lower dental arch, an imaginary line drawn anteroposteriorly through the middle of the lower denture should pass between the lower central incisors (Figure 18-57). The maxillary and mandibular midlines fail to coincide in most adults with natural teeth, however, so the prosthodontist must attempt to set the artificial teeth to coincide with this imaginary midline.

The application of these principles regarding the placement of central incisors and their inclinations may be modified to meet individual needs as indicated by preextraction records.

Harmony of the Teeth with the Smiling Line of the Lower Lip

When a person smiles, the lower

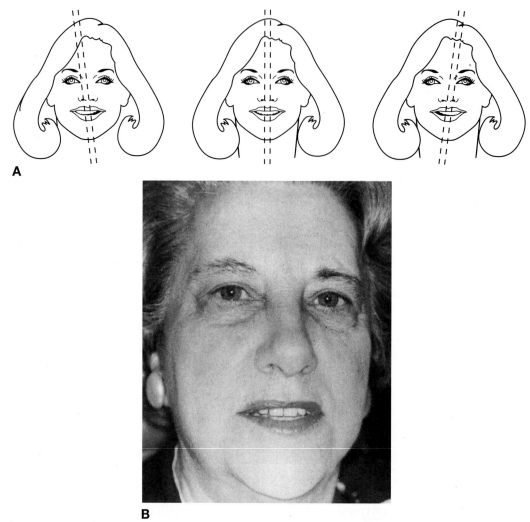

Figure 18-56 The long axes of the central incisors should be parallel to the long axis of the face. **A,** The middle drawing shows that such parallelism provides a necessary harmony of lines. Notice the disharmony of the left and right. **B,** The long axes of the artificial central incisors have been correctly aligned.

lip forms a pleasant curvature known as the smiling line. This can be used as a guide in arranging the upper anterior teeth.

When the line formed by the incisal edges of the upper anterior teeth follows the curved line of the lower lip during smiling, the two lines will be harmonious and will create a pleasing appearance. When the incisal edges of the upper anterior teeth

form a curved line that is not in harmony with, or is opposite in contour to, the line formed by the lower lip during a smile, the contrast of the lines is disharmonious and will be displeasing in appearance (Figure 18-58, *A*).

The vertical position of the upper canines is primarily responsible for the shape of the smiling line. When the canines are so arranged that their incisal

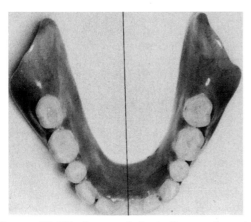

Figure 18-57   Lower anterior teeth correctly positioned, as shown by the imaginary line passing through the middle of this lower denture between the lower central incisors.

edges are slightly shorter than the incisal edges of the lateral incisors, the smiling line will tend to parallel the lower lip as the patient smiles (Figure 18-58, *B*). A reverse smiling line is one of the most frequent causes of artificial-appearing dentures.

Harmony of the Opposing Lines of Labial and Buccal Surfaces   Setting teeth with their long axes parallel to each other is what causes people to dread complete dentures because the appearance is artificial. Many patients are subconsciously irritated by this artificial appearance of dentures and

tend to find other faults with them that would otherwise be overlooked.

A well-balanced painting or drawing must have lines at opposing angles as well as some parallel lines. The same principle applies to having a pleasing picture of the teeth. For example, if the teeth on both sides of the arch were inclined to be parallel to each other, they would make a most unsatisfactory-appearing denture. There should be asymmetrical symmetry in the arrangement of the teeth (Figure 18-59).

The labial and buccal lines must have opposing equivalent angles, or nearly so, for a harmonious effect. If the maxillary right lateral incisor is set at an angle of 5 degrees to the perpendicular, the lateral incisor on the left side should be set 5 degrees to the perpendicular in the opposite direction. The scheme of opposing angles can be carried to the maxillary canines and the mandibular opposing canines (see Figure 18-59). Deviation in angulation may also be arranged in different teeth on the two sides. Extra inclination of a lateral incisor on one side may be balanced by inclination of the opposite canine; asymmetrical symmetry is the objective.

There should be harmony between the labial and buccal lines of the teeth and the lines of the face. Square and ovoid faces should have teeth with lines that are more nearly perpendicular, whereas tapering faces should have teeth with lines that are more divergent from the perpendicular.

An optical illusion may be created for patients who have a nasal deflection. Four of the maxillary

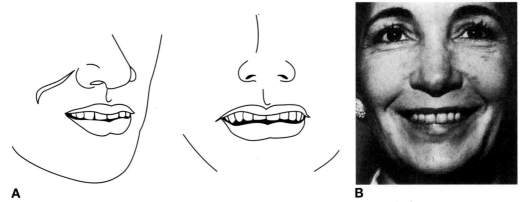

A   **B**

Figure 18-58   Harmony of the line formed by the incisal edges of the upper anterior teeth with that formed by the curvature of the lower lip. **A,** Lines in harmony *(left)* and not in harmony *(right)*. Results are a pleasing and a displeasing appearance. **B,** Notice the harmony in this face.

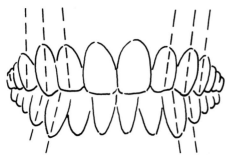

Figure 18-59 Balanced opposing lines. Dissimilarities in the inclination, rotation, and position of the teeth on each side of the midline provide what is called *asymmetrical symmetry,* which is essential for natural-appearing teeth.

teeth can be set at an opposite angle to the deviation, making it less apparent.

Harmony of the Teeth and Profile Line of the Face As a general rule, the labial surfaces of the maxillary central incisors are parallel to the profile line of the face. In prognathic patients with protruding mandibular incisors, the incisal edges of the maxillary teeth are out farther than the cervical ends of the teeth. In the opposite condition (in which the mandibular incisors are retruded to some extent), the incisal edges of the maxillary teeth are inclined lingually more than the cervical ends of the teeth (Figure 18-60).

When the labial of the maxillary central incisors is parallel to the profile line of the face, the lat-

eral incisors should be set at an opposite angle to prevent parallelism from being predominant. For example, in a patient with retrognathic jaw relations whose maxillary central incisors are out at the cervical ends, the lateral incisors could then be depressed at their cervical ends to oppose the line made by the labial surfaces of the central incisors. For the prognathic patient, the incisal edges of the maxillary central incisors often are set labially. The maxillary lateral incisors could then be placed slightly out at the cervical ends to oppose the labial face line of the central incisors.

Most faces are a blend of two or three types of profiles. Arrangement of teeth for a harmonious appearance must be modified accordingly. The predominating facial form can be helpful as a guide for positioning the teeth.

Harmony of Incisal Wear and Age The incisal edges and proximal surfaces of anterior teeth wear concomitantly with age. This is another characteristic of natural teeth that must be incorporated in artificial teeth if they are to appear in harmony with the age of the patient. The incisal edges of denture teeth should always be ground to simulate the wear surfaces that would have developed by the time the patient reached his current age. Therefore a young patient would likely exhibit less incisal wear (Figure 18-61, *A*), and an older one more wear (Figure 18-61, *B*).

A sketch of the anticipated pattern of wear to be placed on the incisal edges of anterior teeth can be

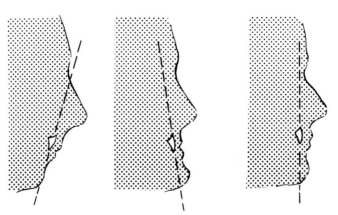

Figure 18-60 The labial face of the central incisor parallels the profile line of the face. Notice how the incisal third of the tooth breaks lingually from the profile line.

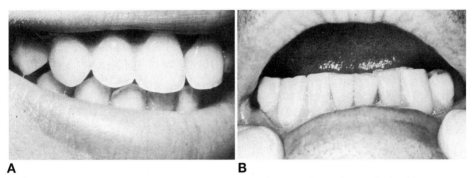

A   **B**

Figure 18-61   The amount of wear on the incisal edges of anterior teeth should concur with the patient's age. **A,** Lack of wear is compatible with youth. **B,** Extreme wear indicates a much older person.

beneficial. The outline form of the artificial teeth is sketched on a piece of paper, and the anticipated changes that are to be created to simulate wear on the incisal edges are depicted on the drawing (Figure 18-62). In general, more lingually placed upper teeth or parts of teeth will wear increasingly, whereas more labially placed upper teeth will wear somewhat less. The greatest amount of wear on the lower anterior teeth or parts of teeth will occur in the more anteriorly placed lower teeth. The simulation of wear on anterior teeth should be logically in harmony with the way it occurs when the upper and lower teeth pass over each other.

Developing incisal wear on artificial teeth during balancing and correcting of the occlusion is a logical approach to this phase of esthetics. Thus wear is placed on the teeth where it would have occurred during function and also where it assists in the mechanics of balancing the occlusion (Figure 18-63).

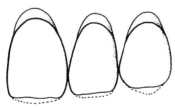

Figure 18-62   A simple sketch by the dentist of the outline form of artificial teeth will be helpful in planning the incisal wear to be incorporated for a particular patient. Dotted line shows the original appearance of the incisal edges of artificial teeth; solid line shows the incisal wear anticipated.

The effect that the form of the tooth creates can be dramatically altered by reshaping the tooth to simulate wear. The same mold of anterior teeth can be altered to help create a young, soft, feminine appearance for one patient or an older, vigorous, masculine appearance for another (Figure 18-64, *A*).

Most patients who need dentures are at an age when the contact areas of their natural teeth have been worn, whether or not the teeth overlap each other. Therefore the artificial teeth should be so altered that they do not have the appearance of ball contact points with large interproximal spaces. If the teeth selected have contact points that resemble those of a young person's teeth, they should be ground to provide a more natural appearance (Figure 18-64, *B*).

Refinement of Individual Tooth Positions

One of the essential factors in satisfying patients with complete dentures is that the dentures be pleasing and natural in appearance. Dentures are not pleasing unless the teeth are arranged in a plan that nature developed. If patients have some anterior teeth remaining, diagnostic casts should be made as preextraction records to be used in selecting and arranging the individual teeth. If dentists use preextraction records in construction of many dentures, they soon will learn nature's scheme in arranging teeth for patients who have lost all teeth before a record was made. With patients for whom no preextraction records are available, dentists can select another cast of natural teeth and follow this arrangement as a guide.

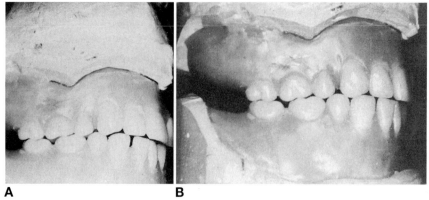

Figure 18-63 **A,** Incisal wear on artificial teeth. **B,** The pattern of wear in **A** has been developed to improve the appearance of the denture and assist in balancing the occlusion. Wear on the upper canine is placed to correspond with wear on the lower canine in a balanced occlusion.

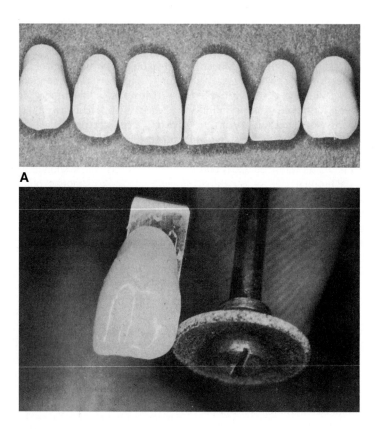

Figure 18-64 **A,** One mold of teeth has been modified so the three teeth on the left depict youth and femininity, whereas the three on the right are suitable for an older masculine individual. **B,** The contact areas and incisal edges of artificial teeth must be modified to provide a natural appearance.

The selection and placing of artificial teeth will not appear natural unless the teeth are set with typical inclinations and rotations that the eye has been accustomed to seeing. These inclinations and rotations can cause the same teeth to appear as oversized or normal. For example, if the canine is rotated so the eye sees only its mesial half, the tooth will look only half as large as it would if its entire labial surface were visible to the eye. Lateral and central incisors, especially in a tapering setup, do not show the entire labial surface when seen from directly in front. This reduction in the amount of surface showing harmonizes with a tapering face.

A beginning point for studying the labiolingual inclination of the maxillary anterior teeth in relation to the perpendicular is shown in Figure 18-65. The labial surface of the maxillary central incisor is parallel to the profile line of the face, which is almost perpendicular. The labial surface of the lateral incisor is angled in at the cervical end more than that of the adjacent tooth. The labial surface of the canine is angled out at the cervical end more than that of any other maxillary anterior tooth. The degree to which the cervical end of the canine extends outward usually harmonizes with the lateral lines of the face. The labial surface of the mandibular central incisor is in at the cervical end more than the labial of the lateral incisor or canine is. The mandibular lateral incisor is out at its cervical end more than the central incisor, so as to be almost perpendicular. The mandibular canine is out at its cervical end to the same degree as the maxillary canine, except at an opposite angle. The labiolingual inclinations of maxillary anterior teeth are intended to serve only as guidelines from which variations must be made if the individual patient's teeth are to appear natural.

A beginning point for studying the anterior teeth from the labial aspect in their mesiodistal inclination is shown in Figure 18-66. The maxillary and mandibular central incisors are almost perpendicular, whereas the laterals are inclined distally at their cervical ends more than any other anterior tooth. The canines are inclined toward the distal at their cervical ends more than the central and less than the lateral incisors are.

A beginning point for studying the rotational positions of the anterior teeth from an incisal aspect is shown in Figure 18-67. The maxillary central incisor is slightly rotated from parallelism with the line of arch contour. The lateral incisor is rotated so its distal surface is turned lingually a considerable angle from the line of arch contour. The canine is rotated so the distal half of its labial surface points in the direction of the posterior arch. The mandibular incisors have a rotational position that generally parallels the arch contour.

A beginning point for studying the superoinferior position of the six anterior teeth in relation to the incisal plane is shown in Figure 18-68. The maxillary lateral incisor and canine are slightly above the level of the incisal plane.

All these positions of anterior teeth from the various aspects serve only as beginning points and must be varied into harmonious irregularities that are not

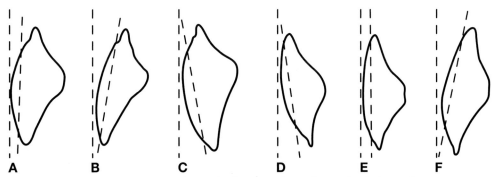

Figure 18-65   Normal labiolingual inclinations of anterior teeth relative to the perpendicular. **A,** Maxillary central incisor. **B,** Maxillary lateral incisor. **C,** Maxillary canine. **D,** Mandibular central incisor. **E,** Mandibular lateral incisor. **F,** Mandibular canine.

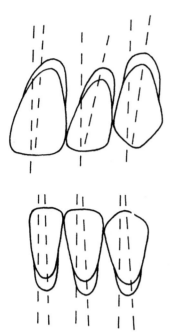

Figure 18-66   Mesiodistal inclination of anterior teeth relative to the perpendicular.

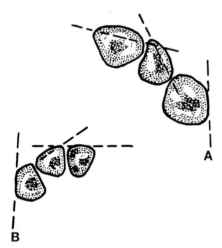

Figure 18-67   Incisal views of anterior teeth showing their angle of rotation. Maxillary (**A**) and mandibular (**B**).

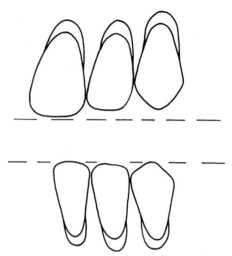

Figure 18-68   Superoinferior positions of anterior teeth relative to the incisal plane.

foreign to any that nature has established. For example, a maxillary canine is seldom in at the cervical end and will appear completely artificial if this irregularity is attempted. The patient cannot point out the exact cause of the unnaturalness but will be aware that something is wrong. Although these are the beginning positions for studying teeth in ideal alignment, dentures with teeth set precisely in these positions also will look artificial. Irregularities are essential to esthetics.

A number of irregularities are found so frequently that they appear natural when reproduced. To reduce the artificiality of dentures, the dentist should make the teeth somewhat irregular. When this is done, a study of the common irregularities of maxillary anterior teeth will show (1) a slight lapping of the mesial surfaces of lateral incisors over the central incisors; (2) a depressing of the lateral incisors lingually so the distal surface of the central and the mesial surface of the canine are labial to the mesial and distal surfaces of the lateral; (3) a rotating of the mesial incisal corner of each lateral incisor lingual to the distal surface of the central while the distal surface of the lateral remains flush with the mesial surface of the canine; and (4) placement of the incisal edge of each lateral higher than that of the central incisor and canine.

Irregularities of the central incisors may be developed by overlapping of the labial incisal angle of one central incisor on the adjacent central incisor, by placing one central incisor slightly lingual to the other central incisor without rotation, and by placing one central slightly labial to and longer than the other.

The maxillary canine may be placed labially in the dental arch, giving this tooth considerable prominence. However, the canine must maintain a rotational position that does not expose the distal half of its labial surface to the eye when viewed from immediately in front. The canine must never be depressed at its cervical end. Rather, its labial surface should be more or less parallel to the side of the face when viewed from the front.

The mandibular anterior teeth can be made slightly irregular, with much effectiveness, if the irregularities are harmonious with nature's frequent irregularities. A setup that decreases the artificial appearance is one in which both central incisors are forward and rotated mesially, one or both lateral incisors are lingual to the arch curve and slightly longer than the adjacent teeth, and the mesial surfaces of the canines overlap the distal surfaces of the lateral incisors (Figure 18-69).

To overlap teeth in rotational positions and at the same time avoid excessive labiolingual irregularities, the dentist must grind the lingual side of the proximal surface of the overlapping tooth. The overlapping contacts in natural teeth have been worn by the movement of the teeth on their contact points in function. Therefore to simulate worn natural overlapping, the dentist must grind the more labially placed of two overlapped teeth on its lingual contact area.

Harmony of Spaces and Individual Tooth Position The use of spaces between teeth can be effective for emphasizing individual tooth posi-

tions and creating a natural-appearing arrangement of teeth. A space usually is not desirable between the upper central incisors unless one existed between the natural teeth. Even then, if the space was large, a smaller space in the denture can create a similar effect and be more pleasing (Figure 18-70, *A*). Spaces between central and lateral incisors, between lateral incisors and canines, and between canines and premolars are effective irregularities that are visible, particularly when seen from the side (Figure 18-70, *B* and *C*). The location of spaces should be chosen carefully to maintain proper balance in the overall composition. Spaces must be designed so they can be self-cleansing.

Concept of Harmony with Sex, Personality, and Age of the Patient

Frush and Fisher presented the concept that creating the illusion of natural teeth in artificial dentures is based on the elementary factors suggested by the sex, personality, and age of the patient. Femininity is characterized by curved surfaces, roundness and softness in the form of the dentition, and a prominent smiling-line alignment of the anterior teeth. Masculinity is characterized by boldness, vigor, and squareness in the dentition and a straightness of the incisal line of teeth. The personality spectrum is divided into delicate, medium, and vigorous, with connotations of personality variations in the masculine or feminine classifications. It is related to the molds, colors, position of teeth, and

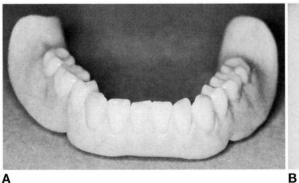
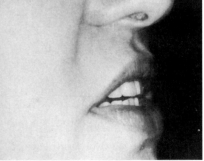

A   **B**

Figure 18-69 **A,** Notice the mesial rotation of the central incisors, the rotation and position of the lateral incisors, and the mesial aspect of the canines overlapping the distal of the lateral incisors. **B,** These mandibular anterior teeth appear natural in the patient's mouth.

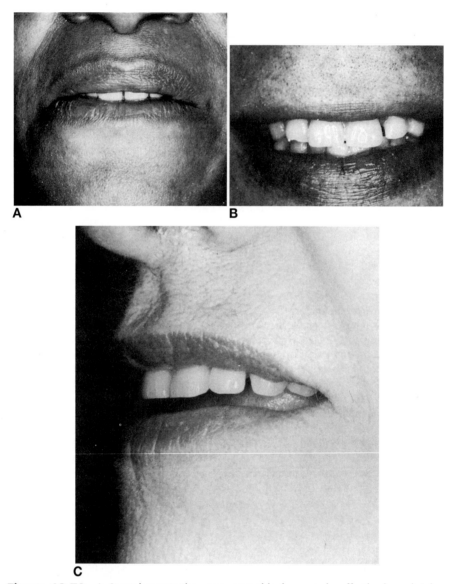

Figure 18-70 **A,** Space between the upper central incisors can be effective in maintaining the identity of a patient if it was present between the natural central incisors. **B,** Space between the central and lateral incisors helps create a natural appearance in the arrangement of artificial anterior teeth. **C,** Space between the lateral incisor and canine provides a good esthetic effect when seen from the side. However, it is not visible when seen from the front. (Compare with Figure 18-56, *B.*)

form of the supporting matrix for the teeth. Age is depicted in dentures by worn incisal edges, erosion, spaces between teeth, and variations in the form of the matrix around the cervical end of a tooth.

Individual tooth form and position also are related to these concepts. The size and position of the central incisors dominate the arrangement of the six upper anterior teeth. Rotation of the distal surfaces anteriorly and placement of one central incisor bodily ahead of the other make the appearance of these teeth more vigorous (Figure 18-71, *A*). Smaller lateral incisors with rounded incisal angles appear more feminine than larger ones (Figure 18-71, *B*). Rotation of the lateral incisors will harden or soften the composition. Canines are positioned to complete the smiling line, rotated so their mesial surface faces anteriorly, abraded according to physiological age, set with the cervical end out, and aligned with the long axis in a

vertical direction when viewed from the side (Figure 18-71, *C*).

The concept of the influence of sex, personality, and age provides additional information for developing harmony between the composition of tooth arrangement and the patient. Dentists must take full advantage of all concepts to create dentures that restore the natural appearance of their patients (Figure 18-72).

Correlating Esthetics and Incisal Guidance

The best plan of occlusion to enhance stability of complete dentures is one with a shallow incisal guidance inclination. The reduction in vertical overlap of the anterior teeth may detract from the appearance of dentures because it is likely to place the maxillary anterior teeth too high or the mandibular anterior teeth too low in the oral

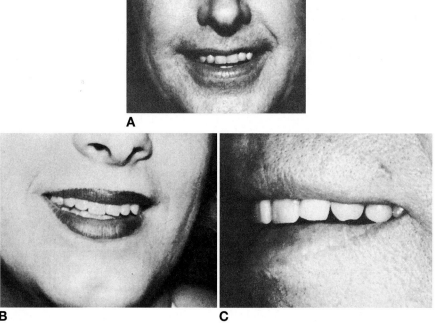

Figure 18-71   **A,** The central incisors dominate this arrangement of artificial anterior teeth. **B,** The rounded incisal edges and relative sizes of the upper lateral incisors provide a composition that is feminine in appearance. **C,** Notice the location of the upper left canine relative to the smiling line. Wear on this tooth is compatible with the patient's age. Notice also the anteriorly facing mesial surface and the vertical long axis of this tooth.

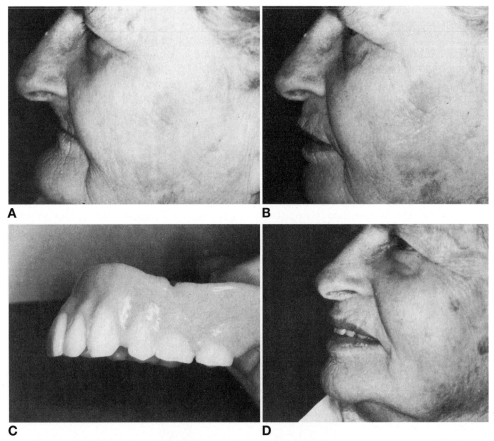

Figure 18-72 **A,** Total lack of support of a patient's face. Notice the prominent chin. **B,** The lips have been restored to a natural position, accompanied by an improved appearance of the chin and restoration of the mentolabial sulcus. **C,** The upper anterior teeth are arranged on an incline relative to the upper lip. Notice their distance in front of the residual alveolar ridge. **D,** The lips move naturally because the muscles that control facial expression have been restored to their proper physiological length. The teeth also appear natural because of their correct size, form, color, and arrangement.

orifice. The simplest way to overcome this difficulty and still maintain a pleasing esthetic appearance would be to increase the horizontal overlap (Figure 18-73). However, if this is done, the lip support or the occlusal vertical dimension will be changed. These procedures may not be feasible if the esthetics and mechanics are to be protected.

The dentist can reduce the vertical overlap of anterior teeth by increasing the interridge distance. However, this must not be done to the extent that it would encroach on the interocclusal distance.

A compromise involves slightly shortening the upper and lower canines while maintaining the full length of the incisors. In this situation, occlusal balance in the protrusive position may not be possible, although it can be achieved in the lateral occlusions. Protrusive balance is less important than lateral balance because incision is performed consciously. The patient can control the amount and direction of force applied when biting into food. On the other hand, chewing is done at a subconscious level. Patients do not think of the

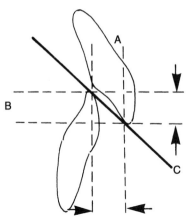

Figure 18-73   Vertical (**A**) and horizontal (**B**) over-laps. **C,** Incisal guidance angle.

amount and direction of the force they apply. Consequently, they cannot protect themselves from forces that would dislodge their dentures. The angle of incisal guidance for lateral occlusion must be adjusted so the posterior teeth contact at the same time that the upper and lower canines are end to end.

Even when the vertical overlap of the anterior teeth must be severe for proper esthetics, the opposing anterior teeth should not be in contact when the posterior teeth are in CO (Figure 18-74). Such contact will eventually cause excess pressures from occlusion of the anterior teeth when the residual ridges resorb and the vertical dimension of occlusion is decreased. Excessive force usually cannot be tolerated by the anterior part of the resid-

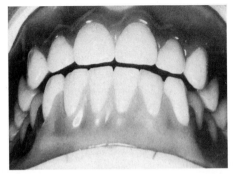

Figure 18-74   Opposing anterior teeth should not contact when the posterior teeth are in centric occlusion.

ual ridges and will likely cause increased resorption of bone and development of hyperplastic tissue in this region.

PATIENT ACCEPTANCE OF THE ARRANGEMENT OF ANTERIOR TEETH

Patients must be given the opportunity to observe and approve the final arrangement of the anterior teeth at the try-in appointment. The dentures should not be completed until approval is obtained. Even when patients indicate that they "do not care how their teeth look," they must be given full opportunity to inspect and approve the arrangement. These patients often become extremely concerned with their appearance when they begin to wear the dentures. Patients should not be permitted to observe the trial dentures in the mouth until the dentist is satisfied with the composition as it is created. The premolars should be in the proper arch form, and the wax denture bases should be carved to approximate the final form. Initial reactions of patients can be longlasting, and an unsatisfactory reaction to a partially completed arrangement of anterior teeth may cause continued problems even though the final appearance of the dentures is perfectly satisfactory.

Because the dentures will be seen most often by other people during normal conversation, patients should first observe themselves in this situation. The patient is positioned 3 to 4 feet (1 to 1.3 m) in front of a large mirror with the trial dentures in the mouth and given the opportunity to observe the dentures during normal conversation and facial expression. The reaction at this time can be critical to the eventual success of the dentures, so this phase must not be done hurriedly or haphazardly. The patient should be encouraged to bring along the most critical family member or friend to assist in evaluating the appearance of the trial dentures.

The dentist should listen carefully to all comments made by the patient and never dismiss any of them as silly or of no consequence. Some changes that the patient may suggest can be incorporated. However, other suggestions may not be advisable, and it will be necessary to explain that they are not anatomically feasible and would prevent the muscles in the cheeks and lips from properly moving the face. Many patients will be pleased with the

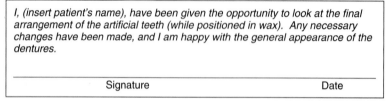

I, (insert patient's name), have been given the opportunity to look at the final arrangement of the artificial teeth (while positioned in wax). Any necessary changes have been made, and I am happy with the general appearance of the dentures.

_____   _____
Signature   Date

Figure 18-75   Patient's statement of satisfaction with the arrangement of artificial teeth.

appearance of the dentures and request few, if any, changes when the position of the artificial teeth approximates that of the natural teeth.

When the dentist and staff and the patient and any critical friends are satisfied with the appearance, it is helpful to have the patient sign a statement that will be placed in the patient's chart (Figure 18-75).

This statement protects the dentist against the occasional patient who will claim that opportunity was not given to view the teeth while arranged in wax or that the requested changes were not done.

Bibliography

Frush JP, Fisher RD: How dentogenic restorations interpret the sex factor, *J Prosthet Dent* 6:160-172, 1956a.

Frush JP, Fisher RD: How dentogenics interprets the personality factor, *J Prosthet Dent* 6:441-449, 1956b.

Frush JP, Fisher RD: Age factor in dentogenics, *J Prosthet Dent* 7:5-13, 1957.

Frush JP, Fisher RD: The dynesthetic interpretation of the dentogenic concept, *J Prosthet Dent* 8:558-581, 1958.

Lombardi RE: The principles of visual perception and their clinical application to denture esthetics, *J Prosthet Dent* 29:358-382, 1973.

Swoope CC: The try-in—a time for communication, *Dent Clin North Am* 14:479-491, 1970.

CHAPTER 19

Speech Considerations with Complete Dentures

Stig L. Karlsson

Speech is a very sophisticated, autonomous, and unconscious activity. Its production involves neural, muscular, mechanical, aerodynamic, acoustic, and auditory factors. Because orodental morphological features also may influence an individual's speech, the dentist should therefore recognize the possible role of prosthetic treatment on speech activity. The specific relationship between dentistry and speech pathology is still emerging. However, considerable clinical experience and research provide a reliable background for addressing this essential topic.

Oral motor functions, such as mastication and speech production, share many common features. They are intimately related because the mouth, lower jaw, lips, teeth, and tongue are used for both activities. Any alteration of these structures will inevitably mediate a disturbance in the system. This may be minor or more substantial in importance, depending on individual responses. Articulatory deficits may be generally classified into three categories: omission of a phoneme, substitutions, and distortions. The latter is the most usual consequence after prosthodontic treatment. Fortunately, the phonetic problems that arise when speaking with new dentures rarely pose serious difficulties. Because most patients' ability to adapt is good, initially experienced speech disturbances will be transient. Nevertheless, the treatment objective is to make complete dentures conform to the individual patient's existing neuromuscular patterns, rather than rely too much on the patient's ability to adapt.

In this chapter, some basic background factors for speech production are described to provide knowledge of possible speech problems induced by the fabrication and wearing of complete dentures.

SPEECH PRODUCTION: STRUCTURAL AND FUNCTIONAL DEMANDS

Controlling the airstream that is initiated in the lungs and passes through the larynx and vocal cords produces all speech sounds. Speech sounds need substantially more air than does quiet exhalation; consequently, subtle adjustments in air flow contribute to variations of pitch and intensity of the voice. The structural controls for speech sounds are the various articulations or valves made in the pharynx and the oral and nasal cavities (Figure 19-1). Each sound is affected by the length, diameter, and elasticity of the vocal tract and by the locations of constrictions along its length.

Because nearly all speech sounds are emitted from the mouth, the nasopharynx (airway into the nose) is closed off from the oropharynx during speech. Closure is performed by an upward lift of the soft palate. A rapid, continuous movement of the entire length of the soft palate takes place during speech. Intimacy of pharyngeal wall contact, as well as magnitude of movement by the soft palate, varies with the nature and sequence of the speech sounds. As the outgoing air passes through the mouth, tongue, lips, and mandibular oscillations modify it. The tongue has a critical impact on speech production and needs optimal mobility to lift, protrude, flatten, form a groove(s), and contact adjacent tissues freely. Jaw and tooth relationships enable the tongue to articulate against the maxillary teeth or alveolus, permit the maxillary teeth and lower lip to make easy contact, and allow the lips to touch.

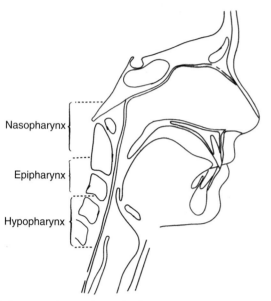

Nasopharynx

Epipharynx

Hypopharynx

Figure 19-1 Schematic picture of the different valves and articulators.

NEUROPHYSIOLOGICAL BACKGROUND

A very complex and imperfectly understood neurophysiological mechanism governs the production of speech. A large number of oral mechanosensitive receptors (tactile and kinesthetic) are involved in its motor control. Therefore all prosthodontic treatment will, more or less, have an influence on speech performance because a great number of these structures will be involved.

Speech production includes large numbers and sequences of innate and learned motor acts produced in rapid sequences of 12 to 16 sounds per second in a rhythmic behavior, similar to chewing. In this context, the theory of "least effort" also has been discussed among researchers in the field. It has been hypothesized that less cortex area is required for processing of skills as they become automatic. Once automatized, speech control becomes localized in certain areas such as the premotor and motor cortex. For the precise movements executed in speech production, the pyramidal motor system has the primary role. Still, there is no convincing evidence to explain fully the mechanisms behind these very rapidly occurring events.

Feedback plays a dynamic and flexible role in the control of most motor events, including sequencing and timing of speech movements. There seems to be a subconscious but learned type of pattern recognition, or feedback, of afferent information used to guide central pattern generators (CPGs) and a central program. The CPGs are thus important in the basic rhythm generation and timing of motor activity. Other neural networks are probably also very active in the rapid transformations of the shape of the oral cavity from one fixed configuration to another. Proprioceptive mechanosensitive afferents will establish the timing of certain aspects of the very fast motor pattern and will, in synergy with cortical information, generate the final motor output and rhythm. A precise coordination between different articulators is essential for the final sound production.

A prerequisite for satisfactory speech sounds and adaptation is an intact general feedback system; that is, orosensory and audio feedback (Figure 19-2), which is regarded as an important mechanism. Gradual hearing loss could be present at older ages, and the process of adaptation of dental prostheses could be impaired. Adaptation after an oral rehabilitation also may create problems in the formation of a new speech motor programming.

It appears that adaptation to complete dentures may be explained by feedback mechanisms related to speech motor programming. Initially, a complete denture wearer attempts to overcome problems related to the new prosthesis by the help of auditory and orosensory feedback during function. After a while, only the patient will be aware of remaining articulatory difficulties, which often are related to certain specific sounds. The listener (dentist) is, however, not able to detect any speech production disturbances. At this stage, there is still sensory stimulation from orofacial afferents to central areas. Finally, if the process of adaptation proceeds, the patient will not be aware of any articulatory difficulties or distortional sounds due to the prosthesis. New speech production central engrams have been established, and adaptation and habituation to the complete denture occur.

SPEECH PRODUCTION AND THE ROLE OF TEETH AND OTHER ORAL STRUCTURES

Because speech production can be used as a guide to position artificial teeth, it is necessary to be

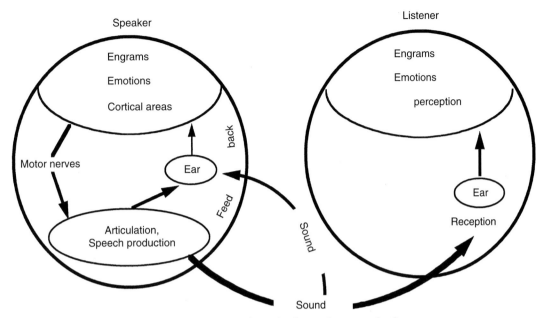

Figure 19-2 Speech production and communication.

familiar with how various speech sounds are produced. Tooth positions are sometimes critical to the production of certain sounds and not at all for others. Because the teeth are being arranged for esthetics, it is not the speech sound itself that is critical but rather, the interrelationships of the tongue, teeth, denture base, and lips. Speech production made by patients at the try-in appointment can never be as accurate as when the processed acrylic resin denture base has been substituted for the trial bases, and the patient has become accustomed to the new dentures. The following definitions and examples provide information for a tabular presentation of various sounds (Table 19-1). Vowels are voiced sounds, that is, the vocal cords are activated by vibration in their production. They are the free emission of a speech sound through the mouth and require subglottic pressure for the production. The vowels in English are *a, e, i, o,* and *u*. Consonants may be either voiced or produced without vocal cord vibration, in which case they are called *breathed sounds*. Consonants are produced as a result of the airstream being impeded, diverted, or interrupted before it is released, such as *p, g, m, b, s, t, r,* and *z*. Most consonants may be classified in pairs that are formed in the same manner, except

that one is breathed and the other voiced. For example, *p* is breathed; *b* is voiced. Consonants also are divided into groups, depending on their characteristic production and use of different articulators and valves. Plosive consonants are produced when an overpressure of air has been built up by contact between the soft palate and the pharyngeal wall and released in an explosive way, such as *p* and *t*. On the other hand, fricatives, such as *s* and *z*, also are called *sibilants* and are characterized by their sharp and whistling sound quality created when air is squeezed through the nearly obstructed articulators. Affricative consonants are a mix between plosive and fricative ones. Nasal consonants are produced without oral exit of air (*m, n,* and *ng*). Liquid consonants are, as the name implies, produced without friction, and finally, glides, that is, sounds characterized by a gradually changing articulator shape.

According to Table 19-1, six different valves exist, of which five may be affected by teeth position.

Bilabial Sounds

The sounds *b, p,* and *m* are made by contact of the lips. In *b* and *p*, air pressure is built up behind the

Table 19-1
English Consonants: Their Position and Modes of Production

Position	Plosives (stops) Breathed	Plosives (stops) Voiced	Fricatives Breathed	Fricatives Voiced	Affricatives Breathed	Affricatives Voiced	Nasals Breathed	Nasals Voiced	Liquids Breathed	Liquids Voiced	Glides Breathed	Glides Voiced
Bilabial	p (pay)	b (bay)						m (man)				w (witch)
Labiodental			f (fan)	v (van)								
Linguodental			th (thumb)	th (there)								
Linguoalveolar	t (to)	d (dot)	s (so)	z (zoo)				n (name)		r (rose)		
Linguopalatal			sh (shoe)	z (vision)	ch (chin)	j (jar)						y (you)
Linguovelar	k (back)	g (bag)	h (who)					ng (bang)				

lips and released with or without a voice sound. Insufficient support of the lips by the teeth or the denture base can cause these sounds to be defective. Therefore the anteroposterior position of the anterior teeth and thickness of the labial flange can affect the production of these sounds. Likewise, an incorrect vertical dimension of occlusion (VDO) or teeth positioning hindering proper lip closure might influence these sounds.

Labiodental Sounds

The labiodental sounds *f* and *v* are made between the upper incisors and the labiolingual center to the posterior third of the lower lip. If the upper anterior teeth are too short (set too high up), the *v* sound will be more like an *f*. If they are too long (set too far down), the *f* will sound more like *v* (Figure 19-3).

However, the most important information to be sought while the patient makes these sounds is the relationship of the incisal edges to the lower lip. The dentist should stand alongside the patient and look at the lower lip and the upper anterior teeth. If the upper teeth touch the labial side of the lower lip while these sounds are made, the upper teeth are too far forward, or the lower anterior teeth are too far back in the mouth. In this situation, the relationship of the inside of the lower lip to the labial surfaces of the teeth should be observed while the patient is speaking. If the lower lip drops away

from the lower teeth during speech, the lower anterior teeth are most probably too far back in the mouth. If, on the other hand, imprints of the labial surfaces of the lower anterior teeth are made in the mucous membrane of the lower lip or if the lower lip tends to raise the lower denture, the lower teeth are probably too far forward, and this means that the upper teeth also are too far forward.

If the upper anterior teeth are set too far back in the mouth, they will contact the lingual side of the lower lip when *f* and *v* sounds are made. This may occur also if the lower anterior teeth are too far forward in relation to the lower residual ridge. Observing from the side and slightly above the patient will provide the necessary information for determining which changes should be made.

Linguodental Sounds

Dental sounds (e.g., *th* in this) are made with the tip of the tongue extending slightly between the upper and lower anterior teeth. This sound is actually made closer to the alveolus (the ridge) than to the tip of the teeth. Careful observation of the amount of tongue that can be seen with the words *this, that, these,* and *those* will provide information as to the labiolingual position of the anterior teeth. If about 3 mm of the tip of the tongue is not visible, the anterior teeth are probably too far forward (except in patients with a Class II malocclusion), or there

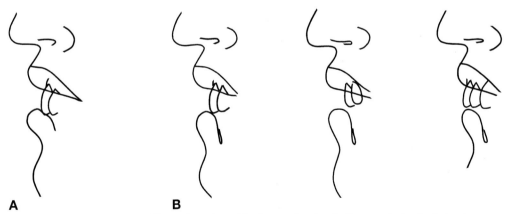

A   **B**

Figure 19-3   Effects of tooth positioning on *f* and *v*. **A,** Upper anterior teeth too long. During the pronunciation of *f*, they will contact the lower lip in a position similar to *v*, and the sounds may sound alike. **B,** Effects of anteroposterior positioning of the teeth from left to right are correct, too far posterior, and anterior.

may be an excessive vertical overlap that does not allow sufficient space for the tongue to protrude between the anterior teeth. If more than 6 mm of the tongue extends out between the teeth when such *th* sounds are made, the teeth are probably too far lingual.

Linguoalveolar Sounds

Alveolar sounds (e.g., *t, d, s, z, v,* and *l*) are made with the valve formed by contact of the tip of the tongue with the most anterior part of the palate (the alveolus) or the lingual side of the anterior teeth. The sibilants (sharp sounds) *s, z, sh, ch,* and *j* (with *ch* and *j* being affricatives) are alveolar sounds because the tongue and alveolus form the controlling valve. The important observation when these sounds are produced is the relationship of the anterior teeth to each other. The upper and lower incisors should approach end to end but not touch (Figure 19-4). A phrase such as "I went to church to see the judge" will cause the patient to use these critical sounds, and the relative position of the incisal edges will provide a check on the total length of the upper and lower teeth (including their vertical overlap).

More important, a failure of the incisal edges to approach exactly end to end indicates a possible error in the amount of horizontal overlap of the anterior teeth (Figure 19-5). This test will reveal the error but will not indicate whether it is the upper teeth or the lower teeth that are incorrect labiolingually.

From a dental point of view, the *s* sound is the most interesting one because its articulation is mainly influenced by the teeth and palatal part of the maxillary prosthesis. Clinical experience suggests that *s* and *t* can cause most problems in a prosthodontic context. In nearly all languages of the world, *s* is a common speech sound. Some languages (e.g., Finnish and Spanish) have diverging *s* pronunciation, but generally the interlanguage quality variation is small. On the other hand, the interindividual variation in articulatory details may be great because of individual variation in teeth, palate, lower jaw, and tongue shape and size. Given this variation, different speakers have to shape the detailed *s* gestures differently to achieve a similar *s* quality. The following phonetic properties, however, are common to all *s* sounds:

Articulatory Characteristics

1. The tip of the tongue is placed far forward, coming close to but never touching the upper front incisors.
2. A sagittal groove is made in the upper front part of the tongue, with a small cross-sectional area.
3. The tongue dorsum is flat.
4. Normally, the mandible will move forward and upward, with the teeth almost in contact.

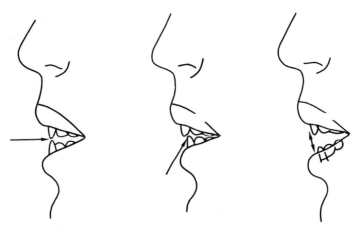

Figure 19-4 Vertical length of the anterior teeth during sibilant production from left to right are correct, excessive, and inadequate vertical overlap.

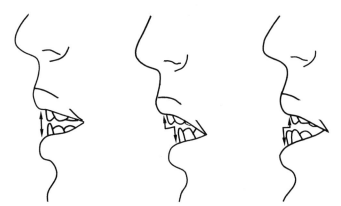

Figure 19-5   Horizontal relation of the anterior teeth during sibilant production from left to right are correct, excessive, and deficient overlapping.

Acoustic Characteristics

1. The comparatively strong sound energy is concentrated to a high-frequency range, with a steep energy cutoff at about 3 to 4 kHz.

Auditory Characteristics

1. The sound is fairly loud, with a light, sibilant (sharp) quality.

The *s* sounds can be considered dental and alveolar speech sounds because they are produced equally well with two different tongue positions, but there can be some variation even behind the alveolus. Most people make the *s* sound with the tip of the tongue against the alveolus in the area of the rugae, with but a small space for air to escape between the tongue and alveolus. The tongue's anterior dorsum forms a narrow groove near the midline, with a cross section of about 10 mm^2. The size and shape of this small space will determine the quality of the sound. Part of the sibilant sound is generated when the teeth are being hit by a concentrated air jet. If the opening is too small, a whistle will result. If the space is too broad and thin, the *s* sound will be developed as an *sh* sound, somewhat like a lisp. The frequent cause of undesired whistles with dentures is a posterior dental arch form that is too narrow.

Creation of a sharp *s* requires accuracy of the neuromuscular control system, for the creation of the groove and directioning of the air jet. Even small deviations of only 1 mm will influence the quality. For example, if the tip of the tongue touches the upper front teeth, the result will be a lisped sound. The fact that the teeth play an important part in articulating this sound often has been neglected, and the oral aerodynamics involved are still an unexplored area.

Linguopalatal and Linguovelar Sounds

The truly palatal sounds (e.g., those in *year, she, vision,* and *onion*) present less of a problem for dentures. The velar sounds (*k, g,* and *ng*) have no effect on dentures, except when the posterior palatal seal extension encroaches on the soft palate.

METHODS FOR SPEECH ANALYSIS

A number of methods are available for speech analysis, with some more useful for the dentist than others. There are basically two categories: perceptual/acoustic analysis, and kinematic methods for movement analysis.

When patients have severe speech pathology problems, their clarity and pronunciation should preferably be analyzed by a speech pathologist. It would be valuable to do this before starting prosthodontic rehabilitation, just to establish a basis for future comparisons and, if possible, identify problems.

An acoustic analysis is based on a broadband spectrogram recorded by a sonograph during the uttering of different phrases containing key phrases. By doing this, an objective opinion of the performance of certain sounds may be achieved.

Kinematic analysis includes such methods as ultrasonics, x-ray mapping, cineradiography, opto-electronic articulatory movement tracking, and electropalatography (EPG). Some of these methods play an essential part in both experimental and routine clinical evaluations of speech defects and treatment effects. They also could be a useful tool for assessment of tongue contact positions and movements. A number of these methods are very exclusive and not aimed for routine examinations, whereas others, such as cineradiography, may have undesirable side effects. EPG is used for registrations of tongue contact patterns during speech production and a mapping of the contacts could be achieved (Figure 19-6).

None of these methods is, however, aimed for use in routine practice but rather after the failure of conventional means to improve an impaired speech production.

PROSTHETIC CONSIDERATIONS

Speech problems usually are identified immediately after prosthetic treatment. When compared with younger individuals, older complete denture wearers experience greater difficulties in adapting their speech to new prostheses and also need longer time to regain their natural speech. A frequent cause is impaired auditory feedback, and therefore a simple auditory test might be useful in such patients to make a proper diagnosis. It also is important to listen to and analyze patients' speech sounds before the rehabilitation starts and even more important to inform patients that temporary speech sound deterioration may result from the oral rehabilitation treatment.

Speech adaptation to new complete dentures normally takes place within 2 to 4 weeks after insertion. If maladaptation persists, special measures should be taken by the dentist or by a speech pathologist, if the problem continues. Particular attention should be paid to patients with long experience of wearing complete dentures. When new prostheses have to be made for these patients, certain difficulties in learning new motor acts may delay and obstruct the adaptation. Consequently, a virtual duplication of the previous denture's arch form and polished surfaces, especially the palate of the maxillary denture, will ensure a minimal period of postinsertion speech adaptation. Old dentures may be of guidance when designing new ones and, if necessary, a virtual copy of the denture could be made. This procedure will frequently solve a problem that may arise due to speech and adaptation difficulties.

A prudent way to overcome possible problems is to study the profile form and lip line of the patient's face, which often is representative of the natural anterior tooth inclination. In such a situation, it would be logical to assume that this profile parallels a correct positioning of the anterior teeth, both for speech production and harmony in esthetics. If the teeth are too far lingual, the *t* in *tend* will sound more like a *d*. If they are too far anterior, the *d* will sound more like a *t*. The palate of a denture base that is too thick in the area of the rugae could have the same effect.

A cramped tongue space, especially in the premolar region, forces the dorsal surface of the tongue to form too small an opening for the escape of air. The procedure for correction is to thicken the center of the palate so the tongue does not have to extend up as far into the narrow palatal vault. This allows the escape way for air to be broad and thin.

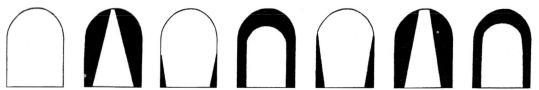

Figure 19-6 Typical electropalatography diagrams for the sounds in *oh sadist*. Shaded area represents the contact between tongue and palate. Note the sagittal groove created when the *s* sound is uttered.

A lisp with dentures can be corrected when the procedure is reversed and a narrow concentrated airway is provided for the *s* sound.

About one third of patients make the *s* sound with the tip of their tongue contacting the lingual side of the anterior part of the lower denture and arching itself up against the palate to form the desired shape and size of airway. The principles involved in such a palatal valve are identical to those involved in the other tongue positions. However, the mandibular denture can cause trouble. If the anterior teeth are too far back, the tongue will be forced to arch itself up to a higher position, and the airway will be too small. If the lingual flange of the mandibular denture is too thick in the anterior region, the result will be a faulty *s* sound. It can be corrected when the artificial teeth are placed in the same position that the natural teeth occupied and the lingual flange of the mandibular denture is so shaped that it does not encroach on the tongue space.

When the vertical dimension is established during the maxillomandibular registration, speech can be used for guidance to assess a correct VDO. Such a procedure is recommended by many dentists, but a dentist using this method needs longtime experience and knowledge to perform properly. During the pronunciation of the *s* sound, the interincisal separation, vertical distance, should average 1 to 1.5 mm. This also is referred to as the *closest speaking space*.

In a recent study, influence of alterations of VDO and palatal configuration on three consonants, *k*, *c*, and *s*, was investigated. It was concluded that malformation of the palatal parts of the denture influenced speech production more than differences in VDO did.

SUMMARY

Speech difficulties as a sequel of oral rehabilitation with complete dentures is generally a transient problem. When encountered, the difficulties may not be easily solved. Therefore efforts should be made to avoid them by pretreatment records or assessment of speech and provision of information to patients about likely initial deviations from normal speech, immediately after the oral rehabilitation. If persistent difficulties to pronounce certain sounds or other speech disorders persist for more than 2 to 4 weeks, the dentist is recommended to follow this protocol:

1. If the patient has a previous complete denture experience, compare the new set with the old one to diagnose possible design differences of significance for speech production. If, on the other hand, a remaining natural dentition is to be converted into a complete denture, a transfer of the original position of the natural teeth to the denture should facilitate adaptation.
2. Listen to the patient and then try to produce the very same distorted sound yourself. Observe the position of your own articulatory structures, tongue, lips, mandible, and so on, when producing this sound and transform them to the patient, thereby making it possible to identify the structures hindering a correct speech production.
3. Make the necessary modifications; soft wax might be helpful.
4. Have the patient's hearing checked. An auditory deficit will prolong the adaptation period and render it more difficult.
5. If the reported/perceived problem cannot be resolved by dental methods, the patient should be referred to a speech pathologist.

Bibliography

Abbs JH, Connor NP: Motorsensory mechanisms of speech motor timing and coordination, *J Phonetics* 19:333-342, 1990.

Benediktsson E: Variation in tongue and jaw position in "s" sound production in relation to front teeth occlusion, *Acta Odontol Scand* 15:275-281, 1958.

Bladon RA, Nolan FJ: A video-fluorographic investigation of tip and blade alveolars in English, *J Phonetics* 5:185-193, 1976.

Fletcher SG, Neuman DG: (s) and (f) as a function of lingual palatal contact place sibilant groove width, *J Acoust Soc Am* 89:850-858, 1991.

Grillner S: Possible analogies in the control of innate motor acts and production of sound in speech. In Grillner S, Lindblom B, Lubker J, Persson A, editors: *Speech motor control*, Oxford, 1982, Pergamon Press.

Hardcastle W, Gibbon F, Nicolaidis K: EPG data reduction methods and their implications for studies of lingual coarticulation, *J Phonetics* 19:251-266, 1991.

Ichikawa T, Komoda J, Horiuchi M et al: Influence of alterations in the oral environment on speech production, *J Oral Rehabil* 22:295-299, 1995.

Jacobs R, Manders E, Van Looy et al: Evaluation of speech in patients with various oral implant-supported prostheses, *Clin Oral Impl Res* 12:167-173, 2001.

Lindblad P, Karlsson S, Heller E: Mandibular movements in speech phrases. A syllabic quasiregular continuous oscillation, *Scand J Log Phon* 16:36-42, 1991.

Lindblom B, Sundberg J: Acoustic estimations of the front cavity in apical stops, *J Acoust Soc Am* 88:1313-1317, 1990.

Lundqvist S, Karlsson S, Lindblad P et al: An electropalatographic and optoelectronic analysis of (s) production, *Acta Odontol Scand* 53:372-380, 1995.

Lundqvist S, Lohmander-Agerskov A, Haraldson T: Speech before and after treatment with bridges on osseointegrated implants in the edentulous upper jaw, *Clin Oral Impl Res* 3:57-67, 1992.

McCord JF, Firestone HJ, Grant AA: Phonetic determinants of tooth placement in complete dentures, *Quintessence Int* 25:341-345, 1994.

Petrovic A: Speech sound distortions caused by changes in complete denture morphology, *J Oral Rehabil* 12:69-79, 1985.

Runte C, Lawerino M, Dirksen D et al: The influence of maxillary central incisor position in complete dentures on /s/ sound production, *J Prosthet Dent* 85: 485-495, 2001.

Seifert E, Runte C, Riebandt M et al: Can dental prostheses influence vocal parameters?, *J Prosthet Dent* 81:579-585, 1999.

Shadle HC: The effect of geometry on source mechanisms of fricative consonants, *J Phonetics* 19:409-424, 1991.

Stevens KN: Airflow and turbulence noise for fricative and stop consonants: statistic considerations, *J Acoust Soc Am* 50:1180-1192, 1971.

CHAPTER 20

Waxing and Processing the Dentures, Their Insertion, and Follow-up

Rhonda F. Jacob, George A. Zarb, Charles L. Bolender

SECTION I: WAXING AND PROCESSING THE DENTURES

WAXING AND POLISHING SURFACES

Three principal surfaces are involved in the functional stability of dentures: the basal or impression surface (often called the *intaglio surface*), the occlusal surface of the teeth, and the polished surfaces. The latter is defined by the width of the border, the buccolingual position of the teeth, and the fullness given the wax to obtain convexity or concavity both facially and lingually. These three surfaces of the denture are positioned in harmony with facial form and the anatomy and physiological movements of the tissues and muscles of the oral cavity. Appropriate position of the dentition and waxing of the polished surface contours and border thickness should be determined at the try-in appointment. This will give the patient and the dentist the opportunity to evaluate esthetics, phonetics, and comfort. Ideal position of the prosthetic dentition has been discussed in previous chapters, but this chapter discusses the details of the final form of the polished surface as it relates to achieving optimal phonetics and enhanced stability and retention.

The form of the polished surfaces of a denture influences its stability and retentive quality. In addition, it influences denture esthetics. The denture bases between the teeth and the border should be shaped in such a manner as to aid retention by the mechanical directional forces of the muscles and tissues. Generally speaking the contours are full on the buccal aspect of the denture but are quite concave on the palatal and lingual surface

because of the functional and "at rest" space requirements of the tongue.

Because the mandibular denture rarely achieves the desired retention and has a limited surface area compared with the maxillary denture, the tongue and cheek muscles can easily dislodge it. Muscles of the cheek and tongue approximate the external denture surface and exert forces on the lateral inclined planes of the dentition and the polished surfaces. Figure 15-1 suggests action of the cheek and tongue in gripping a bolus of food. This action may be described by the illustration of a patient chewing a small grape, with the tongue and cheek holding the grape in place over the occlusal surfaces of the teeth while closing pressure is exerted on it. In addition, a horizontal force is exerted along the occlusal plane by the tongue and cheek.

A further study of Figure 15-1 suggests these muscular forces on the inclined planes of the polished surfaces that can serve as a mechanical aid or a detriment to retention. For instance, when the lingual and buccal borders of a mandibular denture are being shaped, they can be made concave to conform to the tongue and cheek so their muscles will grip and tend to seat the denture. In the opposite situation in which the lingual and buccal surface are made convex beyond the confines of the border, the inclined plane forces resulting from pressures of the tongue and cheeks will tend to unseat the denture. The correct buccolingual position of the teeth is important because lateral forces are also exerted on the dentition during function. Teeth positioned too buccally or too lingually allow the musculature of the cheek or tongue to create unfavorable forces on the inclined plane of the surface of the teeth and the polished denture. These forces will tend to unseat the denture. The contours of the polished surface begin at the gingival collars of the prosthetic dentition. A buccal position of the teeth would likely not allow an adequate concavity of the denture base between the gingival collar and denture border; the muscle action of the cheeks would tend to unseat the mandibular denture.

The buccal surface of mandibular dentures in the first premolar region should be vertical to concave in shape so as not to interfere with the action of the modiolus, connecting the facial muscles with the orbicularis oris muscle. This connecting point of muscles can displace the mandibular denture if the polished surface inclines toward the cheek or if the dental arch in the premolar region is too wide. The lingual flange of the mandibular denture should have the least possible amount of bulk, except at the border (which must be quite thick). This thickness is under the narrower portion of the tongue, and it greatly enhances the seal by contacting the mucolingual fold.

In the maxillary denture, the speech of the patient will be handicapped unless the dentist develops a contour comparable to that of the palate before the natural teeth were lost. The thickness of the vertical walls of the maxillary alveolar area will vary with the loss of bone from the residual alveolar ridge. The horizontal palatal bones and the midline of the palate experience minimal resorption in the edentulous patients. Therefore the thickness of the palatal surface of the maxillary denture should be waxed to a uniform thickness of 2.5 mm. Thus when the processed resin is smoothed and polished, the palate will be as thin as possible and yet sufficiently thick to provide adequate strength.

In the maxillary denture, additional care should be taken with the contours of the palatal alveolar surface in the area of the premolars and canines. Airflow for speech sounds is greatly affected by the contact or approximation of the lateral tongue in these areas. There should be a gentle concave contour of the denture base extending from the palatal surface of these teeth to the horizontal shelf of the palate. If this contour is a deep concavity or a near right angle between the vertical alveolar process and the horizontal shelf, the lateral border of the tongue will not control air during speech. Particularly, the *s* sound will be distorted, sounding more like a "sh." Fricative sounds of *f* and *v* may

also be distorted. Wax should be flowed along the junction of the alveolar ridge and the horizontal shelves to create a gentle concave curve. Patients can also be given water during the try-in of the dentures. With a slightly wet mouth, they can be asked to speak. If water escapes from the lips, wax should be added in the area of the premolars and canines on the offending side. When these ideal contours are created, the technician must be advised not to alter these contours during the final wax-up or finishing of the denture.

If the technician is using a laboratory technique that routinely removes the palate of the trial-base before final wax-up of the maxillary denture, the final contours of the junction of the alveolar process and the horizontal palate is left to the technician. The technician may create too much concavity in the final wax-up resulting in "slurring of speech" when the patient wears the final denture. The dentist and technician must be aware of the bulk required in this area. Although most of these contour considerations are addressed at the try-in appointment, they may have to be refined further when preparing the dentures for processing; therefore there is this reemphasis on fine-tuning the polished surfaces while still in wax.

WAXING THE POLISHED SURFACES

Before the addition of wax to finalize the wax-up, it is important to evaluate the prosthetic occlusion. Wax shrinks when it loses temperature; therefore it is not uncommon for teeth to move slightly out of occlusion. This is particularly visible when viewing from the posterior of the articulator into the lingual aspect of the dentition. Often the lingual aspect of the teeth needs to be lifted to meet the occlusal plane. Use of the metal occlusal plane is useful to evaluate that the teeth are set in harmony with each other and the metal occlusal plane.

The wax surfaces around the teeth are known as the *art portion* of the polished surface and should, for esthetic reasons, imitate the form of the tissues around the natural teeth. Any fancy or artificial festooning is distinctly out of place. A slight projection of the root to follow the individual tooth can be made, however. The upper part of the polished surface, known as the *anatomical portion,* should be formed in such a way as to lose none of the origi-

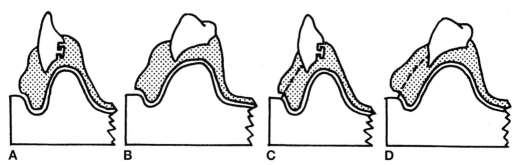

Figure 20-1   **A** and **B,** The amount of wax to be added. **C** and **D,** The correct reduction to enhance both stability and esthetic result.

nal border width of the impression. An excess of baseplate wax is added on the buccal and labial surfaces of the mandibular and maxillary trial dentures and along the cervical collars of the teeth. The wax is cut back to the outer border of the cast (Figure 20-1), and then the small end of a knife is held at a 45-degree angle to the tooth surface to form the wax gingival margin (Figure 20-2). Care should be taken to expose the complete clinical crown of the incisors. This adds to the esthetics because most adult natural dentition reveals the teeth to the cemento-enamel junction (CEJ). Also, the less acrylic resin that is visible around the teeth, the more natural the appearance is. The common tendency is to cut the line too straight from interproximal to interproximal, not leaving enough wax in

the interproximal spaces (Figure 20-3). This will lead to food traps in the final denture, making them less self-cleansing during eating. It is well to have a surplus of wax along the gingival line and then to retrim when a complete view of the entire waxing is possible. Triangular markings can be placed as a guide to the length and position of the root indications, as long as it is kept in mind that the root of the maxillary canine is the longest, the root of the lateral incisor is the shortest, and the root of the central incisor is a length between these two (Figures 20-4 and 20-5). On the mandibular denture the root of the canine is the longest, the root of the central incisor is the shortest, and the root of the lateral incisor is between these two. The wax is scraped out of these triangular areas, after which the root indications will become manifest (Figure 20-6). The sharp and rough indications are now rounded with a large scraper and the spatula (Figure 20-7). They should not be overemphasized.

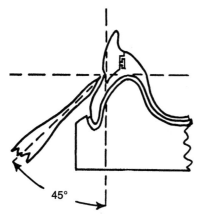

Figure 20-2   The angle at which the wax knife should be held for cutting the gingival line.

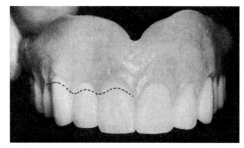

Figure 20-3   Gingival line cut with the proper contour. The dotted line shows incorrect cutting.

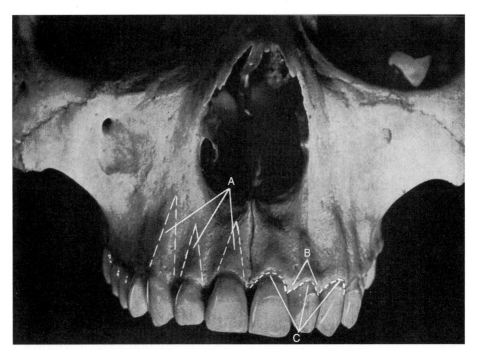

Figure 20-4 *A,* Root indications on the skull. *B,* Continued gingival prominences. *C,* contour of the gingival line.

The lingual surface of the mandibular denture may be made slightly concave without extending the depth of the concavity under the lingual surface of the teeth. A projection of the tooth beyond the polished surface acts as an undercut into which the patient's tongue will slip, thereby causing the den-

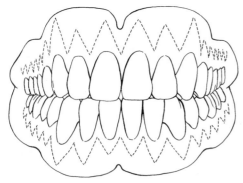

Figure 20-5 Location and lengths of root indications to be made in wax.

ture to be unseated and also allowing food to accumulate (Figure 20-8).

In the maxillary denture, palatal festooning restores part of the palatal surface of the tooth that is not supplied in artificial teeth. Wax is added and carved on the artificial teeth to imitate the normal palatal contours of each tooth (Figures 20-9 and 20-10).

FORMATION AND PREPARATION OF THE MOLD

After the trial dentures have been waxed, they are prepared for flasking. An ejector-type (three-piece) flask is used to facilitate removal of the denture after processing without danger of breaking the denture. The pieces of the flask are usually referred to as the *drag* (bottom), *cope* (middle portion that will capture the teeth of the denture), and the *cap* (which is the thin top of the flask). Dental stone is used to invest the dentures and create the mold within the flask. A limited number of steps are necessary to create the mold, but optional steps are

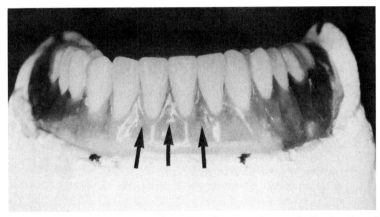

Figure 20-6   Preliminary removal of wax from between the root indication lines *(arrows)*.

often taken during the investing procedure to allow the multiple portions of the stone mold to "fall apart" during deflasking. This offers ease in deflasking the denture and decreases the risk of fracturing the denture or teeth during removal of the denture from the flask (divesting). These optional steps are described as such.

The denture with master cast is placed in the flask to establish its height in relation to the height of the drag of the flask (Figure 20-11). The cope of the flask is placed in position to ensure that the teeth do not project beyond the top of the flask.

Ideally, approximately $^1/_8$ to $^1/_4$ inch (3 to 6 mm) of space should be available between the occlusal surface of the teeth and the top of the flask. If the teeth are too high, the cast must be reduced in thickness. The artificial rim of the cast (land area) should be flush with the drag of the flask to prevent possible breakage of the cast in later separation of the two halves of the flask (Figure 20-12).

The distal ends of the lower cast may be high in relation to the remainder of the cast and extend close to the posterior edge of the flask. This condition causes the distal ends of the cast to be at an

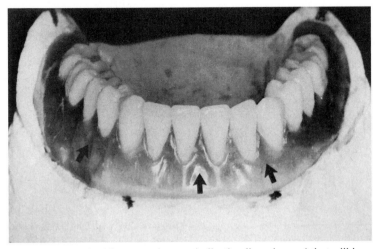

Figure 20-7   Depressions between the root indication lines *(arrows)* that will be smoothed with the wax spatula.

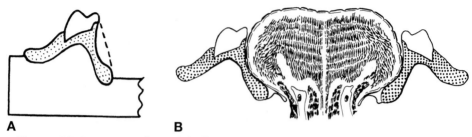

Figure 20-8 **A,** Proper form of the lingual polished surface contour. **B,** Position of the tongue relative to the lingual surface of the denture base is accommodated in the concavity designed in the denture's lingual polished surface.

acute angle to the rim of the flask. Thus the distal ends are vulnerable to breakage when the flask is separated; care should be taken to avoid creating an undercut or too vertical a surface in this area when the cast is invested.

A mix of artificial stone is placed in the bottom half of the flask, and the cast, which has been painted with separating medium (Figure 20-13), is placed down into the stone until its rim is nearly level with the top edge of the flask. The stone is leveled between the edge of the cast and the rim of the flask.

After separating medium has been applied to the exposed stone in the flask, a core of artificial stone 2- to 4-mm thick is developed around the labial and buccal surfaces of both wax dentures, on the lingual surface of the lower wax denture, and the palatal surface of the upper. The top of the cores should be 2 to 3 mm below the occlusal plane of the teeth (Figure 20-14). V-shaped grooves are placed in the cores so they will separate with the top half of the flask. This step is arbitrary. It allows easier divesting of the denture and decreases the risk of breakage of the denture. However, many technicians do not create this incremental making of the mold in the cope.

Separating medium is applied on the exposed surfaces of the core, and the top half (cope) of the flask is set in position. The two flask halves must

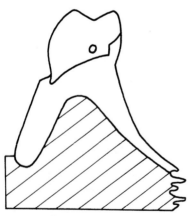

Figure 20-9 The normal lingual contour of artificial posterior teeth is established during the waxing procedure.

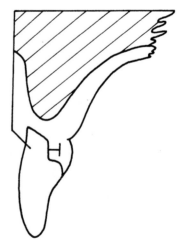

Figure 20-10 The lingual contour of the upper central incisor is reestablished in the waxing procedure. This particular contour will aid phonetics and provide a natural feel to the patient's tongue.

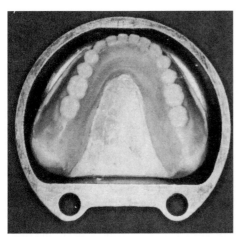

Figure 20-11   The lower wax denture pattern and its cast in the bottom half of the lower flask. Beveling of the posterior height of the land area can reduce the risk of creating an undercut in this area when investing the cast.

meet exactly. Then a mix of artificial stone is poured up to the level of the incisal edges of the anterior teeth and the tips of the cusps of the posterior teeth (Figure 20-15). The exposed stone is painted with separating medium, the flask is completely filled with artificial stone, and the cap of the flask is set in

position. Some technicians do not expose the tooth surfaces with this pour of stone, but rather place one complete pour of stone up to the superior level of the cope and then place the cap. If the teeth are exposed and an additional thin pour of 2 to 3 mm is used, this pour will easily be separated during the divesting procedure, and the technician will be aware of the position of the teeth when using any mechanical devices to break away the stone mold. This "protective" step might be especially useful when easily breakable porcelain teeth are used on the denture. The flask is placed in boiling water and allowed to remain 4 to 6 minutes to soften the wax. Then it is removed from the water, and the drag and cope portion are "opened" from the side opposite the greatest undercut. The wax is removed, and the residual wax is washed out with a stream of boiling water. When the water has been drained from the flask, the mold is washed again with boiling water containing a powdered detergent and then with clean boiling water. Liquid detergents have a greater tendency to leave a residue, which is undesirable, especially with acrylic resin teeth, and solvents such as chloroform are not used because of their chemical contamination of the mold, thereby negatively effecting polymerization of the acrylic.

After the stone is dry, but while still hot, the inside of the mold and the cast are painted with a tinfoil

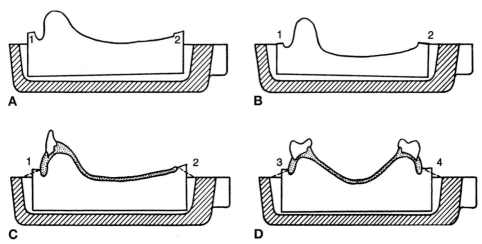

Figure 20-12   First half of flasking of the maxillary trial denture. **A,** Cast too high in areas *1* and *2*. **B,** Areas *1* and *2* at a favorable level. **C,** Areas *1* and *2* should be beveled. **D,** Areas *3* and *4* to be beveled.

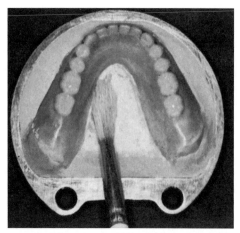

Figure 20-13 Separating medium applied with a camel hair brush on the exposed stone of the land.

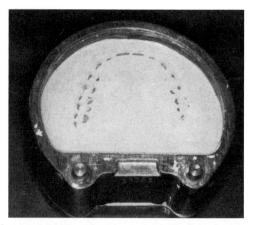

Figure 20-15 After the upper half of the flask has been put in place, a heavy mixture of dental stone is poured to the level of the tips of the cusps.

substitute with a camel hair brush (Figure 20-16). The tinfoil substitute must not come in contact with the teeth or pool in the mold around the teeth. It is allowed to dry, and a second coat is painted on the inside of the mold. The flask is allowed to cool to room temperature. When acrylic resin teeth are used, the exposed surfaces of the teeth must be free of wax and tinfoil substitute and any other debris. Residue on the teeth is the main cause for adhesive failure.

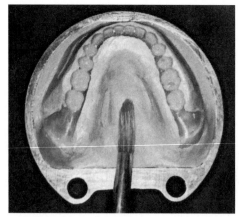

Figure 20-14 Labial, buccal, and lingual cores with v-shaped grooves coated with a separating medium.

PACKING THE MOLD

An acrylic resin dough is made by mixing the powder (polymer) and liquid (monomer) in accordance with the manufacturer's directions. Monomer is a sensitizer that can cause an allergic contact eczematous reaction on the skin or mucous membrane. Consequently, it is advisable to wear rubber gloves and work under proper ventilation. When the monomer is completely polymerized, it rarely elicits an allergic reaction. When the mixture has reached a doughy consistency, it is placed between two plastic sheets and formed into a roll that is flattened about $1/4$ inch (6 mm) thick, and pieces are cut and systematically placed over the teeth in the flask (Figures 20-17 and 20-18, *C*). If there are severe undercuts in the anatomical portion of the edentulous ridge (in the drag of the flask), a small portion of resin may be placed in these undercut areas also. The flask is closed in a press with a sheet of separating plastic between the two halves until they are almost in approximation. Then the flask is opened, the excess flash resin is cut away precisely at the denture border, and additional resin is added at any places where no flash was evident (Figure 20-18). This trial packing procedure is repeated until the mold is filled and no flash is formed. It is usually not necessary to continue to add resin after the first trial pack; however, repeated

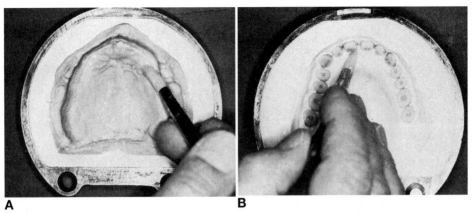

Figure 20-16   **A,** The flask has been separated and the wax removed. The tissue surface of the upper cast is painted with a tinfoil substitute. **B,** All wax has been removed, and the teeth are in their proper places in the mold. The stone is painted with a tinfoil substitute, which must be kept out of contact with the teeth.

packs reveal a need to continually remove the flash. Then the flask is closed completely without the separating sheet. The slightest discrepancy in closure of the two halves of the flask will cause an error in the occlusion.

The flask is transferred to a spring clamp for processing. The clamp is closed tightly but not fully compressed. This will allow the resin to expand upon processing and then finally contract while still under pressure. Most methylmethacrylate denture resins are processed for 9 hours in a cooling bath of water held at a constant temperature of 165° F (73.5° C).

However, acrylic resins can be processed at temperatures of 135° to 180° F. Distortion is reduced when the resin is processed at or below the manufacturer's recommended temperature. However, the amount of monomer remaining in the cured resin clearly affects the degree of cytotoxicity of the denture base material. Potentially more monomer will be present at the processing temperatures. The flask must cool to room temperature before deflasking begins. It is crucial that sufficient time be allowed for cooling inside the flask. If this precaution is not taken, increased distortion of the resin will occur.

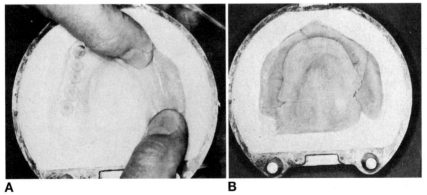

Figure 20-17   **A,** A section of the dough is placed in the mold for the upper denture. It is carried to place with cellophane to prevent contamination. **B,** The dough has been distributed throughout the upper mold.

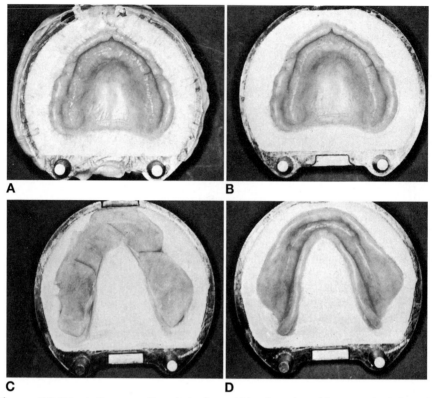

Figure 20-18 **A,** Excess acrylic resin in the mold has been forced between the halves of the flask during the initial trial packing. **B,** Excess resin in the upper mold removed through a series of trial packings. **C,** The dough is distributed throughout the lower mold. **D,** Flash should extrude from the entire periphery of the denture. If it does not extrude on the first pressing, that area requires the addition of more dough. Trial packing with excess removal should continue until no more flash appears.

PRESERVING THE ORIENTATION RELATIONS

Deflasking is usually carefully completed with an air chisel, and the processed dentures are left on the casts. The casts and dentures are returned to the mountings on the articulator, and the processing changes are observed. Usually the change is noted by observing the occlusal pin on the anterior guidance platform and is often in the realm of 1 to 2 mm. Minor processing changes are usually corrected at this time. However, new interocclusal records and final adjustment of the dentition will be done at insertion time. It should be noted that adjusting the occlusion after processing and at delivery could sacrifice too much tooth stock.

The upper cast is attached to the upper mounting, and a record of its relationship to the articulator is made in plaster on the remounting jig. Fast-setting plaster is spread on the jig, and the teeth of the upper denture are pressed into the plaster while the cast is in its keyed position on the articulator (Figure 20-19). This index can also be made after the final waxup, just before investing the maxillary denture.

SHAPING AND POLISHING THE CURED RESIN BASES

The dentures are removed from the artificial stone casts. The feather edges of the denture base material are removed with files, scrapers, and burs.

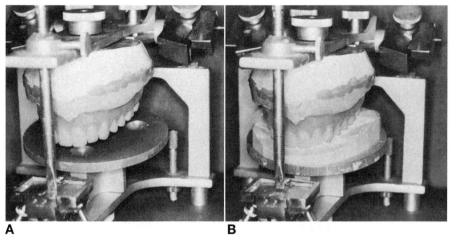

A   **B**

Figure 20-19 **A,** The upper cast and processed upper denture are returned to the articulator mounting and attached with sticky wax. The remounting jig is positioned on the lower member of the articulator. **B,** The upper denture is closed into the plaster on the remounting jig so the occlusal surfaces of the teeth will make an imprint in plaster. This will permit the denture, after removal from the artificial stone cast, to be repositioned in proper relation to the upper member of the articulator.

The feather edges around the gingival line of the teeth are cut down by means of chisels and knives to conform with the desired contour; care is taken not to cut acrylic resin teeth. With burs, stones, chisels, and sharp scrapers, the surface is shaped until it is smooth and clean. No plaster and no deep scratches should remain before polishing. Any difficulty during polishing of the dentures is due to their not being properly prepared for polishing.

A rag wheel and felt cone with pumice are good for smoothing the palatal portion of the upper denture. A single-row brush wheel and a rag wheel about ¼ inch (6 mm) in width are used with pumice to smooth the labial and buccal surfaces of the denture without destroying the contour. A final high polish is given to all the surfaces with a rag wheel and polishing material (tripoli, tin oxide, and water).

CONSTRUCTION OF REMOUNTING CASTS

Remounting casts serve as an accurate, convenient, and time-saving method of reorienting the completed dentures on the articulator for occlusal corrections. All undercuts on the tissue surface of the dentures are filled with wet tissue paper, clay, or wet pumice (Figure 20-20, *A*). Block-out should be only at the undercuts. Most internal denture anatomy should remain to support the dentures during occlusal adjustments. Remount casts that only duplicate the flanges often allow the dentures to rock or shift during the occlusal adjustments.

Fast-setting plaster or artificial stone is poured into the denture. After the plaster has set, the excess is trimmed down to the border (Figure 20-20, *B*) and the dentures are removed from the casts. The casts are examined to ensure that the grooves formed by the border of the dentures are not deeper than 1 mm to allow accurate seating of the dentures (Figure 20-20, *C*).

With the remounting jig and index positioned on the mandibular member of the articulator, the maxillary denture and remounting cast are placed in the plaster indentations. The maxillary remount cast is attached to the maxillary member of the articulator by means of fast-setting plaster (Figure 20-21).

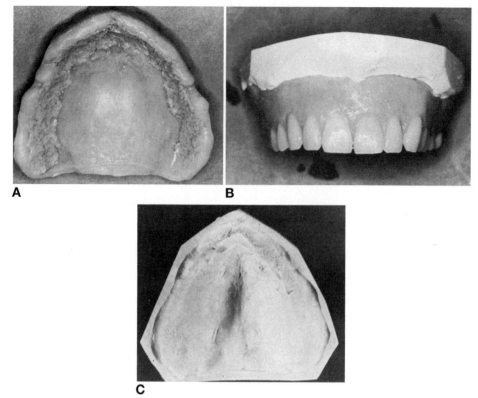

Figure 20-20 **A,** Undercuts are eliminated from the tissue surface of the denture when they are filled with wet tissue paper. Only block out the undercut areas, not the entire denture ridge. Too much block-out will allow the cast to "rock" during occlusal adjustments. **B,** Upper remounting cast poured in the upper denture. **C,** Upper denture removed from the upper remounting cast. All the block-out material should be removed, and the denture should fit accurately on the cast.

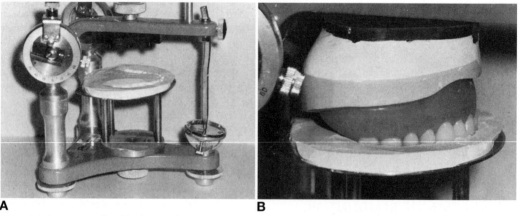

Figure 20-21 **A,** Occlusal index previously made on the Dentatus articulator before the waxed-up maxillary denture was removed from the original mounting. **B,** Remounting cast attached to the mounting ring on the upper member of the articulator with fast-setting plaster.

CRITIQUING THE FINISHED PROSTHESES

The moment new dentures are placed in a patient's mouth, all of the procedures involved in denture construction are subject to review and reevaluation. The choice of materials, the technical and clinical effectiveness of procedures used, and the skill in carrying out the procedures are exposed to three evaluations. These are by the dentists who rendered the service, the patients who are to use the dentures, and the friends and family of the patients who will be viewing the dentures.

Dentists' Evaluations

Evaluations made by dentists should be the most critical because these are the professionals who know the potentialities and limitations in the treatment of the patient. Dentists must recognize deficiencies in the prosthodontic service provided. Some of these may become manifest at delivery, and some may become evident during follow-up examinations. If dentists are not knowledgeable about the type of observations that should be made and are not critical of the results of the treatment, they are not rendering a truly professional service. If dentists cannot find anything that they would change in treating the same patient again with complete dentures, they are not being as critical of their own efforts as they should be. The maintenance of quality of prosthodontic service depends on a constant vigilance and self-discipline. A critical evaluation by the dentist of every prosthodontic service rendered will tend toward a constant improvement of the service.

Patients' Evaluations

Patients' evaluations of their new dentures are generally made in two phases. The first is the reaction to the completed dentures when they are first placed in their mouth. This can range from enthusiastic acceptance to fear and apprehension.

The patient's frame of mind will greatly depend on the dentist's tempering the patient's expectations, but it may be affected by previous experiences in denture wearing and by comments of other people. If adequate diagnoses were made before any treatment was started, all misconceptions and inaccurate information should have been discussed. Limitations in denture wear as a result of the patient's particular anatomy and function will have been addressed. It is especially important to spend adequate time at the try-in appointment to avoid patient dissatisfaction at insertion. If confidence cannot be earned and established before the day the dentures are placed in the mouth, the treatment after this time will be more complicated. Skilled practitioners will have demonstrated to their patients that they are treating them professionally and that they have used the utmost care in the clinical and technical procedures involved in fabricating their dentures.

Friends' Evaluations

When patients leave the dental office with their new dentures, it is generally with mixed emotions. They want their friends to notice their improved appearance; they hope their friends and relatives will compliment them and confirm their judgment and choice of dentist; and they still wonder how they will progress with eating and speaking. If people comment about the new teeth, some patients may wonder if the teeth look natural; if they do not comment, the patients may wonder if their friends are just being kind. The evaluations by friends may not be accurate. Friends cannot know how the dentures feel. They cannot judge the efficiency of the dentures in eating and speaking. They cannot know the difficulties encountered by the dentist because of the poor anatomical foundation. They cannot understand the possible lack of coordination of the patient or the ineptness of some patients in attempting to follow instructions or to use the dentures. The patients themselves may recognize these difficulties as partly their responsibility, but the comments of friends may cause them to blame the dentist for problems that may have been beyond the dentist's control. Such well-meaning friends can add to a patient's difficulties because they have not been exposed to the information supplied to the patient by the dentist. The way to guard against patients being misinformed by their friends is to take the lead and make certain that patients have been correctly informed. This process is a continuing one and should start at the time the diagnosis is made. Enlisting the aid of a patient's most critical friend or relative in critiquing the appearance at the try-in or having this person available during the many denture appointments can be very helpful.

TREATMENT AT THE TIME OF DENTURE INSERTION

There are certain technical procedures that must be carried out to ensure a successful prosthodontic service. Inaccuracies in the materials and methods used to get the dentures to this stage must be recognized and eliminated before the patient wears the dentures. The inaccuracies may be the result of (1) technical errors or errors in judgment made by the dentist, (2) technical errors developed in the laboratory, or (3) inherent deficiencies of the materials used in the fabrication of the dentures.

Ideally the patient should be instructed to keep any previous dentures out of the mouth for 12 to 24 hours immediately before the insertion appointment. This is essential if the new dentures are to be seated on healthy and undistorted tissues. If the tissues are being distorted by old dentures, the new dentures will not seat perfectly, even if they fit perfectly. Improper seating of dentures at this time can cause the appearance of errors in occlusion or fit that would not exist if the tissues were undistorted. Adjustments of any type to correct such apparent errors, if made at this time, may be unnecessary and can cause irreparable damage to the dentures. This caution is predicated on the requirement that the patient be without any dentures for 24 hours (sometimes longer) to get the tissues healthy before the final impressions are made.

As mentioned in Chapter 18, many patients will find leaving the dentures out of their mouth for 12 to 24 hours an unreasonable request. An acceptable alternative is to have the existing dentures relined with a soft temporary material to minimize tissue distortion problems.

ELIMINATION OF BASAL SURFACE ERRORS

Before the placing of dentures in the patient's mouth, the dentures should be inspected to be sure that there are no imperfections on the tissue surface, the polished surface is smooth, the denture flanges have no sharp angles and are not too thick, and the denture borders are round and smooth with no obvious overextension. If carefully border-molded impressions have been made, the flanges and borders should require little if any alteration. The dentist's objective should be to make the impressions and casts so perfectly that there is no doubt in the mind of the technician as to the form and extent of borders and flanges when the dentures are trimmed and polished.

Using a magnifying glass, in addition to digitally inspecting the denture bases, can be effective in locating and correcting such irregularities. All denture borders, especially the frenal notches, must be examined carefully for sharp edges. Sharp borders in the frenal notches must be carefully rounded before the initial placement of the dentures. The use of pressure indicator paste is essential to evaluate the accuracy of tissue contact. It is especially helpful when bilateral undercuts on the residual ridge interfere with the initial placement of dentures or when pressure spots were present in the final impression. The paste is brushed on the tissue surface of the denture base in a thin layer so the brush marks are visible and run the same direction. In this manner, tissue interferences during placement of the dentures or excessive pressure on the residual ridge can be more easily interpreted than without the paste. The painted surface may be sprayed with a silicone liquid or wetted with water. The denture is carefully placed in the mouth and pressure is applied by the dentist on the teeth to reveal any pressure spots in the denture base that would displace soft tissue (Figures 20-22 and 20-23). The marks in the paste indicate where the denture base should be adjusted to relieve the interference (Figure 20-24). Pressure indicator paste should be used for every new denture, and any necessary adjustments should be made before proceeding with the occlusal adjustment.

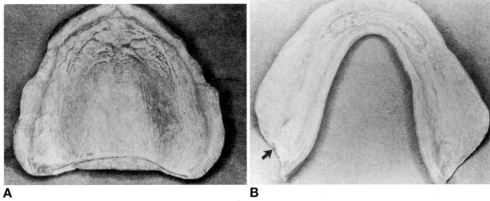

A   B

Figure 20-22   **A,** Marks showing through the pressure indicator paste reveal the location of pressure spots exerted by the denture on areas that are not primary stress-bearing areas. The spot in the region of the left hamular notch also was present on the final impression. The posterior palatal seal bead is visible through the pressure indicator paste and shows that the desired seal is being provided. **B,** Pressure areas visible through the alveolar groove anteriorly in both canine areas and the retromolar fossa *(arrow)*. These should be relieved because they are not allowing the denture to seat; therefore there is little disruption of the surface texture of the neatly applied pressure paste. This reveals that there is no contact on the remainder of the denture-bearing surface, particularly not in a primary stress-bearing area for the mandibular denture.

Despite the methods used to make or finish the borders, overextension may occur, causing tissue trauma if not corrected. A thick layer of paste can be applied to an incremental area of the denture border. The entire border should not be painted because the paste will be smeared in some areas upon placing it in the mouth. The denture should be placed in the mouth, avoiding any inadvertent contact of the disclosed area. After complete seating of the denture, the dentist can "border mold"

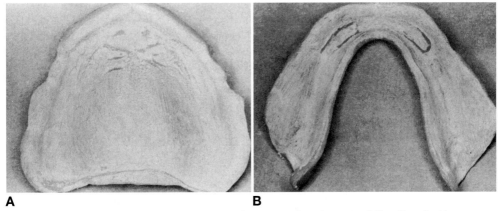

A   B

Figure 20-23   **A,** The pressure spots in Figure 20-22 have been carefully relieved with a no. 8 round bur. A minimum of denture base material was removed. **B,** The severely undercut area of the retromolar lingual flange must be carefully disclosed on the periphery and internal aspect of the periphery. Each side should be evaluated independently so as not to disturb or displace the paste on insertion. The denture should be slightly twisted and pulled forward when evaluating this area because the denture can be expected to move under function. This thin lingual mucosa surface is very vulnerable to ulceration with denture movement.

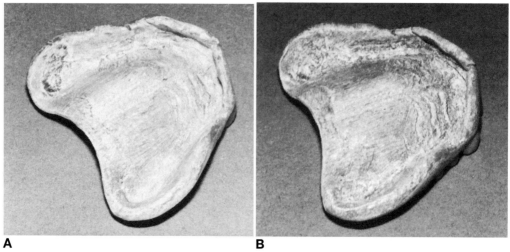

A **B**

Figure 20-24 **A,** Interference in the left posterior buccal flange area is noted before seating the maxillary denture in its correct position. **B,** After careful adjustment, a new recording of the indicator paste indicates proper seating of the denture.

that area of the border. On removal of the denture, any pressure area or overextension will be visible. These areas can be adjusted; this adjustment ensures that border tissues and frena are not displaced.

ERRORS IN OCCLUSION

Maxillomandibular relations are bone-to-bone relations and as such represent the status between two solid objects: the maxillae and the mandible. These bones are covered by mucosa and submucosal tissues, which are resilient and displaceable. Errors in occlusion might not be apparent unless specific procedures are used to test for them. Because of tissue displaceability, some dentists have considered that the dentures will settle into the tissues and small errors in occlusion will correct themselves. If this is true, it is done at the expense of the health of soft tissues and eventually at the expense of bone because bone is a more plastic tissue than mucosa. Bone, in time, will change to relieve soft tissues of excess pressure. Thus failure to correct occlusion before the patient wears the dentures can cause destruction of the residual alveolar ridges.

Errors in occlusion can result from a number of factors. These include a change in the state of the temporomandibular joints (TMJs), inaccurate maxillomandibular relation records by the dentist, errors in the transfer of maxillomandibular relation records to the articulator, ill-fitting temporary record bases, change of the vertical dimension of occlusion on the articulator, incorrect arrangement of the posterior teeth, failure to close the flasks completely during processing, or use of too much pressure in closing the flasks. Occlusion errors may be the result of unavoidable changes in the denture base material (Figure 20-25). Acrylic resins shrink when they change from a moldable to a solid form. They have a high coefficient of thermal expansion, and in cooling after polymerization they shrink, causing dimensional changes. The greatest amount of change occurs when the dentures are removed from the casts. Further change may occur if too much heat is generated in polishing the dentures. Subsequently, the acrylic resin absorbs water while in use, resulting in expansion. Processing changes are inevitable, though some can be minimized by careful handling of the materials and prostheses by the dentist and laboratory technician.

Some of the errors in occlusion can be corrected after deflasking the master casts with the

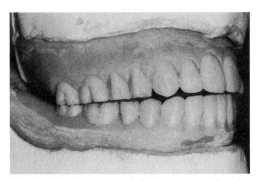

Figure 20-25   Processed dentures are replaced on the articulator while still on their casts. The changes that occurred in processing of the acrylic resin have caused errors in the occlusion.

processed dentures still on them, in their original mountings in the articulator, and modifying the occlusal surfaces of the teeth by selective grinding (see Figure 20-25). This will eliminate most of the errors caused by processing changes. However, it will not eliminate errors produced by the impressions or jaw relation records, nor will it eliminate errors that develop when the dentures are removed from the casts or are polished. Therefore new interocclusal records should be made at the time new dentures are first inserted in the patient's mouth. Denture base acrylic resins absorb water and saliva. This absorption causes a 1% to 3% expansion and can alter the relationships of the cusps' inclined planes. After finishing of the dentures, the prostheses should be maintained in water so this dimensional change occurs before the final occlusal refinement that is accomplished at the insertion appointment. To avoid dimensional and occlusal changes, patients should be advised to store dentures in water.

Checking for Occlusion Errors

The technique to determine whether there are errors in occlusion is not difficult, but it does require the willingness to see an error. Given the myriad of reasons for occlusal discrepancies, dentists must assume that an error exists and work to find it. If they simply tell the patient to close their jaws and then observe the occlusal contact, the error in occlusion will unlikely be detected. The

dentures may shift on the ridges, the soft tissue supporting the dentures may distort or be displaced, or the mandible may move into an eccentric position; the occlusal error will be obscured, at the expense of tissue damage. To observe the error, the dentist should guide the mandible into centric relation (CR), while supporting the lower denture intraorally. The patient is instructed to close until the first "feather touch" is felt on the posterior teeth. At the first contact, the patient is instructed to open and repeat this closure, stopping the instant tooth contact is felt; then the patient is instructed to "close tight." This procedure will reveal errors in CR by the touch and slide of teeth on each other (see Figure 18-1). The amount of occlusal error and the location of the deflective contacts will be determined after the dentures have been remounted in the articulator. They are usually minute, and their accurate localization requires remounting. If articulating paper is used in the mouth to locate interceptive or deflective occlusal contacts, shifting of the denture bases, tissue distortions, or eccentric closures by the patient, as well as the presence of saliva, can prevent the articulating paper marks from accurately recording errors. Much of the selective grinding done in the mouth according to articulating paper marks made actually increases the amount of error in the occlusion. Occlusion errors are ideally detected and corrected when the dentures are accurately mounted in the articulator.

INTEROCCLUSAL RECORDS FOR REMOUNTING DENTURES

The dentures must be remounted on the articulator by means of accurate interocclusal records (CR and protrusions are necessary for this procedure) for the selective grinding necessary in perfecting the occlusion. When new accurate interocclusal records are made and the completed dentures are remounted on the articulator, the errors in occlusion are easily visible, easily located, and easily corrected by selective grinding. Properly made interocclusal records will not cause the denture bases to slip or rotate in relation to their bony foundations. Furthermore, on the articulator, the dentures will be firm on their remount casts. The points of contact and errors of occlusion can be observed visually, with magnification if desired, and articulating paper marks are quite easily made on the dry teeth.

There is another advantage to making these corrections without the patient present. The interocclusal records, of course, are made in the patient's mouth; from the patient's standpoint this is just another step in the construction of the dentures. On the other hand, if the grinding of occlusion is attempted in the presence of the patient, the operation may appear to the patient to be one of correcting an error made by the dentist. Thus there is a psychological advantage in doing the selective grinding in the laboratory.

INTEROCCLUSAL RECORD OF CENTRIC RELATION

Two pieces of wax wafer (e.g., Aluwax) are placed over the mandibular posterior teeth. A thickness is chosen to eliminate the danger of making contact with the opposing teeth when biting pressure is exerted. The teeth must be completely dry and the wax pressed firmly on them to eliminate voids. The two thicknesses of wax are sealed with a warm spatula (Figure 20-26). The maxillary denture is placed in the patient's mouth, and just the Aluwax portion is immersed in a water bath of 130° F (54° C) for 30 seconds (Figure 20-27). Both the temperature and the time are critical in achieving a uniformly softened wax. The Aluwax retains heat longer than baseplate wax, thereby providing time for the next step.

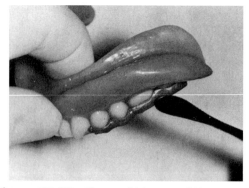

Figure 20-26   The two thicknesses of Aluwax are sealed with a warm spatula.

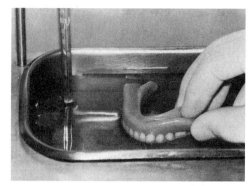

Figure 20-27   The Aluwax is immersed in 130° F (54° C) water for 30 seconds.

The occlusal surfaces of the maxillary teeth are lightly lubricated with petroleum jelly, and the maxillary denture is firmly seated in the mouth. The mandibular denture is then seated with the index fingers bilaterally positioned on the buccal flanges. The mandible is guided into CR by placing the thumbs on the anteroinferior portion of the chin in such a way that some guidance is directed toward the condyles. The patient is guided in a hinge movement, closing lightly into the wax. As contact with the wax approaches, the fingers are slightly raised from the buccal flanges and the patient is instructed to close into the wax until a good index is made (Figure 20-28). Care must be taken to prevent the patient from penetrating the wax and making tooth contact; a minimal amount of occlusal pressure should be exerted. Because the wax slightly distorts when the mandible is opened, this "drag" of the wax can be reduced by having the patient open only a few millimeters on the arc of closure and "tap" lightly into the wax.

The mandibular denture is carefully removed from the mouth and placed in ice water to chill the wax thoroughly (Figure 20-29). Next, the dentures are removed from the ice water and dried. The imprint of the opposing teeth must be crisp and about 1 mm deep, with no penetration of the interocclusal wax record by opposing teeth (Figure 20-30). If there is direct tooth contact through the wax, there is the possibility that the bases sifted and an incorrect record was made. The record must be repeated.

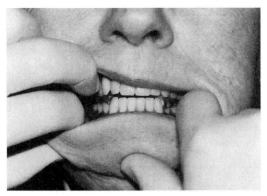

Figure 20-28   The mandible is guided into centric relation with the thumb on the anteroinferior part of the chin and the index fingers lightly seating the mandibular denture in a downward and forward direction. The patient is instructed to close lightly into the softened wax. Then the patient should be instructed to gently "tap-tap" into the wax in the hinge motion, before removal of the denture from the mouth.

The Aluwax is thoroughly chilled before the dentures are returned to the patient's mouth and the patient is guided into CR, as previously described. The record is acceptable if there is no tilting or torquing of the dentures from initial contact to complete closure (Figure 20-31). Underlying soft-tissue displacement may cause a slight movement of the bases and must be taken into account when evaluating the contact. If the record does not satisfy these criteria, the procedure must be repeated.

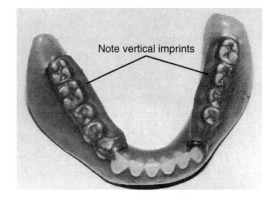

Note vertical imprints

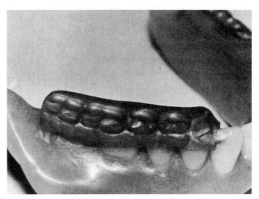

Figure 20-30   The occlusal record is approximately 1 mm deep and free of any penetration by the underlying teeth. The imprint of the opposing teeth is vertical with no evidence of a slide *(arrows)*.

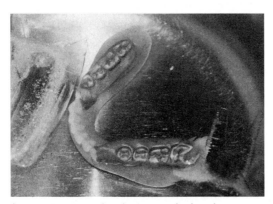

Figure 20-29   The Aluwax attached to the mandibular denture is chilled in ice water.

REMOUNTING THE MANDIBULAR DENTURES

The maxillary denture will have been mounted in the articulator by means of the remount occlusal index (see Figure 20-21), which will have preserved the face bow orientation of the dentures. As a result, the horizontal condylar setting recorded at the try-in appointment should be valid, and it is not necessary to repeat the face bow or protrusive record.

After the dentures and wax are chilled and thoroughly dried, the mandibular denture is positioned on the remount cast (Figure 20-32). Next, the maxillary denture teeth are carefully positioned in the wax index and secured with a drop of sticky wax in

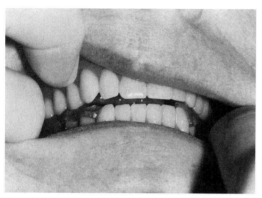

Figure 20-31 Checking the accuracy of the chilled interocclusal wax record. There should be no tilting or torquing of the dentures from initial contact to complete closure.

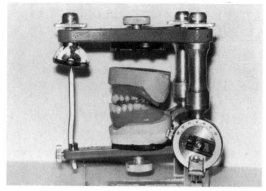

Figure 20-33 The maxillary teeth are secured to the wax index with a drop of sticky wax in the canine and second molar areas and secured with fast-setting plaster.

the canine and second molar regions bilaterally (Figure 20-33). (Sticky wax can be used to secure both dentures to their remount casts, if necessary.) The incisal pin should be adjusted to allow for the thickness of the interocclusal wax record by raising the upper member of the articulator about a millimeter and dropping the incisal pin. The condylar controls must be locked into centric position. Plaster is used to secure the mandibular denture to the lower member of the articulator.

VERIFYING CENTRIC RELATION

The CR record should be verified for accuracy before any tooth adjustments. The Aluwax is used, and the CR recording is repeated. After chilling and drying of the wax record, the dentures are returned to the articulator. With the articulator locked in CR, the maxillary teeth should fit precisely into the new wax record (Figure 20-34). If all the teeth drop simultaneously into the wax record, the mounting is correct. If the opposing teeth do not fit exactly into the indentations in the new record, either the original mounting was incorrect, or the patient gave an incorrect relation when making second record. To

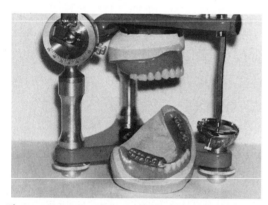

Figure 20-32 The mandibular denture with the wax interocclusal record attached is positioned on and secured to the mandibular mounting cast with sticky wax. The maxillary denture has been previously positioned on the upper member of the articulator with the occlusal index (see Figure 20-21) and secured to place with sticky wax.

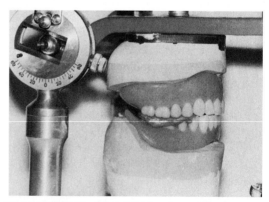

Figure 20-34 The original cast mounting is verified when the maxillary teeth fit precisely into the wax index on the articulator with locked centric controls.

evaluate this, the dentist returns the dentures with the chilled wax record to the mouth and evaluates the accuracy, as previously described. If the record still appears correct in the patient's mouth, the original CR registration or mounting was incorrect. In this situation, the mandibular cast should be separated from the mounting ring and the cast remounted according to the second interocclusal wax record. The new mounting is again checked in the same manner to validate its correctness.

PROTRUSIVE INTEROCCLUSAL RECORD (OPTIONAL)

The original face bow orientation of the dentures can be preserved by means of the remount occlusal index; thus the optimal condylar setting recorded at the try-in appointment should still be valid. If there is any question as to the accuracy of the original condylar setting, a new protrusive record is made (Figure 20-35). As previously stated in the chapters related to articulators and lateral excursive records, precise lateral records are difficult to record because of denture instability and tissue resiliency. Therefore most clinicians agree that average lateral condylar settings are sufficient for denture construction.

Eliminating Occlusal Errors in Anatomical Teeth

Final correction of occlusal disharmonies is made at this time by means of methodical selective grinding that will give simultaneous contact around the arch in CR occlusion and in eccentric movements and also maintain tooth form. Unlike occlusal philosophies in natural dentition, it is desirable for working and balancing contacts to occur simultaneously. The goal is for balancing side contacts to appear across the arch and within the tooth on the working side of the arch. During evaluation of contacts and selective grinding, tooth contacts will prevent other teeth around the arch from making contact. The goal is to maintain the integrity of the "stamp" or central bearing cusp tips in both arches (maxillary lingual and mandibular buccal cusps) and allow all cusps to move through the "sluce ways of the opposing dentition" (working and balancing grooves and mesial and distal inclines). The

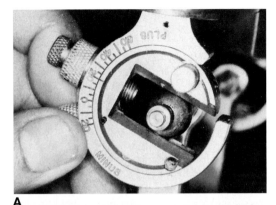

A

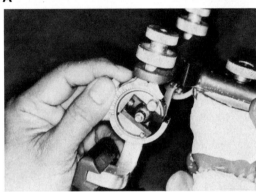

B

Figure 20-35 **A,** Protrusive interocclusal records in place, and the horizontal condylar guidance loosened and rotated to a neutral position. **B,** The horizontal condylar guidance is adjusted so both dentures stay seated on their plaster mountings and in the protrusive interocclusal records. Lateral condylar guidance is usually set at an average position for denture fabrication.

central bearing cusp tips are not reduced, but rather the opposing fossae are made deeper. Also, if the "high" contact is on the central bearing cusp inclines, the cuspal inclines can be reduced, thereby gradually moving the contact more toward the bearing cusp tip. In lateral excursions, if a central bearing cusp is "high," creating simultaneous contacts of other teeth, the opposing fossa can be widened. Balancing cusp tips and inclines are adjusted similarly, but adjustments to the cusp tips can be accomplished if needed, without the risk of decreasing vertical dimension of occlusion. CR occlusion is established first with the condyles in their locked position. During this CR grinding procedure, the incisal guide pin is relieved of contact on the incisal guidance table to allow for the slight reduction in vertical dimension that must necessarily take place. Articulating ribbon of minimum thickness is used for marking contacts of the teeth because thicker articulating paper gives deceptive contacts. Ribbon is interposed between the teeth, and markings are obtained by tapping the teeth together in the CR position. This can be recorded on both sides at the same time. After the first few taps on the articulating paper, only a few high contacts appear (Figure 20-36). Representative occlusal errors and adjustments are depicted in Figure 20-37. Grinding is done with small stones or a number 8 round bur. The marking process and the grinding are repeated until all except the anterior teeth contact in CR. Ideally all bearing cusps of the maxillary and mandibular posterior teeth will make simultaneous contact. However, it is not uncommon for one or two bearing cusps not to make contact after establishing the final CR occlusion. It is not necessary to continue adjusting until these cusps make contact because that aggressive adjustment

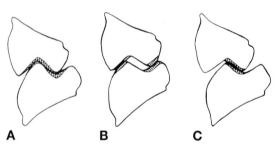

Figure 20-37   Correction of errors in centric occlusion. Grind the shaded areas. **A,** Teeth too long. **B,** Teeth too nearly end to end. **C,** Too much horizontal overlap.

will sacrifice the established vertical dimension of occlusion. The final articulating marks should remain on the dentition to maintain a reminder of the CR contacts during the upcoming adjustment of lateral excursions.

After the CR contacts have been established, the pin is placed in contact with the incisal guide table and is kept in contact throughout the remainder of the adjustment procedure. One of the articulator condyles can be released to allow a unilateral working movement. With a different color articulating ribbon, the ribbon is placed over the teeth on both sides, the articulator is moved into a working lateral position, and the contacts are marked on both sides for the same lateral movement (Figure 20-38). Care is taken not to grind on working cusp tips or the opposing fossae contact of the working cusp tips that were established in CR occlusion and remain marked with the original color ribbon. Grinding to correct lateral occlusion is limited to altering the lingual inclines of the maxillary buccal cusps and the buccal inclines of the mandibular lingual cusps on the working side and the lingual inclines of the mandibular buccal cusps on the balancing side (Figure 20-39). Because the lateral wings of the incisal table are set very shallow (often between 0 and 5 degrees), initially the pin will rise away from the table during lateral movements. Adjustments as previously described should continue until the pin remains on the table during lateral excursions. This marking and grinding procedure is repeated for the right lateral movement (Figures 20-40 and 20-41). Three types of occlusal errors can exist in adjustment of CR and

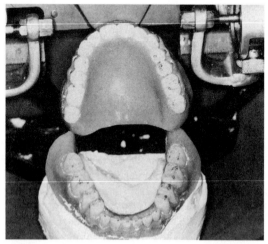

Figure 20-36   Articulating paper marks made in centric relation show interceptive or deflective occlusal contacts in centric occlusion. Grinding should be done only in fossae and not on cusps.

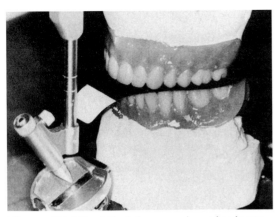

Figure 20-38   Articulating paper is used to locate deflective occlusal contacts in left lateral occlusion. Notice the position of the incisal guide pin, which has resulted from movement of the articulator into a left working position.

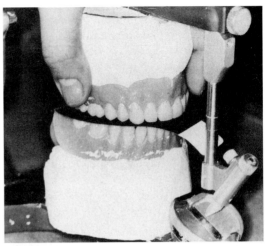

Figure 20-40   The articulator is moved between right lateral occlusion and centric occlusion, with articulating paper between the teeth to locate deflective occlusal contacts in the lateral excursion. Notice the position of the pin on the incisal guidance table.

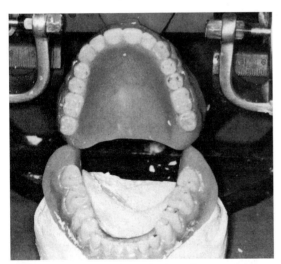

Figure 20-39   Marks on the buccal cusps of the maxillary teeth and the lingual cusps of the mandibular left posterior teeth indicate contacts in left lateral occlusion. These surfaces are ground to develop uniform contacts. The lingual cusps of maxillary teeth and the buccal cusps of mandibular teeth are not ground, even though they show marks from the articulating paper.

as many as eight errors in excursive movements. The types of interceptive occlusal contacts and the necessary adjustments are depicted in Figures 20-42 through 20-44. In most instances the lateral movement of the incisal guide pin need not exceed 3 mm. This amount of lateral movement usually moves the posterior cusp tips in an end-to-end position and meets the functional demands of the patient.

Inasmuch as denture teeth are fastened together as a unit, it is permissible to relieve the centric contact of the four incisors. This relief may be made at the time of setting the teeth, which will permit the use of a vertical overlap without increasing the incisal guide angle. Depending on the amount of anterior horizontal overlap, it will often be necessary to adjust the palatal aspect of the maxillary incisors and the length and cuspal inclines of the mandibular canines and incisors. Interceptive lateral and protrusive contacts in the anterior area must be eliminated. The sacrifice of tooth structure is usually accomplished on the mandibular anterior teeth so as not to compromise maxillary esthetics, although incisal wear patterns on the maxillary anterior teeth can be very natural appearing. The dentist may choose to make anterior adjustments on both arches.

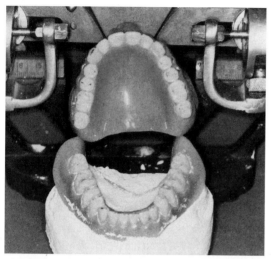

Figure 20-41   Articulating ribbon markings in right lateral excursion. Marks on the buccal cusps of maxillary right posterior teeth and the lingual cusps of mandibular right posterior teeth indicate the contacts in right lateral occlusion. These surfaces are ground to develop uniform contacts. The lingual cusps of the maxillary teeth and the buccal cusps of the mandibular teeth are not ground, even though they show marks from the articulating paper. (These marks should overlay the previous colored marks representing the central bearing contacts.)

If the grinding has been done in right and left lateral and intermediate movements, grinding in protrusion will also have been accomplished; however, a straight protrusive movement should be evaluated. Again, the dentist may wish to use a

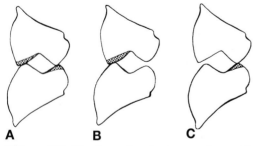

Figure 20-42   Correction of errors on the working side. Shorten interfering cusps as indicated by the shaded areas. **A,** Buccal and lingual cusps too long. **B,** Buccal cusps too long. **C,** Lingual cusps too long.

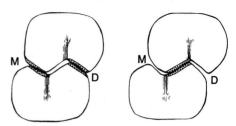

Figure 20-43   Correction of errors in the mesiodistal relationship. Grind where areas are shaded. *D,* Distal surface; *M,* mesial surface.

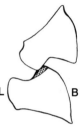

Figure 20-44   Eliminating deflective occlusal contact on the balancing side. Grind the lingual incline of the mandibular buccal cusp. *B,* Buccal surface; *L,* lingual surface.

third colored ribbon to protect the central bearing contacts and to note what "new" protrusive contacts have occurred that may be severely lifting the anterior pin from the incisal guide table. Usually only few teeth reveal a heavy discluding contact and require adjustment. Testing with articulating ribbon should show uniform protrusive contact throughout the arches of the maxillary and mandibular dentures (Figure 20-45).

Carborundum paste should not be indiscriminately used to eliminate errors in the occlusion of cusped teeth. Aggressive use of the paste could decrease vertical dimension and the sharpness of the cusps. If carborundum paste is used, smoothing of minute irregularities must be limited to only a few gliding movements of the articulator (Figure 20-46).

Eliminating Occlusal Errors in Nonanatomical Teeth

Previous chapters of this text describe several different tooth arrangements. Lingualized occlusion can be

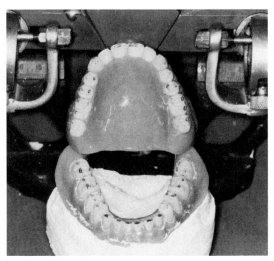

Figure 20-45 Markings made by movements in all directions indicate uniform contacts.

established by a variety of tooth designs and even with differing tooth molds in opposing arches. Nonanatomical or so-called functional posterior teeth are frequently set to establish anterior and lateral compensating curves. There can be an attempt to establish some balancing and working contacts in monoplane teeth with a "buccal-lingual tilt" of the posterior teeth with the addition of an anterior-posterior compensating curve. Complete monoplane teeth with a "flat plane" occlusion have gained in popularity. No attempt is made to achieve balanced

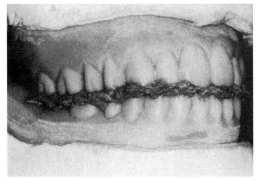

Figure 20-46 Final smoothing can be done by abrasive paste in one or two gliding movements of the articulator.

occlusion in eccentric movements. Some practitioners modify the plane of the second molar in this flat plane design to set this tooth completely out of occlusion, and others use this tooth as the sole tooth set "on a curve" to achieve balance with the premolar area, which tends to remain in contact during excursions. All of the proposed philosophies of teeth arrangement require attention to CR occlusion. The refinement of balancing and working occlusion is often possible across the arch, but it is often more difficult to achieve balancing and working contacts simultaneously within the same tooth as compared with anatomical tooth designs. It may be difficult to achieve excursive contacts in all posterior teeth. There may be only a few working or balancing contacts on each side of the arch. However, because dentures function as a unit, often only these few excursive contacts are adequate for a balanced occlusion. Whatever the occlusal philosophy established at try-in, it should be carried through with the required correction of occlusion at prosthesis insertion.

Examination of the occlusion at the time of denture insertion often reveals one or more discrepancies that may be attributable to teeth coming out of alignment during the final stages of the laboratory procedure. An interocclusal CR record is made in a bite registration material with the opposing teeth just out of contact. As in the insertion appointment of dentures with anatomical teeth, it is recommended that the dentist use remount casts, maintain the original position of the maxillary cast and condylar settings from the try-in appointment, and make a second (verification) CR record before beginning any occlusal adjustments.

After being detected by articulating ribbon between the teeth, gross premature (interceptive occlusal) contacts in CR are adjusted (Figure 20-47). The same procedures are used to locate and remove all interceptive interferences in lateral and protrusive occlusions as the occlusal philosophy dictates. The grinding is done on the occlusal surfaces of teeth that appear to have been tipped or elongated in processing. In the use of monoplane occlusion where an attempt is being made to create balance in eccentric occlusion, there are no cuspal inclines within the tooth anatomy to adjust. One can use the following method of complimentary opposing arch adjustment: in eccentric occlusion, no grinding is done on the distobuccal portion of the

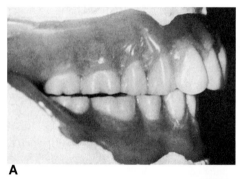

A

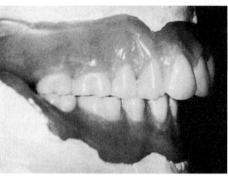

B

Figure 20-47 **A,** Gross interceptive occlusal contact in the premolar region is removed. **B,** Maximal intercuspation now occurs in centric relation.

mandibular second molar; rather, balancing-side grinding is done on the lingual portion of the occlusal surface of the maxillary second molar.

Abrasive paste is placed on the teeth in the articulator. These teeth are milled when the upper member of the articulator moves in and out of protrusive and right and left lateral excursions. A bit more aggressive use of the abrasive paste can assist in creating an almost imperceptible gentle curve in the nonanatomical tooth. Care should be taken not to excessively sacrifice vertical dimension or anterior esthetics with the paste. When the teeth slide smoothly through all excursions, the dentures are removed from the articulator and washed. Spot grinding is done to correct any small discrepancies in CR that remain after the grinding with abrasive paste. The dentist adjusts them after identifying the discrepancy with articulating ribbon, using a light tapping motion with the articulator, and grinding

the marks to ensure even occlusal contact in centric occlusion (CO).

If all occlusal correction steps were properly performed, the contacts achieved in the mouth should be the same as those achieved on the articulator when the dentures are inserted (Figure 20-48). The mounted casts and articulator should be maintained until the adjustment period is over. Finally the remount casts can be sent home with the patient to bring at follow-up visits.

ADVANTAGES OF BALANCED OCCLUSION IN COMPLETE DENTURES

What is the advantage of balanced occlusion in dentures when a bolus of food on one side separates the teeth so that they cannot possibly be in balancing contact on the opposite side? This question has caused many dentists to speculate that balancing occlusion is a fetish of college professors and a few specialists. Many dentures that are delivered are not balanced in excursive movements because a large proportion of the profession is not thoroughly convinced of the value of balanced occlusion in relation to the effort involved in achieving it. If a bolus of food were between the teeth during most of the day, there would not be much merit in having an exactly balanced occlusion. However, teeth make contact many thousands of times a day in both eccentric nonfunctional mandibular movements and centric positions, with no food in the mouth. Even while a person chews food, the teeth cut through to contact every few fractions of a second. A balanced occlusion ensures even pressure in all parts of the arch, which maintains the stability of the dentures.

SPECIAL INSTRUCTIONS TO THE PATIENT

Educating patients to the limitations of dentures as mechanical substitutes for living tissues must be a continuing process from the initial patient contact until adjustments are completed. However, certain difficulties that will be encountered with new dentures and the information related to the care of dentures should be reinforced at the time of initial placement of the dentures. Forewarning makes the

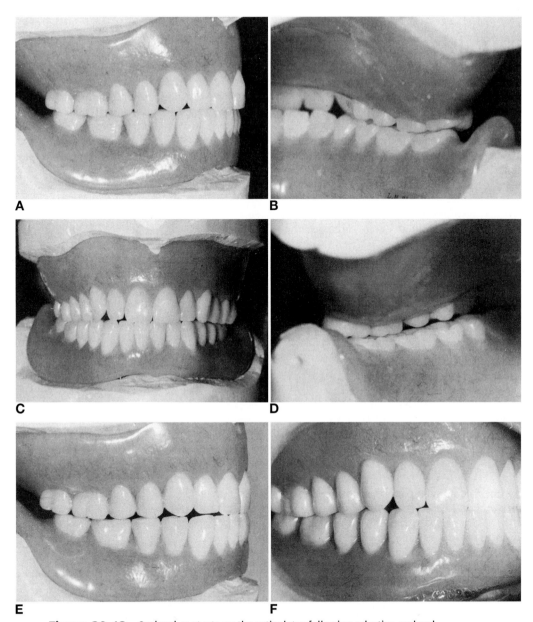

Figure 20-48 Occlusal contacts on the articulator following selective occlusal adjustment. **A** and **B,** Centric occlusion, buccal and lingual views. **C** and **D,** Right lateral occlusion, labial and lingual views. Notice in the lingual how balance has been achieved in the molar region. **E,** Protrusive position. Here, multiple balancing contacts exist because of the shape of the compensating curve. **F,** In this clinical view, notice the uniformity of contacts as established on the articulator (**A**). Color photographs of this patient are presented in Plate 18-1, D to F.

patient more tolerant of problems and less likely to relate them incorrectly to the fit of the dentures. Explanations provided after problems develop often are interpreted as excuses by the dentist for dentures that function less than satisfactorily.

Individuality of Patients

Patients must be reminded that their physical, mental, and oral conditions are individual in nature. Thus they cannot compare their progress with new dentures to other persons' experiences. Denture complaints that are annoying and painful to some patients may be of secondary importance to others. Chewing and speech patterns considered successful by some persons may be interpreted as unsuccessful by others. Patients tend to forget the severity of problems with the passage of time. Many persons indicate that their dentures have always been comfortable, even though they may have had a difficult adjustment period. In addition, adaptability to new dentures is modified by age. Persons who make the adjustment to new dentures during middle age may experience considerably more difficulty with dentures 15 years later, even though the new dentures may be technically superior to the original ones. These remarks can be discouraging to patients with new dentures unless they have been advised of this possibility.

Appearance with New Dentures

Patients must understand that their appearance with new dentures will become more natural with time. Initially, the dentures may feel strange and bulky in the mouth and will cause a feeling of fullness of the lips and cheeks. The lips will not adapt immediately to the fullness of the denture borders and may initially present a distorted appearance. Muscle tension may cause an awkward appearance, which will improve after the patient becomes relaxed and more confident. Patients should be instructed to refrain from exhibiting their dentures to curious friends until they are more confident and competent at exhibiting them. When patients are not careful in following these instructions, they may likely become unfairly critical of the dentures and develop an attitude that will be difficult for the dentist to overcome. During the edentulous or partially

edentulous period, gradual reduction of the interarch distance and collapsing of the lips will have occurred. These changes usually have been so gradual that family and friends were not aware that they existed. Therefore a repositioning of the orbicularis oris muscle and a restoration of the former facial dimension and contour by the new dentures may seem like too great a change in the patient's appearance. This can be overcome only with the passage of time, and patients are advised to persevere during the period.

Some dentists advise patients to change a hairstyle or change glasses along with their new dentures. This allows onlookers to notice the overall change in the face. Often the dentures are not even noticed by the observer as being responsible for the change in appearance, but rather the pleasing change in the overall face will be observed. A change in glasses or hairstyle also allows the patient to respond to the comments with a discussion about the glasses or the hair and not confide about the new dentures, unless he or she wishes.

Mastication with New Dentures

Learning to chew satisfactorily with new dentures usually requires at least 6 to 8 weeks. Patients will become discouraged unless they are aware that this learning period is to be expected. New memory patterns often must be established for both the facial muscles and the muscles of mastication. Once the habit patterns become automatic, the chewing process can take place without conscious effort. The muscles of the tongue, cheeks, and lips must be trained to maintain the dentures in position on the residual ridges during mastication. Patients can be told that "these muscles must learn what they should and should not do."

Patient comfort and mastication may be impaired because of the elicited excess flow of saliva for the first few days after placement of new dentures. However, in a relatively short time the salivary glands accommodate to the presence of the dentures, and normal production of saliva returns.

Patients should begin chewing relatively soft food that has been cut into small pieces. If the chewing can be done on both sides of the mouth at the same time, the tendency of the dentures to tip will be reduced. Patients should be told that during this early period, mastication is best attempted on simple types of food such as crackers, soft toast, or chopped meat and that no attempt should be made to masticate more resistant foods. First-time denture wearers may be advised to eat foods that require little mastication, but those that are ready for swallowing with a simple push of the tongue against the palate. This will give the patients confidence in stabilizing the dentures. Also, during the learning period, patients are advised to avoid observation by friends or members of the family because the patients will be awkward in the beginning phases of chewing and susceptible to embarrassment and discouragement. Kindly but misplaced joking remarks and comments by members of the family may readily lead a patient to become self-conscious about the dentures, and this will be reflected in the attitude toward the dentist and the dentures.

When biting with dentures, patients should be instructed to place the food between their teeth toward the corners of the mouth, rather than between the anterior teeth. Then the food should be pushed inward and upward to break it apart rather than downward and outward as would be done if natural teeth were present. Inward and upward forces tend to seat the dentures on the residual ridges rather than displace them.

Occasionally, edentulous patients have gone without dentures for long periods and have learned to crush food between the residual ridges or perhaps between the tongue and the hard palate. These persons usually experience increased difficulty in learning to masticate with new dentures, and the time for adjustment will likely be extended.

Patients should be told that the position of the tongue plays an important role in the stability of a lower denture, particularly during mastication. Patients whose tongues normally rest in a retracted position relative to the lower anterior teeth should attempt to position the tongue farther forward so it rests on the lingual surfaces of the lower anterior teeth. This will help develop stability for the lower denture.

Speaking with New Dentures

Fortunately, the problem of speaking with new dentures is not as difficult as might be expected. The adaptability of the tongue to compensate for changes is so great that most patients master speech with new dentures within a few weeks. If correct speech required exact replacement of tissues and teeth in relation to tongue movement, no patient would ever learn to talk with dentures. If it were not for the extreme adaptability of the tongue, the necessity of additional bulk over the palate would cause a lasting speech impediment. Even a 0.5-mm change at the linguogingival border of the anterior teeth would cause a speech defect, especially in the production of *s* sounds. Therefore tooth positions that restore appearance and masticatory function usually do not produce phonetic changes that are too great to be readily compensated.

Speaking normally with dentures requires practice. Patients should be advised to read aloud and repeat words or phrases that are difficult to pronounce. Patients usually are much more conscious of small irregularities in their speech sounds than those to whom they are speaking. It should be noted that elderly patients with dentures often have hearing impairments and will have a greater difficulty in changing speech patterns without auditory feedback. An understanding of tongue positions during speech is valuable. Dentists should have an appreciation of tooth position, palatal contours, and lingual contours of the mandibular denture, and these should be technically addressed at try-in and insertion, rather than complete reliance on patient adaptation.

Oral Hygiene with Dentures

Patients must be convinced of the importance of maintaining good oral hygiene for the health of the oral cavity. Plaque, stains, and calculus accrue on dentures and oral mucosa of edentulous patients in a similar fashion as in the mouths of dentulous patients. Dental plaque is an etiological factor in denture stomatitis, inflammatory papillary hyperplasia, chronic candidiasis, and offensive odors, and it must be removed.

Patients should be instructed to rinse their dentures and their mouths after meals whenever possible. Once a day, it is essential that the dentures be removed and placed in a soaking type of cleanser for a minimum of 30 minutes. This time is required for effective killing of microorganisms on the dentures, as well as removal of all stains. Commercial cleaners are quite effective, and leaving the dentures in the cleanser overnight is even better. Before the dentures are placed in the cleanser, they should be brushed gently with a soft brush. Patients need to be instructed that the brushing is required to remove plaque because the soaking will not do so. The dentures should be brushed over a basin partially filled with water or covered with a wet washcloth to prevent breakage in case they are dropped. Patients should be discouraged from using toothpastes because most contain an abrasive material that will wear away the surface of acrylic resin. An inexpensive alternative soaking cleanser is one that can be made up with 1 teaspoon of household bleach and 2 teaspoons of water softener (Calgon) in 8 oz of water. The mucosal surfaces of the residual ridges and the dorsal surface of the tongue also should be brushed daily with a soft brush. This will increase the circulation and remove plaque and debris that can cause irritation of the mucous membrane or offensive odors.

Preserving the Residual Ridges

The residual ridges were not intended to bear the stresses of mastication created by complete dentures. Therefore patients, especially when their general health is somewhat impaired, may expect some irritation and discomfort of the oral tissues. No two patients' mouths will react alike because some tissues tolerate stress better than others. Therefore it is impossible to predict exactly what to expect. Patients must be aware of these varying and unpredictable conditions.

If some irritation of the tissues is experienced, patients are advised to remove their dentures and rest the mouth for a time. It may be harmful to the patients' tissues and their psyche by telling patients that they must keep their dentures in the mouth constantly during this initial adjustment period. They may become highly nervous and fatigued and be unnecessarily discouraged. However, patients are requested to wear the dentures for several hours before an adjustment appointment so any sore spots will be visible and accurate corrections of the dentures can be made. Patients must be cautioned concerning the critical nature of adjustments to the dentures. They must be convinced that the dentist is

the only person qualified to undertake this most important aspect of denture service. Obviously, patients should never attempt to adjust the dentures themselves.

Patients should be told that dentures must be left out of the mouth at night to provide needed rest from the stresses they create on the residual ridges. Failure to allow the tissues of the basal seat to rest may be a contributing factor in the development of serious oral lesions, such as inflammatory papillary hyperplasia, or may increase the opportunity for microbial infections, such as candidiasis. When dentures are left out of the mouth, they should be placed in a container filled with water to prevent drying and possible dimensional changes of the denture base material.

Residual ridges can be damaged by the use of denture adhesives and particularly home-reliners, to compensate for ill-fitting dentures. Patients should therefore be cautioned about this. If these materials are used, patients soon feel insecure without them. Adhesives, and especially home-reliners, can modify the position of the denture on the residual ridge that can result in a change of both vertical relations and CRs or a change in occlusal contacts, which may cause irreparable damage to the residual ridges in a short time.

The special instructions must include directions for continued periodic oral examinations for all edentulous patients. The tissues supporting dentures change with time, and the rate of change depends on both local and general factors. Good dentures eventually become ill fitting and can damage the mouth without the patient's being aware that anything is wrong. Pathosis, which may or may not be associated with the dentures, can develop in the edentulous oral cavity. All edentulous patients should be examined by a dentist at least once a year, and their names should be placed on a recall list for that purpose.

Educational Material for Patients

Because the education of patients is so critical to the success of new dentures, many dentists provide written instructions or other formal educational material that has been developed. In studying the material, patients become aware that dentures are not permanent, that the mouth changes, and most important, that the care they provide themselves may be a deciding factor in the success they experience with dentures. People remember less of what they hear than of what they see. For this reason, it is wise to provide denture-wearing patients with printed information about their new teeth, about the care and cleaning of the teeth, about their use, and most important, about the periodic inspections that will be necessary.

SECTION III: MAINTAINING THE COMFORT AND HEALTH OF THE ORAL CAVITY IN A REHABILITATED EDENTULOUS PATIENT

The complete denture service cannot be adequate unless patients are cared for after the dentures are placed in the mouth. In many instances, the most crucial time in the patient's perception of success or failure of dentures is the adjustment period. The dentist is responsible for the care of the patient throughout this period, and this occasionally requires a number of appointments. The complete cooperation of the patient during the adjustment period is essential. In educating patients, the dentist must explain to them the problems that they are likely to face during the adjustment phase and the procedures that both the patient and the dentist must follow to alleviate these problems. It is important that the dentist and the patient have a clear understanding as to the financial implications of the adjustment period, which reflects the dentist practice management protocol.

TWENTY-FOUR-HOUR ORAL EXAMINATION AND TREATMENT

An appointment for a 1- to 3-day adjustment should be made routinely. Patients who do not receive this attention have more trouble than those who are cared for the first several days after the insertion of the new dentures. This is the critical period in the denture-wearing experience of the patient. When the patient returns for the first adjustment, the dentist can ask, "How are you getting along with the sore mouth?" This invites patients to describe their experiences and soreness, if any. The dentist must listen carefully to the patient and on the basis of these comments can learn approximately where to look for trouble. The statements may also furnish valuable information about esthetic, functional, and mental attitude problems that may be developing.

Examination Procedures

The occlusion should be observed before the dentures are removed from the mouth. To do this, the mandible is guided into CR by placing a thumb directly on the anteroinferior portion of the chin and supporting the mandibular denture intraorally, directing the patient to "open and close your 'lower jaw' until you feel the first feather touch of your back teeth." At the first contact, the patient is directed to open and repeat this closure, "only this time stop the instant you feel a tooth touch and then close tight." If the teeth touch and slide, there is an error in CO. When such an error is detected, the dentures are placed on their remount casts on the articulator, and the occlusion is rechecked there. If the same error is found on the articulator, it requires occlusal adjustment. If there is an error in the mouth and none is found on the articulator, new interocclusal records must be made. The mandibular remount cast is removed from the articulator, and the mandibular denture is remounted before the occlusion is corrected.

After the occlusion has been tested and corrected (if necessary), a thorough visual and digital examination of the oral cavity is performed so the location of sore spots can be determined. The examination begins with the mucosa of the maxillary buccal vestibule and proceeds around through the labial and the buccal vestibules on the other side of the mouth, with careful observation of the frena. The hamular notches and the hard and soft palates are examined for signs of abrasion. The area of the coronoid process is palpated, and the patient is asked if there is any tenderness in this region.

The mandibular dental arch and associated dental structures are systematically examined both visually and digitally. The tissues lining the vestibular spaces and the alveololingual sulci, particularly the mylohyoid ridges and the retromylohyoid spaces, are observed carefully. The sides of the tongue and the mucosal lining of the cheeks must also be inspected.

Adjustments Related to the Occlusion

A number of problems can result from errors in the occlusion. Soreness may develop on the crest of the residual ridge from pressures created by heavy contacts of opposing teeth in the same region. Soreness also may be seen on the slopes of the residual ridge as a result of shifting of the denture bases from deflective occlusal contacts (Figure 20-49). Before unnecessarily shortening or excessively relieving the denture base, the dentist must observe the occlusion carefully in the mouth and on the articulator, giving particular attention to the possibility of heavy balancing-side contacts that could cause rotation of the mandibular denture base. Such occlusion errors are almost impossible to locate in the mouth because of movement of the denture bases on the supporting soft tissues.

Small lesions on the buccal mucosa of the cheek in line with the occlusal plane indicate that the patient is biting the cheek during mastication. This problem usually can be corrected by reducing the buccal surface of the offending mandibular tooth to create additional horizontal overlap, thus providing an escape for the buccal mucosa.

A patient may complain, "My dentures are tight when I first put them in my mouth, but they seem to loosen after several hours." This symptom usually is an indication of errors in the occlusion that can be corrected after new interocclusal records are made,

the dentures are remounted, and the occlusion is adjusted on the articulator. The dentures become loose because the deflective occlusal contacts cause a continual shifting of the denture base, which in turn causes distortion of the tissues in the basal seat. Although this problem may develop by the time of the 1- to 3-day adjustment, it is more likely to be seen a little later on.

Adjustments Related to the Denture Bases

A number of problems with new dentures are related to the denture bases themselves. Irritation to the vestibular mucosa is most often caused by denture borders that are too sharp or denture flanges that are overextended. This is often seen at the hamular notch area, along the mandibular retromylohyoid area, mandibular buccal area, and prominent anterior frena. Before any adjustments are made, a heavy coating of pressure paste in the offending area, with border molding, will determine if the problem is overextension or contact pressure along the bone at the flange extension. Lesions in the region of the hamular notch must be considered carefully. If the irritated tissue is posterior to the notch, the denture base is too long and must be shortened. However, if the soreness is in the notch itself, the posterior palatal seal is likely creating too much pressure, and the inside of the

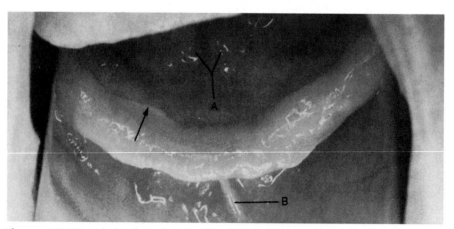

Figure 20-49 A lesion *(arrow)* on the lingual slope of the mandibular residual ridge is likely due to errors in the occlusion that caused the denture base to shift and thus impinge on the mucosa. *A,* Sublingual caruncles; *B,* mandibular labial frenum.

tissue surface of the denture base will need to be relieved very cautiously so as not to loosen border seal. Use the following three steps to evaluate this area with paste: (1) one notch with adjustment, (2) the other notch with adjustment, and (3) then the posterior border length and posterior palatal seal on the denture surface with adjustment. The use of these steps will minimize making an error in reading the pressure paste and overreducing the seal (Figures 20-50 and 20-51). The remainder of denture borders are shortened and rechecked with paste again. Finally they can be polished with pumice and a rag wheel. Irritated frena or paste-disclosed pressure in the notches will require that the notches be deepened slightly (Figure 20-52). Widening of the notch may not be necessary and, if done to excess, could reduce denture retention. The notch is deepened with a fissure bur and polished with a stone or small wheel. Pressure indicator paste should be used to evaluate pressure areas on the basal surface, regardless of whether sores or ulcerations are evident. It should be applied and read in the same way as described during the insertion phase. When pressure areas are found, they need to be adjusted and the entire denture disclosed again. It will be common that additional pressure areas will present, and need relieving. Finally the contact will be uniform throughout the denture. Use of an indelible marking pencil placed on the ulcerative tissue as a pressure transfer should never be used as the only means of tissue recall evaluation. Only focusing on the acute problem will likely move the pressure to another area of the denture, causing another acute ulcer to be dealt with a few days later. Skilled practitioners may use a combination of paste and markers, but the student who watches the faculty use the indelible pencil may incorrectly assume it is the faster and easier diagnostic tool of choice. Students should be encouraged to learn to "read" the subtle but very diagnostic signs derived from correctly manipulated pressure paste (Figures 20-53 through 20-55).

Excessive pressure from the mandibular buccal flange in the region of the mental foramen may cause a tingling or numbing sensation at the corner of the mouth or in the lower lip. This results from impingement on the mental nerve and occurs particularly when excess resorption has caused the mental foramen to be located near the crest of the mandibular residual ridge. A similar situation can occur in the maxillae from pressure on the incisive papilla transmitted to the nasopalatine nerve. The patient may complain of burning or numbness in the anterior part of the maxillae. Relief may be required in the maxillary denture base in this region.

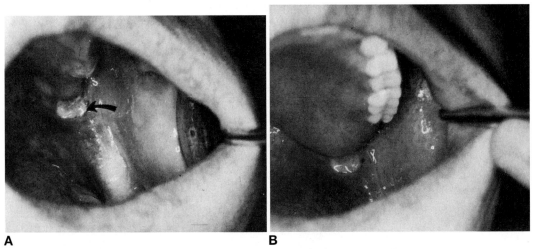

A   **B**

Figure 20-50   **A,** The sore spot *(arrow)* is posterior to the hamular notch, indicating that the denture base is too long in this region. **B,** After adjustment of the denture, notice that the spot is posterior to the border.

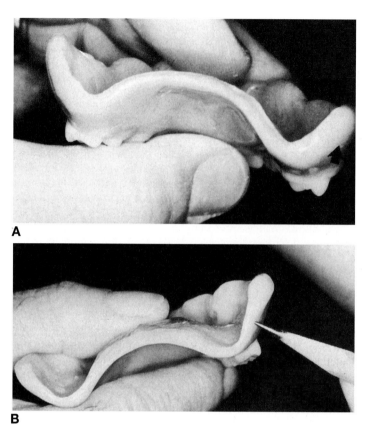

Figure 20-51 **A,** The distobuccal flange of this maxillary denture is too thick below the border *(arrow).* Using paste along the border periphery and thickness of the flange in this area reveals the pressure created in the hamular area. **B,** This flange is of proper thickness.

Patients may return for the initial adjustment appointment complaining that their dentures cause them to gag. This problem may actually be related to the dentures themselves, or there may be a psychological component. When the problem is den-

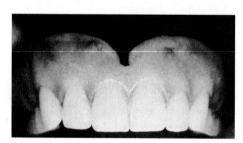

Figure 20-52 Labial notches must be sufficiently deep, with borders that are rounded and smooth.

ture related, usually the maxillary denture is the culprit, although on occasion the mandibular denture or both will be involved. Most often, the gagging relates to the posterior border of the maxillary denture. The border may be improperly extended, or the posterior border seal may be inadequate (Figure 20-56). Gagging often occurs when the posterior border seal is disrupted as the tissue distal to the vibrating line moves upward and downward during function. When the vibrating line has been properly located, it is not necessary (and usually not desirable) to extend the posterior border of the maxillary denture more than 2 mm beyond this point. If the posterior palatal seal is inadequate, modeling compound can be added to reshape this part of the maxillary denture and help alleviate the situation. Then the modeling compound can be

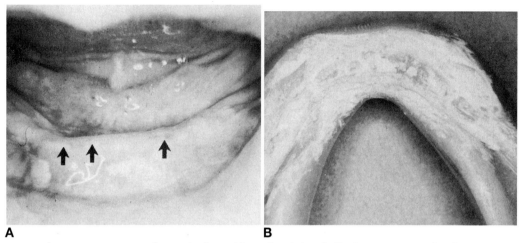

A   B

Figure 20-53   **A,** Spiny projections of bone *(arrows)* underlie the mucosa covering the crest of this mandibular residual ridge. **B,** Pressure spots in the indicator paste show where relief will be needed. The denture base will be adjusted with a no. 8 round bur.

replaced with acrylic resin. The occlusion may also be a factor because shifting of the denture bases affects the posterior palatal seal.

On occasion, patients will state that the maxillary denture comes loose when they open their mouth wide to bite into a sandwich or to yawn. Generally, this complaint indicates that the disto-buccal flange of the maxillary denture is too thick and interferes with normal movements of the coronoid process (see Figure 20-51). The borders of the

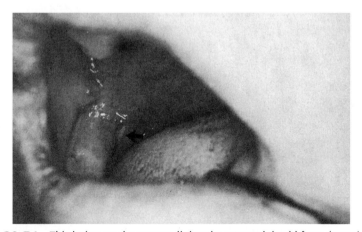

Figure 20-54   This lesion on the mucosa lining the retromylohyoid fossa *(arrow)* was caused by excessive length and pressure from the denture base. Pressure paste that is placed in this area will likely rub off the border as well as reveal a pressure area along the bony mandible just internal to the flange. Both the flange and basal surface will require adjustment. Often patients will complain of soreness when they swallow or state that they feel as if they have a sore throat. Complaints of soreness during swallowing also are frequently related to irritation in the region of the mylohyoid ridges.

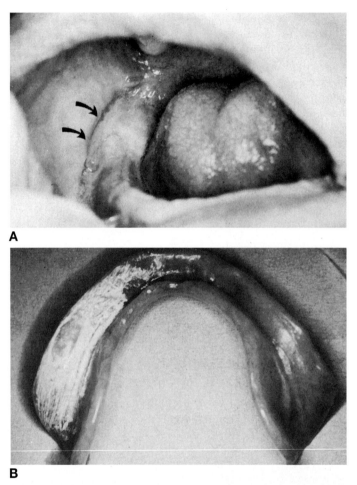

Figure 20-55 A, This line of irritation *(arrows)* was caused by an overextended buccal flange of the mandibular denture. Pressure paste that is placed on the flange edge of the flange only will reveal the area causing the problem. It should be repeatedly checked and adjusted until none of the paste rubs off the denture. **B,** The pressure spot in indicator paste represents the part of this denture base that has been placing excessive pressure on the buccal shelf and is not related to the length of the flange causing the ulcers in **A.**

maxillary buccal flanges should properly fill the buccal vestibule. However, the distal corners of the denture base below the borders must be thin to allow the freedom necessary for movement of the coronoid process.

Again, in discussions with patients, it may be revealed that the maxillary denture tends to loosen during smiling or other forms of facial expression.

Excessive thickness or height of the flange of the maxillary denture in the region of the buccal notch or distal to the notch may cause this problem (Figure 20-57). As the buccal frenum moves posteriorly during function, it encroaches on a border that is too thick, and the denture becomes loosened. Reduction of the width of the border posterior to the maxillary buccal notch often will relieve this problem.

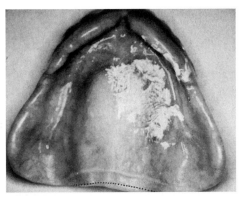

Figure 20-56 Overextended posterior border of a maxillary denture. When the border was shortened to the approximate length indicated by the dotted line, the denture no longer caused the patient to gag.

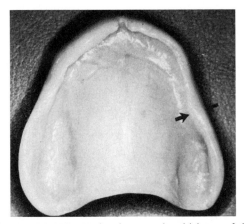

Figure 20-57 Notice the excessive thickness of the right buccal border in the region of the buccal notch *(arrows)*. The buccal frenum, moving posteriorly over this border during facial expression, can loosen or unseat a maxillary denture. This area can be discerned from patient complaint and pressure paste on the border.

SUBSEQUENT ORAL EXAMINATIONS AND TREATMENTS

Dentures require inspection and sometimes further adjustment after they have been used by the patient. During the first several weeks, the acrylic resin absorbs water. This can result in small changes in the size and shape of the dentures. Even though the

alterations are small, they may be sufficient to change the occlusion. Minute changes in the occlusion can create discomfort by making the dentures shift or slide in function. Soreness reported by patients in this situation is most likely on the lingual side of the mandibular ridge in the region of the canine and first premolar and is most likely due to deflective occlusal contact between the last molar teeth diagonally across the mouth, often between the balancing inclines of the mandibular second molars.

In most instances, the occlusal error can be observed and corrected by placement of the dentures in their original remount casts on the articulator. If, however, the bases have so changed that they no longer fit the remount casts the way they did originally, it will be necessary to make new remount casts and new interocclusal records. The remount jig record will permit the maxillary denture to be remounted without making a new face bow transfer record.

After the new records are made, the occlusion is corrected by selective grinding with the same procedure as was used at the time of the dentures' insertion. It is interesting that the occlusal changes will likely be small, but the soreness they produce is very real and disturbing. Dentists should not succumb to the temptation to grind from the denture base without determining the real cause of the trouble.

Sometimes generalized irritation or soreness of the basal seat will develop. Although this condition may be attributable to a number of factors (such as an excessive vertical dimension of occlusion, nutritional or hormonal problems, or unhygienic dentures), it more likely is due to the occlusion. As indicated previously, errors in occlusion should be suspected whenever a patient states that the dentures are "tight when I first put them in my mouth in the morning but seem to loosen later in the day." A collection of calculus on the teeth on one side of the denture also indicates the need for correcting the occlusion.

Certain symptoms at an adjustment appointment suggest an insufficient interocclusal distance. The patient may comment, "After I've worn the new dentures for several hours, my gums get sore and the muscles in the lower part of my face seem tired." On removal of the dentures, the mucosa of the basal seat often will exhibit a generalized irritation. These symptoms indicate that when the patient's mandible is in the resting position, there is not sufficient space between the opposing teeth to allow the supporting structures of the residual ridge and the involved muscles to rest normally. If this is true, several options exist. Sometimes creating a small amount of additional interocclusal distance will solve the problem, and the dentist can do this by returning the dentures to the articulator and grinding the artificial teeth to reduce the vertical dimension of occlusion; esthetics and the amount of clearance between the anterior teeth are the limiting factors in this procedure, and another 1 to 1.5 mm of interocclusal distance can thus be created. Other times it may be necessary to reset the artificial teeth of one or both dentures; the decision as to which teeth should be moved is based on esthetics and the vertical dimension of occlusion. Finally, in some instances, the dentures will have to be remade.

Periodic Recall for Oral Examination

When patients are judged to be successfully treated and the necessary adjustment appointments after denture insertion are completed, patients are instructed to call for an appointment if they have any problems. Patients with some of the more difficult problems should be scheduled for appointments periodically, perhaps at 3- to 4-month intervals. This will help their morale and may tend to eliminate their seeking adjustment appointments on a weekly basis or even more often.

Every denture-wearing patient should be in a recall program, just as any other dental patient is. The dentist should not hesitate to inform a patient that occlusal corrections, relining, new dentures, or other fairly involved procedures may be necessary as changes in the mouth continue to occur. A 12-month interval is the suggested time between recall appointments for most patients with complete dentures.

Bibliography

Johnstone EP, Nicholls JI, Smith DE: Flexure fatigue of 10 commonly used denture base resins, *J Prosthet Dent* 46:478-483, 1981.

Spratley MH: An investigation of the adhesion of acrylic resin teeth to dentures, *J Prosthet Dent* 58:389-392, 1987.

CHAPTER 21

Single Dentures

Alan B. Carr

As mentioned earlier, the edentulous state can be considered equivalent to the absence of a body part with specific morphological functional and psychological sequelae. This chapter discusses the patient with a single edentulous arch. For such a patient, the clinical challenge is one of appreciating the biomechanical differences in the supporting tissues for the two arches and applying the appropriate management procedures to produce and maintain the conditions necessary for long-term treatment success. In this chapter, a basic treatment protocol is also described.

SINGLE EDENTULOUS ARCH

The prevalence of the condition in which one edentulous arch opposes a natural or restored dentition is common, and it has been estimated that in some patient populations mandibular canines are retained for the longest time—four times longer than other teeth. After the mandibular canines, the next longest-lasting teeth are mandibular incisors. This documented arch discrepancy in tooth survival suggests that the maxillary arch exhibits earlier tooth loss. The reasons for the loss of the maxillary teeth before the mandibular teeth are unclear and are influenced by a combination of factors. One major factor might be the dental profession's perception of the ease of construction of maxillary dentures compared with mandibular ones and the comparative functional success of maxillary versus mandibular complete dentures. It is therefore important for the clinician to have an appreciation of some oral conditions that may predispose this specific patient population to complications after treatment with conventional complete dentures. Such an understanding will help the clinician determine when preservation of useful maxillary teeth is warranted over their extraction. Because mandibular anterior teeth are preserved the longest, most of the discussion in this chapter focuses on the oral condition in which the maxillary arch is edentulous and opposed by a natural or restored mandibular dentition.

CHALLENGE OF VARYING SUPPORT

The qualitative and quantitative difference between natural tooth and complete denture support has been emphasized earlier in this book. The difference is one of adaptability versus maladaptability: the natural dentition is capable of sophisticated responses to occlusal demands that largely preserve functional capability, whereas mucoperiosteal bone support is incapable of such favorable adaptation. Unfavorable responses exhibit a spectrum of severity for varying population groups. For example, the postmenopausal white female is more likely to exhibit a rapid and severe morphological change in the denture-bearing tissues than a younger white male who has been edentulous for the same length of time. However, even with the same patient population, the group ability to adapt to comparable morphological features differs among patients. In other words, for a group of patients in the same age, sex, and racial category, the patient response to complete denture use will be variable. This does not appear to be the case for patients with fixed prostheses in whom treatment response appears to be more predictable. Consequently, managing the replacement of the missing maxillary dentition must take into account the variation in opposing arch support and provide for an optimum distribution of occlusal forces to minimize the negative effects in the compromised edentulous arch. This will demand an understanding of factors that magnify the inherent risk of regressive changes in the edentulous arch. Early identification of these factors and their likely impact on complete denture prognosis must be addressed with the patient.

DIAGNOSIS AND TREATMENT PLANNING

The commonly cited long-term goal in prosthodontics is the preservation of that which remains. This demands an appreciation of occlusal biomechanics as referred to in Chapters 16 and 17. Salient considerations include: (1) acceptable interocclusal distance, (2) stable jaw relationship with bilateral tooth contacts in retruded closure, (3) stable tooth quadrant relationships with axially directed forces, and (4) multidirectional freedom of tooth contact throughout a small range (within 2 mm) of mandibular movements. These characteristics of a physiological occlusion are frequently encountered in fully dentate mouths. They also can be almost invariably achieved when treating fully edentulous patients. However, when only one arch is edentulous, tooth positions in the dentate arch may preclude such objectives being reached. Unfavorable

force distributions may then cause adverse tissue changes that compromise optimum function. It is therefore important to identify such clinical changes and to correct them.

These changes include: (1) extensive morphological changes in denture foundation that can result in arch relationship or occlusal plane discrepancies, (2) jaw relationship extremes, and (3) excessively displaceable denture-bearing tissue. Routine morphological changes occur after tooth extraction and result in a generally smaller maxilla when compared with the dentulous state. This creates a horizontal discrepancy between the arches anteriorly and posteriorly (Figure 21-1) and makes it difficult to direct occlusal forces to the denture-bearing surfaces because the support is at a distance from the denture tooth position. The best strategy for correcting this discrepancy posteriorly is to place the teeth in a reverse horizontal overlap or crossbite arrangement. However, such a correction procedure for the anterior discrepancy is not possible because of the esthetic impact on the maxillary lip of such a tooth position.

Changes in the denture foundation also can occur because of longstanding uncontrolled occlusal forces (Figure 21-2). This elicits a combination of morphological and spatial changes, for example, a maxillary complete denture opposed by

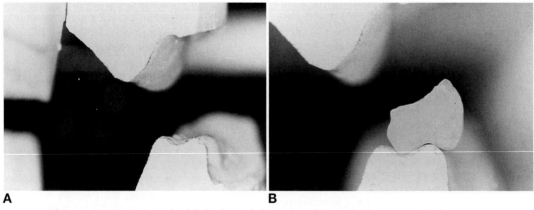

A   **B**

Figure 21-1 **A,** Posterior left horizontal ridge–opposing tooth discrepancy. Notice the location of the mandibular molar is directly beneath the maxillary vestibule. **B,** Same location with the maxillary molar denture tooth placed in normal intercuspation. Notice the distance from the tooth to the ridge and the potential for tilting to result, given the lack of support directly beneath the denture tooth.

Continued

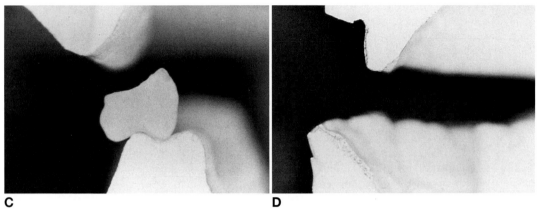

C   **D**

Figure 21-1 *cont'd* **C,** The same location; however, the maxillary denture tooth is placed in a reverse horizontal occlusion and in such a position presents less of a tilting potential on mastication. **D,** A sagittal view of the anterior region of the same mouth reveals the horizontal discrepancy between the mandibular incisors and the opposing maxillary anterior ridge.

anterior mandibular teeth only or by a mandibular arch restored with a Kennedy Class I removable partial denture that has not maintained the denture support. Both conditions are characterized by occlusal forces that are concentrated exclusively on the premaxillary region. When such a force distri-

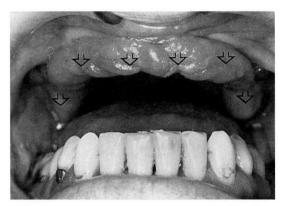

Figure 21-2 The entire maxillary denture-bearing ridge area has been replaced by mobile, hyperplastic tissue. Its surgical removal will result in a nonretentive prosthesis because the vestibule will be virtually obliterated. This morphological predicament has partly resulted from the complete maxillary denture's opposing an intact natural dentition after many years of denture wearing.

bution is allowed to go uncorrected, the premaxillary region undergoes destructive changes that allow displacement of the denture superiorly, and the resultant change in the occlusal plane can allow a downgrowth of the maxillary tuberosities. If not addressed through the necessary preprosthetic surgery, as well as provision and maintenance of posterior occlusion, such a combination of changes in the maxillary arch may predispose new prostheses to failure because of the inability to prescribe a normal occlusal plane and denture foundation that provide optimum occlusal force distribution and support around the arch.

Extremes of jaw relationship also make it difficult to place the denture teeth in a position that allows the denture-bearing area to be in line with the occlusal support. This is most often the situation with a Class III skeletal relationship, and the dilemma is similar to the previously mentioned arch discrepancy seen with the normal postextraction ridge changes. The most common procedure for addressing the problem is to place the posterior teeth in a reverse horizontal overlap or crossbite relationship. The anterior teeth, however, cannot be placed lingual to the mandibular teeth, and the potential for dislodgement with anterior tooth contact is problematic.

The dilemma posed by excessively displaceable tissue is one of differential support capability to the same load. The forces of occlusion are resisted by the mucoperiosteum, which allows some movement of the denture base by virtue of its resiliency. When tissue changes allow excessive displacement in one area but not in another, the movement of the prosthesis under load is greater in the region of greater tissue displacement, with resultant dislodgement.

Conditions in the opposing arch also can predispose the patient to problems with a single complete denture. The most common condition is an irregular occlusal plane (Figure 21-3). This often is seen as a tilting or extrusion of teeth after the extraction of a mandibular first molar, and the second and third molars exhibit an anterior inclination and possibly a superior position compared with the normal relationship. This results in an irregular occlusal plane and consequent unfavorable force distribution. Assessment of the irregularity present in an occlusal plane is necessary to guide the required selective grinding. It can be achieved with a template or curved occlusal plane such as that used in setting denture teeth. When placed on the dental arch, this device rests on the teeth that are most prominent in the vertical plane and can be used to determine the selective grinding of the most prominent teeth to ensure that a sufficient number of teeth are in contact. This provides a uniform reduction but may not meet the needs of a specific denture arrangement for stable cross arch balance.

CLINICAL AND LABORATORY PROCEDURES

In the case of a single maxillary denture, a final impression is made of the maxillary arch, and an opposing impression is made of the mandibular arch. If a cast metal base (nonprecious or gold alloy) is prescribed, this is now made in a full palatal coverage design with mesh extensions over the edentulous ridges and extending to the posterior palatal seal area. A maxillary occlusion rim is fabricated, and if bilateral or tripod stable centric stops can be established on this rim, a centric relation (CR) record is made in wax or fast-setting plaster. When stable centric stops are not feasible because of a reduced mandibular dentition, a partial mandibular occlusion rim must be used for the

CR record. A face bow registration is made, and the casts are mounted on a semiadjustable articulator. The condylar guidances on the articulator are set either to an average value or to settings provided by protrusive records. The incisal guidance is set at the angle considered necessary for the denture's occlusion. Horizontal settings will allow for shallow inclines and a more stable denture during eccentric contact movements. Esthetics will influence the angle of the incisal guide because the vertical position of the anterior teeth varies with the amount of vertical overlap used.

The teeth are arranged with the proper inclinations and vertical overlaps but without following the exact occlusal plane of the opposing natural teeth when their arrangement is not ideal. As mentioned before, a nonideal occlusal plane is frequently encountered because of the loss of some teeth and the shifting of adjacent teeth. For example, because the mandibular first molar is the most frequently missing tooth, resultant drifting of the second and third molars creates steep inclines in the occlusal plane. If the maxillary teeth were to be positioned into a maximum intercuspation relationship with these molars, the result would be horizontal movement of the denture base on closure, which would tend to dislodge the denture. Consequently, the maxillary molars should not be placed into maximum intercuspation with teeth exhibiting steep inclines; rather, the denture teeth are prepared with reduced inclines to diminish lateral stress and encourage occlusal stability by directing occlusal forces vertically toward the supporting tissues.

The teeth placed in the hard baseplate–wax occlusion rim are then evaluated on the articulator in eccentric positions. Modifications to tooth position are made to provide stable cross arch balance within a functional range of eccentric movement (2 mm). In deciding the best possible denture tooth positions, given the opposing tooth positions, the dentist may find that the best option is to alter the natural tooth contours through selective tooth reduction. The denture arrangement is completed, and the necessary natural tooth modifications are accomplished on the opposing stone cast, with care taken to mark the location and extent of modification. When it is clinically determined that natural tooth modification can be carried out, the modifi-

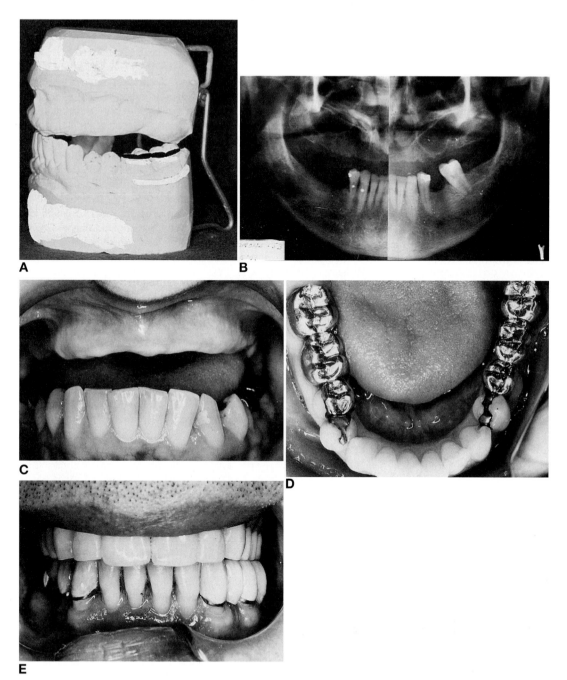

Figure 21-3 Extrusion of the mandibular molars in both **A** and **B** will require modification of their coronal shape to ensure an optimally stable occlusal scheme. In **C** and **D,** the mandibular posterior teeth have been restored to rectify drifting and extrusion of teeth, a disruption in the occlusal plane. A similar clinical and laboratory strategy ensured a balanced occlusion in **E.**

cation is accomplished at the final prosthesis insertion appointment. If, however, it is determined that the natural tooth modification that is required to ensure a stable denture prosthesis would result in perforation of the enamel and a restoration of the natural tooth is necessary, discussion with the patient as part of the overall treatment plan will be required. It also may be observed that the required tooth positions will place the maxillary prosthesis at risk of fracture because of required occlusal relations coupled with prosthesis design. If this is suspected, a cast metal base should be recommended for the patient.

After denture tooth placement is accomplished and if an opposing fixed or removable partial denture is part of the treatment, it is finalized at this stage. The most predictable control of the occlusion can be provided if the prostheses are fabricated and inserted at the same time. After verification of the occlusal requirements on the articulator and at the wax trial denture stage, the prosthesis is processed and completed. At insertion, the tissue surface is checked for fit and retention, the borders are checked for proper extension, and the occlusion is checked for duplication of the articulator mounting. Significant occlusal discrepancies should be adjusted after a clinical remount procedure. Any necessary minor adjustment of the natural dentition is accomplished with the adjusted stone cast as a guide. With a thin articulating paper to record the steep inclines that require adjustment, the teeth are marked, checked against the cast markings, and reduced to the predetermined inclination. Preliminary adjustment can be accomplished with a diamond bur, followed by fine adjustment with a fine carborundum or similar stone. The adjusted contacts are again checked against the stone cast to verify completion of the CR adjustments. Next, simulated excursive movements are performed and adjusted with the same procedure. The objective at this stage is to provide smooth excursive movement within a 2-mm functional range with cross arch tooth contacts to ensure prosthesis stability. Completion of the occlusal refinement involves careful pumicing of the occlusal surfaces. If the clinician chooses to allow the patient to complete the refinement by using an intraoral paste (carborundum paste) as the patient goes through excursive movements, care must be taken

to prevent excessive adjustment to the CR position.

POTENTIAL ADVERSE TREATMENT OUTCOMES

Two of the most common adverse sequelae of treatment using a single complete denture include natural tooth wear (Figure 21-4) and denture fracture. The use of maxillary porcelain denture teeth, especially when adjusted during the occlusal correction phase, can lead to rapid wear of the opposing natural or restored dentition. Teeth restored with various cast restorations are often less resistant to the wear from unglazed porcelain, and the best strategy is to use new generation acrylic/composite resin denture teeth in conjunction with periodic examinations. This is the most practical approach given the average life expectancy of the conventional completed denture. If the clinician desires to estab-

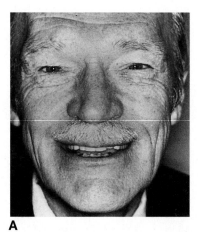

A

Figure 21-4   A and B, An increased interocclusal distance (therefore a collapsed vertical dimension of occlusion) resulted from the consequences of unfavorable occlusal relationships in this elderly patient. The biological price of such an unserviced, long-term prosthetic experience frequently manifests itself as advanced residual ridge resorption in both maxillary and mandibular edentulous segments, plus a perpetuation of adverse concentration of anterior stresses as evidenced by severe tooth wear matching the concentrated hyperplastic ridge replacement in the opposing arch

Continued

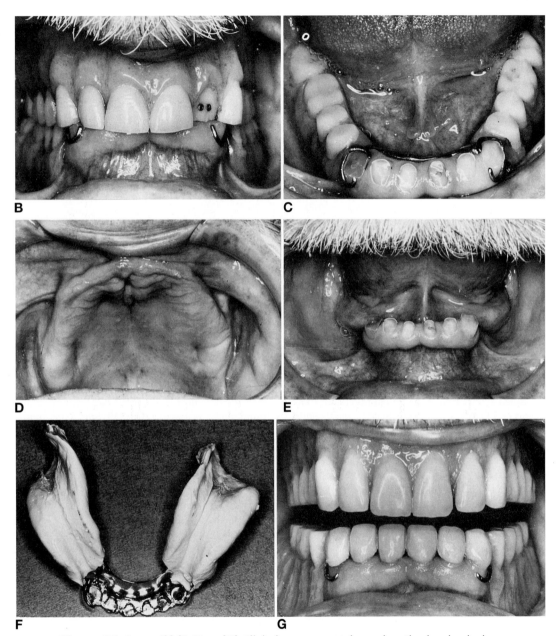

Figure 21-4 *cont'd* (**C, D, and E**). Clinical management demands optimal occlusal relations, which were readily incorporated into a removable partial overdenture/RPD type of mandibular prosthesis opposing a complete maxillary denture. **F to I,** Optimal esthetics and function were restored to preclude further morbidity.

Continued

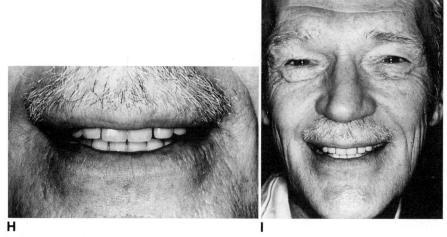

H   I

Figure 21-4 *cont'd*

lish similar material occlusal surfaces and the single denture opposes cast restorations, there are techniques to follow that allow the use of cast metal for the production of the denture occlusion.

Because the single denture is often opposed by a full or near full complement of natural teeth, a common complication is fracture of the denture base. Specific conditions that encourage such fracture include heavy anterior occlusal contact, deep labial frenal notches (especially when in conjunction with midline diastema), and high occlusal forces due to strong mandibular elevator musculature. Careful attention to the occlusion, an adequate denture base thickness, and control of the denture labial notch are frequently the only necessary requirements to prevent fracture. When the clinician is unable to control these factors or is suspicious that fracture potential is high, a cast metal base is best used to resist deformation and fracture.

Considerations during maintenance visits for the patient with a single denture include verification of the occlusal contacting relationships that provide stable occlusal forces in CR and eccentric contact positions. Also, the condition of the supporting tissues should be evaluated, and when the tissues exhibit changes that would encourage excessive movement, measures should be taken to reduce movement and the potential for dislodgement.

RATIONALE FOR IMPLANTS IN THE EDENTULOUS MAXILLA

As described earlier, change in the denture-supporting tissues is variable but inevitable. The major tissue change is an irreversible bone loss resulting from both local and systemic effects. Such morphological change in the maxillary denture-bearing foundation can lead to difficult functional stability problems. Even for those patients who have demonstrated remarkable skill in manipulating biomechanically challenging prostheses, the need to improve the denture foundation to ensure better functional stability often arises.

Providing improved stability to a prosthesis through the use of dental implants allows both enhanced function and a reduction in the irreversible bone loss that led to the instability. Well-distributed implants used to stabilize an overdenture prosthesis design have been shown to be an effective treatment modality for the edentulous maxillary arch (Figure 21-5).

MANDIBULAR SINGLE DENTURE

The single mandibular denture opposing a restored complete or partial maxillary dentition poses an even greater challenge to the clinician. The situation often is compounded by severe residual ridge resorption of the edentulous mandible, which makes con-

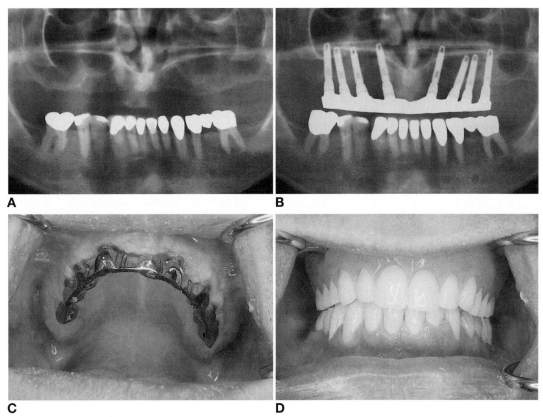

A **B**

C **D**

Figure 21-5 Composite illustrations of an edentulous maxilla in a patient struggling with maxillary denture stability due to the combination of an intact mandibular natural dentition and a regressing edentulous maxilla. Placement of implants allowed construction of an overdenture with enhanced functional stability. **A** and **B,** Panoramic radiographs of an edentulous maxilla before and after placement of eight well-distributed implants with a connecting bar that supports the overdenture prosthesis. **C,** Clinical view of the implant connecting bar. **D,** Overdenture prosthesis in occlusion with natural mandibular dentition.

ventional treatment nearly impossible (Figure 21-6). The edentulous mandible is always at a disadvantage because of a limited quantity of mucosa, the amount of denture border adjacent to moveable mucosa, and the impact of occlusal forces from the moving mandible contacting the static dentate maxillary arch. These conditions frequently make conventional treatment unwise and have been best addressed through the use of endosseous dental implants to provide retention and support for the mandibular complete denture and to retard residual bone resorption.

When the clinician is unable to provide the option of endosseous dental implants, treatment with a single denture should proceed only after a clear discussion of the potential for problems, given the clinical findings, between the patient and clinician. The clinical and laboratory procedures are very similar to those described earlier in this chapter. However, many clinicians think that the use of a resilient liner in the mandibular denture is beneficial. With such a procedure the dentist attempts to provide a stress-reducing element in the denture base to resist the forces of functional and parafunctional loads.

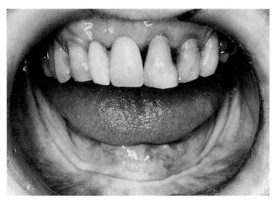

Figure 21-6 The mandibular denture-bearing area has been adversely affected by long-term wear of a complete lower denture opposing a partially edentulous maxillary dentition restored with a removable partial denture.

SUMMARY

The patient who requires a single denture opposing a natural or restored dentition challenges the clinician even more than the completely edentulous patient does. This is due to the biomechanical differences in the supporting tissues for the opposing arches. Certain conditions must be evaluated and corrected early in treatment to provide for a more stable prosthesis. The unique biomechanical features of the patient with a single denture have been emphasized, and methods for controlling denture tooth and opposing tooth position to maximize stable functional relationships have been presented.

Bibliography

Denissen HW, Kalk W, van Waas MA et al: Occlusion for maxillary dentures opposing osseointegrated mandibular implants, *Int J Prosthet* 6:446-450, 1993.

Hansen CA, Clear K, Wright P: Simplified procedure for making gold occlusal surfaces on denture teeth, *J Prosthet Dent* 71:413-416, 1994.

Jacobs R, van Steenberghe D, Nys M, Naert I, et al: Maxillary bone resorption in patients with mandibular implant-supported overdentures or fixed prostheses, *J Prosthet Dent* 70:135-141, 1993.

Kelly E: Changes caused by a mandibular removable partial denture opposing a maxillary complete denture, *J Prosthet Dent* 27:210-215, 1972.

Kiener P, Oettertli M, Mericske E et al: Effectiveness of maxillary overdentures supported by implants: maintenance and prosthetic complications, *Int J Prosthodont* 14:133-140, 2001.

Koper A: The maxillary complete denture opposing natural teeth: problems and some solutions, *J Prosthet Dent* 57:704-707, 1987.

Schneider RL: Diagnosing functional complete denture fractures, *J Prosthet Dent* 54:809-814, 1985.

CHAPTER *22*

The Retention of Complete Dentures

Kenneth Shay

Optimal outcome of complete denture treatment depends on the successful integration of the prosthesis with the patient's oral functions plus psychological acceptance of the dentures by the patient. These parameters require that patients perceive their dentures as stationary or well retained during function and that the prostheses and their effects on the face meet the esthetic and psychodynamic requirements of the patient. In this chapter, the factors involved in achieving denture retention (the resistance to removal in a direction opposite that of insertion) are reviewed, and the role that a denture adhesive agent may play in the context of the patient's adjustment to and acceptance of the dentures is discussed.

FACTORS INVOLVED IN THE RETENTION OF DENTURES

Interfacial Force

Interfacial force is the resistance to separation of two parallel surfaces that is imparted by a film of liquid between them. A discussion of interfacial forces is best broken into separate comments on interfacial surface tension and viscous tension.

Interfacial surface tension results from a thin layer of fluid that is present between two parallel planes of rigid material. It is dependent on the ability of the fluid to "wet" the rigid surrounding material. If the surrounding material has low surface tension, as oral mucosa does, fluid will maximize its contact with the material, thereby wetting it readily and spreading out in a thin film. If the material has high surface tension, fluid will minimize its contact with the material, resulting in the formation of beads on the material's surface. Denture base

materials vary in their surface tension (also termed *wettability*), with processed materials displaying greater wettability than autocured products. All denture base materials have higher surface tension than oral mucosa, but once coated by salivary pellicle, their surface tension is reduced, which promotes maximizing the surface area between liquid and base. The thin fluid film between the denture base and the mucosa of the basal seat therefore furnishes a retentive force by virtue of the tendency of the fluid to maximize its contact with both surfaces.

Another way to understand the role of surface tension in denture retention is through capillary attraction, or capillarity. Capillarity is what causes a liquid to rise in a capillary tube because in this physical setting the liquid will maximize its contact with the walls of the capillary tube, thereby rising along the tube wall at the interface between liquid and glass. When the adaptation of the denture base to the mucosa on which it rests is sufficiently close, the space filled with a thin film of saliva acts like a capillary tube in that the liquid seeks to increase its contact with both the denture and the mucosal surface. In this way, capillarity will help to retain the denture.

Interfacial surface tension may not play as important a role in retaining the mandibular denture as it does for the maxillary one. Interfacial surface tension is dependent on the existence of a liquid/air interface at the terminus of the liquid/solid contact: if the two plates with interposed fluid are immersed in the same fluid, there will be no resistance to pulling them apart. In many patients, there is sufficient saliva to keep the external borders of the mandibular denture awash in saliva, thereby eliminating the effect of interfacial surface tension. This is not so in the maxilla. Interfacial

437

viscous tension refers to the force holding two parallel plates together that is due to the viscosity of the interposed liquid. Viscous tension is described by Stefan's law.[*] For two parallel, circular plates of radius *(r)* that are separated by a newtonian (incompressible) liquid of viscosity *(k)* and thickness *(h)*, this principle states that the force *(F)* necessary to pull the plates apart at a velocity *(V)* in a direction perpendicular to the radius will be

$$F = \frac{(3/2)\pi kr^4}{h^3} V$$

The relationship expressed by Stefan's law makes it clear that the viscous force increases proportionally to increases in the viscosity of the interposed fluid. The viscous force drops off readily as the distance between the plates (i.e., the thickness of the interposed medium) increases. The force increases proportionally to the square of the area of the opposing surfaces. When applied to denture retention, the equation demonstrates the essential importance of an optimal adaptation between denture and basal seat (a minimal *h*), the advantage of maximizing the surface area covered by the denture (a maximum *r*), and the theoretical improvement in retention made possible by increasing the viscosity of the medium between the denture and its seat. It also explains why a slow, steady displacing action (small *V*) may encounter less resistance and therefore be more effective at removing a denture than is a sharp attempt at displacement (large *V*).

In application, interfacial forces are further enhanced through ionic forces developed between the fluid and the surrounding surfaces (adhesion) and the forces holding the fluid molecules to each other (cohesion).

Adhesion

Adhesion is the physical attraction of unlike molecules for each other. Adhesion of saliva to the mucous membrane and the denture base is achieved through ionic forces between charged salivary glycoproteins and surface epithelium or acrylic resin. Through its promoting contact of saliva to both oral tissue and denture base, adhesion works to enhance further the retentive force of interfacial surface tension.

Another version of adhesion is observed between denture bases and the mucous membranes themselves, which is the situation in patients with xerostomia (sparse or absent saliva). The denture base materials seem to stick to the dry mucous membrane of the basal seat and other oral surfaces. Such adhesion is not very effective for retaining dentures and predisposes to mucosal abrasions and ulcerations because of the lack of salivary lubrication. It is annoying to patients to have denture bases stick to the lips, cheeks, and tongue. An ethanol-free rinse containing aloe or lanolin, a water-soluble lubricating jelly, or a saliva substitute containing carboxymethylcellulose (CMC) or mammalian mucin can be helpful in this situation. For patients whose mouths are dry because of irradiation or an autoimmune disorder such as Sjögren's syndrome, salivary stimulation through a prescription of 5 to 10 mg of oral pilocarpine three times daily can be very beneficial if the patient can tolerate the likely adverse effects of increased perspiration and (occasionally) excess lacrimation.

The amount of retention provided by adhesion is proportionate to the area covered by the denture. Mandibular dentures cover less surface area than maxillary prostheses and therefore are subject to a lower magnitude of adhesive (and other) retentive forces. Similarly, patients with small jaws or very flat alveolar ridges (small basal seats) cannot expect retention to be as great as can patients with large jaws or prominent alveoli. Thus the dentures (and therefore the impressions that serve as the patient analogue for their fabrication) should be extended to the limits of the health and function of the oral tissues, and efforts should be made at all times to preserve the alveolar height to maximize retention.

Cohesion

Cohesion is the physical attraction of like molecules for each other. It is a retentive force because it occurs within the layer of fluid (usually saliva) that is present between the denture base and the mucosa and works to maintain the integrity of the interposed fluid. Normal saliva is not very cohesive so that most of the retentive force of the denture-mucosa interface comes from adhesive and

---

[*]Stefan J, Sitzberger K: *Akad Wiss Math Natur* 69:713, 1874.

interfacial factors unless the interposed saliva is modified (as it can be with the use of denture adhesive).

Thick, high-mucin saliva is more viscous than thin, watery saliva, yet thick secretions usually do not result in increased retention because watery, serous saliva can be interposed in a thinner film than the more cohesive mucin secretions. Stefan's law makes it clear that if all other factors are equal, then an increase in fluid viscosity cannot be accompanied by an equal increase in film thickness if displacement force is to be kept the same.

Oral and Facial Musculature

The oral and facial musculature supply supplementary retentive forces, provided (1) the teeth are positioned in the "neutral zone" between the cheeks and tongue and (2) the polished surfaces of the dentures are properly shaped (see Chapter 15). This is not to say that patients must hold their prosthetic teeth in place by conscious effort but that the shape of the buccal and lingual flanges must make it possible for the musculature to fit automatically against the denture and thereby to reinforce the border seal (Figures 22-1 and 22-2). One of the objectives in impression making and arch form design is the

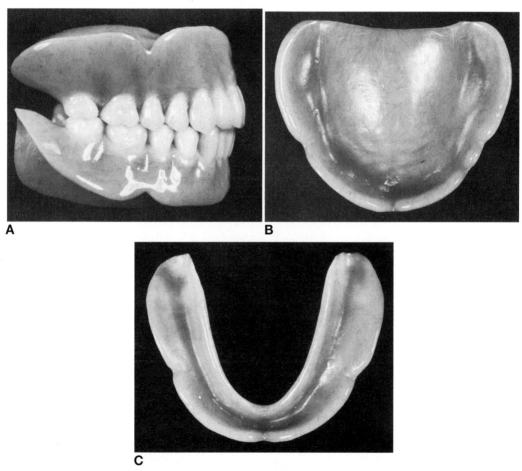

A

B

C

Figure 22-1 Complete dentures have three surfaces that must harmonize with the oral biological environment. **A,** The dentures' polished surfaces are so contoured as to support and contact the cheeks, lips, and tongue. **B** and **C,** The impression or basal surfaces are fitted to the basal seats. *Continued*

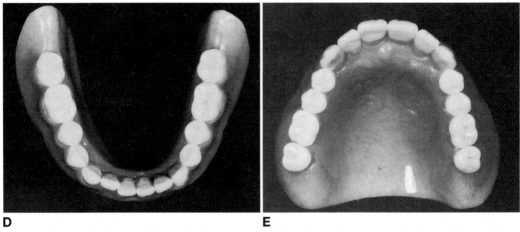

D   **E**

Figure 22-1 *cont'd* **D** and **E**, The occlusal surfaces of one denture must fit those of the opposing denture.

harnessing of a patient's unconscious tissue behavior to enhance both retention and stability of the prostheses. If the buccal flanges of the maxillary denture slope up and out from the occlusal surfaces of the teeth and the buccal flanges of the mandibular denture slope down and out from the occlusal plane, the contraction of the buccinators will tend to retain both dentures on their basal seats.

The lingual surfaces of the lingual flanges should slope toward the center of the mouth so the

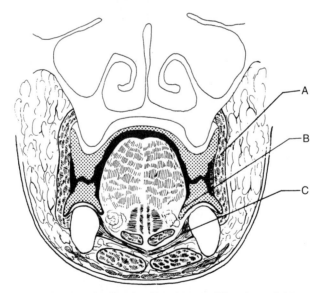

Figure 22-2 Frontal section showing dentures properly filling the available space. *A,* The buccinator. *B,* The lingual flange and border are placed under the tongue. *C,* The mylohyoid ridge. Notice that both upper and lower dentures are so shaped that the action of the tongue and cheeks tends to seat rather than unseat them. If posterior artificial teeth are too wide buccolingually, the form of the dentures will be changed and the tongue and cheeks will tend to unseat them.

tongue can fit against them and perfect the border seal on the lingual side of the denture. The base of the tongue is guided on top of the lingual flange by the lingual side of the distal end of the flange, which turns laterally toward the ramus. This part of the denture also helps ensure the border seal at the back end of the mandibular denture. Strain-gauge measurements of the retentive forces exerted by patients' tongues demonstrate significant increase when the flange, particularly in the anterior, is so configured.

The base of the tongue also may serve as an emergency retentive force for some patients. It rises up at the back and presses against the distal border of the maxillary denture during incision of food by the anterior teeth. This is done without conscious effort when the experienced denture wearer bites into an apple or sandwich or other food. It is seldom that a patient needs to be taught how to do this. For the oral and facial musculature to be most effective in providing retention for complete dentures, the following conditions must be met: (1) the denture bases must be properly extended to cover the maximum area possible, without interfering in the health and function of the structures that surround the denture; (2) the occlusal plane must be at the correct level; and (3) the arch form of the teeth must be in the neutral zone between the tongue and the cheeks.

Atmospheric Pressure

Atmospheric pressure can act to resist dislodging forces applied to dentures, if the dentures have an effective seal around their borders. This resistance force has been called *suction* because it is a resistance to the removal of dentures from their basal seat, but there is no suction, or negative pressure, except when another force is applied. (Suction alone applied to the soft tissues of the oral cavity for even a short time would cause serious damage to the health of the soft tissues under negative pressure).

A suction cup pressed against a pane of glass stays in place because the rubber of the squeezed cup elastically seeks to return to a larger shape, thereby causing air pressure within the cup to be less than the pressure outside the cup. A denture cannot be distorted like a suction cup, but oral mucosa can be. When a force is exerted perpendicular to and away from the basal seat of a properly extended and fully seated denture, pressure between the prosthesis and the basal tissues drops below the ambient pressure, resisting displacement.

Retention due to atmospheric pressure is directly proportionate to the area covered by the denture base. For atmospheric pressure to be effective, the denture must have a perfect seal around its entire border. Proper border molding with physiological, selective pressure techniques is essential for taking advantage of this retentive mechanism.

Undercuts, Rotational Insertion Paths, and Parallel Walls

The resiliency of the mucosa and submucosa overlying basal bone allows for the existence of modest undercuts that can enhance retention. Although exaggerated bony undercuts or less overt ones covered by thin epithelium may compromise denture retention by necessitating extensive internal adjustment of the denture, less severe undercuts of the lateral tuberosities, maxillary premolar areas, distolingual areas, and lingual mandibular midbody areas can be extremely helpful to the retention of the prosthesis.

Some "undercuts" are only undercut in relationship to a linear path of insertion or relative to a presumed vertical path of insertion. However, if the undercut area is seated first (usually in a direction that deviates from the vertical) and the remainder of the denture base can be brought into proximity with the basal seat on rotation of the prosthesis around the undercut part that is already seated, this "rotational path" will provide resistance to vertical displacement. One common example of this is to be found in the area inferior to the retromolar pad, into which the distolingual extensions of the mandibular base can be introduced from the superior and posterior before rotating the anterior segment of the denture down over the alveolar process. The opposite sequence is common in the maxilla, where a prominent or even undercut anterior alveolus may dictate an insertion path that begins with seating the anterior in a posterior and superior direction and ends with rotation of the posterior border over the backs of the tuberosities. This concept increases in importance as other retentive mechanisms decline in strength. For instance, in a patient who has undergone loss of normal anatomical contours due to tumor resection or trauma, surgically created relative undercuts may mean the difference between prosthetic success and failure.

Prominent alveolar ridges with parallel buccal and lingual walls may also provide significant retention by increasing the surface area between denture and mucosa and thereby maximizing interfacial and atmospheric forces. Prominent ridges also resist denture movement by limiting the range of displacive force directions possible. Very flat ridges may bear dentures that display strong resistance to displacement perpendicular to the basal seat, due to interfacial and atmospheric forces. However, these same prostheses are very susceptible to movement parallel to the basal seat, analogous to sliding a suction cup along a pane of glass or sliding apart two glass pieces separated by intervening fluid.

Gravity

When a person is in an upright posture, gravity acts as a retentive force for the mandibular denture and a displacive force for the maxillary denture. In most cases, the weight of the prosthesis constitutes a gravitational force that is insignificant in comparison with the other forces acting on the denture, but if a maxillary denture is fabricated wholly or partially of a material that increases its weight appreciably (e.g., a metal base or precious metal posterior occlusal surfaces), the weight of the prosthesis may work to unseat it if the other retentive forces are themselves suboptimal. Increasing the weight of a mandibular denture (through the addition of a metallic base, insert, or occlusal surfaces) may seem theoretically capable of taking advantage of gravity. Anecdotal evidence suggests that this may indeed prove beneficial in the mandible in cases where the other retentive forces and factors are marginal, although a controlled study of 12 subjects failed to find subjective or objective benefit. Curiously, another report focusing on maxillary denture base materials in patients with xerostomia found strong patient preference for metal-based (and therefore heavier) prostheses in the upper arch.

ADJUNCTIVE RETENTION THROUGH THE USE OF DENTURE ADHESIVES

Complete denture treatment needs to be customized for each patient's particular needs. Successful treatment combines exemplary technique, effective patient rapport and education, and familiarity with all possible management options to provide the highest degree of patient satisfaction. Commercially available denture adhesives are products that have the capacity to enhance treatment outcome. This reality is compellingly underscored by two facts: (1) consumer surveys in the United States reveal that approximately 33% of patients with dentures purchase and use one or more denture adhesive products in a given year and (2) denture adhesive sales in the United States exceeded $200 million in 2001 (12% more than for denture cleaners and nearly twice the spending on dental floss). Dentists need to know about denture adhesives for two reasons: (1) to be able to educate all denture-wearing patients about the advantages, disadvantages, and uses of the product because adhesives are a widely used dental material and patients rightfully expect their dentists to be accurately informed about over-the-counter oral care products and (2) to identify those patients for whom such a product is advisable and/or necessary for a satisfactory denture-wearing experience.

In this chapter, *denture adhesive* is used to refer to a commercially available, nontoxic, soluble material (powder, cream, or liquid) that is applied to the tissue surface of the denture to enhance denture retention, stability, and performance. It does not refer to insoluble patient-directed efforts at improving denture fit and comfort, such as home reliner kits, home repair kits, paper or cloth pads, or other self-applied "cushions," many of which have been anecdotally linked with incidents of serious soft-tissue damage, alterations in occlusal relations and vertical dimension of occlusion, and exacerbated alveolar bone destruction. Included in this second category are thin wafers of water-soluble material that are adherent to both basal tissue and denture base and that lack the ability to flow and therefore do not have the capacity to direct uneven and point pressures against the bearing tissues.

Components and Mechanism(s) of Action

Denture adhesives augment the same retentive mechanisms already operating when a denture is worn. They enhance retention through optimizing interfacial forces by (1) increasing the adhesive and cohesive properties and viscosity of the medium lying between the denture and its basal seat and (2) eliminating voids between the denture base and its basal seat. Adhesives (or, more accurately, the hydrated material that is formed when an adhesive comes into contact with saliva or water) are agents that stick readily to both the tissue surface of the denture and the mucosal surface of the basal seat. Furthermore, because hydrated adhesives are more cohesive than saliva, physical forces intrinsic to the interposed adhesive medium resist the pull more successfully than would similar forces within saliva. The material increases the viscosity of the saliva with which it mixes, and the hydrated material swells in the presence of saliva/water and flows under pressure. Voids between the denture base and bearing tissues are therefore obliterated.

Denture adhesive materials in use before the early 1960s were based on vegetable gums (e.g., karaya, tragacanth, xanthan, and acacia) that display modest, nonionic adhesion to both denture and mucosa and possessed very little cohesive strength. Gum-based adhesives (still commercially available) are highly water soluble, particularly in hot liquids such as coffee, tea, and soups, and therefore wash out readily from beneath dentures. Allergic reactions have been reported to karaya (and to the paraben preservative that the vegetable derivatives require), and formulations with karaya impart a marked odor reminiscent of acetic acid. Overall, the adhesive performance of the vegetable gum–based materials is short-lived and relatively unsatisfactory.

Synthetic materials presently dominate the denture adhesive market. The most popular and successful products consist of mixtures of the salts of short-acting (CMC) and long-acting (polyvinyl methyl ether maleate], or "gantrez") polymers. In the presence of water, CMC hydrates and displays quick-onset ionic adherence to both dentures and mucous epithelium. The original fluid increases its viscosity and CMC increases in volume, thereby eliminating voids between prosthesis and basal seat. These two actions markedly enhance the

interfacial forces acting on the denture. Polyvinylpyrrolidone ("povidone") is another, less commonly used agent that behaves like CMC. Over a more protracted time course than necessary for the onset of hydration of CMC, gantrez salts hydrate and increase adherence and viscosity. The "long-acting" (i.e., less soluble) gantrez salts also display molecular cross-linking, resulting in a measurable increase in cohesive behavior. This effect is significantly more pronounced and longer lived in calcium-zinc gantrez formulations than in calcium-sodium gantrez. Eventually, all the polymers become fully solubilized and washed out by saliva; this dissolution is hastened by the presence of hot liquid.

Other components of denture adhesive products impart particular physical attributes to the formulations. Petrolatum, mineral oil, and polyethylene oxide are included in creams to bind the materials and to make their placement easier. Silicone dioxide and calcium stearate are used in powders to minimize clumping. Menthol and peppermint oils are used for flavoring, red dye for color, and sodium borate and methylparaben or polyparaben as preservatives.

Some Objective and Subjective Responses to Denture Adhesive

With the exception of uncommon allergic reactions to either karaya or paraben, as just mentioned, there have been no reports of tissue reactions to denture adhesive products. For example, before 1990, a few of the commercially available denture adhesives contained very low levels of benzene, which is regarded as a carcinogen. These products were recalled by the Food and Drug Administration. Today's adhesives are either free of benzene or contain trace amounts considered to be harmless. Commercially available formulations in the United States must pass laboratory animal tests of skin and eye sensitivity and oral toxicity before they are acceptable for sale to the public. Clinical studies of mucosal tissues underlying adhesive-bearing dentures reveal lessened inflammation in patients who perform adequate denture hygiene daily. Dentists must ensure that they are cognizant of any sequelae that may be associated with the prescription of all materials used in routine dental practice.

Incisal bite force exerted by well-fitting dentures overlying well-keratinized ridges with favorable anatomical features (square arch form; broad, prominent alveoli without undercuts; mild or absent frena) is improved significantly with the use of an adhesive. More interesting, incisal bite force of well-fitting dentures overlying inferior basal tissues (tapering arch form, little or no keratinization, spiny or absent alveolar ridges, frena extending to ridge crests) can be increased to the range of the adhesive-bearing dentures overlying ideal basal tissues. The frequency of dislodgment of dentures during chewing also is markedly decreased with the use of adhesive. Vertical, anteroposterior, and lateral movements (short of full dislodgment) of new and old maxillary dentures retained on their mucosal seats under chewing and speech function can be decreased between 20% to 50% for up to 8 hours after placement of denture adhesive and up to 4 hours after placement of the mandibular denture.

Objective comparison of chewing performance fails to show an improvement after use of adhesive, although subjects report increased confidence and security in chewing with the use of denture adhesive. Not all products are the same, and patients can tell them apart: subjects are able to identify preferred adhesive characteristics and products in comparison trials of different formulations. Improvement in chewing efficiency during adjustment to new dentures progresses further in patients who use a denture adhesive product.

Patient response to the use of these materials is not universally positive. Some patients object to the "grainy" or "gritty" texture of powder or to the taste or sensation of semidissolved adhesive material that escapes from the posterior and other peripheries (often due to use of excessive quantity or use in an inadequate prosthesis). Others object to the difficulties encountered in removing adhesive from the denture and the oral tissues, as well as to the cost of the material.

Indications and Contraindications

Scientific evidence favoring the support of routine and safe use of adhesives is lacking, yet clinical experience indicates that prudent use of adhesives to enhance the retentive qualities of well-made complete dentures is sound clinical judgment.

Denture adhesives are indicated when well-made complete dentures do not satisfy a patient's perceived retention and stability expectations. Irrespective of the underlying reasons (e.g., psychological, occupational, morphological, and functional) for a patient's reported dissatisfaction the dentist must recognize that a patient's judgment of the treatment outcome is what defines prosthodontic success. Such maladaptive patients are clearly candidates for an implant-supported prosthesis (see Chapter 25). However, health, financial, or other considerations can preclude this, and then a well-organized protocol of functional do's and don't's may be the best palliative measure the professional can offer. Specific patient populations who can benefit from this strategy include patients with salivary dysfunction or neurological disorders and those who have undergone resective surgical or traumatic modifications of the oral cavity.

Patients who have xerostomia due to medication side effects, a history of head and neck irradiation, systemic disease, or disease of the salivary glands have great difficulty managing complete dentures because of impaired retention and an increased tendency for ulceration of the bearing tissues. The use of denture adhesive can compensate for the retention that is lacking in the absence of healthy saliva and can mitigate the onset of oral ulcerations that result from frequent dislodgments. Patients with xerostomia must be educated, however, that the adhesive-bearing denture will need to be deliberately moistened (e.g., with water from the tap) before it is seated in the otherwise dry mouth to initiate the actions of the material.

Several neurological diseases can complicate the use of complete dentures, but adhesive may help to overcome the impediments imposed. Cerebrovascular accident (stroke) may render part of the oral cavity insensitive to tactile sensation or partially or wholly paralyze oral musculature. Adhesives can assist in helping these patients accommodate to new dentures or to prostheses that were fabricated before the stroke but that the patient is now unable to manage because of lost sensory feedback and neuromuscular control. Orofacial dyskinesia is a prominent side effect of phenothiazine-class tranquilizers (e.g., fluphenazine, trifluoperazine, thioridazine, or thiothixene), other neuroleptic drugs (e.g., haloperidol), and even gastrointestinal medications (e.g., prochlorperazine and metoclopramide). This movement disorder, sometimes termed *tardive dyskinesia* because it is often a late-onset side effect of dopamine-blocking drugs, is characterized by exaggerated, uncontrollable muscular actions of the tongue, cheeks, lips, and mandible. In such situations, denture retention, stability, and function may be a virtual impossibility without adjunctive retention, such as that made possible with denture adhesive.

Patients who have undergone resective surgery for removal of oral neoplasia or those who have lost intraoral structures and integrity due to trauma may have significant difficulty in functioning with a tissue-borne prosthesis unless denture adhesive is used, even if rotational undercuts have been surgically created to resist displacement of the prosthesis.

It must be emphasized that a denture adhesive is not indicated for the retention of improperly fabricated or poorly fitting prostheses.

Patient Education

It is incumbent upon dentists to educate patients with dentures about denture adhesives: their use, abuse, advantages, disadvantages, and available choices. The major information resource for a patient should be the dentist and not magazine and television advertisements or the testimonials of relatives and acquaintances.

The choice between cream and powder is largely subjective, but certain facts may underscore a patient's selection. Powder formulations, as a rule, do not confer the same degree of "hold," nor do their effects last as long, in comparison with comparable cream formulations. However, powders can be used in smaller quantities, are generally easier to clean out of dentures and off tissues, and are not perceived as "messy" by patients. Furthermore, the initial "hold" for powders is achieved sooner than it is with cream formulations.

Obtaining the greatest advantage from the use of an adhesive product is dependent on its proper usage (Figures 22-3 to 22-7). For powder and cream products, the least amount of material that is effective should be used. This is approximately 0.5 to 1.5 g per denture unit (more for larger alveolar ridges, less for smaller ones). For powders, the

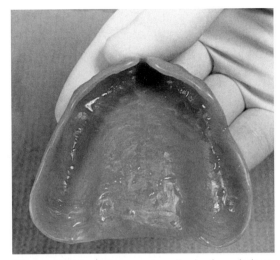

Figure 22-3 Before powder adhesive formulations are applied, the denture must be cleaned and then thoroughly moistened.

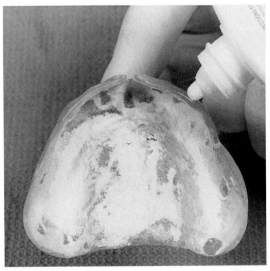

Figure 22-4 The moistened denture surface is then covered with a slightly excess coating of the powder.

clean prosthesis should be moistened and then a thin, even coating of the adhesive sprayed onto the tissue surface of the denture. The excess is shaken off and the prosthesis inserted and seated firmly. If the patient has inadequate or absent saliva, the

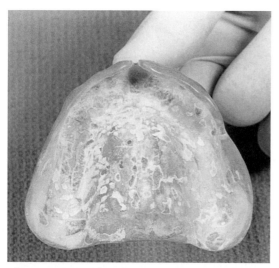

Figure 22-5 When the excess powder is shaken off, a thin, even coat remains.

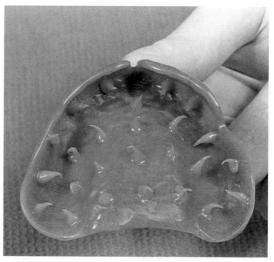

Figure 22-7 An alternative application procedure for cream adhesive. To the clean and dried denture, small dots of product are placed at 5-mm intervals. If adhesive is expressed around the periphery of the denture in function, the dots should be distributed farther apart.

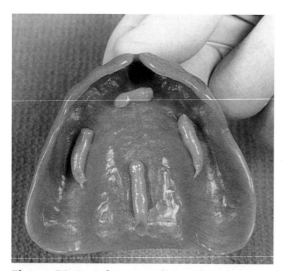

Figure 22-6 Before cream denture formulations are applied, the denture must be cleaned and then thoroughly dried. Most manufacturers recommend the distribution of product as shown. For the mandibular denture, a series of thin beads at the crest of the ridge is recommended. If adhesive is expressed around the periphery of the denture in function, a lesser quantity should be used.

sprayed denture should be moistened lightly with water before being inserted. For creams, two approaches are possible. Most manufacturers recommend placement of thin beads of the adhesive in the depth of the dried denture in the incisor and molar regions; an anteroposterior bead should be placed along the midpalate in the maxillary unit. However, more even distribution of the material can be achieved if small spots of cream are placed at 5-mm intervals throughout the fitting surface of the dried denture. Regardless of the pattern selected, the denture is then inserted and seated firmly. As with powders, use of denture adhesive cream by patients with xerostomia requires that the adhesive material be moistened with water before inserting the denture.

Patients must be instructed that daily removal of adhesive product from the tissue surfaces of the denture is an essential requirement for the use of the material (Figure 22-8). Removal is facilitated by letting the prosthesis soak in water or soaking solution overnight during which the product will be fully solubilized and can then be readily rinsed off. If soaking is not possible before new adhesive

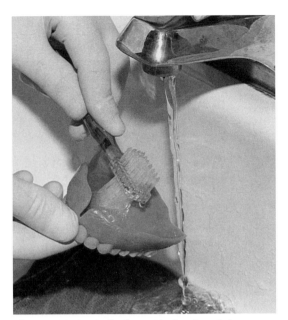

Figure 22-8 Daily thorough cleaning of the denture is essential. Removal is facilitated by running warm or hot water over the tissue surface of the denture while scrubbing with a suitable hard-bristle denture brush. The sink should be partially filled with water, or a washcloth or towel should be placed in the sink beneath the denture to prevent accidental damage in the event the prosthesis is dropped during cleaning.

material needs to be placed, removal is facilitated by running hot water over the tissue surface of the denture while scrubbing with a suitable hard-bristle denture brush. Adhesive that is adherent to the alveolar ridges and palate is best removed by rinsing with warm or hot water and then firmly wiping the area with gauze or a washcloth saturated with hot water.

Finally, patients need to be educated about the limitations of denture adhesive. Discomfort will not be resolved by placing a "cushioning layer" of adhesive under the denture. In fact, pain or soreness signals a need for professional management. A gradual increase in the quantity of adhesive required for acceptable fit of the denture is also a clear signal to seek professional care. In all cases, denture patients need to be recalled annually for oral mucosal evaluation and prosthesis assessment, but they also need to be edu-

cated about the warning signs that should alert them to seek professional attention between the check-ups.

Professional Attitudes toward Denture Adhesive

Denture adhesive products can improve patient acceptance of and comfort and function with dentures. They are, however, regarded frequently as unesthetic and an impediment to a dentist's ability to apprise accurately the health of a patient's oral tissues and the true character of denture adaptation. The fact that ill-fitting dentures often are retained by large amounts of adhesive material has regrettably led many dentists to presume a correlation between denture adhesive and severe alveolar ridge resorption, although recent surveys of denture faculty at U.S. dental schools suggest that these misgivings about the material may no longer be as strong as they once were.

If a correlation did indeed exist between denture adhesive use and increased alveolar ridge resorption, it would provide a strong basis for cautioning patients against the use of adhesives, yet there is no scientific basis for presuming this alleged correlation.

Denture adhesives themselves are not capable of exerting forces that would accelerate resorption. Adhesives are liquid materials that are no more capable of directing forces than is saliva. There is no mechanism through which adhesives can "exert" forces to further accelerate resorption; as fluids, adhesives will transmit occlusal forces evenly to the basal tissues, just as would an intimately fitted acrylic base. If they fail to do so in one or more areas, the patient will experience discomfort and seek professional attention.

Denture adhesives merely reduce the amount of lateral movements that dentures, even well-fitting dentures, undergo while in contact with basal tissues. Admittedly, this benefit can mislead a patient into ignoring his or her need for professional help when dentures actually become ill fitting. This is an inherent risk when using any form of adjunctive therapy. However, it should not preclude prudent clinical strategies. Denture adhesives are an integral part of a professional service, and their adjunctive benefits must be recognized.

Bibliography

Aydin AK, Terziogly H, Ulubayram K et al: Wetting properties of saliva substitutes on acrylic resin, *Int J Prosthdont* 10: 473-477, 1997.

Berg E: A clinical comparison of four denture adhesives, *Int J Prosthodont* 4:449, 1991.

Boone M: Analysis of soluble and insoluble denture adhesives and their relationship to tissue irritation and bone resorption, *Compend Contin Educ Dent* (4):S22-S25, 1984.

Grasso J, Gay T, Rendell J et al: Effect of denture adhesive on retention of mandibular and maxillary dentures during function, *J Clin Dent* 11:98-103, 2000.

Hummel SK, Marker VA, Buschang P et al: A pilot to evaluate different palate materials for maxillary complete dentures with xerostomic patients, *J Prosthodont* 8:10-17, 1999.

Kapur KK: A clinical evaluation of denture adhesives, *J Prosthet Dent* 18:550, 1967.

Miller WP, Moneith B, Heat R: The effect of variation of the lingual shape of mandibular complete dentures on lingual resistance to lifting forces, *Gerodontology* 15:113-119, 1998.

Ohkubo C, Hosoi T: Effect of weight change of mandibular complete dentures on chewing and stability; a pilot study, *J Prosthet Dent* 82:636-642, 1999.

Shay K: Denture adhesives: choosing the right powders and pastes, *J Am Dent Assoc* 122:70-76, 1991.

Slaughter A, Katx RV, Grasso JE: Professional attitudes toward denture adhesives: a Delphi technique survey of academic prosthodontists, *J Prosthet Dent* 82:80-89, 1999.

Tarbet WJ, Boone M, Schmidt NF: Effect of a denture adhesive on complete denture dislodgement during mastication, *J Prosthet Dent* 44:374, 1980.

Tarbet WJ, Grossman E: Observations of denture-supporting tissue during six months of denture adhesive wearing, *J Am Dent Assoc* 101:789, 1980.

Tarbet WJ, Silverman G, Schmidt NF: Maximum incisal biting force in denture wearers as influenced by adequacy of denture-bearing tissues and the use of an adhesive, *J Dent Res* 60:115, 1981.

Vinton P, Manly RS: Masticatory efficiency during the period of adjustment to dentures, *J Prosthet Dent* 5:477, 1955.

Zissis A, Yannikakis S, Jagger RG et al: Wettability of denture materials, *Quintessence Int* 32:457-462, 2001.

CHAPTER 23

Maxillofacial Prosthodontics for the Edentulous Patient

Rhonda F. Jacob

Maxillofacial prosthodontics focuses on optimizing the rudimentary functions of speech and swallowing. These functions are disrupted because of congenital, organic, traumatic, or surgical abnormalities involving the oral cavity and related anatomical structures. Modifying routine dental procedures, the dentist creates static prostheses to fill voids created by missing tissues or to approximate organs with suboptimal function. Although rehabilitation of these rudimentary functions often is considered the primary goal by the health care provider, no less important to the patient is restoration of normal esthetics and mastication. These prostheses can be critical requirements to improve quality of life for individuals whose rehabilitation will be a lifelong proposition. Normal function may not be achieved, but optimal function should always be attained, and normalcy should always be sought.

ANATOMICAL AND PHYSIOLOGICAL CONSIDERATIONS: NORMAL FUNCTION

The superior aspect of the oral cavity includes the hard and soft palate. As the beginning of the upper aerodigestive tract, the oral cavity serves to move air for speech and respiration and food and liquids for nutrition. The hard palate is the static "roof" of the oral cavity and the "floor" of the nasal cavity and maxillary sinuses. It serves to separate the oral cavity from the nasal cavity as required for speech, respiration, and swallowing. The soft palate is a dynamic separator of the oral cavity and nasal cavity.

During respiration, an individual either inspires or expires through the nose or the mouth, but never both simultaneously. During expiration, air passes from the lungs, through the pharynx, and then through the oropharynx. Either the air then passes behind the soft palate into the nasopharynx, the nasal cavity, and out the nose, or the soft palate elevates to block the nasopharynx and the air passes out the oral cavity. During inspiration, the air passes in the opposite direction, through either the nasal cavity or the oral cavity.

For appropriate separation of these cavities during speech, respiration, and swallowing, the soft palate elevates in the middle third to separate the oropharynx and nasopharynx. The soft palate musculature extends from the pharynx at the level of the palate, inferiorly to the tonsillar area. The right and left muscles of the soft palate attach to the distal aspect of the hard palate and then intermingle on the entire midline length of the soft palate, forming an aponeurosis. Simultaneous contraction of these bilateral muscles causes the midline elevation of the soft palate. As the soft palate elevates, the pharyngeal wall simultaneously moves anteriorly and medially at the level of the soft palate elevation, which is in line with the plane of the hard palate. The sphincter formed by the soft palate and pharyngeal wall tightly closes and prevents any passage of liquid or food into the nasopharynx during deglutition. During phonation, the soft palate also elevates, and the pharyngeal wall moves anteriorly and medially; however, the movement of both structures is usually less dramatic than the sphincteric movement that occurs in swallowing. These functional movements of the soft palate and pharyngeal walls during speech and swallowing are called *velopharyngeal closure* (Figure 23-1). In the English

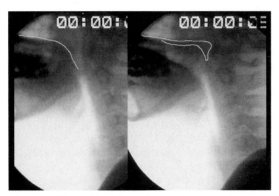

Figure 23-1 These lateral videofluoroscopic frames show the "at-rest" position of the soft palate *(left)* that postures against the base of the tongue and leaves the nasopharynx open for respiration. During swallowing *(right)*, the soft palate sharply elevates as the pharyngeal wall constricts, thereby forming a sphincter that separates the nasopharynx and oropharynx.

language, there are very few sounds that require air to travel from the oral cavity, behind the soft palate, and escape from the nose. These "nasal sounds" are *n, m,* and *ng* and resonate in the nasal cavity before exiting the nose. All "oral sounds" require that air be impounded in the oral cavity by the elevation of the soft palate and closure of the pharyngeal walls.

The inferior aspect of the oral cavity includes the tongue, muscles, and tissues of the floor of mouth, and the mandible. These inferior structures act in concert during speech. The tongue acts as the primary articulator. Airflow and the sounds emanating from the larynx are modulated through specific sites of contact and approximation of the tongue with the hard palate, the soft/hard palate junction, and the dentition. Accurate and rapid tongue movements are required for intelligible articulation.

During mastication, the tongue constantly moves the food bolus on the occlusal surfaces. It finally forms the food into a mass and pushes the mass posteriorly against the hard palate and into the oropharynx. The soft palate simultaneously elevates as the pharynx squeezes. The pharyngeal squeeze pushes the food into the esophagus.

FUNCTIONAL DEFICITS OF SPEECH AND SWALLOWING

There are a myriad of functional interactions in the oral cavity, nasal cavity, nasopharynx, and oropharynx that influence speech and swallowing. Disruption of any of these interactions can lead to deficits in speech and swallowing. These disruptions result from congenital malformations, central nervous system trauma, or surgery. They are seen as tissue loss, muscular denervation, or both. The most common congenital deficit is a cleft palate, seen as missing tissue in the hard and/or soft palate. Central nervous system deficits result from head injuries and cerebrovascular accidents. Tissues remain intact but are centrally denervated. Surgery for neoplastic disease results in tissue loss and local denervation; in addition, closure of the surgical site often tethers remaining tissues and restricts their movement.

When a patient has disruption of velopharyngeal closure or defects in the hard palate, air escapes inappropriately from the nose in nonnasal speech sounds. The patient is said to have hypernasal speech. As the volume of air that inappropriately escapes from the nose increases, the patient becomes more hypernasal until his or her speech becomes unintelligible. During swallowing, these same functional defects allow reflux of food and liquids into the nasal cavity. In the case of velopharyngeal inadequacy, dysfunction of the pharynx or soft palate may be the cause. When the soft palate is partially resected, the bilateral synchronous movement of the right and left muscles is disturbed. Unilateral soft palate function will not close the sphincter. Limited movement of any of the walls of the pharynx will not close the sphincter. Lack of adequate movement of the pharynx or the soft palate may result from surgical resection of these structures, causing lack of tissue, surgical scarring, or denervation of muscles. Head trauma or stroke can centrally denervate the soft palate or pharynx.

When the tongue or its contiguous structures in the inferior aspect of the oral cavity are resected, tissue loss, denervation of tongue muscles, or tethering of the tongue from surgical closure of the floor of the mouth inhibits the appropriate tongue-palate contact necessary for articulation. Loss of

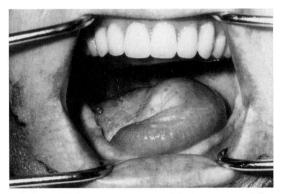

Figure 23-2 After a right partial glossectomy, this patient's residual tongue was used to cover the exposed mandible and right floor of the mouth. It is not possible for the patient to move the tongue or any food bolus laterally onto the occlusal surfaces of her teeth.

lateralization of the tongue inhibits movement of the food bolus onto the teeth, and mastication is impaired (Figure 23-2). Loss of elevation and "curling" of the tongue will inhibit moving the food bolus into the oropharynx to initiate the swallow.

MAXILLOFACIAL PROSTHODONTICS

When patients have disruption of the rudimentary functions of speech and swallowing, as previously described, various intraoral prostheses are made to compensate for loss of function. There are particular prosthetic considerations that are universal for edentulous maxillofacial prosthesis, and these will be addressed before individual prostheses are discussed.

Facial Form

Patients who have received trauma or surgical resection for neoplastic disease to the face or oral structures can be expected to have altered facial contours. This is due to scarring and tissue contracture, lack of bony support for the soft tissues of the face, and tissue edema. The patient and clinician should expect that it may take several months after an operation or trauma for the soft tissues to reach a final, stable position. These changes necessitate fabrication of interim prostheses and repeated

prosthesis adjustments to conform to soft tissue changes. Constant wearing of an interim prosthesis may slightly decrease tissue contraction and collapse, but this decrease is minimal. Because of lack of retention in an edentulous prosthesis, contracture of tissues and prosthesis overextension will unseat the prosthesis. When making an intraoral prosthesis, the clinician is very cognizant of the need to support the lips and cheeks, but soft tissue support and esthetics must be compromised to achieve prosthesis retention and stability.

Loss of Vertical Opening and Altered Mandibular Movements

Surgical resection, or trauma to oral cavity structures, can lead to loss of vertical opening of the mandible and altered mandibular range of motion. When there is surgical resection of the posterior aspect of the hard palate for neoplastic disease, the muscles of mastication are frequently detached from the maxilla or they are partially resected. This operation most often involves the medial and lateral pterygoid muscles. Trauma to the mandible in the area of the muscles of mastication also can damage the muscles. Trismus is the immediate result of muscular trauma, and the patient will have decreased vertical opening and range of motion of the mandible. As the area heals, the patient usually is given manual exercises to improve range of motion and opening. As time progresses, the traumatic muscular injury may become fibrotic and scarred. A decreased vertical opening often will be present in these patients and can make oral hygiene, prosthetic treatment, and manipulation of a food bolus difficult.

Partial resection of the posterior mandible removes the ipsilateral temporomandibular joint (TMJ) and its muscles of mastication and allows the remaining mandible to function on the opposing joint and muscles. Unilateral joint and muscle control causes mandibular deviation and altered range of motion. The medial pull of the ipsilateral pterygoid muscles pulls the mandible toward the side of the resection. The muscles on the floor of the mouth that are attached to the remaining mandibular body rotate the chin inferiorly, causing loss of anterior vertical overlap. When the patient attempts to occlude, the mandibular body is positioned lingually to its appropriate position, and the anterior mandible is positioned inferiorly.

Processed Bases

Processed bases have definite advantages in the patient with a maxillofacial prosthesis. Numerous soft tissue and bony undercuts exist after an oral cavity surgery or maxillectomy that may be used as prosthetic-bearing surfaces. When conventional record bases are made, the undercuts are blocked out to allow removal of the record bases from the master cast. Blocking out of these undercuts can result in lack of tissue contact of the record base with the periphery and the bearing surfaces within the surgical site (Figure 23-3). Without bearing surface contact, the occlusal plane and the centric relation (CR) record often are inaccurate. Using processed bases and denture adhesive in both the maxillary and mandibular prostheses will aid in achieving accurate records. Without peripheral extension of the base, it is difficult to set teeth in the appropriate buccal position, and it is not possible to discern how much additional lip and facial support may be gained from the teeth. Processed bases will allow the clinician to judge prosthesis retention and position of soft tissues supported by the base. At the try-in appointment, the patient and the clinician will be able to arrive at the ideal tooth position to con-sider esthetics, speech, retention, and stability of the prosthesis given the less than ideal postsurgical intraoral and extraoral tissue contours.

Border Molding the Velopharyngeal Area: Patient Movements

Border molding the velopharyngeal area includes making an impression to restore missing tissues of the soft palate and pharynx. Missing tissues may include portions or all of the soft palate or surgery to the pharyngeal wall. After placement of the impression material, the patient is asked to swallow. The greatest restriction of the size of the pharyngeal extension of the prosthesis occurs during the swallow; thus it is important to perform this function while the material is the least viscous. The patient will then open and close the mouth, move the mandible from side to side, turn the head from side to side, place the chin down to the chest, move the head from side to side, and extend the head backward.

Border Molding Peripheries of Maxillary Resections and Hard Palate Defects: Patient Movements

The hard palate is a static structure. Border molding its bony margins requires no special patient

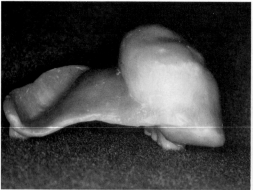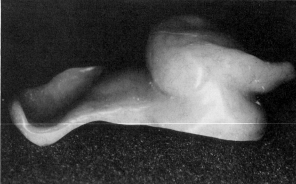

Figure 23-3 The conventional trial base *(left)* has been blocked out at the peripheries of the maxillary resection to allow removal from the master cast. The processed base *(right)* made from the same master cast allows maximum tissue contact and stability for the arrangement of teeth and jaw relationship records.

movements. Border molding the posterior and lateral area of a maxillectomy requires that the patient go through head and mandible movements similar to border molding the velopharyngeal area. Mandibular movement has the greatest effect on the lateral and posterolateral borders. Swallowing is important to move the cut edge of the soft palate at the posteromedial margin of the prosthesis.

Testing the Prosthetic "Seal" between the Oral Cavity and the Nasal Cavity

Drinking liquids is the usual test for prosthetic closure of an anatomical defect in the soft or hard palate. If the patient drinks in an upright position, water should not reflux into the nasal cavity. Placing the head downward will allow gravity to carry the liquid into the nasal cavity as well as the esophagus: the patient will need to keep the head upright when swallowing. Patients state that reflux is a particular problem when eating soup or drinking from a fountain because in both of these instances, the patient has the chin and head tucked. It is unlikely that most patients will be able to drink from a straw, even though the "seal" may adequately stop reflux of liquids.

Listening to speech sounds is the usual way to test for appropriate separation of airflow from the oral cavity and nasal cavity. There are particular sounds that are very sensitive to airflow. To test for possible hypernasality, have the patient say the word "beat" with the prosthesis in position. Pinch the patient's nares closed and have him or her say "beat." There should be no nasal air escape when saying this word, and there should be no difference in the sound of this word with or without the nares pinched together. If there is a difference in the sound of the word "beat" with and without pinching the nares, air is inappropriately escaping around the prosthesis periphery. Also, if the word "beat" sounds more like "meat," there is inappropriate air escape. Patients will report that they are misunderstood when using words that start with *B;* rather, the listener thinks that patients are using the letter *M.* To test for hyponasality, or lack of air escape through the nose on nasal sounds, have the patient say the phrase, "Momma made lemon jam." If the air is not allowed to escape from the oral cavity through the nose, the phrase will sound more

like "Bobba, bade lebon jab." These are the speech sounds of a person with the common cold and indicate that air is not escaping through the nose as it should on nasal sounds. In this regard the prosthesis may be too large or overextended; however, creating hyponasal speech with an obturator is uncommon. It is more likely that the obturator is satisfactory, but that the patient really is congested in the nasal passages.

MAXILLARY OBTURATOR PROSTHESIS

An obturator prosthesis is required for patients who have undergone tumor resection of the hard palate for neoplasms that originate in the paranasal sinuses or superior aspect of the oral cavity. Resection of the hard palate causes disruption of articulation and airflow during speech production and allows nasal reflux during deglutition. The obturator prosthesis serves to restore continuity of the hard palate and separate the nasal cavity and maxillary sinus from the oral cavity. This prosthesis also is used for hard palate defects in the patient with a cleft palate.

The patient who undergoes maxillary resection is rehabilitated in three phases. Each phase requires an obturator prosthesis that supports the patient through various stages of healing. These three prostheses are surgical obturator, interim obturator, and definitive obturator.

Surgical Obturator Prosthesis

The surgical obturator serves some rudimentary goals: (1) to support the surgical packing placed in the resection cavity created by removal of the walls of the maxillary sinus and (2) to restore continuity of the hard palate. This prosthesis allows the patient to take oral nutrition immediately postoperatively and, if the swallowing mechanism is not disrupted by extensive surgery to the pharynx, precludes use of a nasogastric feeding tube. Speech is generally quite normal with this prosthesis also. This prosthesis will be in service for approximately 5 to 10 days.

The patient must have a presurgical dental examination, and a maxillary cast must be made. This will be used to make the surgical and interim prosthesis. The clinician will also plan treatment for the patient for necessary preprosthetic surgery to remove epuli, reduce pendulous tuberosities, and relieve bony undercuts. Ideally, these are performed concurrently with the tumor resection.

A baseplate with routine denture extensions or an existing well-fitting denture may be used for the surgical obturator. The clinician should be aware, however, that if an existing denture is used, the patient usually expects that the denture will be used for the interim prosthesis also.

If the tumor is altering the normal contours of the hard palate, the cast should be altered to restore appropriate palatal contour. No other alteration of the cast is needed. The clinician should not attempt to delineate the exact posterior surgical margin on the soft palate, lateral surgical margins into the infratemporal fossa or pharynx, or superior margin into the sinus cavity. Appropriate design of the prosthesis allows fabrication of only one prosthesis. Extension of an acrylic resin prosthesis beyond the confines of the oral cavity would likely be overextended and require major adjustments in the operating room before it could be inserted. The packing placed superiorly into the surgical site will be supported by the baseplate and obturate any discrepancies between the surgical margins and the prosthesis borders.

Edentulous surgical obturators must be secured by circumzygomatic wires, sutures, or bone screws. Retentive holes for zygomatic wires are placed bilaterally with a no. 8 round bur in the premolar area through the prosthesis flanges. For the prosthesis to be sutured in position, the same bur is used to drill six holes in the periphery of the anterior and lateral flanges (Figure 23-4). A single bone screw may be placed through the vomer bone, through a predrilled hole in the midpalate at the junction of the premaxilla and hard palate. This hole should be drilled from the oral side of the palate and angled posteriorly (with the oral side of the hole anterior to the intaglio side of the hole) to allow manipulation of a screwdriver in the patient's mouth. The bone screw should be freely movable in the predrilled hole, but the diameter should not be large enough for the head of the screw to pass through (Figure 23-5). The hole should be countersunk to recess the head of the screw away from the patient's tongue. If the hole is not drilled with an oversized diameter, the screw often binds on the prosthesis as it engages the vomer bone. A self-

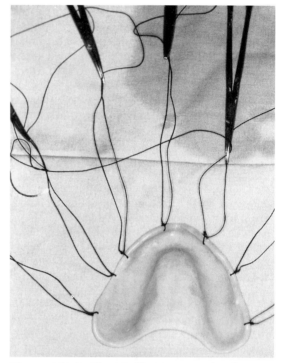

Figure 23-4   The 2-0 silk sutures are placed through the predrilled holes at the periphery of the obturator, knotted, and tagged with a hemostat before being placed into the mouth and suturing into the patient's vestibule.

tapping screw may be sharp enough to be placed directly into the vomer, but a "starter hole" drilled in the vomer aids placement of the screw. As a precaution, the screw should be covered with a tissue conditioner material to keep it in the denture in the unlikely event that it works loose from the bone. If the midpalate is crossed during the operation, the vomer will not be present. Two bone screws can then be placed in the residual alveolar process at antagonistic angles. Rarely is a starter hole necessary in the alveolar process. The maxillary sinus that has not been operated on may be entered with the screws, but healing is uneventful when the screws are removed. Removal of the bone screw and sutures is easily accomplished in an outpatient setting. Removal of zygomatic wires should be done with the surgeon's assistance and usually requires an operating room setting.

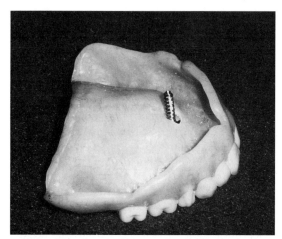

Figure 23-5 A 14- to 16-mm palatal bone screw can be placed into the vomer of the edentulous maxillectomy patient. The hole should be drilled in the midline with sufficient space to allow the screw to move freely in the hole, but not allow the head of the screw to pass through.

Interim Obturator Prosthesis

The interim obturator is delivered when the surgical obturator is removed. The prosthetic goals are to restore deglutition and speech by restoring palatal contours and separating the nasal cavity, maxillary sinus, and nasopharynx from the oral cavity. The patient and dentist understand that this prosthesis will be altered considerably as the patient heals and facial contours change. This prosthesis will be in service for approximately 2 to 6 months. A baseplate without dentition or the patient's existing denture can be used for the maxillectomy in the edentulous patient. Retention of the edentulous obturator prosthesis is always a problem. The dentist should be certain that the border extensions and palatal tissue contact are optimal for maximal contact on the intact maxilla. Relining the existing denture may be required before modifying the surgical area. Denture adhesives usually are required. Constant adjustments and relining are necessary because even slight border overextension in the edentulous maxillofacial prosthesis will unseat the prosthesis. Keeping the prosthesis hollow in the surgical site will decrease weight and aid retention.

The prosthesis is modified with an intermediate denture liner to conform to the periphery of the surgical site. The bulb portion should be kept hollow during the relining procedure to limit the weight of the prosthesis. The material is added to the periphery in incremental fashion as when border molding any removable prosthesis. An ideal material should have enough body to support itself during the initial impression procedure and for several weeks (Figure 23-6).

As the patient heals, the periphery of the surgical site will become smaller. The material can be reduced with a carbide bur and readapted with the addition of more liner. The primary areas requiring readaptation are the posterolateral and the anterior borders. The greater the volume of bone resected, the greater the amount of postsurgical soft tissue contracture and the more time it will take before the surgical site is stable. As the tissue contracts, the prosthesis borders will be overextended, and the patient will have difficulty seating the prosthesis. The intermediate denture liner borders should then be relieved and resurfaced. The patient may return, complaining that there is discomfort on the nonsurgical area of the maxilla or that the prosthesis is no longer retentive. Adjustments should not be made to the nonsurgical side of the prosthesis because the problem is likely to be tissue changes in the

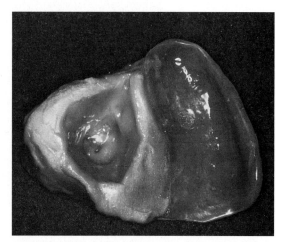

Figure 23-6 The edentulous baseplate is border molded with a low-viscosity tissue conditioner material that can be relieved and modified as facial contracture occurs (Tru-Soft, Henry J. Bosworth, Skokie, Ill).

surgical area shifting the entire prosthesis. The prosthesis must be worn constantly, removed only for cleaning of the surgical site or prosthesis. If the patient removes the prosthesis nightly, the tissue changes will be rapid, and the patient will not be able to seat the prosthesis after only a few days. These contour changes are usually a combination of edema and tissue contracture.

When the surgical site is changing shape less rapidly (in approximately 1 month), the prosthesis can be flasked, replacing the denture liner material with acrylic resin. For the prosthesis to be delivered in the same day, autopolymerizing resins usually are used. One should not keep the prosthesis overnight; major tissue changes of the entire surgical border can occur, requiring relief of the periphery and another relining impression. Over time, slight tissue changes will continue, exemplified by increased nasal reflux and hypernasal speech. These usually occur at the medial junction of the prosthesis and cut edge of the soft palate. These isolated areas can be addressed with tissue conditioning material or chairside autopolymerizing resin as needed.

The clinician and patient should be aware that using the existing maxillary denture as an interim obturator prosthesis will be successful only for 2 to 3 weeks, and then a new prosthesis or resetting of teeth usually is required. If the resection includes any of the premaxillary area, facial collapse is pronounced (Figure 23-7). The original border extension and the teeth will soon be overextended in a horizontal direction. The flange must be reduced, and the anterior teeth will need to be reset more palatally. The posterior teeth also may require palatal repositioning, but the problem is most evident in the anterior area. In addition, repeated relining of the prosthesis, while attempting to maintain occlusion with a mandibular denture, is very difficult. For patient satisfaction, it may be necessary to remake the maxillary and mandibular prostheses or reset teeth more than once during the healing process. The patient must understand that mastication is rarely restored in the interim phase because of the constant transition of the tissues and fit of the dentures. These necessary modifications must be factored into the treatment plan and may be beyond the available time and finances of many patients.

For this reason, an alternative edentulous interim obturator prosthesis is a simple baseplate. It will restore speech and deglutition and satisfy most patients if they understand that complete dentures

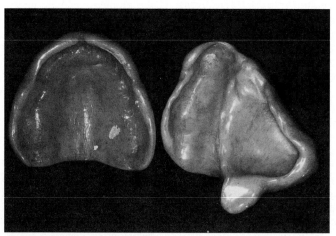

Figure 23-7 The patient's original denture has normal anatomical borders *(left)*; however, the obturator prosthesis relined at 4 weeks after surgery *(right)* has markedly altered contours in the anterior of the prosthesis because of facial contracture. A tray extension over the soft palate into the pharynx was added to support an impression of the pharynx in function, which was necessary because the patient's velar movement was inadequate in the weeks after surgery (see Figure 23-11).

are the goal when postsurgical healing is complete. The surgical baseplate can be border molded and relined with a tissue conditioner material on the nonsurgical side. This step stabilizes the prosthesis, and then the surgical site may be relined. The baseplate can be flasked as a wax pattern. The relined baseplate is then removed from the flask during the boil-out procedure and replaced with resin. This technique ensures a well-fitting baseplate during the interim obturator phase. Subsequent relining will be necessary in the surgical site.

Definitive Obturator Prosthesis

This prosthesis is fabricated when tissue healing and contraction are complete. When irradiation follows surgery, resolution of radiation mucositis also is necessary. Proceeding with a definitive prosthesis before tissue contours are stable may require major adjustments that will involve changing tooth positions or gross adjustments to the prosthesis periphery. It may be 2 to 6 months postoperatively before the tissues are stable.

Preliminary impressions are made with irreversible hydrocolloid. It is desirable to capture the periphery and height of the surgical site in the preliminary impression so that maximum extension of the definitive impression tray is possible (Figure 23-8). It is not necessary to block out the surgical defect with gauze to prevent the impression material from entering this space. (The only time the opening to the sinus needs to be protected is when the opening is a fistula.) Some impression materials lack body and therefore do not "carry" into the surgical defect without adding wax or compound support into the defect or injection of the material with a large custom syringe. There are irreversible hydrocolloids with considerable viscosity. These give good border extensions for edentulous and maxillofacial impressions without support from the tray or need to inject the material. This significantly reduces operator time.

Decreased vertical opening is often a problem in the patient undergoing a maxillectomy because of surgical trauma and fibrosis of the muscles of mastication in proximity to the maxillary resection. It may be difficult to carry impression material into the surgical defect because of the limited oral opening, but because of the lack of dentition, the clini-

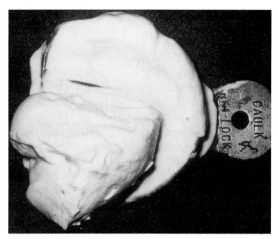

Figure 23-8   It is desirable to capture the total maxillary cavity in the preliminary impression for adequate extension of final impression trays. It is not necessary to "block out" the cavity with gauze (Supergel, Harry J. Bosworth, Skokie, Ill).

cian usually has enough access in the oral cavity despite the decreased opening.

A maxillary custom impression tray extended into the maxillary defect will decrease operator time when fabricating the final impression. The preliminary cast should be "blocked out" to allow space for compound and wax/impression material. Undercuts in the cast also must be blocked out before making the tray, or after the final impression is poured, the tray will not separate from the master cast. Border molding the nonsurgical side and making the final impression before border molding the surgical site ensures that the tray is reseated in a consistent manner when the surgical site is impressed. The clinician should always be aware that manual seating pressure of the tray during border molding and impression making should be obliquely directed against the remaining alveolar ridge and not against the midpalate as is done when seating a normal maxillary denture tray. Seating against the midpalate often causes the tray to rotate into the surgical site and away from the residual alveolar ridge without operator awareness.

Compound is incrementally added to the tray to record the periphery of the surgical site. The clinician must support the tray during these movements because the patient must perform a variety of movements to shape the compound. The clinician should constantly look at the anatomical form and landmarks of the surgical site to determine that the compound is not underextended. There is commonly a soft tissue undercut at the junction of the oral mucosa and skin graft that lines the maxillary cavity called a *cicatricial line* or *scar band*. The clinician should see this anatomical landmark and the cut edge of the soft palate in the compound. If the impression tray moves during the patient's movements, an area of compound is overextended. The clinician must find this area of overextension and readapt it before proceeding any further. With partial maxillectomy procedures, some bony walls of the maxillary sinus may remain. When these walls have been grafted with skin, it is possible to use them for vertical support. They should be captured in the border molding of the surgical site. At completion of border molding, the compound can be slightly relieved and an impression wax painted over the surface or a final impression material used. The advantage of using wax is that areas of pressure will show through the wax and the compound can be further relieved. The easiest method of using the wax is to cover the relieved compound, quickly dip the area in the warm water bath, place it in the mouth, and have the patient go through the border molding movements.

Maxillary and mandibular processed bases and denture adhesive are used to ensure maximum stability and soft tissue support. The clinician should manually stabilize the least stable base when making the record and watch very carefully for shifts of the bases. In the case of a patient undergoing a maxillectomy, this would be the maxillary base. If the bases shift, the record should be remade. Because of the instability of the obturator prosthesis, monoplane occlusion is recommended for the completely edentulous patient.

Because of facial contracture on the surgical side, it often is necessary to place the anterior teeth in an end-to-end or reverse horizontal articulatim situation. The facial position of the anterior teeth may be verified at the try-in appointment Esthetics and lip support are often compromised to aid retention. An end-to-end occlusion in the posterior teeth should be avoided. Horizontal overlap is necessary to avoid cheek biting. When decreased vertical opening is seen in these patients, interocclusal space at maximum opening may be only 1 to 1.5 cm. The clinician may choose to slightly close the vertical dimension of occlusion to allow the patient more functional space; however, lip and cheek biting may become a problem, and attention to horizontal overlap is very important. Decreased vertical dimension of occlusion also can lead to periodic angular cheilosis that requires treatment.

The palatal contour should be evaluated in an obturator prosthesis. The contour on the surgical side should mimic that of the nonsurgical side. Making these contours too low constricts the tongue, which will then lift the prosthesis into the surgical site during speech and swallowing. Making the contour too high will not allow proper tongue/palate contact during speech, affecting articulation and the impounding of air in the oral cavity. If the posterior teeth were placed in reverse articulation bite, it may be necessary to remove the palatal half of these teeth. The height of the palate may be examined visually and with pressure indicator paste. The patient should be asked to swallow and speak. The paste can be checked for uniform contact of the tongue. If additional acrylic resin is needed to refine the palatal contours, this may be added when the teeth are processed onto the base.

At insertion of the prostheses, it is not necessary to perform a clinical occlusal remount procedure because processed bases were used and a laboratory remount was done at deflasking. Final evaluation of the prostheses fit should be done. Evaluating pressure areas and border extensions is best done with a combination of pressure-indicating paste and tissue-conditioning material. The pressure paste is effective for the intaglio surface of the prosthesis but often smears on insertion or removal of the prosthesis, and therefore accurately interpreting the pressure areas on the obturator portion of the prosthesis is quite difficult. A fast-setting, contrasting-color, tissue-conditioning material is ideal (Softone, Harry J. Bosworth, Skokie, Ill.). The obturator portion should be lightly coated with petroleum jelly. The material should be mixed with enough body so it will not flow off the prosthesis. The patient should swallow and go through all head and jaw movements. A uniform, thin, functionally formed coating of material remains with obvious "show through" of the acrylic resin in pressure areas.

Denture adhesive can be used to aid in retention, and the prosthesis extension into the surgical site can be made hollow to decrease the weight of the prosthesis. Some clinicians leave the hollowed area open superiorly, and some clinicians choose to place a cap from the superior aspect or the palatal aspect. Placing a cap precludes any reflux of food or liquids into the extension and the need for the patient to clean this area of the prosthesis.

Troubleshooting an Obturator Prosthesis

Lack of Retention   Overextension of borders in an interim prosthesis is the result of soft tissue changes, and the prosthesis borders will need to be relieved and relined. Adhesives are almost always required for any edentulous obturator prosthesis. The patients should be advised to masticate as little as possible on the defect side because this tends to unseat the prosthesis. Retention is a very difficult problem for the edentulous patient. When planning the treatment for a patient with poor dentition, before maxillectomy, the plan should be to save teeth for denture retention. Severely carious teeth are often problematic because of cost of root canals, need for crown lengthening, and the lack of vertical opening after surgery and postoperative radiotherapy. For this reason grossly decayed or peridontally involved molars are of limited value. However, saving some anterior teeth that have at least 50% bone remaining with limited soft tissue pockets can create adequate retention and last many years. Often, eventual loss of single-rooted teeth in the irradiated maxilla will heal uneventfully. If only one to two teeth are remaining, an overdenture with magnetic attachments can be considered. These attachments, in addition to adhesive, can serve patients very well. This is true for the patient undergoing a maxillectomy and a mandibulectomy (Figures 23-9 and 23-10).

Nasal Reflux   Explain to the patient that the prosthesis cannot function as a "cork in a bottle," and some reflux is to be expected. An upright head position is required during swallowing. Check the palatal contours with pressure indicator paste. A palatal form that is too low constricts the tongue and unseats the prosthesis. Check the tissue adaptation at the posteromedial and posterolateral margins (at the prosthesis/soft palate junction). Place petro-

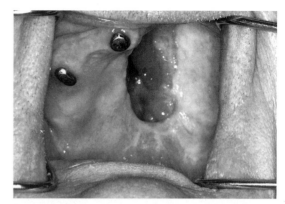

Figure 23-9   This patient had two teeth with recession and wear. Both teeth were reduced without need for root canals. A ferrous metal was used to create copings.

leum jelly on the prosthesis surface and functionally disclose the area with a viscous tissue conditioner, as previously described. If the tissue conditioner material is thick and successfully decreases reflux, this area should be addressed for a relining procedure. When the required relining area is only 1 to 2 cm and the remainder of the obturator portion is well fitting, a chairside relining should be considered. Cut finish lines to demarcate the area indicated by the tissue conditioner. These finish lines will confine the relin-

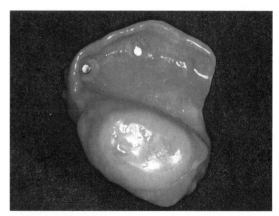

Figure 23-10   The magnets were incorporated in the denture. This magnetic system was in service for over 10 years until the patient died of cardiac arrest.

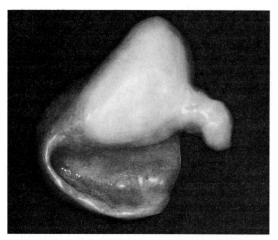

Figure 23-11   This patient who underwent a maxillectomy had lack of appropriate velar movement after surgical contracture of the velum. A pharyngeal extension was added to the prosthesis to obturate the pharynx and correct hypernasality.

ing material. An autopolymerizing relining resin or a light-cured composite resin material can be added and border molded in the patient's mouth. Conversely, if the tissue conditioner material is quite thin and indicates a well-fitting prosthesis, the seal cannot be improved.

Hypernasality   When reflux has been minimized but hypernasality exists, one should consider that the velopharyngeal closure may be compromised from surgery. The soft palate may elevate, but there may not be enough elevation to close the nasopharynx. If the resection also includes a portion of the soft palate, the remainder may be too short to contact the pharyngeal walls. The clinician should attempt to add a pharyngeal extension, as in the soft palate obturator prosthesis, over the inadequately functioning soft palate to obturate the pharynx (Figure 23-11).

SOFT PALATE OBTURATOR PROSTHESIS

A soft palate obturator or speech aid prosthesis is required for patients who have a resection of their soft palate or have a soft palate deficit from a cleft palate. Absence of soft palate tissue disrupts speech

and swallowing by allowing nasal escape of air during speech and nasal reflux during swallowing. An immediate surgical soft palate obturator prosthesis usually is not inserted. If the pharynx is obturated with any rigid material or a tissue-conditioning material in the operating room, the extension will invariably be overextended, and the patient will experience postoperative pain in the pharynx when he or she awakens and resumes swallowing and movement of the head. Even small, arbitrary acrylic resin extensions made on a surgical cast to support a surgical gauze packing placed in the pharynx will likely be overextended in some areas with the postoperative sphincteric closure of the pharynx.

A pharyngeal extension can be added to a denture prosthesis or baseplate within a few days after resection. When only the soft palate is resected, patients will resume swallowing with minimal discomfort; however, if the resection is more extensive, patients may not resume normal swallowing immediately because of additional surgical involvement of the pharynx. They may require nasogastric tube feeding or gastrostomy until they can swallow without aspiration. In these situations, the obturator's major function will be to restore speech.

A posterior extension is added to a denture prosthesis to contact the patient's pharyngeal wall when it closes during speech and swallowing. The extension should be made at the level of the hard palate and at the level of the most active movement of the pharyngeal sphincter. This movement can be visualized by asking the patient to say "ahh" or by stroking the posterior wall with a mirror handle, initiating a gag reflex. Often a prominent muscular ridge on the pharyngeal wall, called *Passavant's ridge*, is present when the patient says "ahh" (Figure 23-12). This ridge has been called a compensatory mechanism because it is present in most patients with cleft palates and has been seen to increase and become more obvious with time in patients with cleft palates and resected soft palates.

A small acrylic resin posterior projection can be added to the denture as a tray to support the impression material. A viscous tissue conditioner material or compound can be added. The patient should go through the necessary movements to capture the functional movements of the pharynx at the area of most movement. The impression should be examined for contact with the pharynx bilaterally and

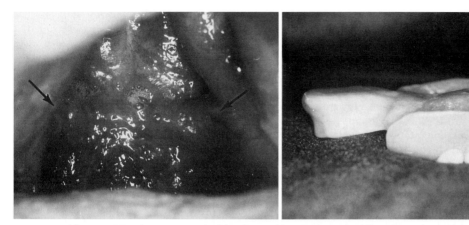

Figure 23-12 Passavant's ridge *(arrows)* is prominent in this patient who had undergone a total soft palate resection. The pharyngeal obturator prosthesis is approximately 1 cm in height, and the ridge is evident in the posterior contour of the prosthesis.

posteriorly. If any of the acrylic resin tray projects through the material, it should be generously relieved and that portion of the impression remade. The inferior extent of the pharyngeal extension should be at or slightly below the inferior aspect of the pharyngeal sphincter. The overall height of the extension should not be more than 1 cm. This will successfully cover the area of pharyngeal constriction without adding excessive weight. The compound may be relieved and covered with impression wax. If the clinician wants the wax to flow during the impression, the wax-coated extension will need to be quickly dipped in a hot water bath before insertion, or the patient will need to wear the prosthesis for approximately 30 minutes while repeatedly going through swallowing and head movements. The clinician may test the final impression for closure of the nasopharynx in swallowing by asking the patient to drink water. Hypernasality and hyponasality may be tested at this time. Ideally, airflow in speech should be appropriate.

Troubleshooting the Soft Palate Obturator Prosthesis

Prosthesis Feels Too Long The patient complains that they "feel the prosthesis in the back" of their pharynx. They also may describe that they have difficulty initiating a swallow reflex. The prosthesis should be disclosed with a functional tissue conditioner rather than pressure indicator paste. A paste does not reveal the overextension as accurately as tissue conditioner. If the patient continues to complain, it may be necessary to reduce the entire extension and make a new functional impression.

Hypernasality Evaluate for appropriate tissue contact in swallowing using a tissue conditioner. If a uniformly thin coating is evidenced but hypernasality persists, the difference in pharyngeal wall constriction in swallowing versus speech is the problem. During swallowing, pharyngeal constriction is usually more pronounced than in speech. As the difference between pharyngeal function in swallowing and speech becomes greater, the more likely it is that the patient will have hypernasal speech. It usually is not possible to add more material to the extension, or the patient begins to complain of overextension. Increased "compensatory" pharyngeal constriction may be seen as time passes. This compensatory movement may decrease or even eliminate hypernasality, but predicting this compensation for an individual patient is not possible.

PALATAL AUGMENTATION PROSTHESIS

During speech, swallowing, or mastication, the tongue contacts the palate and teeth to move the food bolus and articulate speech sounds into language. When the tongue or contiguous oral cavity structures are resected for neoplastic disease, the deficits in tongue function are related to loss of tissue bulk, denervation, and tethering of the remaining portion of the tongue. Hypoglossal nerve damage causes the tongue to deviate toward the affected side on protrusion, and the tongue tip may not elevate. If the remaining tongue is used to surgically close the oral cavity wound, it will be sutured to the cheek, impairing range of motion and posturing it in an abnormal position. When mandibular deviation occurs in a nonreconstructed partial mandibulectomy patient, the tongue deviates with the mandible and does not make appropriate tongue/palate contact.

Clinical Examination

Patients with any of the preceding surgical findings should be considered for a palatal augmentation prosthesis. Look for normal range of motion of the tongue, evaluate if food collects on the palate or pools in other areas of the oral cavity, ask patients if they aspirate when they eat, and finally, listen for articulation errors. These errors may include slurred speech on the *s* and *sh* sounds and lack of intelligibility with *k, g, t, l,* and *d*. If it has been some time since the operation and if the patients have not been wearing dentures, they may have accommodated to the lack of tongue mobility and are making tongue/palate contact by inappropriate "overclosure" of the mandible. The only obvious clinical finding in this "overclosed" patient may be abnormal range of motion of the tongue and perhaps a slight dysarthria.

Attachments of the tongue and floor of mouth soft tissues to the mandible may preclude making dentures. The ridge may be entirely covered with the tongue flap or with bulky tissue brought from distant sites, such as the pectoralis or rectus muscle. Thinner tissues, such as from the forearm, may be used for reconstruction, but if these are freely movable over the mandible, a stable mandibular denture may not be possible.

Informing the Patient

Patients should be aware of the difficulties of wearing a mandibular denture without normal tongue range of motion. If they are experienced denture wearers, they will probably accommodate better than the first-time wearer. Patients will equate receiving dentures with an advancement of their diet to more solid foods; however, mastication may not be possible. Lateral tongue movement and an ability to elevate the tongue to the height of the mandibular occlusal table are necessary for mastication; some patients will not have lateral motion. Patients who have accommodated to the altered tongue function by overclosure of the mandible should be aware that delivering dentures and restoring the correct vertical dimension of occlusion will require an augmentation prosthesis. A period of learning new compensatory speech and swallowing mechanisms will be necessary. These individuals may be very disappointed with the immediate difficulties experienced with their new prostheses and the apparent "backward" step in their rehabilitation. Adhesives for the mandibular denture usually are required. Speech and swallowing therapy are necessary to optimize function. Finally, the decision may be not to deliver a mandibular denture because of mandibular retention problems. Maxillary prostheses with anterior teeth and an augmentation for function and esthetics may be the definitive prosthodontic care.

Usual denture fabrication techniques should be used. The vertical dimension will be established by looking at facial form and speaking space. The sounds may be quite distorted, but the relationship of the maxillary and mandibular anterior teeth when the patient attempts the *s* sound should be normal. At the try-in stage, the augmentation may be added. A processed maxillary base is suggested because the bulk of acrylic resin needed in the palate could cause considerable processing distortion if the base and augmentation are processed simultaneously.

If a speech and swallowing therapist is available, he or she can assist in evaluating the contours. The area of loss of tongue bulk should be correspondingly augmented on the palate with baseplate wax. Additions should include evaluation with pressure indicator paste, looking for uniform tongue contact. The tongue may not be able to move to all quadrants of the mouth, so there may not be an impression of the tongue on the entire surface of the augmentation. Placing a tissue conditioner material on the palatal surface of the denture can be used to create a functional impression of the residual mobile tongue made during swallowing. This technique usually will achieve an improvement in articulation also.

Fine tuning for subtle changes in articulation and air flow (needed for such sounds as *s, sh,* and *t*) usually is better accomplished with small additions and subtractions of wax after the gross contours needed for swallowing are established. These minute refinements are more difficult to accomplish if tissue conditioner material, rather than baseplate wax, is used to form the initial swallowing contacts. Specific target sounds to assess anterior and posterior contact are used. Posterior sounds include *k* and a hard *g.* If these sounds are not distinct, the posterior palate must be lowered. The tongue tip may not be centered in the palate because of tethering or deviation toward the surgical side due to hypoglossal nerve damage. Additional wax may need to be added to allow the most elevated portion of the tongue (if the tongue tip no longer elevates, this new area of elevation in the body of the tongue becomes the tongue tip) to make definite contact for the *t* and *d* sounds. As for the routine denture wearer, a lisp may be present during the *s* and *sh* sounds. During these sounds, the normal tongue does not contact the anterior palate, but rather it curls and approximates the palate in the midline to create an air channel. A narrow channel forms the *s* sound, and the same channel is made wider by flattening the tongue for the *sh* sound. Patients undergoing glossectomy may not be able to curl the tongue or approximate the anterior palate in the midline. Placing a groove in the anterior palate may create the necessary air channel. This groove will not necessarily be in the midline but must coincide with the deviation of the anterior tongue.

Patients with the best results will have most of their tongue remaining and have a tongue tip that is not tethered, although they may have speech errors in connected speech. The impaired tongue will not be able to move to all positions of the mouth rapidly; therefore the patient must slow the rate of speech. Despite the best prosthodontic efforts, patients with greater range-of-motion deficits may be able to eat only pureed foods or a liquid diet, and they may continue to have errors in certain target sounds.

MANDIBULAR RESECTION PROSTHESES

Special maxillofacial prostheses for the mandible usually are required because of surgical resection for neoplastic disease. A discontinuity resection of the mandible implies that a portion of the mandible is resected, and the condyle-to-condyle continuity of the mandible is disrupted. A marginal mandibulectomy implies that a margin of bone is resected, but the continuity of the mandible is maintained. Usually, the margin of resection is at the superior aspect and is involved with epithelial neoplasms of the mouth.

Marginal Mandibulectomy Prostheses

A marginal mandibulectomy can be restored with a complete mandibular denture provided the soft tissue reconstruction over the mandible is not grossly mobile or compressible. If the tongue or floor-of-mouth tissues are sutured over the mandible to the cheek, the tissue mobility will unseat the denture (Figure 23-13). Thin microvascular flaps from the forearm are commonly used in the floor of mouth over the mandible, but these tissues do not attach to the bone and are also too mobile for denture stability (Figure 23-14). The ideal closure is a split-thickness skin graft placed over the bone and sutured to the buccal and lingual tissues. The skin

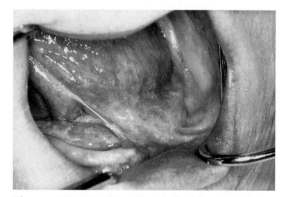

Figure 23-13   This patient had a left marginal mandibulectomy and floor-of-mouth resection. The remaining tissues of the floor of the mouth and buccal tissues of the cheek were closed primarily over the mandible, precluding fabrication of a stable denture.

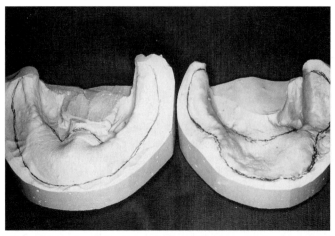

Figure 23-14   This patient had a free soft tissue flap from the forearm placed over a marginal mandibulectomy, replacing missing soft tissue of the floor of mouth and mandible. The right cast reveals the contour changes after connective tissue debulking 1.5 cm of soft tissue; however, because the flap does not attach to the mandible, the tissue is very mobile, and the patient could not successfully wear dentures.

graft will attach to the marrow bone and behave similarly to attached gingiva. The mobile lingual and buccal tissues are separated by nonmobile skin over the mandible (Figure 23-15). This skin-grafted mandible will respond well to radiotherapy also. Surgeons should be encouraged to use a skin graft on marginal mandibulectomies, unless consider-

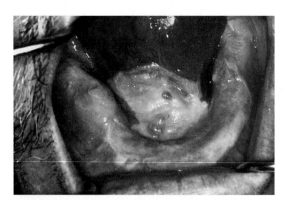

Figure 23-15   This patient had a marginal mandibulectomy and floor-of-mouth resection that was reconstructed with a split-thickness skin graft from the thigh. Given the excellent posterior mandibular height and nonmobile tissue in the anterior mandible, the patient did very well wearing conventional dentures.

able soft tissue is required to restore gross resection of the tongue and floor of mouth. If a skin graft is not used for primary reconstruction, secondary debulking of the movable flap and placement of a skin graft often are necessary before making a mandibular denture. Processed bases are advantageous.

Discontinuity Mandibulectomy Prostheses

Mandibular discontinuity resections are usually in the lateral aspect of the mandible and result from epithelial lesions in the oral cavity overlying the mandible. Recently, predictable use of microvascular bone grafts has allowed immediate reconstruction of mandibular resections, and delayed particulate bone grafts can be used; however, this reconstruction is not available in all institutions, and not all patients are candidates for these secondary complex operative procedures. These unreconstructed lateral resections will continue to require prosthetic rehabilitation.

A custom border molded tray should cover the available mandibular body. There is often a desire to extend the denture beyond the mandible into the resected area to gain a broader area of contact or to support the lip. The soft tissues in the resected area should be scrutinized because they usually move when the tongue moves or when the patient opens the mouth. These movements will unseat the prosthesis. If the tongue is "pulled" to the surgical side with the surgical closure, a deep anatomical space is created on the posterior lingual aspect of the remaining mandible. Because the tongue lacks mobility, this space does not change. Extension of the denture flange into this space improves denture stability. A processed base will allow a thorough evaluation of the base stability before the addition of teeth.

Making maxillomandibular relationship records for this patient is challenging. Patients do not have a condylar hinge movement. Because of unilateral muscle attachments to the intact mandible on the nonsurgical side, as the patient opens the mouth, the chin and midline deviate as much as 1 to 2 cm to the surgical side. As the patient closes the mouth, the anterior mandibular path is not vertical, but rather it follows a diagonal path toward the nonsurgical side. At final closure, the patient usually reaches the vertical dimension of occlusion with the mandible positioned palatal to the maxillary teeth. Besides the problem of unilateral muscle attachments, there often is scarring in the surgical area that also prevents the mandible from returning to its presurgical relationship with the maxilla.

When shaping the maxillary rim, it may be necessary to decrease the upper lip support slightly so as not to accentuate the Class II appearance of the patient. This appearance occurs as a result of the deviated and recessed chin point. Do not "push" the mandible laterally to achieve normal maxillary/mandible horizontal overlap. It is unlikely that the patient will be able to achieve this relationship during function. Patients should move the mandible toward the surgical side using their own muscles of mastication. This patient-generated position is used as the centric occlusion (CO) position. The patient undergoing a lateral mandibulectomy has proprioception for a "repeatable position" within an occlusal area, but it will not be an exact repeatable position as is seen in a CR position of the nonresected mandible. Adapt the occlusal wax rims in harmony with this position.

Vertical dimension of occlusion should be determined by assessing lip competence, facial appearance, and speaking space. Normal lip closure often

is compromised in these patients because of bisecting of the lower lip during surgery, damage to the marginal mandibular branch of the facial nerve and lack of bony support; therefore it is important that the patient can close the lips without straining to prevent loss of liquids or food bolus. Lip closure and an unstrained facial appearance may be the best determinant of the correct vertical dimension of occlusion. Closest speaking space may be a helpful parameter, but because of possible articulation problems and mandibular deviation, this parameter may deviate greatly from normal.

After the occlusion rims are formed for horizontal alignment and equal contact in CO position, the interocclusal record may be made. Using any material with resistance will cause the mandible to rotate as the denture encounters the resistance. Using a plaster for the recording material requires that the patient maintain a position until the material sets. Maintaining a mandibular position without occlusal contact or moving the mandible to a specific location often is difficult for a patient with a partial resection. An alternative is to have the patient close repeatedly and observe the repeatable occlusal table "area." The occlusal rims should be adapted to coincide with this position to offer maximum maxillomandibular wax rim contact. Make large notches on the buccal of the occlusal rims. Have the patient lightly close into the maximum rim contact and then inject impression plaster along the buccal surfaces of the two occlusion rims (Figure 23-16). In this manner, the patient's mandible is in its most stable position, and the vertical dimension of occlusion is accurate.

Mount the processed bases on remount casts. Use of a face bow to achieve a relationship of the condyles to the maxilla is not an issue in the patient with a resection because the condylar function is unilateral. However, mounting the maxilla in the correct relationship to the upper member of the articulator will give the clinician an appreciation for the rotation of the mandible. When the relationship of the mandible with the maxilla is viewed, the deviation toward the surgical side, the medial rotation of the mandibular body, and the inferior rotation of the chin point will be evident. Monoplane occlusion is recommended to allow patients freedom

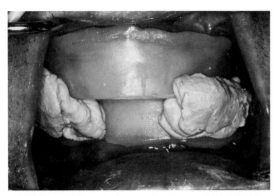

Figure 23-16   For interocclusal records, impression plaster is injected along the buccal surfaces of the occlusion rims while the patient is sitting upright and his mandible is in the postsurgical centric occlusion position.

to function in an occlusal area. Given the medial mandibular rotation, it is likely that the posterior mandibular teeth may be positioned on the buccal shelf, which is now the functional ridge crest. Placing the anterior teeth more buccal than the vestibule will decrease the Class II appearance but usually serves to decrease denture stability. If processed bases are used, this tooth position can be assessed at the try-in appointment. If the bases become less stable when positioning the mandibular anterior teeth, the teeth should be set more lingually. The mandibular plane will coincide with the maxillary plane. Because of the inferior rotation of the anterior mandible, the vertical height of the mandibular denture in this area may be considerably more than the posterior denture height. Vertical overlap of the anterior teeth may be considered. Because incising or movement of the mandible into a normal "s position" during speech is unlikely in this patient population, vertical overlap may not unseat the denture in function. During the try-in stage, anterior vertical overlap can be assessed in relation to denture stability and its benefit to speech.

For proper maxillary buccal corridors to be achieved, the maxillary teeth are set in the appropriate buccal/lingual position. Because of mandibular deviation, it may be necessary to place a flat occlusal platform palatal to the maxillary teeth on the nonresected side to achieve occlusal contact.

Making a sloped platform to guide the mandible farther toward the nonresected side and achieve a more normal occlusal buccal/lingual alignment usually unseats the mandibular denture rather than moves the mandible. A sloped platform should be avoided in the edentulous patient, unless it is a sloped platform that corresponds to the slope of the path of closure.

Placing prostheses and establishing a vertical dimension of occlusion may alter tongue/palate contact. The patient should be considered for a palatal augmentation prosthesis. It may be formed at the try-in appointment or added later. After processing on the teeth, the dentures are returned to the remount casts, and a laboratory remount is done.

Troubleshooting Prostheses for the Patient with an Edentulous Mandibulectomy

Unstable Mandibular Denture   Stability of the base should be evaluated with processed bases at the time of maxillomandibular relationship records before placement of wax rims. Overextension onto movable tissue will unseat the prosthesis. Overextensions should be reduced before making records. If the prosthesis is unstable at the try-in appointment, inappropriate tooth position may be unseating the prosthesis. Denture adhesive often is necessary.

Inability to Chew or Inability to Chew beyond a Soft Diet   Tongue lateralization is very important for moving a food bolus onto the teeth. Patients with partial mandibulectomies often have impaired range of motion of the tongue. A liquid diet or a soft diet that is washed down with liquids may be all that the patient can accommodate despite the insertion of dentures. Hard food substances require considerable masticatory power that the edentulous mandibulectomy patient lacks. The patient should be educated to these possible limitations before the prostheses process is begun.

Prostheses for Bone-Grafted Mandibles

Restoration of continuity with bone grafting offers a major advantage by maintaining the condyles in the appropriate relationship to each other and to the maxilla, thereby negating mandibular deviation. A repeatable CR position can be achieved. For improvement of prosthetic rehabilitation, an adequate volume of bone and soft tissues overlying the bone graft must not be bulky, compressible, or movable. These soft tissue difficulties usually are seen when soft tissue flaps are required to replace considerable intraoral soft tissues resected with the tumor. Secondary preprosthetic surgical procedures often are necessary to alter these soft tissues. The ideal situation would be debulking of the flap and placement of a split-thickness skin graft over the mandibular graft (Figure 23-17). Routine prosthodontic procedures with processed bases are used. As previously described, in the patient with a partial mandibulectomy, selecting the anterior tooth position and vertical dimension of occlusion so as not to hinder lip competence is important. The need for a palatal augmentation prosthesis also should be assessed.

MAXILLOFACIAL IMPLANT-SUPPORTED PROSTHESES FOR THE EDENTULOUS PATIENT

The edentulous patient with a maxillofacial prosthesis will arguably benefit from implants more than a patient with any other removable prosthesis. The loss of bilateral bony support in either arch, the lack of tongue mobility to stabilize mandibular dentures, movable soft tissue/bone attachments in the oral cavity, and need to use the prosthesis to support facial contours can lead to prosthetic compromise or failure, without the use of dental implants.

Despite these decided advantages, implants are not widely used in this patient population. Adjuvant radiotherapy often is required in the patient with head and neck cancer, which can hinder osseointegration of the implants. A few reports have been published of hyperbaric oxygen therapy administered to assist in osseointegration in the irradiated patient, but this method of treatment is expensive, time-consuming, and geographically unavailable to some patients. Many patients are unwilling to undergo the secondary surgical procedures needed to prosthetically prepare the oral cavity soft tissues and place the implants. Until it is quite certain that patients are disease free, physicians and dentists are unwilling to embark on these additional surgical procedures. The shortest elapsed time from cancer resection to insertion of the implant prosthesis in patients at my institution was 14 months. These individuals had the minimal number of secondary operations and no adjuvant therapy. In most individuals, the time frame was much longer.

The complications seen in patients with routine implants also are seen with this patient population. Because so few patients have been treated, experience is limited. Loss of implants or implants placed that cannot be used because of soft tissue complications or malposition appear to be more common in the patient with a maxillofacial prosthesis compared with the patient with a routine implant. Just as in the insertion of dentures in the patient with a maxillofacial prosthesis, insertion of an implant prosthesis will not ensure that a normal diet will be achieved or that any advancement in diet will occur. Lack of tongue control or a dysfunctional swallow reflex will not be changed with the delivery of an implant prosthesis. This method of retention may not be a panacea. The use of implants in the maxillofacial patient should be encouraged (Figures 23-18 through 23-22).

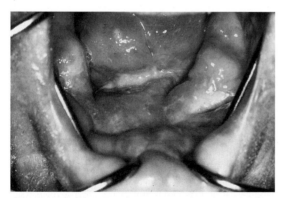

Figure 23-17   This patient has had an anterior free fibular bone graft. The intraoral soft tissue contours are bulky and freely mobile over the bone graft. No anterior vestibule exists. A debulking of the tissues, including epithelium and connective tissue down to the periosteum, and placement of a split-thickness skin graft will improve denture support.

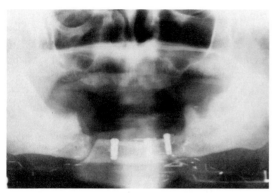

Figure 23-18   Radiograph of the fibular graft and three implants placed in the patient in Figure 23-17.

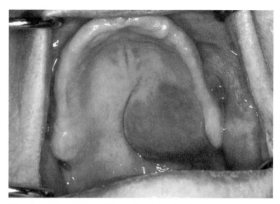

Figure 23-20   This patient had a large benign pleomorphic adenoma requiring total soft palate resection, left alveolar resection and total hard palate resection. The right anterior and right posterior alveolus remained.

LABORATORY PROCEDURES

Boxing and Pouring Impressions

Because of the unusual three-dimensional shapes of some of the maxillofacial prostheses and because impression wax is sometimes used, boxing the impression with a thick half plaster and half pumice mixture may be preferred to using a wax-beading technique. Excess water in the mix can be removed with paper towels and the plaster/pumice material positioned around the impression. The

pumice is then trimmed to create the appropriate land area, boxed with wax, coated with a separating medium, and poured.

Using Processed Bases: Adding Teeth, Adding Palatal Augmentations, or Relining Obturators

During flasking, the entire processed base should be covered with stone except where the addition of new acrylic resin or teeth is desired. This includes pouring stone into the intaglio surface of the prosthesis. Do not block out any undercuts with pumice or wax. This will make the deflasking procedure easier but will also leave some of the acrylic resin of the processed base unsupported. This unsupported area of the prosthesis may crack when packing the acrylic resin addition or distort when the additional acrylic resin is cured. The additional resin may be processed at a lower temperature from the original curing temperature of the base, or an autopolymerizing denture resin may be used. In the case of final processing of teeth onto a base, the maxillary and mandibular prostheses can be finished and placed on the remount casts that have been maintained on the articulator from the try-in appointment. The final occlusion may be refined and the prostheses inserted without another maxillomandibular relationship record.

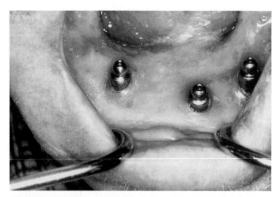

Figure 23-19   The debulking of soft tissues and skin graft were completed, as well as implant placement, in the patient in Figure 23-17. This patient functions very well with an implant-assisted mandibular denture; however, lack of normal tongue movement precludes a diet requiring heavy mastication.

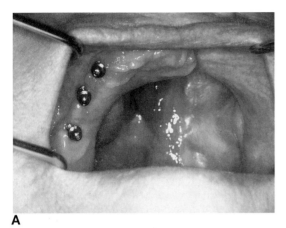

A

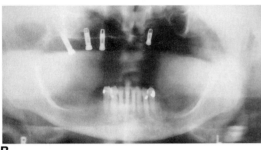

B

Figure 23-21 **A** and **B,** The patient had an iliac crest graft placed with a sinus lift, followed by skin graft vestibuloplasty and placement of four implants. The left anterior implant failed, but the three right posterior 18-mm implants have remained in function for 12 years.

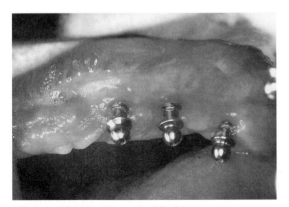

Figure 23-22 The patient had to wear a very unstable maxillary prostheses before uncovering the implants, and the pressure on the buccal bone caused stripping of the threads very early in the clinical course (reversed mirror image).

"Capping" Hollow Obturator Prostheses

Shortcuts in making the lids to cover the hollow obturator portion or shortcuts to sealing the lid and the prosthesis together can be taken, but the final result of shortcuts may be a prosthesis that leaks water around the lid/prosthesis interface. The prosthesis can be "capped" from the palatal side, but one must keep in mind that the lid contours must be in harmony with the remainder of the palate and the patient's tongue. Making a lid for the superior aspect of the prosthesis does not have these contour constraints.

The easiest researched method used at most institutions is the making of a light-cured resin lid (Triad Reline, Dentsply International, Inc., York, Pa.) bonded to the acrylic resin base with the same light-cured resin. After a 1-mm ledge around the internal periphery of the hollow obturator portion is created, the hollow obturator can be filled with a thick mix of plaster and pumice. The superior surface should be slightly convex to allow making a convex lid. The ledge should be exposed. Laboratory foil is adapted to the ledge and the dried plaster/pumice surface. A few drops of cyanoacrylate glue onto the plaster/pumice will secure the foil. The light-cured resin can be adapted over the foil and pressed into the ledge. The entire prosthesis and lid should be placed in the curing unit. After curing, the lid can be removed. The impression of the ledge should be visible in the undersurface of the lid. (Sharp detail is not necessary, but enough of the ledge impression should be present to delineate the borders of the lid.) The lid is then trimmed. The plaster/pumice is removed from the hollow prosthesis. Monomer is used to clean the lid and the prosthesis ledge, and the bonding agent is applied to the ledge and lid. An approximately 2-mm wide strip of light-cured resin is placed around the 1-mm ledge, and the lid is manipulated into position by hand. Excess material will flow at the peripheries of the lid. This can be adapted to the periphery of the lid/obturator portion with a cotton-tipped applicator and monomer. The prosthesis is cured, and the excess material at the margins of the lid is trimmed with laboratory burs. Before insertion of the prosthesis, the entire obturator prosthesis should be submerged in a pressure pot, held under water with a weight and 30 lb of pressure applied to the pot for approximately 1 minute. The

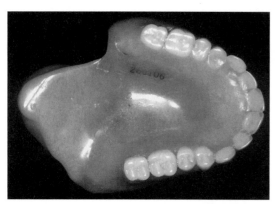

Figure 23-23 This very large hollow prosthesis was required to obturate the hard and soft palate, opposing a mandibular Kennedy Class I partial denture.

prosthesis should then be removed and shaken to check for water inside the sealed obturator. If water is present, continuing to shake the prosthesis or placing it under pressure again in a dry pressure-pot will force the water through the area of the lid that is leaking. Usually, the leak is in a very small area and limited to one or two places. The leaking areas can be opened with a no. 8 round bur, then water is blown out of the bulb (at least two holes are necessary to blow the water out of the hollow prosthesis) and the holes sealed with a small amount of light-cured resin. Again, the prosthesis should be checked for leaks before final delivery of the prosthesis to the patient (Figure 23-23).

Bibliography

Aramany MA, Downs JA, Beery QC: Prosthodontic rehabilitation for glossectomy patients, *J Prosthet Dent* 48:78-81, 1982.

Beumer J, Curtis D, Firtell D: Restoration of acquired hard palate defects. In *Maxillofacial rehabilitation: prosthodontic and surgical considerations*, St Louis, 1979, Mosby.

Brown KE: Complete denture treatment in patients with resected mandibles, *J Prosthet Dent* 21:443-447, 1969.

Cantor R, Curtis TA: Prosthetic management of edentulous mandibulectomy patients. Part II: Clinical procedures, *J Prosthet Dent* 25:546-555, 1971.

Christensen JM, Hutton JE, Hasegawa A et al: Evaluation of the effects of palatal augmentation on partial glossectomy speech, *J Prosthet Dent* 50:539-543, 1983.

Desjardins RP: Occlusal considerations for the partial mandibulectomy patient, *J Prosthet Dent* 41:308-315, 1979.

Franzen L, Rosenquist JB, Rosenquist KI et al: Oral implant rehabilitation of patients with oral malignancies treated with radiotherapy and surgery without hyperbaric oxygen therapy, *Int J Oral Maxillofac Implants* 10:183-187, 1995.

Jacob RF: Duplication of interim speech aid for definitive impression tray fabrication, *J Prosthet Dent* 68:561-562, 1992.

Jacob RF, Martin JW, King GE: Modification of surgical obturator to interim prosthesis, *J Prosthet Dent* 54:93, 1985.

Jacob RF, Reece GP, Taylor TD et al: Mandibular reconstruction for the cancer patient: microvascular surgery and implants, *Tex Dent J* 119:23-26, 1992.

Jacob RF, Yen TW: Processed record bases for the edentulous maxillofacial patient, *J Prosthet Dent* 65:680-685, 1991.

King GE, Jacob RF, Martin JW et al: Rehabilitation of the nasal and paranasal sinus area. In Thawley S, Panke W, Batasakis J, Lindberg R, editors: *Comprehensive management of head and neck tumors, vol 1,* Philadelphia, 1986, WB Saunders.

Logemann JA: Can data on normal swallowing improve treatment selection. In Myers EN, Barofsky I, Yates JW, editors: *Rehabilitation and treatment of head and neck cancer,* US Department of Health and Human Services, NIH Publications No. 86-2762, Washington, DC, 1986.

Logemann JA, Bytell DE: Swallowing disorders in three types of head and neck surgical patients, *Cancer* 44:1095-1105, 1979.

Martin JW, Jacob RF, King GE: Boxing the altered cast impression for the dentate obturator: plaster and pumice, *J Prosthet Dent* 59:382-384, 1988.

McKinstry RE, Aramany MA, Beery QC et al: Speech considerations in prosthodontic rehabilitation of the glossectomy patient, *J Prosthet Dent* 53:384-387, 1985.

Paprocki GJ, Jacob RF, Kramer DC: Seal integrity of hollow-bulb obturators, *Int J Prosthodont* 3:457-462, 1990.

Robbins KT, Bowman J, Jacob RF: Post-glossectomy deglutitory and articulatory rehabilitation with palatal augmentation prostheses, *Arch Otolaryngol Head Neck Surg* 113:1214-1218, 1987.

Taylor TD, LaVell WE: Dental management and rehabilitation. In Thawley S, Panje W, Batasakis J, Lindberg R, editors: *Comprehensive management of head and neck tumors, vol 1,* Philadelphia, 1986, WB Saunders.

Taylor TD, Worthington P: Osseointegrated implant rehabilitation of the previously irradiated mandible: results of a limited trial at 3-7 years, *J Prosthet Dent* 69:60-69, 1993.

CHAPTER 24

Prolonging the Useful Life of Complete Dentures: The Relining Procedure

George A. Zarb, Rhonda F. Jacob

Both biological supporting tissues and materials used in complete denture fabrication are vulnerable to time-dependent changes. The denture base material may discolor or deteriorate, whereas the artificial teeth can also discolor, fracture, or become abraded. These material changes be rectified; however, irreversible change in the tissues supporting the prostheses can only be partially compensated for. This point was emphasized in Part I as an unavoidable sequela of the edentulous state. Meticulous attention and care in the construction of complete dentures can minimize adverse changes in the supporting tissues and in associated facial structures as well, but it cannot preclude them. Thus the need for "servicing" complete dentures to keep pace with the changing surrounding and supporting tissues becomes mandatory. The clinical efforts that aim at prolonging the useful life of complete dentures involve a refitting of the impression surface of the denture, occlusal correction, and a minor spatial reorientation of the prosthesis. Two techniques are available: (1) reline, a procedure used to resurface the tissue side of a denture with new base material that provides accurate adaptation to the changed denture-foundation area, and (2) rebase, the laboratory process of replacing the entire denture base material in an existing prostheses. The alternative (at some point a necessary one) to this sort of "servicing" is the more expensive periodic remake of the complete dentures.

TREATMENT RATIONALE

The foundation that supports a denture changes adversely as a result of varying degrees and rates of residual ridge resorption (RRR). These changes may be insidious or rapid, but they are progressive and inevitable, and they usually are accompanied by one or more of the clinical changes listed in Figure 24-1. The variable reduction in vertical dimension of occlusion (VDO) and resultant spatial reorientation of the dentures also lead to esthetic changes in circumoral support and, consequently, in the patient's appearance. The changes in occlusal relationships can also induce more adverse stresses on the supporting tissues, which increases the risk of further ridge resorption.

One compelling conclusion that can be drawn from clinical experience and research involving denture-wearing patients is that dentures need regular attention for maintenance purposes. Such attention can be achieved only by patient education and a regular recall schedule. During the recall appointments the dentist reconciles a patient's reported denture experiences with information derived from clinical examination. The magnitude of the observed changes allows a decision to be made as to whether the prescribed servicing of the prosthesis will necessitate a laboratory reline, a rebase, or a remake.

The relining procedure is the most frequently prescribed intervention and involves adding a new layer of processed denture material to the denture base. This can be done without adversely affecting the occlusal relationships or the esthetic support of the lips and face. When minimal or moderate changes are evident, relining is the treatment of choice. A thin layer of impression material is added to compensate for resorptive changes that have occurred in the basal seat. Then, in the dental laboratory, the material is replaced by a new layer of acrylic resin that bonds to the original fitting

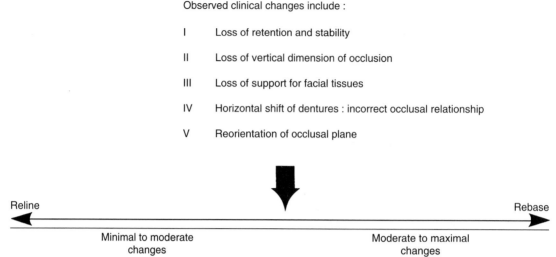

Observed clinical changes include :

I   Loss of retention and stability

II   Loss of vertical dimension of occlusion

III   Loss of support for facial tissues

IV   Horizontal shift of dentures : incorrect occlusal relationship

V   Reorientation of occlusal plane

Reline   Rebase

Minimal to moderate   Moderate to maximal
changes   changes

Figure 24-1 A number of changes can occur in the tissues that support complete dentures. They are more common under mandibular than under maxillary dentures, but they may be encountered under either, particularly when an upper denture is opposed by the natural dentition. The magnitude of the changes is what determines the nature of the resurfacing or refitting prescribed. If a new thin layer of resin is added to the denture base, the resurfacing is called a *reline*. If more material is added (as for a maxillary denture resting on severely resorbed residual ridges), extensive refitting and polymerized material is necessary, and this is called a *rebase*.

surface of the denture. The compensation for the resorbed tissues results in a slightly thicker acrylic resin denture base.

If extensive changes are encountered, the dentist must compensate not only for the reduced supporting tissue but also for the reorientation of the dentures, and this necessitates a simultaneous refitting of the impression surface of the denture with a reorienting of its vertical and horizontal position in the mouth. The resultant bulky denture base will likely require a thinner palatal section in the maxillary denture, that is, the dental laboratory description of a rebasing procedure. This reorientation of the dentures may require that the clinician use various materials and techniques to stabilize the denture in position before making the impression of the entire basal seat.

Relines can be done simply, accurately, and inexpensively. However, rebasing a complete denture involves all the problems of making new dentures, and the teeth cannot be moved around as easily as when a new denture is made. Consequently, a rebase prescription may be regarded as an inferior clinical

alternative to the more expensive and time-consuming decision to make new dentures. Therefore at times a clinician may choose to reline one prosthesis but choose to remake its counterpart rather than rebase it. Socioeconomic realities and common sense dictate that these techniques must be provided frequently, and clinical experience certainly justifies their use.

DIAGNOSIS

Patients who have worn dentures successfully for a long time often return for further service because of looseness, soreness, chewing inefficiency, or perceived esthetic changes. These difficulties may have been caused by (1) an incorrect or unbalanced occlusion that existed at the time the dentures were inserted or, more likely, (2) changes in the structures supporting the dentures that are now associated with a disharmonious occlusion. It is essential that the cause or causes of the reported difficulties be determined before any attempt is made to correct them. Therefore a diagnosis of the changes that have occurred must be made before any clinical procedures are started. It is necessary to determine the nature of the changes as well as their extent and location. The dentist must understand what changes are possible and what symptoms illustrate them.

Dentures with built-in errors in occlusion may not need relining. They may only need to have the occlusion corrected. Simple tests of individual denture bases may show that stability and retention have not been lost, even though the patient reports that the dentures are loose. The stability and retention of the bases are examined for each prosthesis independently. The prosthesis is lightly seated against the ridges and moved horizontally and laterally and also moved in an anterior and posterior direction. A well-adapted denture will unlikely move more than 1 to 2 mm, which is consistent with tissue displaceability. Seating the denture on each ridge independently may exhibit rocking. Pushing on the anterior maxillary dentition or pulling on the anterior dentition may cause the denture to unseat with minimal force. Generally, denture movement or rocking indicates the need for a reline procedure.

If this evaluation reveals a stable and retentive prosthesis, the occlusion may be the culprit. In this situation, the supporting tissues may show more irritation or inflammation on one side of the mouth than on the other. The apparent looseness results from uneven occlusal contact. Treatment involves keeping the dentures out of the mouth for 1 to 2 days and then reevaluating the denture with pressure indicator paste. After adjustments, the dentures should be remounted and occlusal adjustment performed. These procedures will eliminate the cause of the oral discomfort and make the dentures comfortable and serviceable without relining.

A change in the basal seats of the dentures usually is revealed by looseness and movement of the prosthesis on clinical examination, general soreness and inflammation, discernible loss of the occlusal vertical dimension and compromised esthetics, or disharmonious occlusal contacts. An examination of the oral mucosa that supports the dentures will disclose the state of its health. When this tissue is badly irritated, occlusal disharmony associated with loss of the vertical dimension should be suspected. Unsatisfactory changes in esthetics indicate a loss of the vertical dimension,

even though the teeth may seem to occlude properly. Overextension of denture flanges can be observed as ulcerations or hyperplastic tissue in the sulci. If the supporting tissue is traumatized, surgical correction to eliminate the hyperplasia may be necessary before relining impressions are made. When gross adjustments of the flanges are required plus addition of tissue conditioner reline, or the patient does not wear the dentures for 1 to 2 weeks, the result is often complete resolution of the soft tissue hypertrophy without surgery.

The amount of change in the occlusal vertical dimension that has resulted from the loss of supporting structure must be carefully noted. The problem is not simply a change in the occlusal vertical dimension; it also can be a change in the horizontal relations of the dentures to each other and to their basal seats. A loss of vertical dimension will automatically cause the mandible to have a more forward position in relation to the maxillae than it would at the original occlusal vertical dimension. This situation can exist even though the jaws are maintained in centric relation (CR) position. What must not be overlooked is the unpredictability of bone morphological changes. This outcome will in turn influence the dentures' positions (Figure 24-2).

Resorption of the bone of the maxillae usually permits the upper denture to move up and back in relation to its original position. Patients may complain of pain in the anterior vestibule below the nose. However, the occlusion also may force the maxillary denture forward. The lower denture usually moves down and forward, but it may move down and back relative to the mandible as resorption occurs. Concurrently, the mandible closes, and the patient's vertical dimension is less when the teeth are in occlusion than the vertical dimension occupied with the teeth in occlusion before the resorption occurred. This movement is rotary around a line approximately through the condyles. Because the occlusal plane and the body of the mandible are located below the level of this axis of rotation, the mandible moves forward as the space between the maxillae and mandible is reduced from that existing when the dentures were constructed originally. Such rotational forward movement of the body of the mandible is not necessarily an eccentric

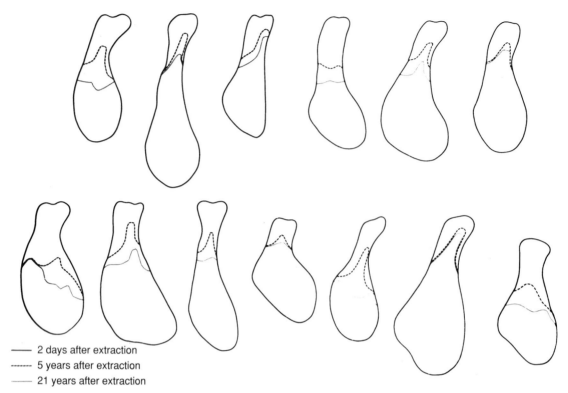

—— 2 days after extraction

------ 5 years after extraction

········ 21 years after extraction

Figure 24-2 Bergman's and Carlsson's research comprised cephalometric tracings from the mandibular symphysis region. They studied 13 patients who had been treated with immediate complete dentures and observed the patients for 21 years after their extractions. All 13 composite tracings underscore the range and unpredictability of the morphological outcome. All patients wore opposing complete maxillary dentures. Clinical judgment regarding the mandibular denture's repositioning for relining purposes requires an understanding of resultant bone resorption outcomes. Comparable information of similar changes in edentulous maxillae is not as compelling.

forward movement of the mandible; rather the CR position of the condyles may be retained despite the apparent forward movement of the mandible when observed in relation to the maxilla.

The effects of this rotary movement vary from patient to patient and appear to result from a complex interaction of several features, particularly the duration and magnitude of bone resorption and the mandibular postural habit. The mandible's rotation may be associated with a number of consequences that frequently occur simultaneously: (1) losing centric relation occlusion (CRO) in the dentures; (2) changing the structures that support the upper denture; (3) forcing the lower denture backward so it impinges on the lower ridge or forcing the lower

denture anteriorly, with an ensuing prognathic appearance (Figure 24-3).

It appears then that mandibular rotation can elicit severe damage in the denture-supporting tissues over a long period of unsupervised denture wear. The stresses are probably augmented by the use of cusped posterior teeth and by the resultant incisal guidance, which now locks the mandibular denture into the maxillary denture. Although proponents of the "noncusp" school of thought frequently indict the other school's choise of "cusped" teeth as accelerating tissue damage in such situations, no research evidence is available to support either school's claim that its tooth choice minimizes changes in the denture-supporting tissues.

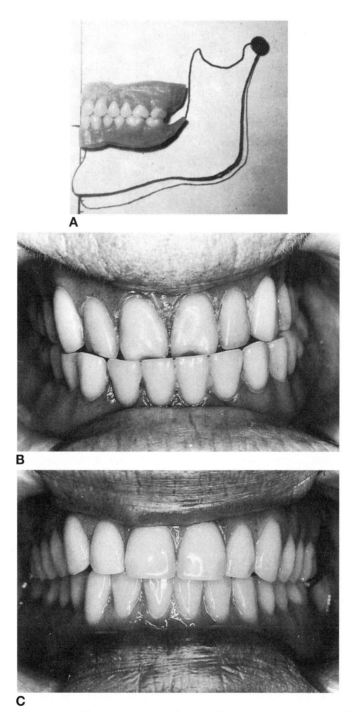

Figure 24-3 **A,** Loss of bone structure under both dentures permits the mandible to move upward a corresponding amount. As the mandible rotates to a closed position without translation of the condyles, it frequently moves forward. The problem is to determine the amount of change that has occurred in both basal seats. The occlusion may not appear to be correct when observed in the mouth of patient **B,** or it may appear deceptively adequate and in patient **C.** The extraoral close-mouthed appearance can be almost identical in both cases.

The horizontal position of each denture in relation to its own supporting ridge must be considered, so a determination can be made as to whether the denture has moved forward or backward because of occlusal forces applied to it. Furthermore, one or both dentures may have rotated in relation to the supporting structures. The occlusion in the mouth cannot therefore be used as a guide to the horizontal repositioning of either denture. A new determination of the vertical dimension of the face must be made by reestablishing a normal interocclusal distance. Again, the principles used in the construction of complete dentures are called on. Examination of the esthetics in profile, as far as the support of the lips in an anteroposterior direction is concerned, will serve to guide the orientation of the dentures in relation to their respective foundations. The relation of the teeth to the ridges must be observed for accuracy. If resorption has been only in the vertical direction (allowing the jaws to approach each other more closely than they should when occlusal contacts are made), the occlusion cannot be correct, even though there has been no anterior or posterior movement of the dentures.

It also must be determined whether remodeling of the jaws has been uniform under both dentures or whether one ridge has been destroyed more than the other. Greater shrinkage in one arch will change the orientation of the occlusal plane. This will cause occlusal disharmony in eccentric occlusions, even though the occlusal vertical dimension has been reestablished by relining. A visual comparison of the size of the ridge with the size of the alveolar groove in the denture will serve as a guide.

PRELIMINARY TREATMENT

It is probable that if the dentures were made by the clinician within the last few years so that resorption may not have been too dramatic, the esthetics of facial profile are only compromised by a few millimeters, and the teeth are still in place over the mandibular ridge, then a reline procedure of both dentures should be successfully accomplished. However, if greater errors in fit, occlusion, occlusal plane, esthetics, and overextension of teeth beyond the ridge are evident, the clinician may be wise to tell the patient that new dentures are necessary or that any changes in the existing dentures will be performed for diagnostic purposes and for the patient's comfort. "Juggling" so many variables in denture rebasing, without having control of the dentition, may end up with a revised denture that requires major modification of the teeth to achieve occlusal harmony. Severe revisions of the dentition often produce poor esthetic results that the patient will not accept.

If the clinician chooses to go forward with existing denture modifications of basal seat and possibly occlusion, some preliminary steps are undertaken before the actual reline procedure. These steps aim at the following objectives: (1) reestablishing the height, orientation, and esthetics of the occlusal plane by manipulation of the mandibular denture (usually, though not necessarily, done first) and (2) relating the maxillary to the mandibular denture while the correct occlusal and esthetic position of the maxillary denture is being established. Both objectives are achieved more or less automatically with a tissue conditioner as a provisional reline material, particularly if the adverse changes to be corrected are mild to moderate. On the other hand, severe changes may necessitate using combinations of compound stops, tissue conditioners, occlusal adjustment, and tooth-colored autopolymerizing augmentation of the denture's occlusal surfaces. This is routinely done to compensate for extensive vertical occlusal changes.

The obvious advantages of using tissue conditioners include simultaneous restoration of a healthy basal seat and the ease with which the liners can be modified for maximal function and cosmetic results.

After making certain that the tissues are healthy, the dentist looks for errors in the occlusion and occlusal vertical dimension that should be corrected, as well as other changes that might be made before the final procedure is undertaken. The implication is that these procedures may take several patient visits over several weeks to obtain healthy tissues and establishment of appropriate occlusion. If the magnitude of the adjustments requires more than minor occlusal adjustments, the clinician may choose to maintain the patient in these "temporary" dentures while new prostheses are fabricated, according to the diagnostic findings determined by working with the patient over the past several weeks.

CLINICAL IMPRESSION PROCEDURES

The clinical relining or rebasing can be achieved by (1) the static impression technique, (2) the functional impression technique, or (3) the so-called chairside technique.

Impression Technique

The static impression technique involves the use of either the closed- or open-mouth relines/rebases variation. In the closed mouth variation, the dentures are used as impression trays and either the existing CRO is used to seat the dentures with lining impression material or else the CR is recorded (in the registration medium of choice) before the impressions are made. Often only the mandibular denture requires reline, and it can be relined against the maxillary denture. It is suggested that the maxillary denture be additionally secured with denture adhesive powder. The mandibular denture is seated as close as the clinician thinks its appropriate position is, and then the patient closes into the selected occlusal position. If the maxillary denture needs relining, it can then be relined against the mandibular denture. Care should always be taken that the posterior borders of the dentures do not make contact during the impression procedures. This can often go unobserved and cause severe occlusal discrepancies at delivery.

In the so-called open-mouth technique, the dentures are used essentially as trays for making the new impressions. Relining/rebasing of both maxillary and mandibular dentures can be done at the same appointment. The existing CO is not used, and a new CRO record is obtained after the impressions are made. This is a demanding and laborious technique. Again, it is assumed that before placing the impression material in the denture, the clinician would have made some type of tissue stops in the dentures with low-fusing compound while placing both dentures in the mouth and maintaining the appropriate occlusal contact, occlusal plane, and esthetic position of the anterior teeth. Establishing these stops, to direct the clinician to the correct placement of each denture against the basal tissues

during the impression procedure, will ensure that the occlusal relationship will be maintained within a reasonable proximity that can be corrected with a remount procedure.

The closed-mouth reline/rebase technique is preferred when the static impression method is used. Several variations have been suggested, all based on the same theme: using the denture as an impression tray with the denture occlusion (corrected in preliminary treatment or stabilized intraorally by wax or compound) and holding the tray steady while the impression material sets. Box 24-1 presents three primary areas that must be addressed and meticulously followed when making a denture

---

Box 24-1

Integral Steps for a Closed-Mouth Reline Technique

Centric Relation

Existing correct intercuspation (CRO) used to stabilize dentures

Wax interocclusal record made at CR

Corrected during reestablishment of a new vertical dimension of occlusion by occlusal adjustment or use of autopolymerizing on the occlusal surfaces of posterior teeth

Denture Preparations

Large undercuts relieved

Hard resin surfaces relieved 1.5 to 2 mm

Tissue conditioner removed or relieved"

Escape" holes drilled, particularly in maxillary base; this will also assist easy removal of palatal portion during laboratory rebase

Denture periphery shortened to create flat border

Impression Procedure

Border molding achieved with preferred material (i.e., low-fusing compound)

Border molding retained from polymerized tissue-conditioning material

Posterior palatal seal achieved with low-fusing compound

Border molding achieved by choosing impression material that is soft and yet viscous enough to support and register peripheral detail (one of the polyether impression materials)

reline impression. Doing so will produce repeatedly good results. Finally, the dentures are sent to the laboratory with an accompanying work authorization form that contains specific directions to the laboratory technician and other information, such as the specifications for alterations, materials, finish, remount casts, and remounting of the upper denture.

For many years, it was thought that the strains inherent in the processed denture base would be released by subsequent processing and cause some degree of warpage. The change in the resin has been reported at 1.5% to 3% by many authors. Certainly the laboratory technicians should attempt to use a low temperature in the heat processing, as opposed to using a boiling technique. However, dentures can be adequately relined with one of the autopolymerizing resins, allowing trial packing to control vertical dimension and thickness of material, without concern for temperature changes and warpage.

When autopolymerizing resin is used, the processed dentures can be ready for insertion on the same day the impressions are made. The protocol described in Part 3 is followed, and occlusal refinement is done intraorally or on the articulator. Follow-up instructions are similar to those provided at the time the new dentures are inserted.

Functional Impression Technique

The functional impression technique is both simple and practical and has gained considerable clinical support. It is technique we routinely use. It depends on a thorough understanding of the versatile properties of tissue conditioners as functional impression materials. The relative ease with which these temporary soft liners can be used as functional impression materials has regrettably led to their abuse and to criticism by many dentists. However, they are excellent for refitting complete dentures when used carefully and meticulously. Improvements in these materials include their retaining compliance for many weeks, their good dimensional stability, and their excellent bonding to the resin denture base.

When a denture needs to be refitted, the patient's complaint or the dentist's oral prosthetic evaluation usually indicates undermined retention, sore spots, and variable denture-bearing tissue hyperemia. The denture is observed intraorally to assess the need for peripheral reduction or extension, and a posterior palatal seal extension is developed with an autopolymerizing resin on modeling compound on maxillary dentures. (Infrequently, if extensive ridge resorption and overt loss of VDO have occurred, three compound stops may be required on the impression surface of the denture to reestablish a proper occlusal relationship or to improve the occlusal plane orientation.) A treatment liner is next placed inside the denture. The lining material should flow evenly to cover the whole impression surface and the borders of the denture with a thin layer. If voids are evident, they should be filled with a fresh mix of liner material. Unsupported parts of the liner may occur on the borders of the denture, and this indicates that localized border molding with stick modeling compound may be needed before the placement of a fresh mix of liner. Occasionally borders are formed that are thin and very flexible, and this too is indicative of inadequate peripheral extension of the denture. Again, the borders must be corrected by border molding with one of the autopolymerizing resins before they are covered with the lining material. Remember: these materials have a tendency to slump during setting unless they are adequately supported. The patient's mandible is guided into a retruded position, which is one of maximum intercuspation, to help stabilize the denture while the lining material is setting. Excess material is trimmed away with a hot scalpel. Most of the materials used for this purpose progress through plastic and then elastic stages before hardening, which can take several days (Figure 24-4). The plastic stage permits movement of the denture base or bases so they are more compatible with the existing occlusion. This also allows the displaced tissues to recover and assume their original position. The patient is instructed regarding care of the prosthesis and its lining material. It should be noted that the actual strength of the processed resin may be weakened by the addition of a tissue conditioner. The processed resin may have to be "reinforced" on the polished denture surface, and the patient should be warned about risk of denture fracture.

Research has shown that a number of denture cleansers and other preparations that may be helpful in the control of plaque on dentures can cause significant deterioration of tissue conditioners in a

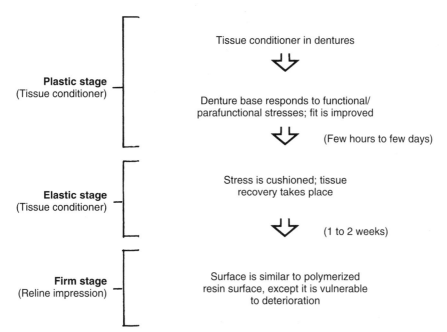

Plastic stage
(Tissue conditioner)

Tissue conditioner in dentures

Denture base responds to functional/
parafunctional stresses; fit is improved

(Few hours to few days)

Elastic stage
(Tissue conditioner)

Stress is cushioned; tissue
recovery takes place

(1 to 2 weeks)

Firm stage
(Reline impression)

Surface is similar to polymerized
resin surface, except it is vulnerable
to deterioration

Figure 24-4   The physical stages of tissue conditioners/treatment liners allow the dentist to use them for different objectives.

short time. Apparently, simple rinsing of the temporarily lined denture and gentle brushing with a soft toothbrush are good interim measures to minimize damage to the lining. Clinical experience indicates that 10 to 14 days should elapse before the material is firm enough to proceed with the clinical reline sequence.

At the next appointment, the temporarily relined denture will usually be well retained, with well-rounded peripheral borders and a healthy-appearing mucosa. It has been observed that the tissue-conditioning materials can create problems when used for impressions. The gradually increasing elasticity of the material in the mouth can lead to a recovery of the compressed material when the load is removed, that is, when the impression is removed from the mouth; thus is the importance of not pouring the cast before the material has reached the firm stage (see Figure 24-4).

Furthermore, these materials tend to deteriorate in some mouths, which precludes their use in this manner. If the dentist has any doubt about the quality of the surface appearance of the hardened liner,

the reline procedure can be carried out as described earlier in the chapter, after the interim treatment liner has been removed or relieved. If the surface or peripheral deterioration is slight, these areas can be trimmed with a carbide bur and the denture or dentures prepared for a secondary, or wash, impression with a light-bodied material.

The stone cast must be poured immediately after removal of the relined denture base from the mouth. The material should not be plastic, or in the "self-flow" stage, because the material's own weight may deform the impression; therefore the use of a new mix of tissue conditioner material as the final impression material is not recommended. It also is possible that the weight of the stone poured into the impression surface will cause distortion of the impression. Maxillary working casts may have to be scored in the selected posterior palatal seal area because the long period of plasticity of the material may not create sufficient displacement action in this area. Alternatively, a thin bead of compound material may be used to augment the posterior palatal seal before making the impression.

The making of a new CRO record and the remount procedure are recommended to ensure an optimal prosthodontic occlusion. Researchers have demonstrated that the functional status of dentures relined with treatment liners used as impression materials is as good as the status of dentures relined by border molding and then refined with a light-bodied impression material.

The recent introduction of visible light–cured (VLC) resin systems has produced promising results when used in a wide range of prosthodontic activities. Biological testing indicates that they are nontoxic and biocompatible. Ongoing research also appears to have improved their properties (such as fit, strength, ability to polymerize without residual components, ease of fabrication and manipulation, patient acceptance, ability to bond with other denture base resins, and low bacterial adherence).

One promising application of VLC resin material is its use for chairside relining. It is used in a similar manner as a tissue conditioner, with all the possibilities of instant modifications because the flow of the material can be regulated by selection of appropriate viscosity, warming and cooling measures in water baths, and partial intraoral polymerization with a handheld curing light. The relined denture is then taken to the laboratory for immediate light-curing of the new layer of material. These materials have been known to be quite brittle, but when supported by the original processed denture base, the VLC material within the denture and at the denture peripheral role has appropriate clinical strength for denture longevity based on the authors' clinical experience. Although long-term clinical results on treatment effectiveness and material integrity maintenance are unavailable, the VLC materials seem to hold considerable promise.

Both the static technique (or versions of it) and the functional impression technique are well accepted and experience-proved procedures. They can be used for simple situations (denture settling is minimal) and complicated situations (excessive tissue changes have taken place). It appears that the choice between the two methods is based on the dentist's skill in manipulating the materials and the patient's convenience.

Chairside Technique

Several attempts have been made to produce an acrylic or other plastic material that could be added to the denture and allowed to set in the mouth to produce an instant chairside reline/rebase. These have met with failure for several reasons: (1) the materials often have produced a chemical burn on the mucosa; (2) the result often was porous and subsequently developed a bad odor; (3) color stability was poor; and (4) if the denture was not positioned correctly, the material could not be removed easily to start again. At this stage of its development, the chairside technique has been of very limited use in clinical practice because of these attendant difficulties, and it is not recommended.

Bibliography

Bergman B, Carlsson GE: Clinical long-term study of complete denture wearers, *J Prosthet Dent* 53:56-61, 1985.

Boucher CO: The relining of complete dentures, *J Prosthet Dent* 30:521-526, 1973.

Braden M: Tissue conditioners. I. Composition and structure, *J Dent Res* 49:145-148, 1970.

Javid NS, Michael CG, Mohammed HA et al: Three dimensional analysis of maxillary denture displacement during reline impression procedure, *J Prosthet Dent* 54:232-237, 1985.

Kazanji MNM, Watkinson AC: Influence of thickness, boxing, and storage on the softness of resilient denture lining materials, *J Prosthet Dent* 59:677-680, 1988.

Klinger SM, Lord JL: Effect of common agents on intermediary temporary soft reline materials, *J Prosthet Dent* 30:749-755, 1973.

Nassif J, Jumbelic R: Current concepts for relining complete dentures: a survey, *J Prosthet Dent* 51:11-15, 1984.

Newsome PRH, Basker RM, Bergman B et al: The softness and initial flow of temporary soft lining materials, *Acta Odontol Scand* 46:9-17, 1988.

Osle RE, Sorensen SE, Lewis EA: A new visible light–cured resin system applied to removable prosthodontics, *J Prosthet Dent* 56:497-506, 1986.

Rantanen T, Sirilä HS: Fast and slow setting functional impression materials used in connection with complete denture relinings, *Suom Hammaslaak Toim* 68:175-180, 1972.

Smith DE, Lord JL, Bolender CL: Complete denture relines with autopolymerizing resin processed in water under air pressure, *J Prosthet Dent* 18:103-115, 1967.

Starcke EN, Marcroft KR, Fischer TE et al: Physical properties of tissue-conditioning materials as used in functional impressions, *J Prosthet Dent* 27:111-119, 1972.

Wilson HJ, Tomlin HR, Osborne J: Tissue conditioners and functional impression materials, *Br Dent J* 121:9-16, 1966.

IMPLANT PROSTHODONTICS

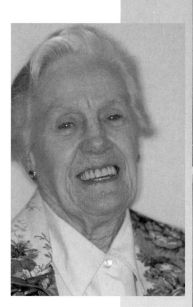

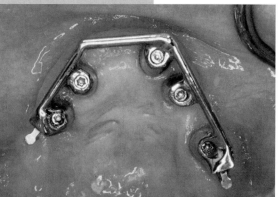

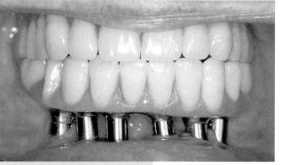

CHAPTER 25

Implant-Supported Prostheses for Edentulous Patients

George A. Zarb, Steven E. Eckert, Regina Mericske-Stern

The applied content of the preceding chapters in Part 3 ensures a satisfactory complete denture experience for most edentulous patients. However, clinical experience confirms the fact that many edentulous patients do not tolerate complete dentures. This is neither an indictment of professional skills nor a condemnation of the patient's response to the dentist's efforts. It must simply be accepted that many patients who wear complete dentures either do not like the experience or encounter difficulty adapting to their prostheses. Other patients may have adapted to dentures for several years but may become maladaptive as a result of regressive tissue changes or systemic health-related considerations. Still others' dentures may be perfectly adaptive, but these patients regret or resent the fact that wearing dentures is their only treatment option, and some patients simply cannot wear dentures at all. The quality of life of all such individuals is profoundly affected by their predicament. Treatment for these patients usually entails considerable efforts of both the clinical-technical and the emotional-supportive variety, albeit with unpredictable results. The dentist may even be tempted to dismiss such patients as having difficult or "impossible" mouths or, worse, as lacking motivation or learning skills. These situations are very frustrating for both parties, especially when it becomes clear that conventional complete denture therapy is not the solution for the patient's edentulism.

MALADAPTIVE DENTURE BEHAVIOR

Diverse reasons are presented in the dental literature to explain the etiology and frequency of chronic inability to wear dentures. In the past it was tempting for clinicians to regard the maladaptive problem as resulting mainly from adverse anatomical changes in the denture-bearing surface. However, clinical experience and some research have also identified physiological and psychological contributions to such a response. Apart from the extensive anecdotal evidence favoring optimized denture construction techniques, the major adjunctive treatment proposed for such patients has been preprosthetic surgery. The goal of this approach is to enlarge the denture-bearing area by deepening the buccal or labial vestibules or augmenting the residual ridge area (see Chapter 8). Implicit in this prescription is the conviction that an enlarged denture-bearing surface will significantly increase the chances of denture stability and therefore patient adaptation. Apart from the inherent morbidity risks associated with such procedures, however, longitudinal assessment of this approach has failed to produce a predictable therapeutic outcome.

Some dentists have understandably pioneered other methods, such as endosseous dental implants, in an effort to treat or preclude maladaptive denture behavior. Implants can serve as substitutes for tooth roots and help provide support and retention for overlying prostheses. They are made out of a variety of biocompatible alloplastic materials and consist of diverse designs, from so-called blades to cylindrically shaped tooth root analogues. They are surgically placed in selected edentulous host bone sites with a prosthetic superstructure subsequently fitted onto transepithelial posts or abutments joined to the buried implants.

The scientific premise in prescribing dental implants is the predictable and safe provision of

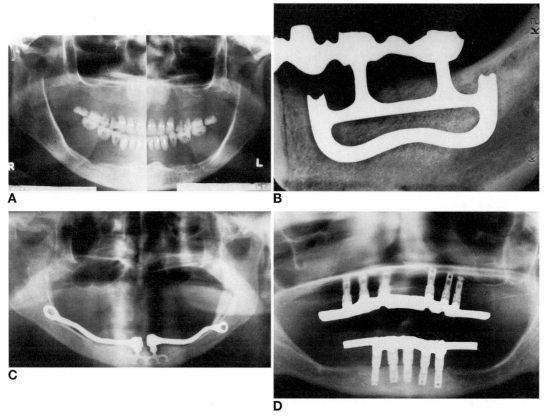

Figure 25-1 Treating the edentulous state with complete dentures presumes that acrylic resin is a reasonable substitute for the absent periodontal ligament and its participation in the maintenance of its surrounding alveolar bone. The shadow between the prosthetic teeth and the underlying bony support in **A** reflects the reduced and profoundly changed support for an occlusion. Attempts to compensate for this inherently compromised support mechanism have included a diversity of implant designs, such as **B** and **C.** Regrettably, this sort of endosseous anchorage yielded unpredictable results because of the high risk of the bone interface changing to a poorly differentiated connective tissue one. The introduction of the osseointegration technique led to a predictable and long-lasting interfacial osteogenesis that ensures predictably favorable and prolonged functional outcomes as in **D.**

alloplastic tooth root substitutes to stabilize and retain a prosthesis (Figure 25-1).

THE SCIENTIFIC ERA IN IMPLANT PROSTHODONTICS

The required evidence-based clinical application of dental implants was ushered in by the osseointegration research work of Per Ingvar Brånemark and his colleagues during the late 1970s and was first presented to the scientific dental community at the 1982 Toronto Conference. Several clinical researchers embarked on clinical trials that involved variations on a theme of inserting machine-turned and machine-threaded cylindrical titanium implants into mandibular and maxillary edentulous sites and using these to support a variety of prostheses designs. Their trials were first conducted in Sweden and subsequently in various teaching centers around the world. The original commercially pure (cp) titanium implants were inserted with a meticulous technique that aimed at creating a direct contact between the implant material and living bone.

Several authors had already hypothesized the induced interfacial osteogenesis (or osseointegration). The belief was that certain implant materials could possess a dynamic surface chemistry that induces histological changes at the implant interface with the host bone site. However, it was Brånemark who first produced laboratory and clinical results that demonstrated the close spatial relationship between titanium and living bone, an interface investigated with radiographs and histomorphometry. The described "osseointegration" suggests a highly differentiated interfacial bone response to the careful placement of cp titanium tooth root analogues. Moreover, this response appears to become organized according to functional demands. Brånemark's clinical technique has now been replicated in several teaching centers in well-designed longitudinal trials and marks a very important advance in this field of implant prosthodontics. Currently, many commercial and some scientific initiatives have also yielded diverse implant designs and materials that have expanded the scope of the technique.

Regrettably, a sort of knee-jerk response to implant replacement of most types of teeth has now emerged. This is alarming for the following important reasons:

1. There is a serious risk of ignoring the merits (functional, esthetic, and financial) of traditional treatment modalities in the management of extensive partial edentulism. Often an exclusive surgically driven treatment plan is proposed; however, efficacy and effectiveness outcomes demand prosthodontically directed treatment rather than an exclusive surgical preoccupation with an implant survival strategy. This reflects a subtle yet profound shift in the required emphasis on what best addresses patient-mediated concerns.
2. The commercial explosion in implant system production has already led to a regression in the scientific rigor required to select scientifically acceptable clinical protocols. Few controlled clinical studies are available

to compare results of different implant designs, materials, or surfaces (Eckert, Parein, Myshin et al., 1997). In fact, too many reports claiming improved outcomes are often based on short-term studies that are wishfully assumed to equate with long-term clinical success. Although historical controls are thought to be useful, study designs are so different that the utility of such controls is limited. The risk of this state of a quasi-scientific anarchy is a return to an anecdotally driven era in implant prosthodontics—thus our preference for prescribing implant systems that reflect scrupulous multicenter and long-term endorsement. Our preferred choices remain the Nobel Biocare and ITI systems. Both are made from cp titanium with different macroscopic and microscopic surface features. Both systems may be used as one- or two-stage surgical procedures. The implants can be either immediately attached to a healing abutment or are else buried submucosally until the time-dependent osseointegration is achieved. The latter will then permit a secondary surgical exposure for prosthetic abutment attachment and subsequent screw-retained or cemented prosthesis loading. Current preliminary yet limited research even suggests the feasibility of immediately loading implants in specific locations, most particularly the anterior edentulous mandible.

PATIENT CONSIDERATIONS

The psychological reactions to various forms of bodily organ loss have been investigated in patients who have undergone procedures such as hysterectomies and mastectomies. However, remarkably little interest has been shown in the psychological reaction to tooth loss. This apparent lack of interest is probably attributable to the prevalence of edentulism and the impressive success enjoyed by the dental profession in treating the condition. Furthermore, edentulism will neither result in death nor likely elicit profound sympathy in a society preoccupied with youthful appearances. The sense of shame and inferiority that many edentulous patients feel is rendered even more poignant by the inability of some of them to tolerate a denture at all.

Patients who cannot wear dentures or who wear them with varying degrees of difficulty usually have one or more of the features listed in Box 25-1. Such patients are candidates for an implant prosthodontic prescription. Also, even the most successful denture wearer frequently regrets his or her dependence on a removable prosthesis and the attendant sequelae associated with its long-term wear. These patients could also be added to the list of treatment candidates because compelling longitudinal research confirms the safety and predictability of implant procedures. It is expected that this advance could very well lead to therapeutic strategies in prosthodontics that considerably reduce the conventional role of removable prostheses.

The objective in prescribing implants is to provide the patient with an analogous attachment mechanism for the lost periodontal ligament (PL) without the latter's vulnerable qualities. The resulting availability of dentist-placed abutment(s) can then be used to support diverse prosthetic superstructure designs. This is achieved through the following:

Box 25-1

Patients' Signs and Symptoms That Frequently Preclude an Adaptive Complete Denture Experience

1. Severe morphological compromise of the denture-supporting areas that significantly undermines denture retention
2. Poor oral muscular coordination
3. Low tolerance of the mucosal tissues
4. Parafunctional habits leading to recurrent soreness and instability of the prosthesis
5. Unrealistic functional prosthodontic expectations
6. Active or hyperactive gag reflex elicited by a removable prosthesis
7. Psychological inability to wear a denture, even if adequate denture retention or stability is present

---

1. *Selection of patients whose systemic health does not preclude a minor oral surgical procedure.* Furthermore, the quality and quantity of the selected edentulous host bone sites must be surgically assessed by a careful and comprehensive radiographic evaluation.
2. *Meticulous surgical protocol.* The predictability of a favorable healing response as manifested by subsequent interfacial tissue differentiation must not be compromised. Surgical judgment and skills have been shown to be successful outcome determinants.
3. *Use of a biocompatible alloplastic material, preferably cp titanium, because it has been shown to yield the best long-term results reported to date.* However, titanium alloys and different surface treatments appear to offer equally good prognosis, at least in the short term.
4. *Implant design that ensures immediate stability and excellent stress distribution.* The screw's cylindrical design appears to be the optimal one; however, preliminary evidence indicates that implants with alternative macroscopic and microscopic design features may be equally good.
5. *Unloaded healing of the implant, although some preliminary evidence supports site-specific immediate loading.*
6. *Ensuring optimal occlusal stress control view; a passive fit of the prosthetic superstructure and correct occlusal relationships.*

The last item in the list is a standard objective in traditional prosthodontics, but the absence of resilient PL support in implant prosthodontics indicates a need for technical accuracy that may very well exceed what is required when using tooth abutments to support cast fixed prostheses.

It should be recalled that the PL's qualitative and quantitative determinants are arguably the gold standard for a dentist-induced attachment mechanism. It is now obvious that the osseointegrated interface is a worthy functional substitute for the PL, even if the area of interfacial attachment is significantly less. On the other hand, a fascinating difference lies in their behavioral nature, given the origins of either interface. The PL is the result of a developmental phenomenon, whereas osseointegration is the result of a carefully planned and, to a larger extent, controlled, healing response. This profound difference accounts for the different pathogenesis of attachment mechanism failure—periodontal disease or loss of osseointegration. Because an induced "ankylotic-like" response is unlikely to be vulnerable to periodontal pathogens, we strongly suspect that implants fail only when the induced healing response is an imperfect one. This is reflected in the fact that most implant failures occur during the prescribed healing interval. Other failures may occur a few months after healing is presumed to be complete or else after a variable period of traumatic occlusal loading when the imperfectly healed interface is overloaded. Infection then becomes the secondary super-imposed insult to the failed or failing interface. This chain of events has regrettably been misunderstood by many dentists who often bring a *PL mind-set* to the fascinating debate on the infrequently encountered postloading or late osseointegration failure.

TREATMENT OUTCOME CONSIDERATIONS

The most important reason for establishing criteria of success in any treatment method is to safeguard the oral health of the public. Each patient who receives implant prosthodontic treatment has the right to know the potential benefits and risks as well as an accurate prognosis of the method. These criteria protect the patient, whose informed consent before undertaking implant therapy should include an awareness of the highest standard of service currently available.

A clinical working definition for osseointegration is "the time-dependent healing process whereby clinically asymptomatic rigid fixation of alloplastic materials is achieved and maintained in bone during functional and parafunctional loading." The definition implies a short list of determinants—asymptomatic, immobile, and time-dependent functions—that underscore treatment outcome criteria reflecting the method's efficacy and effectiveness.

Box 25-2

Determinants of Treatment Outcome in Implant Prosthodontics

The Following Considerations for Successful Outcomes with Implant-Supported Prostheses were Proposed:

1. Implant therapy is prescribed to resolve prosthodontic problems and permits diverse prosthodontic treatments, which in turn may have an impact on the economics of the service. Such prostheses should meet the clinically evolved standards of function, comfort and esthetics. They should also allow for routine maintenance and should permit planned or unplanned revisions of the existing design. Criteria of treatment outcome success for implant-supported prostheses should be assessed in the context of time-dependent considerations for any required retreatment.
2. Criteria for implant success apply to individual endosseous implants and include the following:
   a. At the time of testing, the implants have been under functional loading.
   b. All implants under investigation must be accounted for.

c. Because a gold standard for mobility assessment is currently unavailable, the method used must be specifically described in operative terms.
d. Radiographs to measure bone loss should be standard periapical films with specified reference points and angulations.

The Success Criteria Comprise the Following Determinants:

1. The resultant implant support does not preclude the placement of a planned functional and esthetic prosthesis that is satisfactory to both patient and dentist.
2. There is no pain, discomfort, altered sensation, or infection attributable to the implants.
3. Individual unattached implants are immobile when tested clinically.
4. The mean vertical bone loss is less than 0.2 millimeters annually after the first year of function.

These criteria are still regarded as less than perfect in clinical research circles because they are partially based on fallible resolution levels (e.g., office radiographic imaging) and they do not lend themselves to a range of so-called success norms that are quantifiable. On the contrary, they support a dichotomous, all-or-none diagnosis (e.g., mobile or immobile implant, absent or present interfacial radiolucency, painful or painless). The criteria, however, reflect the outcome of numerous international, scrupulously monitored scientific investigations and have proven to be useful and reliable in the formulation of a yardstick to measure clinical success. Box 25-2 sums up the recommendations of a Consensus Conference on Treatment Outcome Critieria held at the University of Toronto in 1998. We acknowledge their merits and endorse the scope of the proposed and described clinical yardstick package.

Bibliography

Berg E: Acceptance of full dentures, *Int Dent J* 43:299-306, 1993.

Blomberg S: Psychological response. In Brånemark PI, Zarb GA, Albrektsson T, editors: *Tissue-integrated prostheses,* Chicago, Tokyo, 1985, Quintessence Publishing Co.

Brånemark PI, Zarb GA, Albrektsson T: Tissue-integrated prostheses. In *Osseointegration in clinical dentistry,* Chicago, 1985, Quintessence Publishing Co.

Brånemark PI, et al: *Osseointegrated implants in the treatment of the edentulous jaw—experience from a ten-year period,* Stockholm, 1977, Almquist and Wiksell.

Brunski JB, Moccia AF Jr, Pollack SR, Korostoff E et al: The influence of functional use of endosseous dental implants on the tissue-implant interface. II. Clinical aspects, *J Dent Res* 58:1953-1969, 1979.

Carlsson G, Haraldson T: Functional response. In Brånemark PI, Zarb GA, Albrektsson T, editors: *Tissue-integrated prostheses,* Chicago, 1985, Quintessence Publishing Co.

Carmichael RP, Apse P, Zarb GA et al: Biological, microbiological and clinical aspects of the peri-implant mucosa. In Albrektsson T, Zarb GA, editors: *The Brånemark osseointegrated implant,* Chicago, 1989, Quintessence Publishing Co.

Eckert S, Parein A, Myshin HL et al: Validation of dental implant systems through review of literature supplied by system manufacturers, *J Prosthet Dent* 77:271-279, 1997.

van Steenberghe D, Quirynen M, Calberson L et al: A prospective evaluation of the fate of 697 consecutive intraoral fixtures modum Brånemark in the rehabilitation of edentulism, *J Head Neck Pathol* 6:53-58, 1987.

Zarb GA: The edentulous milieu. Toronto conference on osseointegration in clinical dentistry, *J Prosthet Dent* 49:825-831, 1983.

Zarb GA, Albrektsson T: The University of Toronto Symposium Proceedings from Toward Optimized Treatment Outcomes for Dental Implants, *Int J Prosth* 11: 5, 1998.

Zarb GA, Schmitt A: The longitudinal clinical effectiveness of osseointegrated implants: the Toronto study. Part I: surgical results, *J Prosthet Dent* 63:451-457, 1990a.

Zarb GA, Schmitt A: The longitudinal clinical effectiveness of osseointegrated dental implants: the Toronto study. Part II: the prosthetic results, *J Prosthet Dent* 64:53-61, 1990b.

CHAPTER 26

The Science of Osseointegration

Tomas Albrektsson, Ann Wennerberg

Osseointegration, or predictable long-term anchorage of tooth root analogues in bone, is defined as "a time-dependent healing process whereby clinically asymptomatic rigid fixation of alloplastic materials is achieved, and maintained, in bone during functional loading" (Zarb and Albrektsson, 1991). Such stable bone implants have an interface that consists mainly of bone tissue. This attachment mechanism differs from the one retaining the natural dentition because teeth are anchored to their surrounding bone by means of a highly differentiated connective tissue attachment with ordered fibers: the periodontal ligament. To this day, nobody has succeeded in creating and maintaining a replica of a periodontal ligament around an implanted alloplastic tooth root. In fact, past implant efforts ended up anchored in poorly differentiated soft tissues, with unpredictable clinical results. Consequently, typical 5-year survival figures were in the order of 50%. This predicament provided the backdrop for the breakthrough introduction of osseointegrated oral implants in the early 1980s. It became possible to insert oral implants with a favorable predictable outcome, for example, a success rate of more than 90% over a follow-up of 5 years in the anterior region of the mandible. At the beginning of the 1980s, oral implants were prescribed in small numbers and rarely in university clinics. Today, the situation is quite different, and the science and clinical epidemiology underscoring osseointegrated implants are an integral part of most university curricula. The current popular notion that every commercially available osseointegrated implant system will result in a success rate of more than 90% is, however, misconceived. In the absence of scientific evidence, there is a serious risk that some commercially available systems will yield long-term failure as a likely treatment outcome because of adverse reactions to untested implant materials, designs, surfaces, or diverse therapeutic prescriptions. Furthermore, secondary failures have also been reported to occur in previously osseointegrated implants.

Considered in this chapter is the unique self-repairing ability of the surgically prepared bony interface, which, if not unduly disturbed, will remodel sufficiently to carry clinical loads. The specific nature of the osseointegrated interface and its bonding implications are also discussed to provide information about how the osseointegrated interface is sustained or threatened.

OSSEOINTEGRATED INTERFACE

In the past, direct contact (without interposed soft tissue layers) between bone and metallic implants was regarded as impossible to achieve. The operating notion was that a soft tissue interface was inevitable, which in turn implied that the interface was of maximal strength at the time of surgery and thereafter gradually lost holding power. Experimental studies performed at our laboratories by the late 1960s indicated that this notion was not necessarily correct, even if the methodological shortcomings of those days did not allow for definite evidence of direct contact between bone and implant. In the 1980s, when the bone and implant specimen cutting and grinding techniques were developed at the laboratories of Karl Donath in Germany, it was first possible to clearly demonstrate that metallic implants could be anchored in bone without a separating soft tissue interface (Figure 26-1). Subsequent investigations further demonstrated that the bone to metal interface did not achieve ultimate strength at the time of insertion. In fact, the specific interfacial response between host bone and commercially pure (cp) titanium interface developed a stronger attachment with time because of increasing bone formation. After 1 year or longer, depending on the implantation site, full strength is developed over the interface. The unique capacity of bone to remodel in accordance with imposed functional loads appears to be a time-dependent procedure, but the end result is a very strong interface if the implant is not overloaded during its incorporation or interfacial organization. If overloading occurs, this process is compromised, and a poorly differen-

tiated interface will result with ensuing implant loosening.

Knowledge of such basic interfacial reactions guides dentists' clinical decisions. If, for example, an implant is inserted in a previously irradiated maxillary bone bed of poor bone quality and quantity, unloaded periods up to a year or more may be necessary for the remodeling response to result in a "full strength" interface. This situation is in great contrast to oral implants with an inherently compromised anchorage, which constantly run the risk of overload and failure, even if relatively minor forces act over their interface (Figure 26-2). If such soft tissue–anchored implants function at all, they do so within a narrow range of loading.

The bond acting over an osseointegrated implant is probably a biomechanical one (Brånemark, Zarb, Albrektsson, 1985). This means that bone will grow into surface irregularities of the implant with a resultant three-dimensional stabilization. Design characteristics, such as implant threads, represent surface enlargements in the macroscale. Complete bone ingrowth may occur in such macroscopic surface enlargements, provided that a minimum of 100 µm of space is available. However, calcified bone ground substance may invade pores in the 1- to 10-µm of size, and some investigators have even suggested, albeit without proper experimental evidence, that nanometer size defects in the implant

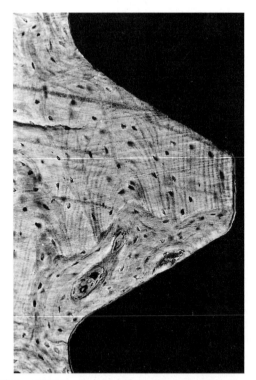

Figure 26-1 A thread of a screw-type implant demonstrates good bone-to-implant contact. The implant was stable in its bed and presumably osseointegrated.

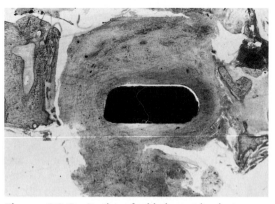

Figure 26-2 Portion of a blade vent implant, surrounded by soft tissue with some inflammation. The implant was mobile, had for years caused pain, and was removed for this reason.

surface may be important for proper load carrying (Figure 26-3). Some investigators have suggested that strong chemical bonds may develop between bone and certain ceramic implant materials and suggested such implants to be "biointegrated." However, there is no conclusive evidence of such chemical bonds, even if they remain theoretically possible. The available evidence for chemical bonds is represented by electron microscopic photographs of tissue coalescence with the implant or an otherwise unexplainable interfacial attachment strength.

Oxidized (anodized) implants have likewise been suggested as being capable of bioactivity (i.e., establishing a chemical bond between foreign material and host tissues). Sul (2002) has recently demonstrated a very strong bone reaction to certain anodized implants with surface-embedded calcium ions. After implantation, calcium cations will move

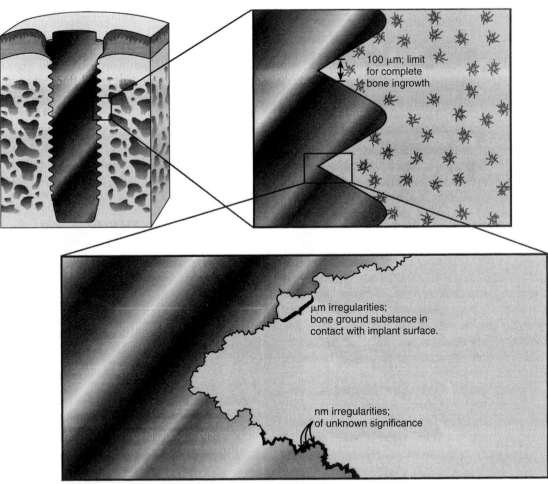

Figure 26-3 Bone tissue including ground substance and cellular components will need pores of a minimal size of 100 μm for ingrowth. Calcified ground substance of bone responds differently to irregularities in the micrometer size that are important for the strength of the osseointegrated response. Implant irregularities in the micrometer range are, to date, of undetermined significance for osseointegration.

from the implant surface toward the extracellular body fluid. Electrostatic ion bonding of calcium ions with polyanionic molecules of bone matrix proteins will follow. The calcium cations will stimulate particular surface receptors and trigger further recruitment of osteoprogenitor cells and osteoblasts through calcium-signaling pathways. Certain anodized implants show a uniquely strong bone reaction that cannot be explained by their surface roughness alone. However interesting these implants are, it must be observed that published clinical scrutiny of such implants is limited to a follow-up period of about 2 years.

FACTORS THAT DETERMINE SUCCESS AND FAILURE OF OSSEOINTEGRATED IMPLANTS

Compelling evidence confirms that a soft tissue interface leads to unpredictable clinical results in contrast to a bone to implant interface. However, it does not necessarily imply that the osseointegrated implant will always remain successful. There are secondary reasons for failure of osseointegrated implants, with overload and infection the most commonly cited. The overload theory reconciles the notion of a primary compromised osseointegration response with the adverse effects of subsequent adverse loading. It also recognizes the potential for adverse loading per se to compromise a favorable osseointegrated response. In the infection theory, the osseointegrated interface has the same vulnerability to periodontal pathogens that the periodontal ligament may have. It appears to be a popular theory among some periodontists but is not subscribed to by us. Whatever the final reason for failure, there is a range of implant- and implantation-related factors that may cause long-term failure. Such compromising factors may be the reason for progressive bone resorption that, in turn, makes implants vulnerable to overload. The starting point in failure may be poor implant biocompatibility with materials that corrode in the body, resulting in leaked-out ions that may secondarily disturb the surrounding bone. Unsuitable implant designs may lead to a relative lack of implant stability, resulting in micromovements, resultant bone saucerization, and subsequent implant loss (Figure 26-4). Implant

surface topography may be too smooth, which results in primary failures, or too rough, which also provide a potential risk of adverse bone reactions and secondary loss of integration. A compromised implant bed (e.g., poor quality or irradiated host bone) may demonstrate a disturbed bone remodeling response, leading to increasing failure rates with time. Improper surgical technique is most likely the cause of primary failures, whereas disturbed loading conditions may result in secondary failures also. These six parameters were first described more than 20 years ago and remain the most relevant ingredients of the successful osseointegration paradigm (Albrektsson et al., 1981).

Implant Biocompatibility

The most commonly used material for oral implants is cp titanium. It has been proven to be the most biocompatible in animal experiments (Sennerby, 1991), supporting the evidence for excellent long-term clinical function with cp titanium devices. Another material used for oral implants, titanium-6aluminum-

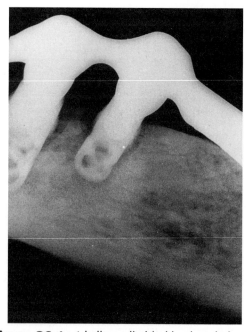

Figure 26-4 A hollow cylindrical implant design that may lead to severe bone resorption.

4vanadium (Ti-6Al-4V) alloy, exhibits in vitro and soft tissue reactions very similar to those reported to cp titanium. However, the development of a bony interface is retarded with Ti-6Al-4V implants compared with the situation for cp titanium. In comparative animal investigations at 3, 6, and 12 months, there were significantly stronger bone reactions to the cp titanium than to the aluminum-vanadium alloy. The reason for this retarded bone formation around the alloy has been suggested to depend on leaked-out aluminum ions that compete with calcium during the early stage of calcification and thereby cause local osteomalacia (Johansson, 1991). Whether these observed differences in early bone response between cp titanium and Ti-6Al-4V are of an exclusive academic nature or are clinically significant is difficult to tell. However, at least in compromised bone beds (e.g., maxillary bone, which has unfavorable bone quality and quantity) where one needs as much bone support as possible for clinical success, cp titanium appears to be the safest alternative.

Hydroxyapatite (HA), one type of calcium phosphate ceramic material, was originally tried as a solid material for use as an oral implant. However, because of the brittle nature of HA and other ceramics, such as aluminum oxides, fractures occur too often for these materials to be suitable as load-bearing devices in their solid form. HA is particularly interesting because there is clear documentation that this specific ceramic results in a more rapid bone response than seen with cp titanium. Unfortunately, such findings from short-term animal experiments alone were regarded as sufficient evidence for introduction of HA-coated oral implants in the mid-1980s. Long-term results with HA-coated implants have been significantly inferior to those cited for cp titanium implants, and some clinicians have incriminated the HA material for the poor clinical outcome. However, one cannot exclude factors other than the HA material for the disappointing clinical outcome, such as the preferred cylindrical implant design. Nevertheless, it is clearly unacceptable to base clinical introduction of a new type of implant on results of short-term animal experiments alone. Gottlander (1994) studied short- and long-term reactions to HA-coated implants in animal models and confirmed the positive short-term reactions reported by other investi-

gators. However, in long-term (6 months) animal experiments, the control cp titanium implants had 50% to 75% more interfacial bone than the HA-coated implants, which was possibly dependent on HA coat loosening, leading to macrophage activation and bone resorption. It is, in fact, quite possible that HA in forms other than plasma-sprayed coats may show more advantageous tissue reactions than the hitherto investigated types of HA-coated implants. With techniques other than plasma spraying for coating metals, it could be possible to use much thinner coats and thereby presumably avoid the adverse reactions seen with the thicker plasma-sprayed coatings. Consequently, HA and other calcium phosphates remain interesting materials that should be promising further.

Implant Design

The vast majority of commercially available implants claiming osseointegration status are cylindrical in shape. Their design may be threaded or else lack similar microscopic retentive/stabilization aspects. Such implants, HA coated or not, have demonstrated primary osseointegration and, in many cases, quite adequate survival at 5 years. Unfortunately, the problem is that no such design has ever been reported to maintain surrounding stable bone levels. Reports indicate a continuing bone saucerization of 1.5 mm during the first year and about 0.5 mm annually thereafter, with even a tendency of an increasing rate of resorption in the few reports of such implants that run over more than 5 years of follow-up (Albrektsson, 1993). This accumulated bone loss may not be dramatic at 5 years but may pose a serious problem thereafter. Some investigators explain the lack of a bone steady state by overload due to micromovements of the cylindrical designs, whereas others incriminate an inflammation/infection caused particularly by the very rough surfaces typical for these types of implants. In contrast, threaded oral implants have demonstrated maintenance of a clear steady state bone height after the first year of function (Figure 26-5).

Implant Surface

The surface may be of importance based on its quantitative or qualitative changes. Quantitative

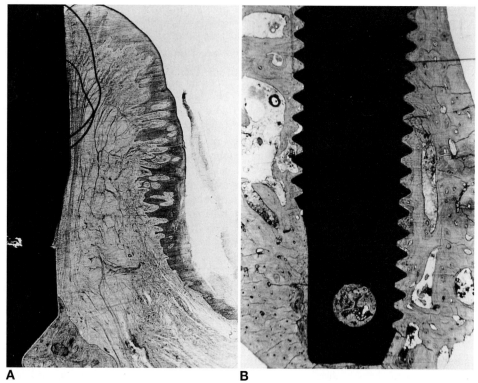

Figure 26-5   Soft tissue penetration **(A)** and bone tissue–anchored portion **(B)** of a postmortem preparation of a threaded implant design with excellent clinical documentation. There are no adverse reactions to the implant seen in the soft or hard tissue.

changes may be exemplified by surface topographical alterations. Qualitative changes refer to new potentially bioactive surfaces best exemplified by oxidized implants or surfaces doped with potentially active substances. Today, new clinical implants are marketed that are either quantitatively or qualitatively surface altered or that are even a combination of the two.

Surface roughness is an implant-related property that has been used extensively in marketing diverse oral implant systems. Because different machining processes result in different surface topographies, several implant manufacturers have machined implants with a turning or milling process, which is a production method that has been the gold standard for many years.

In a series of experimental studies performed in rabbits, as well as in a few human experiments,

moderately rough implants developed the best bone fixation as described by peak removal torque and bone-to-implant contact (Wennerberg, 1996). "Moderately rough" surfaces were produced by blasting to an average height deviation (roughness parameter S_a) of 1.5 µm, an average distance between the individual irregularities of 11.1 µm (S_{ex}) and a developed surface area ratio of 1.5 µm (S_{dr}) (Figure 26-6), and were positively compared with smoother (turned and blasted) as well as rougher-blasted implant surfaces. Very smooth surfaces (S_a values below 0.2 µm), which are in fact only used experimentally for abutment and anchorage studies, will often be surrounded by a soft tissue interface indicative of imminent failure. The reasons as to why rough surfaces (S_a values around and above 2.0 µm) demonstrate less firm bone fixation when compared with less rough surfaces still

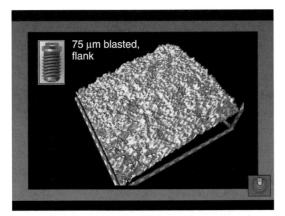

Figure 26-6 A blasted surface with a roughness corresponding to the experimental ideal of 1.5 μm.

need to be investigated (Figure 26-7). The concerns with any surface roughening involve an increased risk of corrosion. However, current knowledge about such increased corrosion appears to be only a theoretical and not a practical problem.

In this context it is worth emphasizing that a careful topographical characterization is essential for a reliable interpretation of the role of implant surface roughness for bone incorporation (Wennerberg and Albrektsson, 2000). There is a need for equipment that can be used to measure arbitrary designs and different surfaces. For example, only some optical instruments such as confocal profilometry

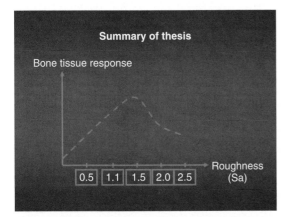

Figure 26-7 Experimentally the strongest bone response has a surface roughness of about 1.5 μm (S$_a$).

amd interferometry can be recommended for threaded implants at this time.

In recent experiments researchers have investigated the possibility of doping surfaces with different kinds of bone-stimulating factors. Such dopings can be done with implants of any surface roughness. A number of these bone-stimulating factors, growth factors, are present in our bodies and serve as important stimuli for the initiation of healing processes. However, external administration of growth factors may not necessarily improve the healing situation. We have doped implants with bone morphogenetic proteins (BMPs) and other growth factors and found no influence on the bone response (Franke Stenport, 2002). One possible explanation of this lack of a positive influence of growth factors may be the fact that we only tried them on regularly placed implants (i.e., a kind of press fit healing situation). However, one cannot exclude a positive influence of external administration of growth factors in gap healing cases, such as a tooth socket.

A rapidly growing number of publications underscore the clinical popularity of certain oxidized implants, and these implants may show strong bone responses quite independently of their surface roughness (Sul, 2002). However, other types of oxidized implants depend mainly on their surface roughness (Sul, 2002). In fact, oxidized implants are manufactured in galvanic element setups (thus the term *anodized*), and the used electrolyte will influence subsequent tissue responses. The clinical use of oxidized oral implants started some 10 years ago, but long-term outcome data are still lacking (for review see Sul, 2002).

In essence, it is still unknown how much bone contact is needed for an implant to be successful. Consequently, the clinical relevance of different surface (roughened and/or anodized) implants can only be verified in controlled clinical studies. However promising these surface alterations are, to date, there is in most cases a lack of supportive data from such studies to verify any clinical superiority of them. In fact, so far, only one surface roughened system has been positively documented in controlled, randomized clinical studies (Gotfredsen and Karlsson, 2001; Engquist et al. 2002).

Implant Bed

A healthy implant host site is required. Patient characteristics, such as age, and history of the proposed host site(s), such as previous irradiation, will affect the outcome of the implantation procedure. It also is believed that a history of smoking may affect the healing response in osseointegration.

Old age per se does not cause poorer implant results. However, extreme young age is a relative contraindication to the insertion of implants. The general recommendation is to await completion of growth before inserting oral implants in young individuals. In selected cases, where strong psychological motivation is present, oral implants may be inserted in children, but then preferably only in the anterior part of the jaw and in combination with overdenture therapy. In selected patients, bone-anchored hearing aids may even be attached to implants when the child is only 2 or 3 years old. The motivation behind treating such young children is to avoid the potential social handicap of severe hearing impairment that cannot be treated in any other way. In the case of facial deformities, insertion of skin-penetrating, bone-anchored implants usually is delayed until the child has reached puberty.

Smoking has been reported to yield significantly lower success rates with oral implants. The mechanism behind this lowered success is unknown, but vasoconstriction may play a role. Continuing substance abuse also may be a contraindication for implant treatment.

Previous irradiation is a relative contraindication for implant treatment (Jacobsson, 1985). After implant therapy is decided, patients treated with irradiation should be transferred to special clinics with sufficient experience with such patients. A 1-year delay after irradiation before inserting implants is recommended. Expected success rates are about 10% lower than for nonirradiated patients. Hyperbaric oxygen treatment in divers' chambers has been shown to improve the outcome in at least one published 5-year clinical follow-up study. If, on the other hand, patients have implants already in situ and osseointegrated when the need arises for therapeutic irradiation, removal of the implants before irradiation is not recommended. There is experimental evidence that osseointegrated oral implants will remain stable in bone despite irradiation, whereas implants that are inserted immediately before irradiation will show a high failure rate.

Surgical Technique

Minimal tissue violence at surgery is essential for proper osseointegration. This objective depends on continuous and careful cooling while surgical drilling is performed at low rotatory rates, with sharp instruments and the use of a graded series of drills. Proper drill geometry is important, as is intermittent drilling, if the bone is of a very dense structure. The insertion torque should be of a moderate level because strong insertion torques may result in stress concentrations around the threads of a screw-type implant, with subsequent bone resorption.

Recent publications suggest the need to expand the surgical parameter to also include surgical skill. It has been noted that individual surgeons' success records may vary in both oral and orthopedic implant placement. Furthermore, at least two surgical reports on outcomes in poor bone quality reveal that technical excellence combined with a modified surgical technique will yield predictably favorable long-term outcomes. Both authors of these reports used machine-turned implants, which were therefore neither surface roughened or oxidized (Albrektsson, 2001)

Loading Conditions

The original recommendation to achieve osseointegration is still valid: a two-stage implant insertion. The implant is first inserted in the bone, and then the soft tissues are sutured back so that the implant will be incorporated in bone under protected conditions. At a second surgical procedure (minimally 3 to 6 months later), the buried implant is exposed and connected to the oral cavity by means of a transepithelial abutment. This procedure guarantees that the implant is well protected during its incorporation in bone when the osseous interface has not been established properly, as evidenced from experimental and clinical studies. Clinical trials with various implant systems have now confirmed the possibility of immediate functional (direct) loading protocols, particularly in the mandible between the mental foramina. However, great caution is recommended with such an immediate loading protocol in the maxilla, particularly if the bone is judged to be of a poor quality. Furthermore, such loading puts a special emphasis on the skills of the surgeon, which is why we recommend newly trained surgeons to only use a two-stage operation. A promising approach for those who prefer a one-stage surgical protocol in combination with direct or rapid loading is to use resonance frequency analysis in an effort to differentiate potentially mobile implants from stable ones.

SUMMARY

It is important to observe that new biomaterials are in need of careful physical and engineering investigations to clarify if they are suitable for implantation. In vitro studies may provide important information, but one must remember that this is related to the controlled laboratory environment, which differs from in vivo testing with its hormonal, blood flow, and loading influences. It is therefore not uncommon that in vivo findings are quite different from those obtained in vitro. Short-term and long-term in vivo experimental studies are imperative before commercial clinical testing of an implant system is initiated. It is only when a biomaterial is found acceptable in such studies that clinical trials should be started. The most important step in the testing procedure remains the controlled, preferably prospective, clinical study that should span an adequate period, which is conventionally at least 5 years.

In the summary of current knowledge about the factors controlling implant function in the body, it is easy to say that the scientific community has made a great number of important findings in the past 25 years. However, researchers may very well be climbing the lower slopes of a mountain of unknown height. Major contributions will be gathered in the future from prospective and controlled treatment outcome studies in patients. The fundamental message in clinical epidemiology is that efficacy without effectiveness usurps the notion of a compelling scientific claim.

References

Albrektsson T: On long-term maintenance of the osseointegrated response, *Aust Prosth J* 7(suppl):15-24, 1993.

Albrektsson T: Is surgical skill more important for clinical success than changes in implant hardware? *Clin Implant Dent Relat Res* 3:174-175, 2001.

Albrektsson T, Brånemark PI, Hansson H-A et al: Osseointegrated titanium implants. Requirements for ensuring a long-lasting, direct bone anchorage in man, *Acta Orthop Scand* 52: 155-170, 1981.

Brånemark PI, Zarb GA, Albrektsson T: *Tissue integrated prostheses: osseointegration in clinical dentistry,* Chicago, 1985, Quintessence Publishing Co.

Engquist B, Åstrang P, Dahlgren S et al: Marginal bone reaction to oral implants: A prospective comparative study of astra tech and Brånemark system implants, *Clin Oral Impl Res* 13:30-37, 2002.

Franke Stenport V: On growth factors and titanium implant integration in bone, PhD thesis, Biomaterials/handicap research, 2002, University of Göteborg.

Gotfredsen K, Karlsson U: A prospective 5-year study of fixed partial prostheses supported by implants with a machined and TiO$_2$-blasted surface, *J Prosthodont* 10:2-7, 2001.

Gottlander M: On hard tissue reactions to hydroxyapatite-coated titanium implants, PhD thesis, Biomaterials/handicap research, 1994, University of Göteborg.

Jacobsson M: On bone behaviour after irradiation, PhD Thesis, Biomaterials/handicap research, 1985, University of Göteborg.

Johansson C: On tissue reactions to metal implants, PhD thesis, Biomaterials/handicap research, 1991, University of Göteborg.

Sennerby L: On the bone tissue response to titanium implants, PhD thesis, Biomaterials/handicap research, 1991, University of Göteborg.

Sul YT: On the bone response to oxidized titanium implants, PhD thesis, Biomaterials/handicap research, 2002, University of Göteborg.

Wennerberg A: On surface roughness and implant incorporation, PhD thesis, Biomaterials/handicap research, 1996, University of Göteborg.

Wennerberg A, Albrektsson T: Suggested guidelines for the topographic evaluation of implant surfaces, *Int J Oral Maxillofac Implants* 15:331-344, 2000.

Zarb GA, Albrektsson T: Osseointegration: a requiem for the periodontal ligament? *Int J Periodont Rest Dent* 11:88-91, 1991 (editorial).

CHAPTER 27

Clinical Protocol for Treatment with Implant-Supported Overdentures

George A. Zarb, Regina Mericske-Stern

Several compelling conclusions can be drawn from the chapters in Part 3:

1. Treatment outcomes with complete dentures depend on both dentist- and patient-mediated considerations. The former include clinical judgment and technical skills, combined with impeccable laboratory technological support. The latter are defined by systemic plus local health and morphological considerations, together with individual adaptive traits.

2. An adaptive denture experience is the treatment goal, and it is frequently achieved. However, an ongoing long-term continuum of adaptation may be unpredictable because of time-dependent anatomical and physiological changes. These include reduced salivary flow, compromised motor skills, severe residual ridge reduction, and an increased tissue vulnerability.

3. The notion of a surgical solution for patients with maladaptive dentures by means of enlargement of the available denture-bearing area (sulcus-deepening procedures, or ridge augmentation, or both) has failed to yield predictable and long-term beneficial results that are morbidity free. Also, this solution does not address the needs of patients who dislike the idea of wearing dentures.

4. The introduction of the osseointegrated implant protocol has eclipsed traditional preprosthetic surgical techniques. It ushered in a new era of versatile, predictable, and virtually morbidity-free implant prosthodontic treatment. Although this development has enhanced the life quality of the treated patients, it also escalated the costs involved in managing the edentulous predicament. The merits of the traditional overdenture technique can therefore be combined with an implant prescription for a cost-effective version of implant-supported prostheses.

5. Clinical experience also shows that many patients who request implant surgery because of denture-wearing problems are really in need of new optimized dentures, at least from an objective clinical point of view. Patients must recognize that implants do not compensate for technically and functionally inadequate dentures.

We therefore regard implant-supported prostheses as a logical outgrowth of the previously noted conclusions and think that they should be considered the standard of service for most edentulous patients, particularly those with maladaptive dentures. However, fiscal realities, particularly in the context of aging populations with fixed incomes, frequently preclude the fixed option. The overdenture choice, on the other hand, could be regarded as more financially accessible and offers virtually similar advantages.

In this chapter we describe the application of the implant overdenture protocol as a routine measure for managing the edentulous predicament.

OVERDENTURES TREATMENT GOALS

Overdentures supported by natural tooth roots have been a long-standing and integral part of treatment planning. However, both their short- and long-term treatment outcome can be unpredictable (see Chapter 10).

Although tooth and implant abutment attachment mechanisms differ, their prosthetic role is quite similar. Both can provide enhanced prostheses retention and stability, and positively influence adjacent bone levels, although periodontal disease and caries are clearly not risk factors for the "ankylotic-like" osseointegrated abutment. In fact, studies of mandibular overdentures retained by implants have shown that bone height is very well maintained in the area where implants were located. It should, however, be pointed out that resorption of the posterior residual ridge was increased when compared with similar sites in patients treated with implant-supported fixed prostheses. It therefore seems prudent to suggest that the younger the edentulous patient, the greater the benefit from implant-supported fixed prostheses to reduce overall long-term residual ridge reduction. On the other hand, overdentures should be recommended routinely for elderly edentulous patients because residual ridge reduction of their basal bone appears to be less vulnerable to residual ridge resorption.

The fabrication of complete dentures, particularly mandibular ones for elderly patients with maladaptive dentures, is complex and difficult. Therefore a simple protocol that may be readily applied to all elderly patients is a prudent objective. Such an approach includes the following considerations:

1. There should be a reduction in the number of prescribed implants: two in the mandible and four in the maxilla. Although mandibular treatment has been extraordinarily successful, the moderate to severely resorbed maxilla is a much bigger treatment challenge.
2. Both patient and tissue stresses should be minimized with a short surgical intervention.
3. Implant abutment availability that ensures denture retention and stability should not compensate for technically and functionally inadequate dentures. Traditional and impeccable complete denture fabrication techniques must be combined with the required surgical protocol to optimize the technique's potential.
4. Esthetic denture design should not be compromised by the location of implants and their connection to retention devices. There is little doubt about the greater ease with which esthetic objectives can be addressed and achieved when using the overdenture technique. This is not easy to accomplish with the fixed prescription, more particularly in the maxilla, when moderate residual ridge resorption has occurred.
5. The dentist should seriously consider managing both the patient's surgical and prosthodontic needs. The educational implications of this conviction are profound ones indeed.

INCLUSION AND EXCLUSION CRITERIA

Implant treatment decisions must be made for each patient according to individual circumstances. The major inclusion criteria underscore the quasi-universal patient eligibility for the method (Box 27-1). Age itself is not an exclusion criterion; however, age-related factors frequently influence treatment planning in elderly patients. Common problems encountered include communication difficulties (e.g., compromised hearing and cognitive skills) with consequent lack of cooperation; the likely need for short appointments; special attention to presurgical measures such as general health status and information; oral hygiene state; and home care provision. Poor general health is often found in elderly patients with consequent deterioration in biological health that is far beyond their chronological age. Therefore medical consultation is frequently required and is of course mandatory for all systemically compromised and therefore high-risk

---

Box 27-1

Inclusion Criteria for Implant Prosthodontic Treatment

Patient desire for implant treatment
Systemic health status, which permits a minor surgical procedure
Sufficient bone quantity to accommodate prescribed implant dimensions
Patient willingness and ability to maintain oral health status

patients, if any suspicion of risk or unclear information is present. The patient's family physician should be routinely consulted.

As mentioned earlier, problems with the wearing of dentures or adaptation to new ones are multifactorial, including age-related considerations. Patient selection criteria must therefore be established with respect to a broad range of local and general aspects. Clinical experience supports the proposed exclusion criteria listed in Box 27-2, but also reveals that patients with a history of cardiovascular disease, osteoporosis, and certain endocrine disorders are all able to undergo a successful implant operation as long as their systemic condition is not a brittle one. Surgical treatment should also be carried out only when the patient's health status allows it and when a patient feels well and is able to undergo the procedure.

PRESURGICAL EVALUATION AND TREATMENT PLANNING

The treatment planning protocol is identical for all edentulous patients and is a result of clinical and radiographic assessments that yield the information contained in Box 27-3. The *clinical oral assessment* provides information about shape, width, and height of the residual ridges and soft tissue conditions. Horizontal and vertical relationships of the residual ridges are examined, and available space for the proposed implants and the planned retention devices is assessed. Most edentulous patients who are treated with implants frequently show advanced reduction of the residual ridges and absence of a wide band of attached mucosa. This does not seem to adversely affect the health of the soft tissue attachment around implants, and gingiva-mucosal grafting is very rarely prescribed. Where necessary, additional bone mapping with a local anesthesia syringe needle helps identify the contours of the maxillary bone. This may be useful because of the thickness of the palatal mucosa, which may disguise the shape of the ridge. This is not necessary for the mandible and is often impossible because the height of the floor of the mouth does not permit easy identification of the lingual shape of the mandibular bone.

Panoramic radiographs are made to overview required bone dimensions, to "scout" anatomical structures, to discover possible pathological findings, and to obtain general information on bone quality or density. The panoramic film is, however,

---

Box 27-2

Exclusion Criteria for Implant Prosthodontic Treatment

Patient's current prosthetic experience is an adaptive one

Residual ridge dimensions do not accommodate preferred implant dimensions

Communication with patient is not possible because of his or her compromised cognitive skills

Patient has a history of substance abuse

General health conditions preclude a minor surgical intervention

Local anesthesia with a vasoconstrictor is contraindicated

Immunosuppressive therapy, prolonged intake of antibiotics or corticosteroids, or brittle metabolic disease history

---

Box 27-3

Specific Objectives of Treatment Planning for a Patient with Implant-Supported Overdentures

To determine the optimum location and number of implants in the context of the morphological aspects of the residual ridge

To design a favorable distribution for occlusal stresses on the implants and the prostheses-bearing tissues

To avoid discrepancies among the design of the dentures, the implants' location, and the dentures' retentive devices

To ensure an optimal esthetic result and hygiene protocol

not entirely reliable, and additional radiographic imaging is frequently required. In the maxilla, loosely structured trabecular or cancellous bone without a dense cortical layer is frequently encountered. As a result, the implants are frequently self-tapped into such bone of compromised quality. In the mandible, dense cortical bone frequently encloses a tightly structural cancellous structure. Templates with metallic markers of known diameter may be used to measure the available bone height on radiographs and to predetermine a favorable location of the implants with respect to the topography of the residual ridge and adjacent anatomical landmarks, such as the mandibular nerve or the maxillary sinus (Figure 27-1). Cephalometric radiographs in particular provide information about faciolingual

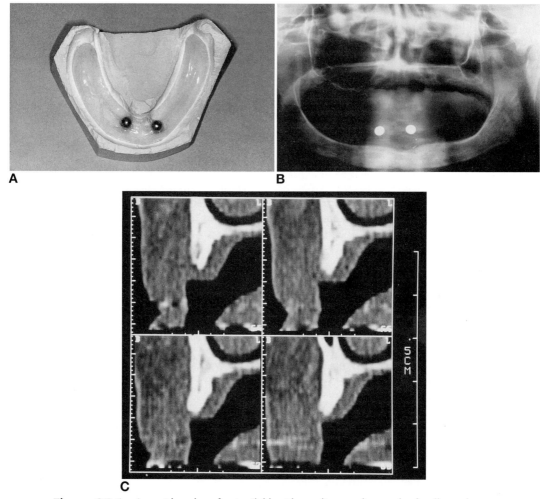

Figure 27-1 Correct imaging of potential host bone sites requires a mix of radiographs, which can be rendered more accurate by using a template with metallic markers of known dimensions (**A**). These markers will show up on a frontal (**B**) or sagittal image and allow for measurement adjustments in bone height or width. Required sagittal views of anterior edentulous zones are provided by means of cephalometric films or, less frequently, computed tomograms (**C**).

dimensions, plus the lingual aspect of the residual mandibular bone and the shape of the maxillary ridge. Tomographic images are rarely used for mandibular interforaminal implant placement; however, they often are needed for maxillary treatment.

Examination of existing dentures helps the dentist decide whether they are adequate for temporary use during the postsurgical healing phase. This is a routine measure with the two-stage surgical protocol. However, the transmucosal aspect of the Bonefit-ITI implants during the healing can be a problem because the effort to prevent inadvertent loading in patients who are unwilling to remain without dentures during the whole healing period may not be easily controlled. New or optimized dentures can be made before surgery if stability of old dentures cannot be achieved by minor adjustments. Old dentures are also examined regarding their esthetic merits, plus the presence of loss of vertical dimension of occlusion.

The following two planning concerns of major prosthodontic treatment must also be considered:

1. Number of implants prescribed and their location
2. Preferred denture retention devices

The number of implants placed for overdenture support differs in the mandible and the maxilla and is influenced by residual jaw shape. Maxillary overdentures require the placement of a minimum of three to four implants, which are usually joined with a connecting bar. In selected patients, two implants are used; however, the dentist must realize that divergent implant axes, a curved shape of the ridge, and unfavorable bone quality are specific contraindications to the placement of only two maxillary implants. In maxillary ridges, short bar segments connecting multiple implants are suggested because a segmented bar is more likely to follow the ridge without encroaching on the palatal space (Figure 27-2). Implant length should preferably be 10 mm or longer, and several implants should be prescribed when resorbed host bone sites preclude placement of 10-mm or longer fixtures.

Mandibular overdentures appear to be adequately supported by two implants. When the anterior mandibular ridge shows a slight curvature or a

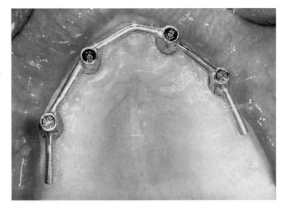

Figure 27-2   The maxilla's ridge contour is reflected in a segmented bar soldered to four implant abutments. Retentive clips can engage any or all of the five available segments, ensuring good retention, optimal prosthetic teeth placement, and nonrestriction of tongue space.

straight line, a bar will connect the two implants on its shortest distance and preferably parallel to the patient's arbitrary hinge axis (Figure 27-3, *A*). The interimplant distance should preferably exceed 12 mm to provide sufficient space to accommodate retentive components. When a pronounced curvature of the mandibular ridge is encountered, the placement of more than two implants is recommended. This arrangement will, however, virtually convert prostheses support from an implant/ridge one to a near exclusive implant support (Figure 27-3, *B*). A shorter design of the bar segments will not interfere with the profile of the ridge.

Patients with advanced mandibular residual ridge resorption will only accommodate shorter implant lengths, and, consequently, more than two implants must be placed. In such situations, three or preferably four implants should be prescribed to achieve sufficient intraosseous support.

Guidelines for selecting retentive devices are discussed at the end of the chapter.

SURGICAL PROCEDURE AND THE OSSEOINTEGRATION PHASE

The surgical protocol is well documented, and the aim is to place the implants into predetermined host sites that address prosthodontic design objectives.

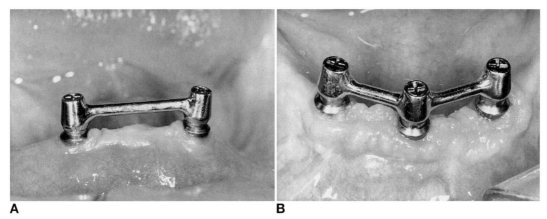

A   **B**

Figure 27-3   A, Mandibular overdentures have been shown to perform well when supported by only two implants. These prostheses are implant/ridge supported and can be so designed when implants are placed as far apart as possible between the mental foramina. Use of a bar that allows for rotation of the prosthesis around the interimplant axis can be achieved if anterior residual ridge shape is parallel to an arbitrarily determined hinge axis that is only slightly curved. **B,** Residual ridge curvature (as opposed to the "flat" one in part **A**) usually necessitates placement of three or more implants to preclude the splinting bar's encroachment on tongue space. However, a trade-off occurs if the bar's segments follow the ridge contour; the prosthesis is then virtually entirely implant supported. The same effect probably results even if alternative retentive mechanisms are prescribed.

Therefore a surgical template or guide is recommended to ensure optimal implant alignment and location, and this is facilitated by duplicating the previous denture and trimming it as needed. The patient's informed consent is obtained, and appropriate premedication is prescribed. The operation is carried out as atraumatically as possible, with the patient under local anesthesia. Postoperative phase is almost always uneventful and is ensured by means of standard analgesia medication plus use of ice packs and chlorhexidine mouth rinses. After 7 to 10 days, depending on the wound healing process, the sutures are removed, and the dentures are provisionally refitted with a tissue conditioner. The one-stage implants should also be protected from contact with the relined denture base, and therefore the dentures are relieved overlying the implants' location. The soft reliner must be changed at regular intervals, and patients are instructed to remove their dentures while sleeping to avoid trauma to the healing sites. Patients also are instructed about careful hygienic procedures with small soft brushes and the use of a mouthwash containing chlorhexidine to facilitate plaque removal.

A healing phase of 3 to 4 months for mandibular implants and 6 months for maxillary implants is usually observed with a longer interval prescribed for compromised bone quality sites. Published research suggests that the healing process is a very individual response that may be accelerated or delayed in different sites in different patients. The dentist may be tempted to shorten the healing interval, but this approach may be an imprudent one, and we strongly recommend the previously mentioned guidelines.

PROSTHODONTIC PROTOCOL

Implant-supported and implant-retained complete dentures resemble the clinical situation of overdentures supported and retained by specially prepared natural tooth roots. Despite a lack of a periodontal ligament and its periodontal receptors, the ankylotic-like osseointegrated attachment appears to provide adequate sensorimotor feedback system through receptors in the oral mucosa, bone, temporomandibular joint, and muscle spindles. As a result, coordinated chewing activity in edentulous and dentate subjects appears to be quite similar. It seems that the masticatory stability of implant-supported overdentures during function compensates for the absence of a periodontal ligament. Patients with implants report high-functional satisfaction and a sensation that they have their natural teeth.

Denture Design

The design and fabrication of implant-supported overdentures follow the previously described principles of fabricating complete dentures as described in Part 3. Stability and retention of complete dentures are enhanced by provision of a well-fitting denture base and properly extended flanges. Where desired by the patient, the denture base may be slightly reduced in its extensions because of the overdenture's relative immobility. This is usually the case with patients who object to prosthesis bulk. The replacement of lost tissue and the restoration of facial support are provided by the denture base and the established vertical dimension of occlusion. These also become very important for patients with intraoral defects resulting from maxillofacial deficits that are caused by congential anomalies, trauma, or oncological surgical resections.

The arrangement of anterior teeth follows basic guidelines as determined by facial esthetic needs, whereas the arrangement of posterior teeth contributes to retention and stability of the dentures. Individual patient preferences frequently can be fulfilled, but anterior teeth positions should not interfere with the circumoral musculature. It is presumed that a stable occlusion is likely to contribute to the protection of implants from overloading.

Clinical and Laboratory Procedures

Prosthodontic treatment planning will result in implant- and tissue-supported overdentures, although a distribution of certain implant locations may lead to exclusive implant abutment support. The impression technique is a crucial first step. The preliminary impression is made with alginate in metal stock trays. The custom acrylic resin trays require openings for accommodating the transfer copings, which are placed on the implants. The final impression is made, it is removed from the mouth, and laboratory implant analogues are connected to the transfer copings. The master cast is poured with the analogues in place. The subsequent clinical/laboratory protocol is identical to that used for complete denture fabrication. An exception is the inclusion of the selected retentive elements in the fitting surface of the prostheses. For example, whenever a clip bar mechanism is used, the bar (1) follows the shape of the ridge, (2) respects the position of the prosthetic teeth, and (3) provides access for oral hygiene procedures. The bar is cast, soldered to the prosthetic copings, and tried in the mouth. The same orientation index is used to cast a metal framework, should this be indicated, after final soldering of the bar. The female parts of bar clip assembly are fixed directly in the denture base during the laboratory processing procedures (Figure 27-4). Some clinicians prefer to use a metal framework embedded in the acrylic resin denture base. In this case the female components should not be soldered to the metal framework. They are retained in the denture base with acrylic resin to facilitate future changes or repairs. Step-by-step clinical and laboratory procedures for fabricating the implant-supported overdenture are shown in Box 27-4.

Guidelines for Selecting Retentive/Anchorage Devices

Several methods for securing retention and stability of overdentures are available. They are arguably equally efficient. However, certain considerations influence the choice of retaining element. These include: (1) number of supporting implants and their distribution over the ridge, (2) length of the bar segments, (3) type and size of the single attachment or bars, (4) number of female retainers, and (5) degree of reduction of the residual ridge. Much empirical discussion exists regarding the benefits of different retentive mechanisms (resilient versus rigid) (Box 27-5). A resilient retention mechanism is widely recommended for anchorage of overdentures to implants. The assumption is that this will protect implants from overload. However, recent results of comparative in vivo measurements of patients with two mandibular implants supporting an overdenture do not reveal a preference of one type of anchorage device or retention

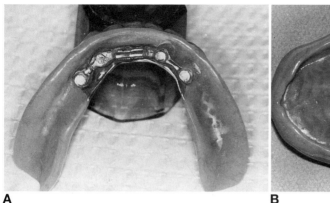
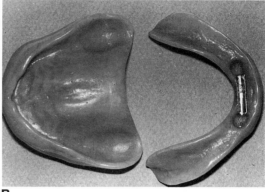

A   **B**

Figure 27-4 The acrylic resin prosthesis may (**A**) or may not (**B**) be reinforced with a Stellite alloy framework; this appears to be a subjective decision, although it clearly has economic implications. The retentive clips (sometimes referred to as the *female parts of the clip bar*) are processed and "fixed" in the acrylic resin denture base. This will make any future clip replacement requirements a relatively easy procedure.

Box 27-4

Step-by-Step Prosthodontic Procedures

One
- Preliminary impression with irreversible hydrocolloid for custom tray fabrication

Laboratory: custom trays with openings over implants' location

Two
- Abutment components selected (may include additional prosthetic copings)
- Mounting of transfer copings
- Full arch or two-stage impression with custom tray

Laboratory: master cast with implant analogues, wax occlusion rims

Three
- Jaw relation records
- Tooth selection

Laboratory: mounting the casts on the articulator, preliminary tooth setup

Four
- Verification of occlusal records
- Esthetic and functional assessment of tooth setup with the patient

- Indexing of setups to allow for optimal bar design

Laboratory: corrections as determined at try-in appointment; bar fabrication

Five
- Complete try-in, obtain consent of the patient
- Try-in of bar assembly, correction of casting if a passive fit is not obtained

Laboratory: final corrections, preparation for processing the denture: assembly of clip/bar components

Processing the denture, occlusal equilibration on articulator to rectify processing errors

Six
- Delivery of dentures to the patient
- Instruction about handling of the dentures
- Cleaning instructions for implants, retention devices, dentures
- Information about and enrollment in the maintenance care program
- Baseline radiographs for comparative monitoring purposes (optional)

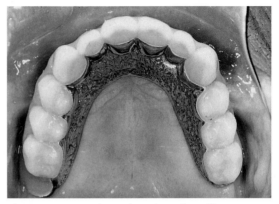

Figure 27-5   A horseshoe-shaped maxillary prosthesis is made out of a combination of prosthetic teeth, Stellite alloy (for strength with minimal bulk), and pink acrylic resin as a substitute for soft tissue reduction and for esthetic support. The undersurface of this prosthesis includes five retentive clips that engage the bar segments shown in Figure 29-3. Note that the clips are retained in the acrylic resin segment to facilitate any future repair needs.

mechanism over another. However, overdentures supported by "unjoined" implants are also reported to be successful.

A popular belief among dentists is that bars may contribute to load sharing. The reported long-term success rate for mandibular implants is quite high, and slightly less so for maxillary implants. Because splinted multiple implants with a bar usually are prescribed for the maxilla, a horseshoe design is possible (Figure 27-5; also see Figure 27-2). As a consequence, this type of maxillary overdenture will resemble a fixed prosthesis with regard to stability and function. Therefore it is understandable that this may not be regarded as a realistic and economic alternative to a tooth-supported overdenture or complete denture, as is the case with mandibular overdentures supported by only two implants.

Indications for Single Attachments   The use of retentive anchors or magnets is the easiest and probably the most cost-effective way to retain dentures by means of implants. This is frequently recommended when implants are placed underneath a patient's presently worn dentures, that is, ones that do not have to be remade. Denture-wearing problems of geriatric patients with impaired manual dexterity may be readily resolved with such retention systems (Figure 27-6). They also may be used

for temporary use after the postsurgical healing phase and before the insertion of technically time-consuming prosthetic reconstructions. It should be pointed out that the belief that spherical attachments may be used to compensate for unfavorable and nonparallel alignment of the implants appears to be a mistaken one.

Indications for Bars   Patients frequently complain about adequate lack of denture retention when single attachments are used—thus our preference for routine use of cast bars. Short distal extensions from rigid bars may additionally contribute to stabilization and prevent horizontal shifting of the dentures. Bars are routinely recommended for maxillary overdentures, atrophic residual ridges in the mandible, and mandibles with more than two implants due to pronounced ridge curvature. When intraoral defects are present, rigid bars are preferred in an effort to minimize overload on adjacent vulnerable soft tissues (Figure 27-7).

MAINTENANCE CARE

The objective of regular recalls for all patients with overdentures is to maintain the health of the oral

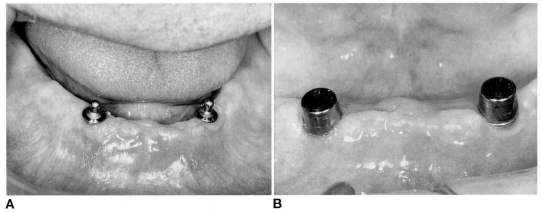

A   **B**

Figure 27-6 A large number of attachment devices have been commercially produced in an attempt to enhance and diversify claims for optimal implant/prosthesis retention. Several of these methods are backed by strong anecdotal support. They include spherical Dalla Bona attachments (**A**) and magnets (**B**).

tissues, particularly the periimplant tissues, and to check the denture for ongoing fit, stability, and occlusion. The dental literature is full of scholarly discussions regarding the merits of periodontal parameters and diagnostic methods borrowed from periodontology. Quite interestingly, they appear to be of limited use in osseointegration, at least with our two preferred implant systems. However, main-

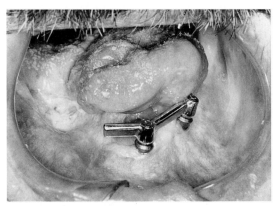

Figure 27-7 A right mandibular resection underscored the need for a stable prosthesis, otherwise precluded by resultant compromised tissues available for retention and stability of a complete denture. The prescription of two implants connected by a rigid bar met this patient's needs for comfortable prosthesis function.

tenance of optimal care to prevent and help diagnose potential problems has proven to be advantageous. Most patients with overdentures who are in special need of oral health care are elderly. These patients frequently possess impaired manual skills and reduced visual capacity. They are likely to have difficulties in following cleaning instructions and therefore rely on their care providers and their professional assistance. They have to be taught individual hygienic procedures that best correspond to their abilities. The wearing of overdentures certainly enhances plaque accumulation and risk of inflammatory soft tissue reactions, but it is not as ominous a concern where successfully osseointegrated implant abutments are used. Periimplant tissues do not appear to be as vulnerable to plaque by-products as periodontal tissues are, yet a variety of *nuisance type* gingival responses may develop and should of course be avoided. When compared with an implant-supported fixed prosthesis, the cleaning of implants and prostheses is certainly easier with removable dentures (Figure 27-8).

Growth of hyperplastic soft tissue around implants and particularly underneath the bars has been observed and recorded. It usually is rectified by a program of vigorous massage and most infrequently by surgical trimming of the excess tissue. The patient's maintenance program also includes checkup and adjustment appointments. The latter

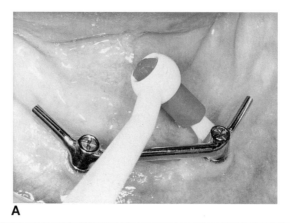

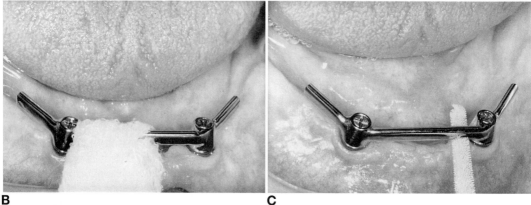

Figure 27-8   Popular adjuncts for ensuring continued soft tissue health including brushing of circumimplant gingival tissue (**A**), deposit-free bar components (note use of a gauze square) (**B**), and stimulation of tissues adjacent to the implants (**C**).

include an assessment of the fit of the denture base to determine the need for relining; an occlusal assessment to establish need for intraoral or "unmounted" occlusal adjustment; a check of female attachment components (loose, broken, lost, or need for activation); and wear and tear of any parts of abutment or retentive elements from contact with the denture base.

The precise response to occlusal transmission of loads to the implants that might lead to bone resorption or loss of osseointegration is unresolved. Research provides evidence that inadequately fitting superstructures (even when not recognized visually) may induce cumulative and adverse stresses on implants, with a risk of adverse bone changes. Therefore a precise, passive fit of denture bases, bars, and attachments is a prerequisite for long-lasting health of the bone surrounding and supporting the implants.

Bibliography

Awad MA, Locker D, Korner-Bitensky N et al: Measuring the effect of intra-oral implant rehabilitation on health-related quality of life in a randomized controlled clinical trail, *J Dent Res* 79:1659-1663, 2000.

Awad MA, Shapiro SH, Lund JP et al: Determinants of patients' treatment preferences in a clinical trial, *Community Dent Oral Epidemiol* 28:119-125, 2000.

Benzing UR, Hall H, Weber H: Biomechanical aspects of two different implant-prosthetic concepts for edentulous maxillae, *Int J Oral Maxillofac Implants* 10:188-198, 1995.

Bryant SR, Zarb GA: Osseointegration of oral implants in older and younger adults, *Int J Oral Maxillofac Implants* 13:492-499, 1998.

Cune MS, de Putter C: Comparative evaluation of some outcome measures of implant systems and suprastructure types in mandibular implant–overdenture treatment, *Int J Oral Maxillofac Implants* 9:548-555, 1994.

Cune MS, de Putter C, Hoogstraten J: Treatment outcome with implant-retained overdentures. Part 2: Patient satisfaction and predictability of subjective treatment outcome, *J Prosthet Dent* 72:152-158, 1994.

Duyck J, Van Oosterwyck H, Vander Sloten J et al: In vivo forces on oral implants supporting a mandibular overdenture: the influence of attachment system, *Clin Oral Invest* 3:201-207, 1999.

Enquist B, Bergendal T, Kallus T: A retrospective multicenter evaluation of osseointegrated implants supporting overdentures, *Int J Oral Maxillofac Implants* 3:129-134, 1988.

Feine JS, de Grandmont P, Boudrias P et al: Within-subject comparisons of implant-supported mandibular prostheses: choice of prosthesis, *J Dent Res* 73:1105-1111, 1994.

Hemmings KE, Schmitt A, Zarb GA: Complications and maintenance requirements for fixed prostheses and overdentures in the edentulous mandible: a 5-year report, *Int J Oral Maxillofac Implants* 9:191-196, 1994.

Humphris GM, Healey T, Howell RA et al: The psychological impact of implant-retained mandibular prostheses: a cross-sectional study, *Int J Oral Maxillofac Implants* 10:437-444, 1995.

Jemt T: Implant treatment in resorbed edentulous upper jaws, *Clin Oral Implant Res* 4:187-194, 1993.

Johns RB, Jemt T, Heath MR et al: A multicenter study of overdentures supported by Brånemark implants, *Int J Oral Maxillofac Implants* 7:513-522, 1992.

Kiener P, Oetterli M, Mericske E et al: Effectiveness of maxillary overdentures supported by implants: maintenance and prosthetic complications, *Int J Prosthodont* 14:133-140, 2001.

Meijer HJA, Starmans FJM, Steen WHA: Location of implants in the interforaminal region of the mandible and the consequences for the design of the superstructure, *J Oral Rehabil* 21:47-56, 1994.

Mericske-Stern R: Oral tactile sensibility recorded in overdenture wearers with implants or natural roots: a comparative study. Part 2. *Int J Oral Maxillofac Implants* 9:63-70, 1994.

Mericske-Stern R, Steinlin Schaffner T, Marti P et al: Periimplant mucosal aspects of ITI implants supporting overdentures: a five-year longitudinal study, *Clin Oral Implant Res* 5:9-18, 1994.

Mericske-Stern R, Zarb GA: Overdentures: an alternative implant methodology for edentulous patients, *Int J Prosthodont* 6:203-208, 1993.

Mombelli A, Mericske-Stern R: Microbiological features of stable osseointegrated implants used as abutments for overdentures, *Clin Oral Implant Res* 1:1-7, 1990.

Narhi TO, Geertman ME, Hevinga M et al: Changes in the edentulous maxilla in persons wearing implant-retained mandibular overdentures, *J Prosthet Dent* 84:43-49, 2000.

Oetterli M, Kiener P, Mericske-Stern R: A longitudinal study on mandibular implants supporting an overdenture: the influence of retention mechanism and anatomic-prosthetic variables on periimplant parameters, *Int J Prosthodont* 14:536-542, 2001.

Palmqvist S, Sondell K, Swartz B: Implant-supported maxillary overdentures: outcome in planned and emergency cases, *Int J Oral Maxillofac Implants* 9:184-190, 1994.

Quirynen M, Naert I, van Steenberghe D et al: Periodontal aspects of osseointegrated fixtures supporting an overdenture: a 4-year retrospective study, *J Clin Periodontol* 18:719-729, 1991.

Smedberg J-I: Studies of maxillary overdentures on osseointegrated implants, *Swed Dent J* 102: 1-49, 1995.

Von Wowern N, Gotfredsen K: Implant-supported overdentures, a prevention of bone loss in edentulous mandibles? A 5-year follow-up study, *Clin Oral Implants Res* 12:19-25, 2001.

Wright PS, Watson RM, Heath MR: The effects of prefabricated bar design on the success of overdentures stabilized by implants, *Int J Oral Maxillofac Implants* 10:79-87, 1995.

Zarb GA, Schmitt A: Osseointegration for elderly patients: the Toronto study, *J Prosthet Dent* 72:559-568, 1994.

Zarb GA, Schmitt A: The edentulous predicament II: the longitudinal effectiveness of implant-supported overdentures, *J Am Dent Assoc* 127:66-72, 1996.

CHAPTER 28

Clinical Protocol: Implant-Supported Fixed Prostheses

George A. Zarb, Steven E. Eckert

Successful osseointegration enables the dentist and the edentulous patient to consider one of two alternatives to the traditional complete denture experience. These alternatives are an implant-supported fixed or an overdenture prosthesis. This chapter reviews some considerations that have an impact on the clinical decision making and protocol for fixed prostheses.

PATIENT SELECTION

Patients who have been shown to benefit most significantly from osseointegration have been those with a maladaptive denture experience. This truism has also led many denture adaptive patients "to trade in" their prosthesis for implant-supported fixed replacements. Consequently, this therapeutic option should be presented to every edentulous patient seeking prosthodontic treatment as an alternative option to complete dentures. Current research suggests that any patient whose systemic health does not preclude a minor oral surgical intervention and whose proposed host bone sites can quantitatively and qualitatively accommodate the dimensions of the dentist's selected implant system and the entailed surgical protocol, as well as afford the procedure's expense, may be regarded as a candidate for osseointegration.

A clinical assessment identical to the protocol articulated in this book's early chapters is carried out. The scrupulous clinical examination is augmented with diagnostic cast and previous prostheses' analysis (Box 28-1). It is then matched by a thorough imaging assessment. Usually, panoramic and cephalometric films provide enough informa-

tion to enable the dentist to determine where implants can be located (Figure 28-1). Occasionally, additional films such as tomograms or computerized tomograms (CAT scans) are requested. More sophisticated imaging techniques offer the surgeon additional information about potential sites for implant placement and may be beneficial in determining situations that are not conducive to implant placement unless bone grafts are placed prior to, or in conjunction with, the implants. The treatment decision is influenced by (1) the magnitude of residual ridge resorption; (2) the relationship to key anatomical landmarks: incisive foramen, nasal cavities, and maxillary sinuses in the maxilla and mental foramina and inferior alveolar canal in the mandible; and (3) the perceived quality of the proposed host bone sites. A validated and predictive classification system for bone quality and quantity that is tied to implant outcomes is still to be developed. However, clinical experience suggests that compromised bone quality and quantity may have an adverse impact on treatment outcomes. This appears to be a somewhat more compelling concern in the maxillary edentulous arch.

PRELIMINARY PROSTHODONTIC DESIGN

The decision to treat an edentulous arch with an implant-supported fixed prosthesis is influenced by the following five crucial considerations:

1. The *number* of the implant abutments. The early, albeit compellingly documented, clinical successes with implant-supported fixed

---

Box 28-1

Considerations for Systemic Local and Prosthodontic Treatment

Medical History Contraindicating Treatment

- Systemic condition that precludes a minor oral surgical procedure (e.g., brittle diabetic, blood dyscrasia, immunologically compromised)
- History of chemical dependency
- History of orofacial irradiation
- Certain psychiatric disorders
- Heavy smoking (possibly)

Local Considerations

- Size of oral opening and interarch space
- Status of opposing dentition, if present (periodontal health, overeruption, occlusal relations)
- Quality and quantity of proposed host sites, which also requires a radiographic evaluation
- Height of smile line (circumoral activity)

Prosthetic Considerations

- Possible shortcomings in appearance, occlusion, and support of previous dentures. Will the presence of implants rectify such problems?
- Relationship of prosthetic teeths' positions to underlying residual ridges. Will a fixed prosthesis resolve the perceived complaints entirely, or will excessive anterior and posterior cantilevering be required?
- Is the desired optimal position and support of the circumoral tissues compatible with the proposed prosthetic teeth placement and the location of the implants' support?

---

prostheses suggested a quasi-general formula: five implants placed between the mental foramina to support a 10- to 12-unit fixed mandibular prosthesis. However, this formula did not address considerations of arch form configuration (flat versus varying degrees of curvature), length of implants, length of cantilevers, and specific considerations regarding diverse occlusal forces plus the configuration of the implant/arch form. The same applies to treatment planning the maxilla, with the additional proviso that six or more implants should comprise a starting point for a fixed design.

2. The *location* of the implants. Implant location is more favorable when its distribution or configuration is a curved rather than a flat one. The former allows for more occlusal units and an optimal cantilever design. A flat implant arch form is probably a better candidate for an overdenture design.

3. The *quality* of the host sites. Clinical experience suggests that loosely textured cancellous bone makes for a potentially vulnerable osseointegrated response. Consequently, careful identification of optimal host site locators is essential, particularly because the loading capacity of individual implants is yet to be determined. The previously mentioned "formula" (five in the mandible, six in the maxilla) was gleaned from published and cumulative clinical experiences, and it has clearly yielded impressive treatment outcomes. Furthermore, current clinical wisdom has refined the formula aided by improved and enhanced technology, for example, self-threading implants with an oxidized surface, plus a range of implants of different lengths. It therefore appears prudent to continue to use a five-mandibular implant abutment design as a starting point for a fixed prosthesis. The length of the prosthetic cantilevers will depend on anticipated patient occlusal activity because most patients exhibit different degrees of magnitude, duration, and frequency of functional loading. However, the profession's current inability to accurately predict the outcome of implants in radiographically determined poor quality bone suggests a need for considerable caution when selecting such sites.

4. The *quantity* of the host bone sites or the amount of residual ridge reduction that has occurred. This is rarely a consideration in the mandible because mandibles measuring less than 10 mm in vertical height in the intermental foramina region are infrequently encountered. It is, however, a frequent problem in the maxilla, where grafting techniques may be required if a fixed prosthesis is planned. Alternative

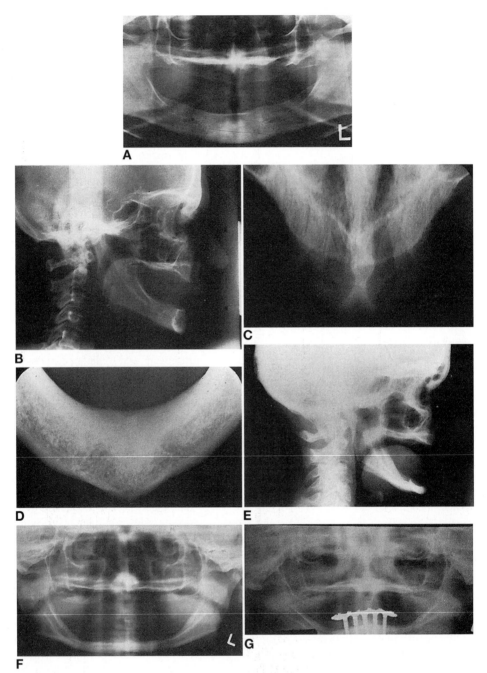

Figure 28-1   A comprehensive radiographic survey of edentulous jaws will enable the dentist to ensure the presence of a healthy host bone site compatible with both quality and quantity considerations. More than one view is necessary if a three-dimensional assessment is to be made (unless there is access to tomography). All three views—panoramic (**A**), cephalometric (**B**), and occlusal (**C** and **D**)—provide magnified dimensions of differing degrees. **E** and **F** are the specific preoperative films, and **G** is the postoperative film of the patient in Plate 1-1.

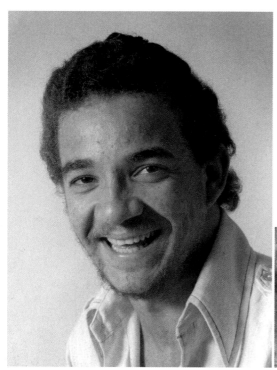
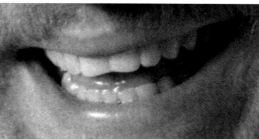

Plate 28-1   These two photographs were provided by a middle-aged patient who desired implant-supported fixed prostheses to replace his present complete maxillary denture and compromised residual mandibular dentition. This is the appearance the patient hoped to achieve after being fitted with his new prostheses. The photographs provide a very useful guide in helping to fulfill esthetic objectives (as described in Chapter 17).

Continued

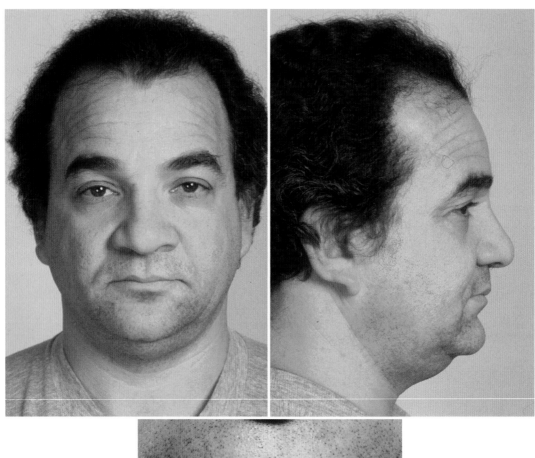

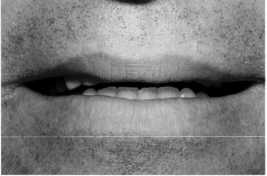

Plate 28-1 *cont'd* Frontal, profile, and circum-oral close-up views of the patient provide current evidence of the need for restoring the patient's desired esthetic appearance of his smile.

Continued

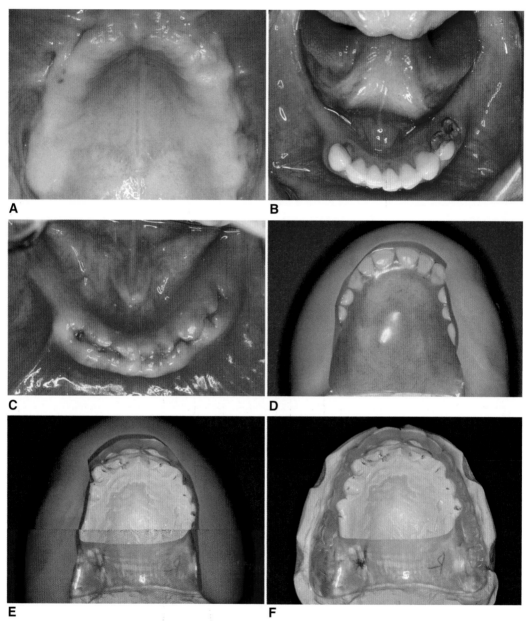

Plate 28-1 *cont'd* The sequence above illustrates the fitting surface appearance of the maxilla (**A**). Pre- and postextraction views of the mandibular supporting areas are shown in **B** and **C**. The recommended approach for a surgical guide's design is illustrated in **D, E,** and **F.** First, the approved set-up is indexed (**D**); then the teeth's positions are replicated in auto-polymerizing resin in the index (**E**). The completed surgical guide is now ready for sterilization and has been trimmed to permit stable seating during the surgical procedure and an easy accommodation of the necessary instrumentation (**F**). Such a surgical template guides the surgeon in optimal implant placement.

Continued

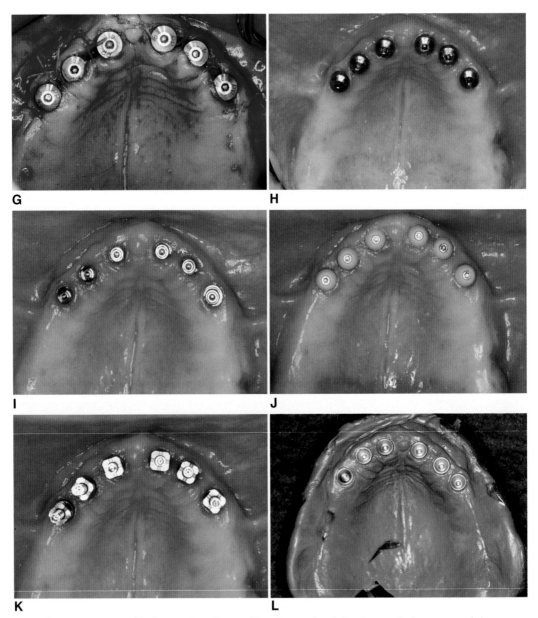

Plate 28-1 *cont'd* The creation of a maxillary impression following surgical exposure of the osseointegrated implants is illustrated in the sequence above. Healing abutments are placed at the second stage surgical procedure in **G,** and following a suitable healing period (**H**), they are fitted with the selected abutments (**I**) and protective plastic copings (**J**). The healing abutments are then fitted with transfer copings (**K**) for the final impression. The last illustration (**L**) shows the tissue surface of the impression in a custom tray, which incorporates the transfer copings.

Continued

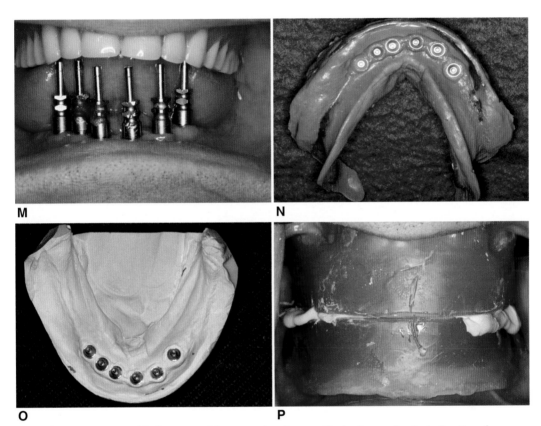

Plate 28-1 *cont'd* The protocol for managing the mandibular impression is similar. Transfer copings are attached to the selected abutments (**M**); the impression is registered (**N**) and poured in stone with laboratory implant analogues fitted into the transfer copings in the final impression (**N** and **O**). This provides for very stable "overdentured" occlusion rims and the making of jaw relation records (**P**) (see Chapter 15).

Continued

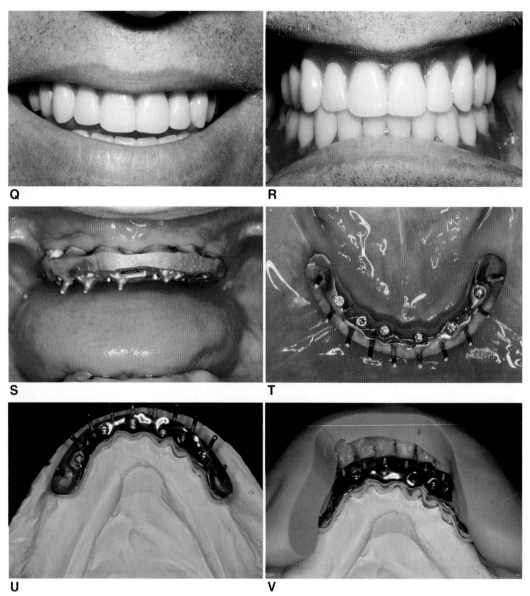

Plate 28-1 *cont'd* In **Q** and **R**, the sequence for ensuring an optimal esthetic try-in of the teeth arrangement is illustrated. Jaw relation records are next confirmed, and the laboratory phase of indexing the set-ups and using the index to design the frameworks in wax and then casting them in the selected metal is completed (**S** and **T**). In **U** and **V**, the silicone putty index is employed to confirm the relationship between the original "tried-in" teeth positions and the cast mandibular framework.

Continued

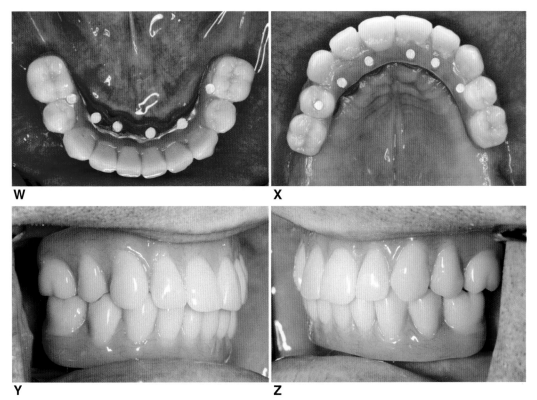

W   X

Y   Z

Plate 28-1 *cont'd* The processed prostheses are retained on the implants via screws and the access holes filled with a choice of one of several materials available for the purpose (**W** and **X**). Lateral views in **Y** and **Z** show shortened dental arch designs for this patient. This protocol has been thoroughly researched in all of its many phases and has yielded extraordinarily favorable and predictable results. It combines the traditional skills and techniques of complete denture fabrication with the availability of substitutes for tooth roots.

Continued

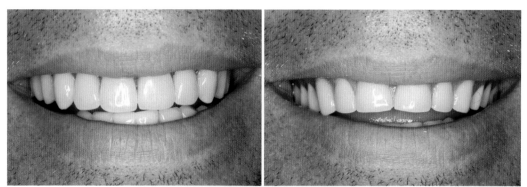

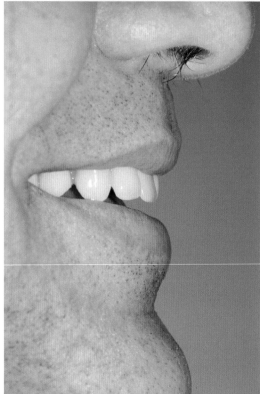

Plate 28-1 *cont'd* The subtleties of the patient's dental appearance are modified as demonstrated in the sequence of illustrations above. In this particular case, the patient's old photographs were used to meet the patient's expectations as suggested in Chapter 17.

surgical approaches include sinus lift procedures and consideration of placement of implants in the zygoma or pterygoid plates. Although both approaches offer exciting possibilities, there is still a lack of well-documented prospective studies to justify their routine prescription.

5. Amount of *circumoral activity* or "generosity" of a patient's smile line. This consideration applies almost exclusively to the maxilla, where both the combination of a high lip line and advanced residual ridge resorption, or conversely, virtually no resorption at all, may indicate challenging problems. The former will require the use of a visible labial flange to compensate for the resorbed tissues. The size and design of such a flange may preclude easy hygiene maintenance and therefore contraindicate a fixed prosthesis. As a rule, patients with extensive vertical and horizontal anterior maxillary bone resorption are candidates for implant-supported overdentures and not fixed prostheses. On the other hand, where little or no resorption is present, a high smile line is not readily reconcilable with ideal implant location and angulation, which lends itself to an optimal emergence profile for the prosthetic teeth. In such morphological situations, the implant abutments cannot be readily located in the anterior part of the maxilla, and, if feasible, are placed in the posterior zone.

PRESURGICAL TREATMENT

The patient is carefully counseled about the proposed treatment. The edentulous mouth is prepared for the osseointegration technique by ensuring tissue health, for example, correction of old prostheses and use of tissue conditioners. Soft and hard tissue lesions that may have an impact on the surgical phase of osseointegration (e.g., hyperplastic tissue, frena, and exostoses) usually are addressed during the surgical osseointegration operation. If there is inadequate bone, surgical procedures designed to generate new bone (so-called site development) may be considered. Once an appropriate site is established a surgical template is prepared, usually with the patient's currently worn prosthesis as a guide.

SURGICAL STAGE(S)

The surgical technique is well described in the dental literature and consists of a sterile procedure in which flaps are raised and holes are carefully and gently drilled into the selected host bone sites. The holes conform to the chosen implants' dimensions and accommodate the threaded tooth root analogues, which are frequently self-tapped into place. The reflected mucoperiosteal flaps are readapted to completely cover the implants if they are to be submerged and unloaded during the healing period. Note that the implants are provisionally sealed with a cover-screw during this interim healing period. This is referred to as the *two-stage surgical procedure*. Alternatively, the implants may be fitted with a "healing abutment" and the flaps readapted around them if the one-stage surgical procedure is selected. In either case, the soft tissues are sutured and the tissues left to heal undisturbed. During the 4- to 6-month healing period, the designated time required for osseointegration to occur in the mandible and maxilla, respectively, the denture is relieved liberally and a tissue conditioner used to refit the denture. When a second-stage surgery is required, transepithelial abutments of selected dimensions are attached to the implants and the prosthodontic procedures started.

PROSTHODONTIC PROTOCOL

The prosthodontic phase of treatment has as its objective the fabrication of a cast prosthesis base (metallic frame) that joins the implants together and provides distal cantilever extensions (Plate 28-1). Artificial teeth and a soft tissue analogue could then be processed onto the framework. This procedure allows for an electively removable prosthesis that could be screwed to the osseointegrated abutments. Other techniques have also been developed to allow the use of screw- or cement-retained metal ceramic prostheses. The discussion of such prostheses' construction is best left to publications that specifically discuss fabrication of implant-supported prosthesis.

The design of the prosthesis, borrowed from both fixed and removable prosthetic protocols, seeks to reconcile traditional principles of occlusion with optimal design for soft tissue health maintenance and esthetics. The clinical protocol used comprises the following stages:

1. Impressions are made in the dentist's material of choice (e.g., a polyether material in a custom tray). An occlusal opening provides access to transfer copings that are screwed to the abutments. The transfer copings are withdrawn in the impression and filled with laboratory analogues. The impression is then poured in artificial stone.
2. A trial denture base stabilized with two prosthetic copings is used to register jaw relation records. Subsequently, the same base is used for a trial arrangement of the artificial teeth. After patient approval and confirmation of jaw relation records, an index of the position of the artificial teeth is made.
3. The proposed framework is designed in the context of the teeth index positions and cast and then surrounded by processed acrylic resin. The metallic frames are cast in a silver-palladium alloy or a Class IV gold alloy. Alternatively, a titanium frame can be employed. The latter technique is currently regarded as being particularly accurate and, moreover, lends itself to employing porcelain for both teeth and soft tissue replacement. Framework design has gradually evolved into a standard that reconciles principles of fixed prosthodontic frame waxing protocols with a predetermined tooth orientation.
4. The framework is tried in the mouth, and where an imperfect or nonpassive fit is noted, the framework is severed. It is reassembled on the implants with the retaining screws and an index and returned to the laboratory for soldering. The soldered, reassembled framework is tried again in the mouth.
5. Processing of the metallic framework and the stock acrylic resin teeth is completed with a commercial acrylic resin; complete denture laboratory technology is used.
6. The completed prosthesis is inserted in the mouth, new jaw relation records are made, and the occlusion is refined on the articulator.

Box 28-2

A Comparison between Presumed Advantages and Disadvantages of the Three Current Therapies Available for Edentulous Patients

Complete Dentures
- Relatively straightforward to fabricate
- Virtually universal in application
- Inexpensive
- A preliminary option for first-time denture wearers
- All the shortcomings of artificial removable prostheses: psychological, tissue morbidity, risk of time-dependent maladaptation
- Lifelong maintenance

Implant-Supported Fixed Prostheses
- Conceptually brilliant and supported by compelling research data
- Limited in application
- Relatively complex to undertake
- Expensive
- Enormous psychological and functional benefits
- A "cure" for patients with maladaptive dentures

- Esthetic outcomes may be difficult and unpredictable
- Maintenance not always easy
- Size of occlusal table has to be reduced

Implant-Supported Overdentures
- Stability, retention, and esthetic problems are readily rectified
- A "cure" for patients with maladaptive dentures without the disadvantages of the fixed approach
- Professional fees are not significantly higher than cost of complete dentures
- Maintenance requirements do not appear to be demanding
- Exhibit minor movement during function and likely to accumulate food debris under the dentures' fitting surface
- Size of occlusal table can be maximized

Each patient is counseled about tissue and prosthesis care. Thereafter, a protocol for annual patient recall is followed.

SUMMARY

The availability of a fixed treatment option is a remarkable advance in prosthodontics. It is one of dentistry's most gratifying treatment modalities, but it demands considerable skill and judgment and a high degree of patient commitment and understanding. It also is quite expensive and comprises very strict inclusion and exclusion criteria as gleaned from this chapter and Chapter 27. A comparison between conventional dentures, implant-supported fixed prostheses, and overdenture treatments will help put these options in perspective (Box 28-2).

Bibliography

Adell L, Lekholm U, Rockler B et al: A 15-year study of osseointegrated implants in the treatment of the edentulous jaw, *Int J Oral Surg* 10:387-416, 1981.

Brånemark PI, Zarb GA, Albrektsson T: *Tissue integrated prostheses: osseointegration in clinical dentistry,* Chicago, 1985, Quintessence.

Brunski, JB: Avoid pitfalls of overloading and micromotion of intraosseous implants (interview), *Dent Implantol Update* 4:77-81, 1993.

Desjardins RP: Implants for the edentulous patient, *Dent Clin North Am* 40:195-215, 1996.

Henry PJ, Tan AE, Uzawa S: Fit discrimination of implant-supported fixed partial dentures fabricated from implant level impressions made at stage I surgery, *J Prosthet Dent* 77:265-270, 1997.

Jemt T: In vivo measurements of precision of fit involving implant-supported prostheses in the edentulous jaw, *Int J Oral Maxillofac Implants* 11:151-158, 1996.

Jemt T, Book K: Prosthesis misfit and marginal bone loss in edentulous implant patients, *Int J Oral Maxillofac Implants* 11:620-625, 1996.

Krekmanov L, Kahn M, Rangert B et al: Tilting of posterior mandibular and maxillary implants for improved prosthesis support, *Int J Oral Maxillofac Implants* 15:405-414, 2000.

Rangert B: Biomechanics of the Brånemark system, *Aust Prosthodont J* 9(suppl):39-48, 1995.

Rangert B, Krogh PH, Langer B et al: Bending overload and implant fracture: a retrospective clinical analysis, *Int J Oral Maxillofac Implants* 10:326-334, 1995.

Rangert B, Sennerby L, Meredith N et al: Design, maintenance and biomechanical considerations in implant placement, *Dent Update* 24:416-420, 1997.

Skalak R: Biomechanical considerations in osseointegrated prostheses, *J Prosthet Dent* 49:843-848, 1983.

White GE: *Osseointegrated dental technology,* Chicago, 1993, Quintessence.

Zarb GA, Schmitt A: The longitudinal clinical effectiveness of osseointegrated implants: the Toronto study. Part I: Surgical results, *J Prosthet Dent* 63:451-457, 1990a.

Zarb GA, Schmitt A: The longitudinal clinical effectiveness of osseointegrated implants: the Toronto study. Part II: The prosthetic results, J Prosthet Dent 64:53-61, 1990b.

Zarb GA, Schmitt A: The edentulous predicament. I. A prospective study on the effectiveness of implant-supported fixed prostheses, *J Am Dent Assoc* 127:59-65, 1996.

CHAPTER 29

Managing Problems and Complications

George A. Zarb, Steven E. Eckert

Active treatment with osseointegrated implants usually spans a period of several months, and it is possible that problems or complications may occur at any time during this phase of treatment. Though insertion of the finished prosthesis marks the end of active treatment, follow-up maintenance and monitoring of the prosthesis, the implants, and the host tissue's response must continue for the life of the patient (Table 29-1).

The dental implant field is inundated with a variety of techniques, designs and, of course, manufacturers' claims. In looking at this broad field the dentist is often confused by the different approaches used to place and restore dental implants. Likewise, the complications that can occur with dental implants seem to be quite varied.

An alternative to evaluation of the differences is to discuss the similarities among bone-anchored implants. All endosseous implants are placed in a surgical procedure, all must be made of a material that is biocompatible and possesses favorable physical and mechanical properties to function as retentive and supporting mechanisms for dental prostheses, and all must undergo a healing process to ensure long-term survival. Although there are variations on surgical techniques and implant materials, these differences are generally minor. The required implant healing interval before occlusal loading, however, can and often does show greater variety.

Implants that are designed to heal to the jawbone may do so after a period of no mechanical trauma. This remains the classic approach used to achieve osseointegration and requires a period of undistributed implant placement beneath the oral mucosa for 3 to 4 months in the mandible and 6 months in the maxilla. At the end of that healing period the second stage of treatment begins, during which the mucosa covering the implant is surgically resected and transmucosal components are connected to the implant. This is the two-stage approach to implant surgery. In contrast to this procedure, some implants are placed in such a way as to allow an attached healing abutment to pass through the oral mucosa at the first stage of treatment. Because there is no mucosa covering the implant, there is no stage II surgery; thus this process is known as a *one-stage approach*. In both situations, efforts are made to avoid functional loading of the implant until the bone has a chance to heal adjacent to the implant and ensure an osseointegrated response.

There is also a current and renewed enthusiasm for the concept of immediate implant loading. This approach uses a rigid connection of implants shortly after their placement within the jaw. Such rigid implant fixation allows the implants to be used to support a prosthesis almost immediately after stage I surgery. These implants are called *immediate load implants*. In another approach, implants are placed as freestanding supporting mechanisms for provisional individual dental prostheses. These single implants are generally not connected to teeth or to other implants but are used to retain provisional restorations that are placed in cosmetic, but not functional load, conditions. This approach is referred to as of an *immediate provisional* implant.

Although it seems that there are many different approaches to implant use, careful scrutiny of the different procedures demonstrates a number of similarities. In the one-stage, two-stage, immediate load, and immediate provisional implant approach there is a period during which the implant must be

Table 29-1
Possible Problems and Complications

Time	Description
Stage I surgery	• Unfavorable implant position/alignment
Post–stage I surgery	• Swelling/ecchymosis
	• Infection
	• Suture remnants, wound dehiscence
	• Neuropathy
Stage II surgery	• Failure to osseointegrate
	• Unfavorable position or angle makes implant unusable
Postprosthodontic insertion	• Prosthodontic complications
	• Soft tissue complications
Delayed complications	• Delayed loss of osseointegration
	• Component fracture
	• Soft tissue complication

protected from functional loading. The first two approaches address this protection by avoiding force transmission to the implant during the early phases of healing. The immediate load approach splints the implants to each other thereby creating a rigid body that is relatively resistant to movement. In the immediate provisional implant therapy the implant is placed under minimal functional load with the assumption that this load will not displace the implant sufficiently to interfere with bone-to-implant healing. Without bone-to-implant healing the long-term survival of the implant is unlikely to occur because the process of osseointegration will be compromised or prevented. This complication, failure to achieve or maintain osseointegration is regarded as the most crucial problem in implant dentistry.

There are numerous ways to categorize the possible complications that can be encountered. They may be referred to as early or late, surgical or prosthodontic, biological or structural, functional or esthetic, or hard tissue or soft tissue related. In this chapter, they are divided under the main headings of surgical or prosthodontic origin. This categorization relates to the phase of treatment rather than the specific type of complication that is encountered. However, it must be emphasized that

complications in one area may affect the other, and, consequently, at times there is no clear differentiation between them.

SURGICALLY RELATED COMPLICATIONS

Endosseous implant surgery can be described as a one- or a two-stage procedure. Both techniques demand placement of the implant within the selected host bone site with a meticulous surgical procedure. A two-stage implant is placed in a position that allows the oral mucosa to be closed primarily over the implant, whereas a one-stage implant is one that passes through the mucosa. Both approaches require primary closure of the oral tissues in the interimplant spaces. Likewise, both techniques require a period of undisturbed healing before the implant can be placed into function.

Surgically related problems can, in turn, be subdivided into chronological order: those related to stage I surgery, to the osseointegration time between the operations, and to stage II surgery. The surgeon will primarily deal with these occurrences; however, it is often the dentist, having made the original diagnosis and treatment plan for the patient, who will be consulted when a problem arises. As the prescribing and referring dentist, the patient's closest association is with him or her. The prescribing dentist must therefore be regarded as that treatment plan's architect and should be aware of the possible complications that may occur during this early phase of treatment. The dentist also should be prepared to deal with the patient's apprehensions and concerns and to make necessary referrals to the surgeon.

Stage I

Any surgical procedure carries with it the risk of bleeding, infection, swelling, and ecchymosis, and surgery for the placement of osseointegrated implants is no exception. A meticulous sterile surgical technique, accompanied with appropriate antibiotic prescription and instruction to the patient regarding hygiene and oral rinses, is the best preventive measure to reduce the chances of these sequelae. Excessive bleeding, if it occurs, is usually noted at the time of surgery or soon after. If observed, excessive bleeding is treated by the surgeon. Swelling is often not at its peak until at least the second day after surgery, but the measures necessary to minimize it must be taken immediately after the surgical procedure. These include the application of pressure packs in the form of rolled sterile gauze and the use of cold compresses or ice packs. A transient and therefore insignificant ecchymosis is also delayed in its appearance and is most likely to occur in patients who have a history of bruising easily. Good preparation and tutoring of the patient will make it easier for him or her to accept this temporary but unfortunate esthetic appearance.

Infection, if it does occur, may be evident within a few days of the surgical insertion of the implants, or it may not be manifested until a few weeks or even a few months afterward. If it is soon after stage I surgery, it will most probably be noted by the surgeon first and treated with a regimen of antibiotic medication. If it is delayed, the patient may consult the referring dentist with a complaint of discomfort or soreness under the prosthesis. In such instances, there will likely be redness and swelling, and in some cases the infection will be accompanied by an exudate. Referral to the surgeon for debridement and cleansing of the site and antibiotic therapy should be done without delay.

Suture removal is sometimes not complete because of swelling or inaccessibility of the suture remnants. It usually is seen as a localized redness or swelling and results in the patient experiencing discomfort when wearing the denture. This mucosal irritation, sometimes mimicking infection, often is ongoing until the offending suture is removed.

Occasionally, especially when there is significant tugging on the sutures through movements of the circumoral muscles or if the sutures loosen early, the incision will reopen. If this occurs within a few days of stage I surgery, the surgeon may choose to close the wound with new sutures. If it occurs later, after the deeper layers of the wound have begun to close, the surgeon is unlikely to resuture choosing to monitor the wound and request that the reinsertion of the denture be delayed 1 to 2 weeks.

In rare instances, damage to the inferior alveolar nerve may occur through a crushing injury during the degloving procedures, or it may occur because of violation of the canal or nerve by the surgical instruments or by the implant itself. With appropriate imaging techniques, paying attention to the details of the anatomy of the surgical field revealed in these images and careful instrumentation will decrease the incidence of this complication. In most instances, the altered sensation will be transient, though the transient time may vary from a few days to several months. If damage to the nerve has been severe, it may be permanent.

At stage I surgery, even when the most advanced imaging techniques are used, unexpected bony morphological deficits or poor bone quality may preclude ideal implant position, angulation, or the number of implants placed. This has obvious repercussions on the final prosthetic design and may lead to a decision to change the prosthodontic prescription. If a fixed prosthesis was originally prescribed, unfavorable implant angle or position could demand a change to a removable prosthesis. Unfavorable implant position or angulation could require change to a different retaining mechanism for an overdenture if a removable prosthesis was initially prescribed. It will sometimes lead to a decision to abort the surgery if it appears that not enough implants can be placed to support an implant-retained prosthesis. The resolution of this complication is covered in other chapters of this book.

Interval between Stage I and Stage II

It is usual for patients to be requested to refrain from wearing their existing prostheses for a short time after implant insertion. At the end of this period, the tissue surface of the denture is relieved sufficiently to allow for the placement of a tissue conditioner or temporary lining at least 1 to 2 mm thick in the region of the implants. An existing denture that is of minimal thickness may be perforated during this reduction unless it is made thicker by the addition of acrylic resin to its polished surface beforehand. Because the surgical incision may be found in the labial vestibule, final resolution of the swelling in the site often is not complete at 2 weeks after surgery. In this situation, it is usually necessary to trim several millimeters from the length of the labial flange to prevent patient discomfort and stress on the incision site. This is true in either arch.

Between the stages of the treatment, the soft liner or tissue conditioner that has been applied to the tissue surface of the denture should be kept in good condition. Doing so will eliminate possible ulcerations caused by the rough and hard flanges of the dentures that develop as the soft liner ages. Soft liners that are old and rough also present a good medium for increased bacterial growth. Keeping the soft liner in good condition can be accomplished either by replacing it every 4 to 5 weeks or by treating the temporary liner and especially the seam between the soft liner and the denture base with a sealant that can be made up using an autopolymerizing acrylic resin powder and a solvent such as 1-1-1 trichloroethane (Box 29-1).

After the sutures are removed and the initial soft tissue swelling has reduced, dehiscence of the cover screw of the implant through the mucosal covering may occur. Experience with one-stage implants demonstrates that implant exposure is not a threat to the success of the implant as long as the site is kept clean. The patient may experience discomfort if the dehiscence of the cover screw is not complete and there is still mucosa partially covering the screw. This tissue can be pinched between the cover screw and the denture base. It can be alleviated by trimming back the soft liner that has been applied to the tissue surface of the denture, thus allowing clearance in the area and preventing the pinching effect.

Box 29-1

Recipe for Varnish for Tissue Conditioner

50 ml 1-1-1 trichloroethane
2 ml autopolymerizing acrylic resin powder
Using a glass bottle with a tightly closing lid, add the autopolymerizing acrylic resin powder to the trichloroethane solvent. This will take a few hours to dissolve completely. The resulting solution should be as viscous as glycerine. If it is found that it is too thick, add solvent; if it is too thin, add powder.
A small amount should be dispensed into a plastic medicine cup and applied to the entire surface of the tissue conditioner, paying special attention to the seam between the denture base and the tissue conditioner.

If a dehiscence occurs where an osteopromotive membrane has been used, this site should be monitored very carefully by the referring dentist and the surgeon. The denture base acrylic resin should be reduced more aggressively in the area to allow an extra thickness of tissue conditioner in an effort to eliminate any possibility of pressure from the denture causing an increase in the size of the dehiscence. The patient should be instructed to keep the site meticulously clean. Antibacterial rinses may prove beneficial. At the first sign of infection, the membrane should preferably be removed.

The time interval between the two surgical procedures often is difficult for the patient because stage I surgery is a major event, and after initial healing, an expected improvement in the denture-wearing experience seems logical. It is important to stress to the patient beforehand that it will not be any easier to wear the denture during the osseointegration phase of treatment and that it may even be a little more difficult. It seems far easier for a patient to deal with this realization if informed before trying to deal with a difficult situation between the surgeries.

Stage II

Stage II surgery usually reveals whether an implant has osseointegrated. There are times, however, when failure to osseointegrate is not detected until the further instrumentation involved in the impression making or even the insertion of the prosthesis itself. If an implant is found to be mobile or tender to percussion or to the stresses of attaching the abutment to it, it should be removed. Experience shows that leaving it in place, with or without antibiotic therapy, will not result in a failed implant becoming osseointegrated. It will merely delay definitive treatment and could result in the development of a larger bone defect (Figure 29-1).

At stage II surgery, the cover screw that protected the internal threads of the implant is removed and replaced with a transmucosal abutment and center screw or with a healing abutment. If the regular abutment is attached at this time, it is important to ensure that the hexagonal female portion of the abutment and the hexagonal male portion of the implant are properly aligned. If this is not the case, there may be a soft tissue reaction or loosening of the compo-

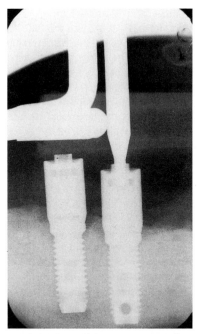

Figure 29-1 The radiolucency surrounding the implant on the left of the radiograph is indicative of an implant that has not osseointegrated. The implant was mobile, and the patient reported mild discomfort when it was tapped. On the right of the radiograph is an implant that has successfully osseointegrated and has no accompanying symptoms or signs of failure.

nents. This particular complication does not occur with the use of the healing abutment because there is no internal hexagon to engage the one at the top of the implant. The healing abutment does, however, seem to have an increased tendency to loosen. Thus care should be taken to tighten it securely to the implant, and the patient should be advised to seek attention immediately if loosening does occur.

Some of the complications encountered at stage I surgery become apparent only at stage II surgery when the implants are uncovered and the abutments are connected. This is especially true of implants that have an unfortunate buccal or lingual inclination or that are spaced too closely. If it is obvious at the time of uncovering that the spacing or the alignment will make it impossible to use the implant to support a prosthesis, the implant may be recovered or "put to sleep" during the surgical procedure.

PROSTHODONTIC-RELATED COMPLICATIONS

One of the earliest complications that can occur after stage II surgery and before prosthesis insertion is loosening of the abutment, whether it is an abutment with a center screw or a healing abutment. This results in an inflamed and painful soft tissue reaction as the soft tissue grows into the space between the components and is pinched each time the patient occludes. Though it can happen with any type of abutment, it seems to occur most frequently with healing abutments. When loosening of the abutment or healing abutment is noted, it is important to evaluate the superior surface of the implant to ensure that there is no soft or hard tissue covering the implant platform. Bone on the implant platform can prevent full seating of the abutment, which will in turn result in component malalignment and a tendency toward increased incidence of component loosening. To reduce this occurrence and to streamline the prosthodontic appointments, the surgeon should leave the chosen final abutments attached to the implants after the final impression for the prosthesis has been made. The top of the abutments should be protected against damage with appropriate healing caps. It must be emphasized that abutments can be damaged from contact with opposing teeth and overlying hard material in the provisional removable prosthesis.

Either immediately after stage II surgery or, if preferred, the week after, the tissue conditioner or the soft liner that had been placed into the patient's existing denture after stage I surgery is removed. The position of the abutments attached to the implants is transferred to the denture with an indelible marker guide, and then the denture is adjusted to allow for a thickness of soft liner above the abutments. Occasionally, the dentist will find that the abutments emerge outside of the borders of the denture, and then either the denture base must be enlarged by the addition of autopolymerizing resin or a change to a very short healing abutment, or to an angled abutment is made.

Selecting the correct height of the abutment is not always an easy procedure because there is usually some swelling present even after stage II surgery. If the selected abutment is too short, the mucosal swelling may lead to the tissue growing over the top of the abutment or healing cap, thereby allowing it to be pinched between the abutment and the relined denture base (Figure 29-2). If too long an abutment is selected, it will be difficult to seat the denture completely without perforating the denture base to make room for the height of the abutment. If the denture is not adjusted sufficiently, the denture base will not be properly seated, and the result will be an opening of the vertical dimension. In some cases, the patient will be able to cope with this increased height; in others, the resulting vertical dimension will be both esthetically and functionally so altered that the patient cannot or will not manage. In all of these scenarios, the problem can be solved by changing the length of the abutments.

The stage I surgical complication of insufficient bone to allow ideal implant position and inclination becomes most apparent at the time of prosthesis fabrication. Once the esthetic and functional try-in of the tooth arrangement has been accomplished and an index of the tooth arrangement has been made, discrepancies between the ideal location and angulation of the implants and the actual location and angulation become evident. Implant manufacturers have been ingenious in their design of components to deal with these situations, but the basic problem remains. Implants that will not be axially loaded by the forces of occlusion may be adversely affected. In that event, steps will have to be taken to reduce to a minimum the magnitude of these forces, either by changing the prescription to a removable prosthesis or by narrowing the occlusal table or by shortening the potential cantilever arms.

Implants that are too close together will make it very difficult for patients with a fixed prosthesis to carry out oral hygiene procedures (Figure 29-3). In the case of the overdenture, implants that are very close together do not leave space for the ideal 1 cm plus length of bar and clip, and when implants are closer than 3 mm, it is difficult to use standard ball attachments. Recent introduction of the smaller ball attachments with gold alloy or titanium keepers has helped to deal with this complication.

Impression

Obtaining an accurate impression for an implant-supported prosthesis is made relatively routine because of the nature of the fit of the impression hardware that has been developed. There are, however, a few complications that may occur. If the implants are close together and also are converging, the impression copings may interfere with each other. If their bulk is not reduced to eliminate

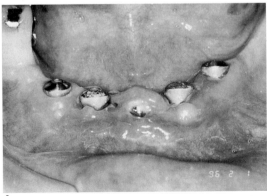 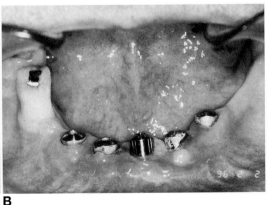

A **B**

Figure 29-2   One week after stage II surgery, the healing abutment, which was attached to the center implant, is partially covered by mucosa. The patient reported acute pain and discomfort as the covering tissue was pinched during wear of his denture (**A**). Replacement of the shorter healing abutment with a longer one eliminated the discomfort and allowed the inflamed mucosa to heal (**B**).

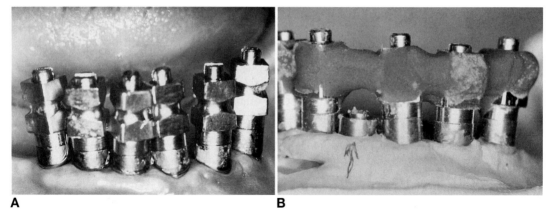

A

B

Figure 29-3 Six implants were inserted into this edentulous mandible where five implants would have been ideal. The proximity of the implants results in a restriction of space for the prosthetic cylinders and difficulty and discomfort in carrying out hygiene procedures (**A**). For the problem to be fixed, the implant marked by the arrow is scheduled to have its abutment removed and to be re-covered with mucosa (**B**).

this contact, the impression is likely to be inaccurate. If there are widely diverging implants, there may be a problem in seating the impression tray over the impression copings and laboratory pins. Impressions will not be accurate if the hexagon of the abutments and the implants are not properly aligned and tightened before the impression is made. It may be prudent to confirm seating of the components with periapical radiographs immediately before making the impression. Radiographs taken by the surgeon after stage II surgery are insufficient for this purpose because abutment screws may have loosened in the interim. Periapical films are suggested because panoramic films will not always reveal problems with the fit of the component parts due to variations of the angles of the implants. If there is even a moderate labial or lingual inclination of the implant, an unseated abutment may not be noted in a panoramic film.

Even if the preceding precautions are taken, there are times when impressions will not be accurate. We recommend fabrication of a confirmation jig, which can be made by attaching impression copings to the abutment analogues on the master cast and then luting them together with acrylic resin or a light-cured material. The jig must be rigid to allow its use in confirming accuracy. For this reason there must be sufficient bulk of acrylic or composite material to ensure rigidity. This jig can

then be used to assess the accuracy of the master model obtained from the original impression. If it does not go into place passively when screwed to the implants in the mouth, the jig can be severed at the offending connection, the sections seated and screwed to the abutments in the mouth, and the parts luted together. The altered jig allows for correction of the master model by drilling out the abutment analogue that was not in the proper place, attaching a new abutment analogue to the impression coping in the jig, and adding new dental stone to secure it. This resulting "altered cast" is then used for fabricating the framework.

Try-in of Tooth Arrangement

At this stage of try-in of the tooth arrangement, the effects of possible compromises made at stage I surgery become evident. Unfortunate inclination or location of implants, whether due to anatomical deficits of the host bone or to operator misjudgment, may make it necessary either to revise the prosthodontic prescription or to use alternate hardware components. A frequent example in the maxillary arch is one or more labially angled implants. An angled abutment will have to be used to avoid having the gold alloy–retaining screw exiting from the labial surface of the prosthetic tooth. This corrects the esthetic concerns, but it does not correct for the nonaxial loading to which the implant will be subjected during function.

As a result of trying to attain both an esthetically pleasing and functionally adequate tooth arrangement, it may become evident that an originally planned fixed prosthetic design will have to be altered to a removable design (e.g., an overdenture). Examples of such cases are implants that have had to be placed in a straight line across the front of the mandible and significant labiolingual discrepancies between the maxillary and mandibular arches.

Framework Try-in

Producing a framework for a fixed implant prosthesis involves several complex laboratory procedures, and occasionally the result is a framework that does not fit passively in the mouth. Sometimes this is visible to the operator; sometimes it is noted only by a response from the patient. This response is most often a small wincing response by the patient or a report of tightness that is alleviated when the "offending" screw(s) is loosened slightly. If either occurs, the framework is severed between the segments that appear to fit passively but are clearly not doing so. Sometimes this will necessitate severing in more than one site to ensure that there is no stress on the components as they are screwed into place. Once it is established that the components fit completely and passively, they are luted together in the mouth with autopolymerizing resin or light-cured composite, and the master model is altered accordingly, as previously described. Then the casting is reassembled through corrective soldering by the laboratory, and a second try-in appointment is scheduled.

Though a nonfitting framework is more likely to occur when there are several abutments being joined together, there also can be discrepancies with bars joining as few as two abutments, especially if the implants diverge significantly from each other.

INSERTION OF PROSTHESIS

Implant-Supported Fixed Prosthesis

Some complications can occur either at the time of or immediately after insertion of the fixed implant-supported prosthesis. A few patients will note masticatory muscle strain and fatigue during the first weeks of wearing a mandibular prosthesis. Counseling the patient to avoid stressing the previously relatively inactive muscles of mastication by initially cutting food into smaller pieces and gradually working up to normal chewing usually resolves this problem. The presence of stable dental prostheses may encourage more rapid chewing, which could result in increased risk of cheek or tongue chewing. Just as counseling is needed to avoid stress to the musculature, patients may benefit from the suggestion that they chew slowly until they are accustomed to their new prostheses.

Potential esthetic problems are hopefully dealt with at the tooth try-in stage of prosthesis construction. The situation is similar to the protocol followed in complete denture fabrication. It must be emphasized, however, that after final insertion, esthetic changes, although feasible, may be more awkward and tedious to be carried out after final processing is complete.

Initial difficulties with speech may be anticipated with a maxillary fixed prosthesis, especially if there is a large difference between the location of the implants and the incisal edges of the prosthetic teeth. The bulk of the prosthesis necessary to reach forward from the implant abutments to the prosthetic teeth can interfere with the tongue during normal speech. Though this problem usually resolves within a few days as the patient's tongue learns to cope, some patients find it necessary to wear an obturator for several months, and very few will wear it indefinitely.

The incidence of speech problems also is increased if the patient's circumoral muscle activity easily reveals maxillary gingival tissue. In these situations, when the upper lip retracts during speech, it will not form an air seal, and there will be a resulting "shshsh" when making the *s* sounds. When there is a high lip line, it may be necessary to add a flange to the prosthesis for speech and esthetics as well. Though the flange solves these problems, it has the potential for creating other problems because oral hygiene is made more difficult.

Implant-Supported Overdenture

Insertion of the implant-supported overdenture is sometimes complicated by the necessity to accommodate both the soft tissue anatomy of the posterior part of the mouth and the implant abutment and hardware connection in the anterior. It may be necessary to remove the otherwise useful extensions into the retromylohyoid space to completely seat the overdenture.

Some patients with implant overdentures find that food will collect under the anterior part of the denture, whether it be retained by a bar and clip assembly or by ball attachments. This is due partly to the relatively inaccurate impression of the anatomy here (remember that the impression tray had to be made wider than usual in this area to accommodate the impression copings and was therefore too wide to achieve an accurate impression of mucosa) and partly to the block-out around the retention hardware that was done before the final processing. A chairside addition of an autopolymerizing acrylic resin to the lingual and labial flanges in this area usually solves this problem.

If a bar and clip assembly is used, the clip may make it very difficult to remove the overdenture, unless it is loosened slightly before the first insertion. It can easily be tightened after the other usual procedures of insertion of a complete denture are completed.

In the first days after insertion of the overdenture, the patient may experience minor denture irritations under the soft tissue–supported area of the prosthesis. This is corrected as the denture is relieved and adjusted in the customary fashion.

POSTINSERTION

During the years of prosthesis wear, there are a number of possible complications that may occur. Some of these are common to both fixed and removable prostheses, whereas others are more specific. The complications fall under the broad headings of biological and prosthodontic mechanical ones (Table 29-2).

Biological complications include failure or loss of integration and soft and hard tissue complications. Because osseointegration appears to result from an induced and controlled healing response, it is not surprising that three fourths or more of all reported implant failures occur during the early healing phase. The remaining failures occur after occlusal loading takes place and are in all likeli-

Table 29-2
Prosthodontic Problems and Complications

Type	Description
Structural	Prosthesis fracture
	Fracture of prosthesis retaining screw
	Fracture of abutment screw
	Fracture of implant
Cosmetic	As perceived by patient and dentist
Functional	Speech problems
	Transient muscle discomfort or temporomandibular disorders

hood caused by an inadequate healing response becoming compromised by subsequent loading demands. Meticulous treatment planning addresses the remote possibility of the small, if inevitable, failures. This will ensure successful prosthodontic treatment outcomes even when fewer implants than hoped for actually osseointegrated. The obvious example would be the conversion of a proposed five-unit fixed prostheses to a two- or three-unit overdenture if two or three implants should fail. Soft and hard tissue problems are also encountered and are a source of some controversy. A periodontic type of mindset considers such changes as a version of periodontal diseaselike sequelae. On the other hand, several researchers, including this book's editors, argue for a mechanical and microbiological cause that challenges the implant's surrounding gingival tissues rather than its ankylotic-like attachment.

Structural

All of the three levels of components of the completed implant-retained system are subjected to repeated stresses of occlusal and parafunctional loading, and it is possible for these stresses to cause fractures of any of these components: the prosthetic retaining screw, the abutment screw, or the implant itself (Figure 29-4). Most common is the fracture of the gold alloy screw, usually at the base of the head of the screw. If the top of the threaded area is accessible, the screw fragment can be removed by carefully touching the outside of the top of the fractured piece, which is remaining in the center screw of the abutment, with a tapered fissure bur in either a slow-speed handpiece or a high-speed handpiece running at very low speed. Another approach is to use a hemostat to grasp the screw fragment and to turn it counterclockwise to remove the screw. If the screw is fractured beneath the top of the abutment, it may be teased out by engaging the top of the screw with an explorer and rotating the explorer tip in a counterclockwise direction. If this proves diffi-cult or if the screw fragment cannot be reached, the entire abutment and center screw can be removed, and the gold alloy screw can then be retrieved on the bench rather than in the patient's mouth.

Cementing a fixed prosthesis would of course preclude fracture of retaining screws, but loosening of the restoration can occur. Cementation is a pop-

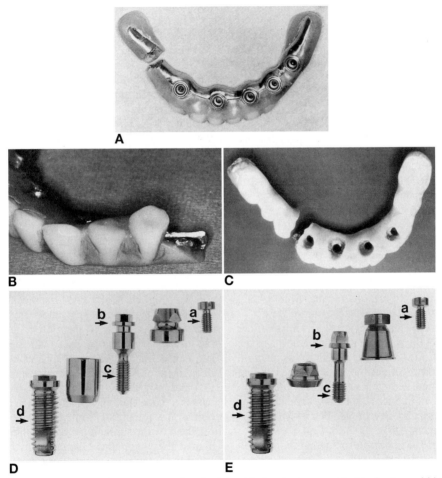

Figure 29-4 Prostheses supported and retained by implants are subject to fracture within the metallic framework (**A**), or the esthetic facing (**B**), or both (**C**). Component fractures are possible at each of the levels of the implant-retained system, whether it be with the original regular tube-shaped abutments (**D**) or with the currently used conical abutments (**E**). The component most likely to fracture is the gold alloy prosthesis retaining screw *a*. The abutment-retaining screw can fail at the head of the screw *b* or at the level of the threaded area *c*, which usually is well within the implant itself. Fracture of the implant *d* is rare, possibly because of the protective nature of the retaining components above it.

Continued

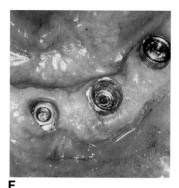

F

Figure 29-4 *cont'd* The clinical photograph
(F) shows two implants with attached abutments. The
abutment-retaining screw in the implant on the right is
intact, whereas the head of the retaining screw in the
middle implant is fractured. On the left of this photograph, the abutment is off because its retaining screw
has fractured at the threaded area, thus illuminating the
retaining function of the screw. Retrieval of an abutment
screw that has fractured within an implant must be done
with great care to avoid damage to the interior threaded
portion of the implant.

ular retentive approach in many clinical circles
because it is presumed to be more "user friendly." It is
argued that fixed prostheses can be easily recemented
when natural teeth are used as abutments. However,
screw-retained prostheses are electively and easily
removable, which we regard as a plus from a long-
term monitoring and maintenance point of view.

Fracture of the abutment screw can occur either
at the level of the hexagonal top portion or at the
spindle or threaded area deep within the implant. In
the case of the fractured hexagonal top, removal
can be accomplished with a tapered fissure bur to
create a slot into which a standard screwdriver is
fitted. The center screw can then be easily reversed
out of the implant.

Removal of an abutment screw that is fractured
farther down its length is more difficult, and great
care must be taken to avoid damaging the internal
threads of the implant. The use of an explorer to
tease the screw out of its seat is described in the
previous paragraph. An abutment screw retrieval or
rescue kit is available to use in cases where removal
is more difficult. The kit contains an end-cutting
tool that grasps the top of the fractured component
when pressure is applied. It is then rotated counter-

clockwise to remove the screw fragment from the
implant. Often this procedure is not as easily
accomplished as this description suggests, especially if the abutment screw fragment seems to
have bonded itself to the interior of the implant.
Another approach is to very carefully prepare a
"well" at the top of the screw fragment with a small
round bur (accompanied by generous irrigation)
and then to use a larger round bur, held either in a
handheld torque driver or in the cutting tool holder
provided in the retrieval kit. The larger round bur is
pressed onto the prepared top surface of the screw
and turned counterclockwise to remove it.

Removal can be further complicated by soft tissue overgrowth or collapse into the space immediately above the implant. Not only does this prevent
a clear view of the top of the fractured abutment,
but also there is often some bleeding because
with a fractured retaining component, the implant-
supported bridge usually is mobile and pinches the
mucosa, causing it to become inflamed.

The instrumentation involved in an attempt to
remove the broken abutment screw must be used
with extreme care to avoid damage to the threads in
the interior of the implant. If the internal threads of
the implant have been damaged, it will be difficult
to insert the replacement abutment screw. In such a
case, the fixture tap, also included in the kit, can
then be used to repair the threads.

The implant itself is also subject to fracture,
though fortunately this is a very rare occurrence.
The two upper levels of the system act as "fuses"
and usually will fracture before damaging stresses
can cause fracture of the implant. If an implant
does fracture, it is usually at the level of the base of
the abutment center screw, and, in most cases, it
happens when the bone level also has reached this
point. The remaining implant fragment must be
removed by the surgeon using a trephine because it
almost always remains osseointegrated.

Whenever component hardware fractures occur,
the implant-supported bridge and its relationship
to the remaining dentition, the occlusal scheme, and
the presence and extent of cantilevers should be
assessed very carefully to determine if it is prudent
to make alterations to prevent further complications.
Long cantilever extensions, especially when implants
have had to be placed in straight-line configurations
rather than in a semilunar arrangement, seem to be

more frequently associated with component fracture. Even with the more desirable arch form implant distribution, a heavy occlusal load on the cantilever portion of the bridge can cause fracture of the gold-retaining screw or even the abutment screw at the most anterior implant.

Bibliography

Brånemark PI, Engstrand P, Lekholm U: Brånemark Novum: a new treatment concept for rehabilitation of the edentulous mandible. Preliminary results from a prospective clinical follow-up study, *Clin Implant Dent Relat Res* 1: 2-16, 1999.

Brown MS, Tarnow DP: Fixed provisionalization with transitional implants for partially edentulous patients: a case report, *Pract Proced Aesth Dent* 13:123-7, 2001.

Buchs AU, Levine UL, Moy P: Preliminary report of immediately loaded Altiva Natural Tooth Replacement dental implants, *Clin Implant Dent Relat Res* 3:97-106, 2001.

Carlson B, Carlsson GE: Prosthodontic complications in osseointegrated dental implant treatment, *Int J Oral Maxillofac Implants* 9:90-94, 1994.

Chow J, Hui E, Liu J et al: The Hong Kong Bridge Protocol. Immediate loading of mandibular Branemark fixtures using a fixed provisional prosthesis: preliminary results, *Clin Implant Dent Relat Res* 3:166-174, 2001.

Eckert SE, Meraw SJ, Cal E et al: Analysis of incidence and associated factors with fractured implants: a retrospective study, *Int J Oral Maxillofac Implants* 15:662-667, 2000.

Eckert SE, Wollan PC: Retrospective review of 1170 endosseous implants placed in partially edentulous jaws, *J Prosthet Dent* 79:415-421, 1998.

Esposito M, Hirsch JM, Lekholm U et al: Differential diagnosis and treatment strategies for biologic complications and failing oral implants: a review of the literature, *Int J Oral Maxillofac Implants* 14:473-490, 1999.

Esposito M, Hirsch JM, Lekholm U et al: Biological factors contributing to failures of osseointegrated oral implants. (I). Success criteria and epidemiology, *Eur J Oral Sci* 106: 527-551, 1998.

Esposito M, Hirsch JM, Lekholm U et al: Biological factors contributing to failures of osseointegrated oral implants. (II). Etiopathogenesis, *Eur J Oral Sci* 106:721-764, 1998.

Froum S, Emtiaz S, Bloom MJ et al: The use of transitional implants for immediate fixed temporary prostheses in cases of implant restorations, *Pract Periodontics Aesthet Dent* 10:737-746; quiz 748, 1998.

Goodacre CJ, Kan JY, Rungcharassaeng K: Clinical complications of osseointegrated implants, *J Prosthet Dent* 81:537-552, 1999.

Hemmings KW, Schmitt A, Zarb GA: Complications and maintenance requirements for fixed prostheses and overdentures in the edentulous mandible: a 5-year report, *Int J Oral Maxillofac Implants* 9:191-196, 1994.

Jemt T: Failures and complications in 391 consecutively inserted fixed prostheses supported by Branemark implants in edentulous jaws: a study of treatment from the time of prosthesis placement to the first annual checkup, *Int J Oral Maxillofac Implants* 6:270-276, 1991.

Levine RA, Clem DS III, Wilson TG Jr et al: Multicenter retrospective analysis of the ITI implant system used for single-tooth replacements: results of loading for 2 or more years, *Int J Oral Maxillofac Implants* 14:516-520, 1999.

Piattelli A, Piattelli M, Scarano A et al: Light and scanning electron microscopic report of four fractured implants, *Int J Oral Maxillofacial Implants* 13:561-564, 1998.

Pilliar RM, Lee JM, Maniatopoulos C: Observations on the effect of movement on bone ingrowth into porous-surfaced implants, *Clin Orthop* (208): 108-113, 1986.

Rangert B, Jemt T, Jorneus L: Forces and moments on Branemark implants, *Int J Oral Maxillofac Implants* 4:241-247, 1989.

Rangert B, Krogh PH, Langer B et al: Bending overload and implant fracture: a retrospective clinical analysis, *Int J Oral Maxillofac Implants* 10:326-334, 1995.

Rangert B, Krogh PH, Langer B et al: Bending overload and implant fracture: a retrospective clinical analysis [see comments] [published erratum appears in *Int J Oral Maxillofac Implants* 1996 Sep-Oct;11(5):575]. *Int J Oral Maxillofac Implants* 10: 326-334, 1995.

Schnitman PA, Wohrle PS, Rubenstein JE: Immediate fixed interim prostheses supported by two-stage threaded implants: methodology and results, *J Oral Implantol* 16:96-105, 1990.

Schnitman PA, Wohrle PS, Rubenstein JE et al: Ten-year results for Branemark implants immediately loaded with fixed prostheses at implant placement, *Int J Oral Maxillofac Implants* 12:495-503, 1997.

Tolman DE, Laney WR: Tissue-integrated prosthesis complications, *Int J Oral Maxillofac Implants* 7:477-484, 1992.

Zarb GA, Schmitt, A: The longitudinal clinical effectiveness of osseointegrated dental implants: the Toronto study. Part III: Problems and complications encountered, *J Prosthet Dent* 64:185-194, 1990.

CHAPTER 30

Implant Prosthodontics for Edentulous Patients: Current and Future Directions

Emad S. Elsubeihi, Nikolai Attard, George A. Zarb

Osseointegration has had a dramatic influence on prosthodontic practice. With its emphasis on scientific rigor, osseointegration now provides expanded treatment management strategies for virtually all partially and completely edentulous patients (Plates 30-1 through 30-5). The clinical yield from osseointegration as summed up in Box 30-1 reflects the results of numerous studies on its efficacy and effectiveness.

In 1990 we reported the results of the first North American long-term prospective implant study in prosthetically maladaptive edentulous patients (Zarb and Schmitt, 1990). One particularly compelling finding was that successful prosthodontic treatment outcomes exceeded individual implant survival ones, and all of the treated patients demonstrated ongoing long-term comfortable and successful prostheses wear. This study and subsequent ones strongly suggested that the provision of a fixed or quasi-fixed (overdenture) prosthesis was the optimal solution to complete denture problems of a functional nature (prosthetic maladaptation). It was concluded that the major determinant of success in wearing removable prostheses was patient-perceived comfort and stability. The latter objective would be readily achieved irrespective of the number of successfully osseointegrated fixtures and underscored the merits of diverse applications of a technique that has arguably revolutionized prosthodontic treatment.

Furthermore, evidence now continues the contribution of osseointegration to a slowing down, or reduction, in the bone resorptive process that would otherwise be likely to occur in the edentulous site(s) of proposed implant placement. Additionally, the documented virtual absence of even minimal morbidity has also become a significant consideration when prescribed surgical and prosthodontic protocols are followed. This encourages the conclusion, albeit a largely anecdotal but very frequently encountered one, that a patient's life quality is significantly enhanced by implant prosthodontics.

Brånemark's pioneering work in osseointegration catalyzed the conclusions in Box 30-1 and quite understandably led to several developmental and research initiatives, which are summed up in Box 30-2. Regrettably, very few of the available systems have been validated in the literature (Eckert, Parein, Myshin et al., 1997), and claims for predictably safe site development tend to remain long on anecdote, if somewhat short on scientifically documented outcomes. As a result both patients and dentists cannot readily answer the basic question that must be asked about any system's or surgical technique's effectiveness evaluation: *Do the proposed biotechnology and interventions lead to more good than harm in those people to whom it is offered?* This has become a dilemma in clinical practice where advertised hype risks outweighing the quality of required long-term evidence, which led to the compelling documented outcomes found in Box 30-1. It is hoped that continued efforts at scientific validation will evolve into the yardstick that dentists and patients will routinely use when making clinical decisions on prescribing implant-supported/retained prostheses and the associated protocols.

It is encouraging to note that significant clinical research initiatives continue to provide a better understanding of treatment outcomes with our preferred implant systems, along with systemic and

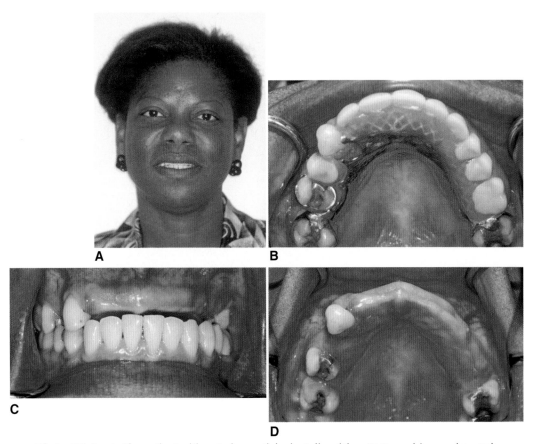

Plate 30-1 **A,** The patient with anterior partial edentulism (Class IV Kennedy) was adequately restored by the use of a removable partial denture (**B**). This patient had always desired a fixed prosthesis, but the length of the edentulous span coupled with inter-arch space considerations precluded a fixed solution (**C** and **D**).

Continued

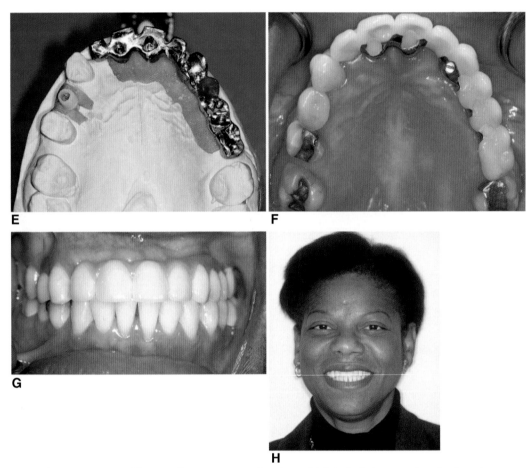

E

F

G

H

Plate 30-1 *cont'd* Scrupulous treatment planning, which included comprehensive imaging of the proposed implant sites (not shown), trial teeth set-up, and patient approval, thorough occlusal analysis and fabrication of a surgical splint, permitted design of a porcelain baked to metal fixed prosthesis (**E, F,** and **G**). The optimized esthetic result (**H**) was achieved via a combination of patient approved prosthetic teeth and a partial labial flange to compensate for ridge morphology deficit and ensure circum-oral support. The extent of the upper lip movement did not expose the junction of gingival replacement material and actual gingival tissues.

Continued

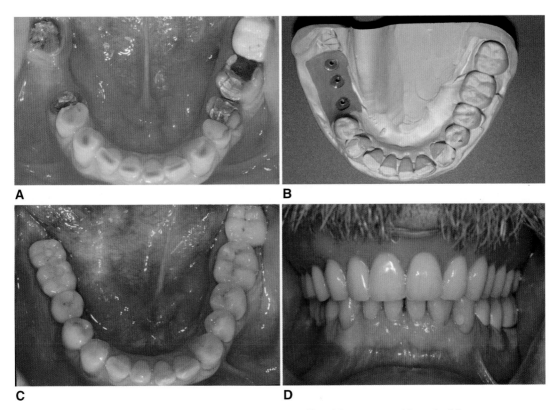

Plate 30-2 **A,** Posterior mandibular partial edentulism (Class II Kennedy) resulted from a failed three unit fixed bridge which necessitated the extraction of both previous abutments. Three osseointegrated implants permitted a new fixed prosthesis (**B, C,** and **D**).

Continued

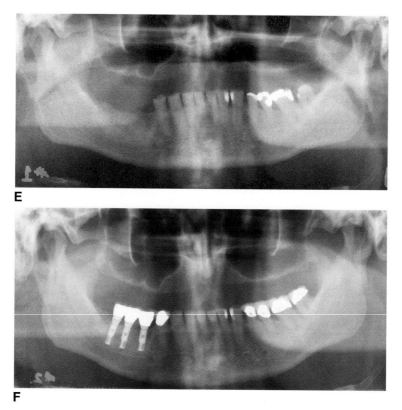

E

F

Plate 30-2 *cont'd* The pre- and post-implant treatment panoramic films shown in **E** and **F** reflect the scope for considering implant prosthodontics for routine partial edentulism involving the posterior zones of either jaw.

Continued

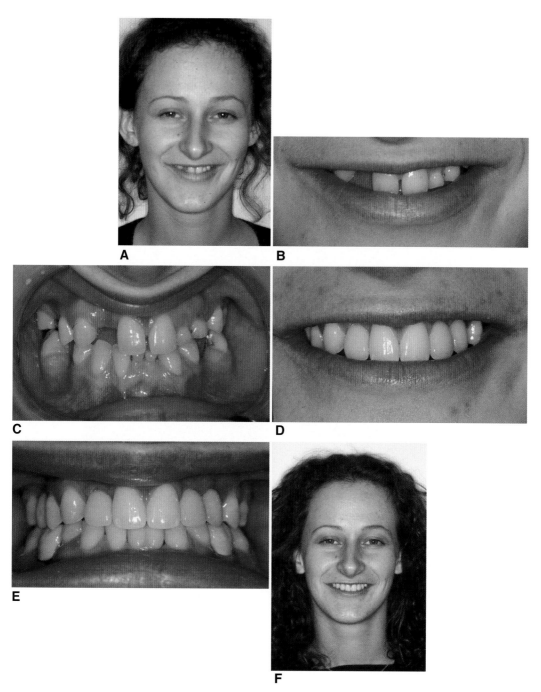

Plate 30-3 **A, B,** and **C,** This patient with oligodontia underwent preprosthodontic orthodontic treatment. The completed prosthodontic treatment as shown in **D, E,** and **F** attests to the versatility of implant prosthodontics for such partially edentulous challenges. This remains the most ecologically prudent treatment, especially for young patients whose natural teeth adjacent to any edentulous span can be spared being prepared.

Continued

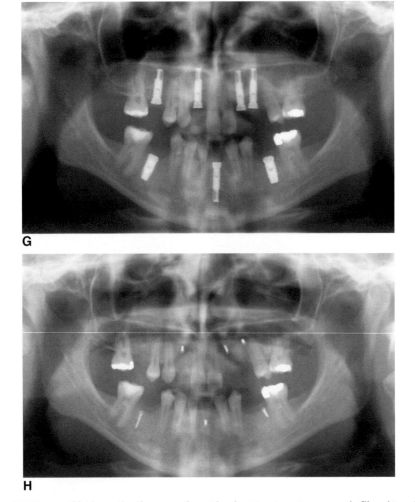

G

H

Plate 30-3 *cont'd* The patient's pre- and post-implant treatment panoramic films (**G** and **H**) reflect the post-orthodontic teeth alignment required to facilitate optimal implant placement, as guided by a suitable surgical guide.

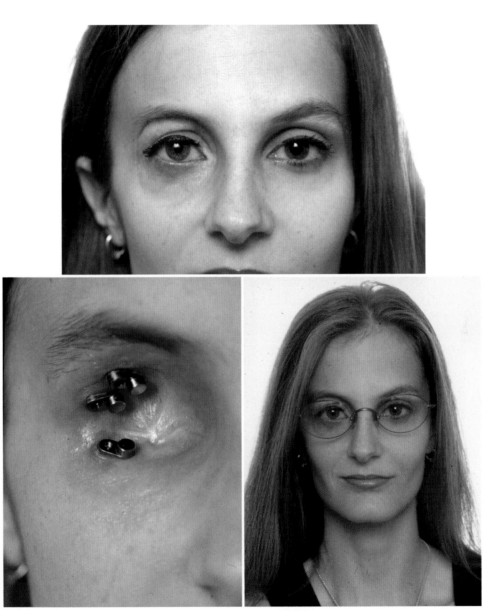

Plate 30-4 The use of miniaturized osseointegrated implants for extra-oral use permits variations on a theme of employing ingenious retentive devices to support and stabilize different types of prosthetic replacements for missing facial parts. The implant-retained prosthetic eye seen above and the implant-retained prosthetic ears seen in Plate 30-5 reflect the ingenuity of prosthodontics at its highest level of clinical skill and artistry.

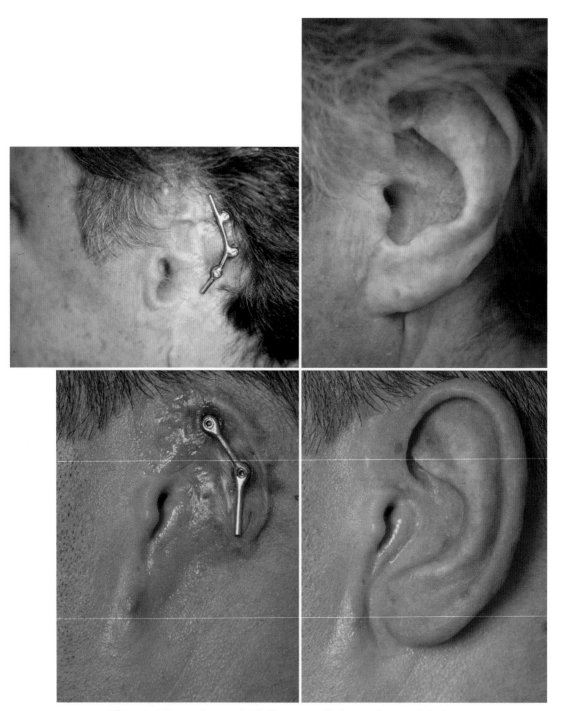

Plate 30-5 Implant-retained silicone prosthetic ears (bars and clips).

Box 30-1

Clinical Yield from Long-Term Prospective Clinical Studies in Osseointegration

1. Enhancement or guarantee of prosthesis retention/stability
2. Retardation in bone reduction
3. Minimal treatment outcome morbidity
4. Enrichment of patients' life quality

Box 30-2

Research Developments

Developments in Implants/Implant Components

Implant material biocompatibility
Implant and component designs
Implant surface characteristics

Developments in Surgical/Prosthodontic Techniques

Surgical technique
Implant placement technique
Site development
Timing of loading protocols

Understanding Patient-Mediated Concerns

Local factors
Behavioral and systemic conditions
Quality of life
Health economic benefits of treatments

local determinants of successful osseointegration (see Table 25-1).

HOST BONE RESPONSE

Long-term studies on the success/survival of dental implants reveal an impressive prosthodontic treatment outcome (Table 30-1). Because osseointegration is essentially a wound healing process, it is presumed that factors that interfere with the healing process may contribute to implant failure. As a result, in some studies investigators attempted to relate implant failure to the status of changes in bone quality or quantity. In other clinical studies researchers attempted to investigate the success rate of dental implants in different systemic conditions that have been shown to adversely affect wound healing and may therefore compromise successful osseointegration (Elsubeihi and Zarb, 2002). Although the results of some of these studies have provided some indications on conditions that can influence osseointegration (Table 30-2), most did not provide conclusive evidence on the impact of systemic conditions on dental implant success. The reason is that most of the reported studies were either case reports or retrospective case series studies of small sample size. This is further complicated by the fact that little is known about local hormonal, metabolic, and cellular processes in the jawbone. The reference section provides more sources of information (Elsubeihi and Zarb, 2002; Sennerby and Roos, 1998; Esposito, Hirsch, Lekholm, et al., 1998).

Smoking

It is estimated that implant failure is about twice as common in smokers as compared with nonsmok-

Table 30-1
Rate and Distribution of Early and Late Implant Failures in Two Studies

	Meta-analysis Study*	University of Toronto†
Total number of implants	2812	1852
Early failure	3.6%	4.21%
Late failure	4.1%	3.66%
Overall failure	7.7%	7.9%

*Meta-analysis of 73 published studies over a 5-year period (Esposito, Hirsch, Lekholm, Thomsen, 1998).
†Data from prospective follow-up studies at the University of Toronto since 1979.

Table 30-2
Summary of Influence of Various Factors on Implant Prosthodontic Treatment Outcomes

Local	Patient-Related Factors		Prosthodontic/Surgical Technique	Implant-Related Factors
	Systemic/Behavioral			
No Demonstrable Negative Effect[*]	Age and gender Controlled diabetes mellitus Controlled cardiovascular disease Controlled hypothyroidism Hereditary ectodermal disease HIV/AIDS Systemic corticosteroid therapy		Incision technique Immediate loading Exposed threads Lack of bicortical stabilization Number of supporting implants	
Possible Risk of Failure Jaw site	Maxilla in postmenopausal women not receiving HRT Vitamin D–dependent rickets Sjögren's syndrome Diphosphonate therapy		Clinician's skill and experience Compromised infection control Lack of initial stabilization Immediate placement in infected extraction sockets Distribution of implants	Implant diameter Implant design[†]
Increased Risk of Failure[*] Compromised bone quantity Compromised bone quality	Cigarette smoking Irradiated maxilla Recent chemotherapy		Lack of antibiotic prophylaxis	Implant length Implant material[†]

[*]Note that with the exception of smoking and diabetes mellitus, the influence of other systemic conditions on implant failure is based on case reports and retrospective studies with small sample sizes.
[†]Implant microscopic and macroscopic characteristics are discussed in Chapter 26.
HRT, Hormone replacement therapy.

ers. Substantial evidence exists to support the conclusion that cigarette smoking is associated with increased risk of implant failure, increased marginal bone loss, and poor periimplant soft tissue health. In general, cigarette smoking has been shown to impair soft tissue wound healing by affecting the circulatory and immune systems and by impairing normal cellular function. Furthermore, it appears that cigarette smoking during adulthood is associated with decreased hip and vertebral bone density later in life in both women and men. However, the exact mechanism by which smoking exerts its negative effect on bone is not yet fully understood. Bone loss occurs if there is an imbal-

ance between the amount of bone resorbed and the amount of bone formed. The available evidence examining whether one or both of these mechanisms contribute to the bone loss associated with smoking is limited. It has been demonstrated that lower bone density at the lumbar spine in smokers was associated with higher serum calcium and urine pyrdinoline levels, which is consistent with increased bone resorption. Furthermore, it was also suggested that increased bone resorption associated with smoking is in part due to decreased production and acceleration of degradation of estrogen leading to early menopause and higher rate of bone loss. On the other hand, histomorphometric investigations suggested that reduced bone formation is responsible for the deficit in bone volume seen in smokers. In vitro and animal studies have shown that several components of cigarette smoke, such as nicotine and aryl-hydrocarbons, can depress osteoblast activity, reduce collagen synthesis, and inhibit osteodifferentiation and osteogenesis. Other components of cigarette smoke, such as carbon monoxide (which binds to hemoglobin to form carboxyhemoglobin) and hydrogen cyanide (which inhibits cellular respiratory enzymes), result in tissue hypoxia and alter tissue healing. The effect of these components on jawbone behavior at the tissue and cellular levels needs to be fully explored.

Irradiation Therapy

Irradiation therapy in which more than 55 gray (Gy) was used has been associated with increased risk of implant failure and soft tissue complications during healing, particularly in the maxilla. It has been suggested that the use of hyperbaric oxygen in these patients can improve success rates, particularly in the maxilla. In addition to the known risk of osteoradionecrosis, experimental evidence suggests that radiation induces cellular changes in bone where osteocytes in the direct pathway of irradiation are killed and the regenerative potential of the periosteum is compromised because of reduced cellularity, vascularity, and osteoid formation potential. Furthermore, blood vessels' patency is reduced leading to diminished hematopoietic turnover.

Osteoporosis

The term *osteoporosis* has been somewhat loosely used in the dental literature and often to imply postmenopausal osteoporosis. Several reports suggest that osteoporosis is not a risk factor for implant failure in the jaws; however, these were limited to case reports and case series studies where the diagnosis of osteoporosis was not confirmed. Interestingly, biochemical analysis of bone derived from human osteoporotic femoral head showed evidence of overhydroxylation of lysine and a consequent reduction in the stabilizing crosslinks of the collagenous framework that has been suggested to contribute to increased fragility of bone. Indeed, mechanical testing of healing femoral

fractures in rats indicated that ovariectomy impairs fracture healing up to 4 weeks after fracture. This returned to normal levels 6 weeks after fracture. The administration of 17-β estradiol during fracture repair also resulted in a dose-dependent increase in the peak force required to break the fracture. These observations may explain the recent findings of increased risk of maxillary implant failure when tested with the reverse-torque method at stage II surgery in osteoporotic patients not receiving hormone replacement therapy. Interestingly, no correlation was found between changes in bone mass in different parts of the skeleton and dental implant failure. This observation underscores the need for a better understanding of the effects of systemic factors on jawbone changes at both the tissue and cellular levels.

Experimental evidence has shown that estrogen depletion leads to a significant loss of bone mass in the edentulous mandible, but not in the dentate mandible, possibly because of the protective effect of masticatory forces (Elsubeihi and Zarb, 2002). The reduction in bone mass of the edentulous mandible of estrogen-depleted animals was associated with an increase in bone turnover where both bone resorption and bone formation rates are increased, with the former exceeding the latter, resulting in bone loss. Evidence at the gene expression, cellular level, and tissue level in other parts of the skeleton further supports these findings.

Several authorities maintain that a clinical diagnosis of osteoporosis per se is not a contraindication for dental implant placement. However, in patients with a diagnosis of osteoporosis and where the local jaw bone quality is judged to be of inferior quality (e.g., Type IV bone, particularly in the maxilla), clinical prudence suggests the following clinical strategy: self-threading implants should be placed with meticulous surgical technique, and an appropriately longer healing period should be allowed before subjecting the implants to high occlusal stresses. The recent introduction of surface-modified self-threading implants may also prove to be of value in these situations. Interestingly, functional loading of healed dental implants in patients may increase the bone mass in the jaws, an observation that is consistent with lack of effect of estrogen depletion on the dentate mandibles of animals.

Other Systemic Conditions

Case reports and retrospective studies with a small patient sample size indicate that there is an increased risk of implant failure in patients with Sjögren's syndrome, patients with vitamin D–dependent rickets, and in patients receiving active chemotherapy and diphosphonate therapy. On the other hand, no evidence of increased risk of implant failure has been demonstrated in patients with controlled diabetes mellitus, controlled cardiovascular disease, controlled hypothyroidism, HIV/AIDS, hypophosphatasia, scleroderma, Erdheim-Chester disease, and hereditary ectodermal dysplasia. It should be emphasized, however, that with the exception of the studies on smoking, diabetes mellitus, and irradiated maxillae, the quality of most reports does not allow for firm conclusions, and further studies are needed.

THE SURGICAL PROTOCOL

Surgical technique and the healing potential of the patient are local determinants of implant success. The aims of the surgical technique are to place and locate the required number of implants (prosthodontically driven) in host sites as atraumatically as possible and to obtain primary stability or implant immobility. This stability is dependent on the surgical technique used, plus the bone quality and quantity of the host site, which in turn determines the length of implant used.

An empirically based classification of bone quality and quantity was proposed by Lekholm and Zarb (1985) and describes commonly encountered variations in jaw morphology or quantity, as determined by clinical examination and radiographic imaging. Bone quality is also described subjectively by the surgeon during the surgical procedure (Figure 30-1).

Bone Quality

Bone quality in the mandible is typically cortical in nature anteriorly and more trabecular posteriorly. Likewise, the maxilla is generally trabecular with minimal cortical bone present in the alveolar process. However, alveolar bone is highly variable, and the transition between anterior and posterior is gradual. Bone quality appears to influence treatment outcomes, with high success rates described

in the anterior mandible and somewhat lower ones observed in the maxilla. This clinical observation catalyzed research to improve success rates for clinical situations where poor bone quality is encountered. Examples include the following:

1. Modification of the surgical technique: underpreparation of host sites and the use of osteotomes. The presumed advantages of such techniques are bone preservation and localized increase in bone density of the osteotomy site.
2. Modification of the implant design: wider diameters, changes in thread design, and introduction of self-tapping implants.
3. Modification of implant topography by introducing roughened surfaces to increase bone to implant contact.

However, the long-term benefits of such modifications, especially those related to surface modification, are still to be determined clinically. To date, long-term prospective studies have revealed predictable prognoses for machined surface implants, even when the implant surface was exposed to oral flora as a result of bone resorption. On the other hand, a rough surface, although reported to induce more initial bone formation, may in the long-term be prone to infection-related problems due to the risk of more enhanced bacterial adhesion. Further research is clearly required to better understand the effects of implant surface topography in situ.

There are currently no specific tools that conclusively determine bone quality before the implant surgical intervention. Although computed tomography remains a helpful diagnostic imaging technique that provides insight into the architecture of the bone, this does not necessarily guarantee successful osseointegration. Further research at the cellular level is also required to determine the various steps of the healing phenomenon and to devise methods of harnessing and improving it (Watzek and Gruber, 2002). Numerous attempts to coat implant surfaces with organic factors (bone morphogenetic proteins [BMPs]) and inorganic materials (such as hydroxyapatite) that stimulate mesenchymal progenitor cell migration and differentiation have also been proposed. Regrettably, published results are still inconclusive. Clinical experience indicated

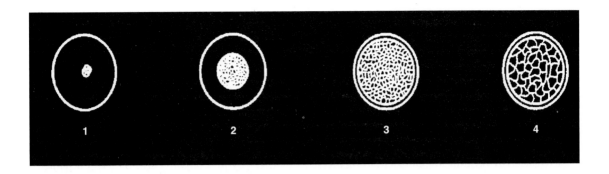

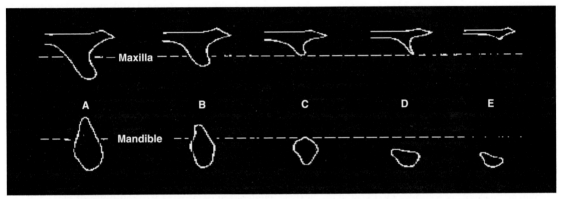

Figure 30-1   Lekholm-Zarb classification of edentulous anterior jawbone quantity and quality. Types *A* through *E* reflect a range of resorptive patterns relative to the presumed demarcation of the alveolar and basal jawbone *(dotted line)*. Quality (Types *1* through *4*) reflects a range of cortical and cancellous patterns, which have been consistently used in planning oral implant treatment.

that implant failure is a localized phenomenon. Site-specific healing potential is yet to be determined both at a morphological and cellular level. Furthermore, if this ability to do so was possible, this does not necessarily guarantee that such parameters would be useful predictors of osseointegration.

Bone Quantity

Ridge reduction is an ongoing and cumulative process, and the resultant residual bone quantity can compromise implant placement. Consequently, several patients who are most in need of implants frequently have compromised bone anatomy. Various surgical endeavors in the edentulous patient have

been suggested for compensatory ridge augmentation, with the gold standard for bone grafting being autogenous bone.

Research has established that a healing phase for the graft is required before implant placement. However, the time required for this intermediate phase before implant placement is yet to be determined conclusively. Currently, the suggested intermediate healing phase is approximately 6 months. Moreover, the impact of these surgical interventions and associated morbidity still needs to be investigated in elderly patients. This is a significant concern because this age cohort will likely be the main recipient of implants.

The need to find alternatives to autogenous bone harvesting has also led to various research initiatives. Basic science research in various animal models demonstrated the bone regeneration capacity of various growth factors such as BMPs, tumor growth factor-β (TGF-β), platelet-derived growth factor (PDGF), and the maintenance of de novo bone under functional loading. A dearth of information remains on the use of these regenerative materials in clinical studies, although short-term results appear to hold promise. The need for minimally invasive preprosthetic surgical techniques to create better host sites for implants remains a serious research priority.

PROSTHODONTIC LOADING

Occlusal forces are the major source of loading on dental implants. The basic tenets of a therapeutic occlusion were originally described by Beyron and underscore the standard determinants of a physiological occlusion in prosthodontic patients (Box 30-3) (Mohl, Zarb, Carlsson, et al., 1988).

These objectives are easily achieved in setting up teeth for complete denture fabrication (see Chapters 16 and 17). However, their effectiveness is also dependent on the quality of available residual ridge support. Occlusal loading potential in the edentulous patient is limited by the health and nature of the oral mucosa and the morphology of the denture-bearing area. As a result, patient successful acceptance of conventional prostheses, notably lower complete dentures, remains a serious treatment challenge and in the past led to numerous ingenious surgical techniques to enlarge the denture load-bearing area.

Initially, patients seeking implant-supported prostheses were treated with a minimum of five to six implants in the anterior mandible and maxilla, respectively. These locations were selected because of likely favorable host site dimensions. The implants' distribution followed the residual arch form so that they were better able to provide mechanical support for the prosthesis, and after a suitable healing period (4 to 6 months), the implants were then restored with a fixed prosthesis.

Efficacy and effectiveness studies on patients with maladaptive prosthetics who were treated with fixed restorations show that these patients were significantly helped with this technique (see Chapter 28). However, it should be realized that this treatment modality is time-consuming and expensive. Therefore we reiterate our conviction that the dramatic impact of osseointegration treatment should include a simpler, less dramatic application of the technique. Since many experienced prosthodontists have long recognized that most patients' denture difficulties can be easily rectified if denture stability is improved, it appears logical that these patients do not necessarily need a conversion of their unstable complete denture into a fixed osseointegrated one. All they appear to need is a source of prostheses stability that can be readily achieved with the presence of two or more overdenture abutments. It is therefore tempting for the prosthodontist to include such an "abbreviated" use of osseointegration in the form of implant-supported overdentures. Such an application offers both practical clinical and financial advantages. The surgical operation becomes a reduced one, both time and money wise, and the approach is kinder to the patient particularly in the context of the patient's state of health or age. Considerable evidence now endorses the functional benefits obtained by patients who wear implant-retained overdentures. These benefits include improved denture stability, expanded scope for aesthetic solutions, enhanced patient confidence and comfort, and retardation of loss of the residual bony ridge height (see Chapter 27).

The initial proposed healing periods for the buried implants were an outgrowth of early trials based on extrapolated observations from orthopedic research. The original Brånemark osseointegration technique required a two-stage surgical approach

---

Box 30-3

Beyron's Determinants of a Physiological/Therapeutic Occlusion

1. Acceptable interocclusal distance
2. Stable jaw relationship with bilateral contacts in retruded closure
3. Freedom in retrusive range of contact
4. Multidirectional freedom of contact movement

with a minimum healing period proposed to obtain durable direct bone to implant contact. This period was suggested to be at least 4 months in the mandible and 6 months in the maxilla.

In the last decade, clinical research has questioned this timing protocol and led to altered immediate or early loading treatment protocols, mainly in site-specific areas. It should be understood that if implants are loaded early, we are not dealing with the biological phenomena of osseointegration per se, but rather with primary mechanical implant stability. The time-dependent secondary implant stability is achieved when bone formation and remodeling at the bone/implant interface is completed. The presumed advantages of the change in time-related loading protocols include the following:

1. Treatment for routine patients with various implant designs, most particularly in the parasymphyseal region of the mandible. This area has the highest reported clinical success rates when compared with the conventional delayed surgical approach.
2. A reduction or elimination of the healing phase before loading of the implants with a resultant reduced time commitment by the patient.
3. One-stage surgery in an effort to reduce the surgical morbidity.

Several published studies suggest that immediate or early loading with fixed or overdenture implant-supported prosthesis is a viable option, at least in the short term. However, the results are far from conclusive, and a number of concerns still need to be investigated to determine the following:

1. The biological implications of reducing the healing time.
2. The true impact of such an approach on the patient's quality of life.
3. The specific protocol of immediate loading to be followed, specifically, the minimum healing time required, the number of implants needed to support fixed or overdenture prostheses, and also the prosthetic design.

4. The long-term success and economic benefits of immediate loading in the context of published treatment outcome criteria that justified use of traditional surgical and loading protocols.

The biomechanics of the healing implant bone interface remains a fascinating if complex concern for various researchers, from tissue engineers to clinical specialists. It appears that time-dependent stress-strain states in mesenchymal tissue influence all differentiation in the various stages of bone healing. This occurs in fractures, in implant-related osteotomies, and in distraction osteogenesis. It must therefore be emphasized that current clinical experiences with different implant-loading protocols (though ingenious and exciting) are based on scrupulous observation exclusively and not on a full understanding of the biomechanics of implant-bone interfaces.

Oral Ecology and Implant Prosthodontics

Ecology is described as that branch of biology dealing with relations of microorganisms to one another and to their physical surroundings. In a broader sense it also includes the relationship between changes in a particular environment and the resulting impact on specific presences or participants. Oral ecological responses to prosthodontic interventions can therefore be regarded as a balance between the implicit invasiveness of any procedure (making crown preparations with subgingival margins, using edentulous ridges for occlusal support, implanting tooth root substitutes) and the host tissue site responses. Consequently, treatment techniques such as the ones mentioned may elicit changes that lead to specific ecological upsets manifested as clinical complications. These include recurrent caries and periodontal disease around a crowned tooth or inflammatory and morphological changes in residual ridges under complete dentures. The development of such adverse ecological shifts are time dependent but also reflect patient- and dentist-mediated judgment and skills. It is therefore quite remarkable to note the very minimal local or systemic morbidity recorded in long-term prospective studies in implant prosthodontics.

One fascinating fact has been the well-recorded observation that osseointegrated implants are very rarely associated with postloading failure. Although clinical skill and judgment, plus optimal patient selection and operating protocols, appear to virtually guarantee favorable long-term treatment outcomes, the choice of implant per se also appears to contribute to clinical success.

When encountered, implant failure after prosthodontic loading has often been attributed to a so-called periimplantitis. This is described as an inflammatory process affecting the tissue around an implant, which results in loss of supporting bone and which has been reported in particular with rough-surface implants. The latter observation may therefore suggest a greater vulnerability for implants with roughened as opposed to machined surfaces extending to their cervical regions, with an analogy with periodontal disease a long-standing temptation. This in turn has led to several hypotheses regarding the etiology of implant failure and a regrettable rigid insistence on a similar periodontitis and pathogenic etiology. It has even led to treatment for periimplantitis based on peri-odontal therapy protocols. A recent literature review (Esposito, Hirsch, Lekholm, et al., 1999) concluded that the treatment of failing implants is still based on empirical considerations often derived from periodontal experiments, from data extrapolated from in vitro findings, or from anecdotal case reports performed on a trial-and-error basis. To date, no compelling data have been presented to justify treating teeth and implants as identical clinical entities. Their attachment mechanisms are different because the tooth's have resulted from an evolutionary process, whereas the implant's is an induced healing response (Figure 30-2). As a result, functional differences between implant and tooth are quite obvious (Table 30-3), yet numerous articles in the periodontal literature and in some microbiological reviews have attempted to advance an argument favoring periodontitis-related bacteria as the cause of implant failure. It appears that the most serious conclusions from such reviews are that the microflora of periimplantitis resemble those of adult or refractory periodontitis and that potential periodontal pathogens that are present in the mouth do not

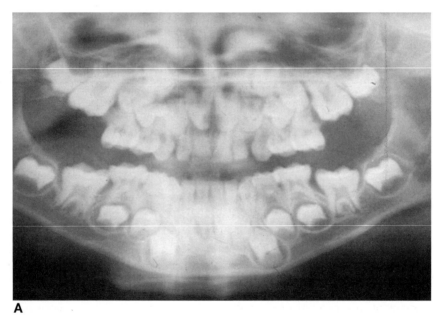

A

Figure 30-2   A, In natural teeth, the structural continuity of tooth and periodontal tissues is the product of a well-integrated series of developmental events.

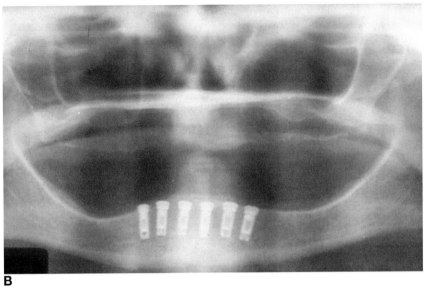

B

Figure 30-2 *cont'd* **B,** In contrast to natural teeth, the structural continuity between an osseointegrated implant and its host site is the result of a wound-healing process and not a developmental one.

Table 30-3 Differences between Teeth and Implants	
Teeth	**Implants**
Attachment mechanism (periodontal ligament) is the result of evolution and has not been replicated	Interfacial osteogenesis (ankylotic-like) is an induced healing response that is readily replicated
Variable mobility is present; increased mobility may be reversible	Immobile (ankylotic-like)
Can be intruded, extruded, or moved	Cannot be intruded, extruded, or moved (ankylotic-like)
In young patients, teeth continue to erupt	In young patients, implants are "left behind" while surrounding tissues change
Proprioception	So-called osseoperception
Has a rich plexus of blood vessels and nerves in the periodontal ligament	A relative absence of such a sophisticated circulation and probably innervation
Data present to show progress of mucosal inflammation to periodontal disease	Similar data are not present

necessarily act as periimplant pathogens. We regard available evidence as circumstantial at best, more particularly because it appears to ignore the likelihood of a compromised healing or osseointegrated response, which could eventually succumb to the diverse and unpredictable magnitudes, frequencies, and durations of occlusal loading. In this context, interfacial cracks may result, and these may eventually coalesce and lead to implant motion and in time a separation at the interface. Secondary infection is then the likely outcome, with complete loss of bony support the inevitable consequence. It is not surprising therefore that failing implants demonstrate a microorganism environment usually associated with periodontal disease. At this stage of our knowledge base it may even be tempting to conclude that the cause of implant failure is multifactorial and perhaps that even genetic factors may play a role. However, our perception is that a reconciliation of the healing process around an implant with the time-dependent nature of the load it is subjected to remains the major determinant of implant success or failure. This conviction does not ignore the fact that pathogenic microorganisms in plaque around teeth or implants may have systemic health implications and that plaque should therefore be controlled.

SUMMARY

Scientifically acceptable treatment outcome time frames for implant loading cover a spectrum of possibilities. This spectrum ranges from over 20 years for machined commercially pure titanium implants and traditional surgical protocols with delayed loading, to virtually immediate loading ones using various surgical methods of host site improvement and implants with roughened surfaces. Time, and even better research that includes economic benefits, will ultimately determine to what extent the complete denture will be eclipsed by the implant-supported prosthesis. In the mean-

time, there is little doubt that both techniques can address the edentulous individual's needs. Both patients and dentists have already benefited enormously from this enriched spectrum of treatment possibilities.

References

Eckert SE, Parein A, Myshin HL et al: Validation of dental implant systems through a review of literature supplied by system manufacturers, *J Prosthet Dent* 77:271-279, 1997.

Elsubeihi ES, Zarb GA: Implant prosthodontics in medically challenged patients: the University of Toronto experience, *J Can Dent Assoc* 68:103-108, 2002.

Esposito M, Hirsch JM, Lekholm U et al: Biological factors contributing to failures of osseointegrated oral implants. II. Etiopathogensis, *Eur J Oral Sci* 106:721-764, 1998.

Esposito M, Hirsch J, Lekholm U et al: Differential diagnosis and treatment strategies for biologic complications and failing oral implants: a review of the literature, *Int J Oral Maxillofac Implants* 14:473-490, 1999.

Lekholm U, Zarb GA: Patient selection and preparation. In Brånemark PI, Albrektsson T, Zarb GA, editors: *Tissue-integrated prostheses: osseointegration in clinical dentistry,* Chicago, 1985, Quintessence.

Mohl ND, Zarb GA, Carlsson GE et al editors: *A textbook of occlusion,* Chicago, 1988, Quintessence.

Sennerby L, Roos J: Surgical determinants of clinical success of osseiointegrated oral implants: a review of the literature, *Int J Prosthodont* 11:408-420, 1998.

Watzek G, Gruber R: Morphological and cellular parameters of bone quality, *Applied Osseointegration Research,* 3:3-10, 2002.

Zarb GA, Schmitt A: The longitudinal clinical effectiveness of osseointegrated dental implants: the Toronto Study. Part II: The prosthetic results, *J Prosthet Dent* 64:53-61, 1990.

Index

Page numbers followed by "f" denote figures, "b" denote boxes, and "t" denote tables.

539